Kraus' Dental Anatomy and Occlusion

Kraus' Dental Anatomy and Occlusion

Second Edition

Ronald E. Jordan, D.D.S., M.S.D.

Dean of the Faculty of Dentistry
University of Manitoba
Winnipeg, Manitoba, Canada

Leonard Abrams, D.D.S.

Clinical Professor of Periodontology
School of Dental Medicine
University of Pennsylvania
Philadelphia, Pennsylvania

Bertram S. Kraus, Ph.D. (Deceased)

Former Director, Cleft Palate Research Center
Professor of Anatomy and Physical Anthropology
University of Pittsburgh
Pittsburgh, Pennsylvania
Director, Dental Research
Elwyn Institute
Elwyn, Pennsylvania

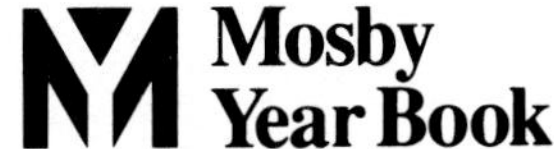

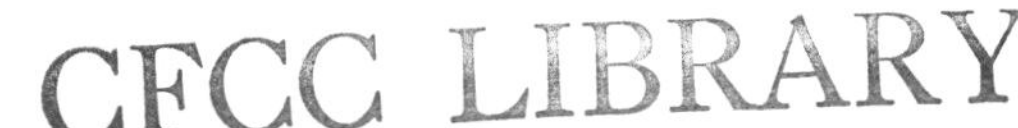

St. Louis Baltimore Boston Chicago London Philadelphia Sydney Toronto

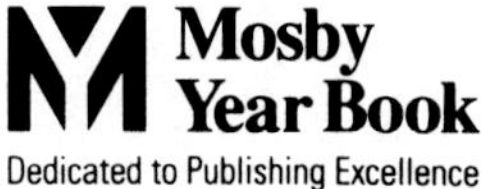

Editors: Walter Bailey/Sandy Reinhardt
Project Manager: Annette Hall
Production: P. M. Gordon Associates

Printed in the United States of America

Mosby–Year Book, Inc.
11830 Westline Industrial Drive
St. Louis, Missouri 63146

ISBN 1-55664-183-4
05828-D

CS/JA/WA 9 8 7 6 5 4 3 2 1

IN MEMORIAM

Bertram Shirley Kraus 1913–1970

Inspiring teacher, gifted researcher, devoted scientist, and noted author of many scientific papers and textbooks. With his foresight and vision, this book became a reality.

His absence from the scientific community has created a void present to this day.

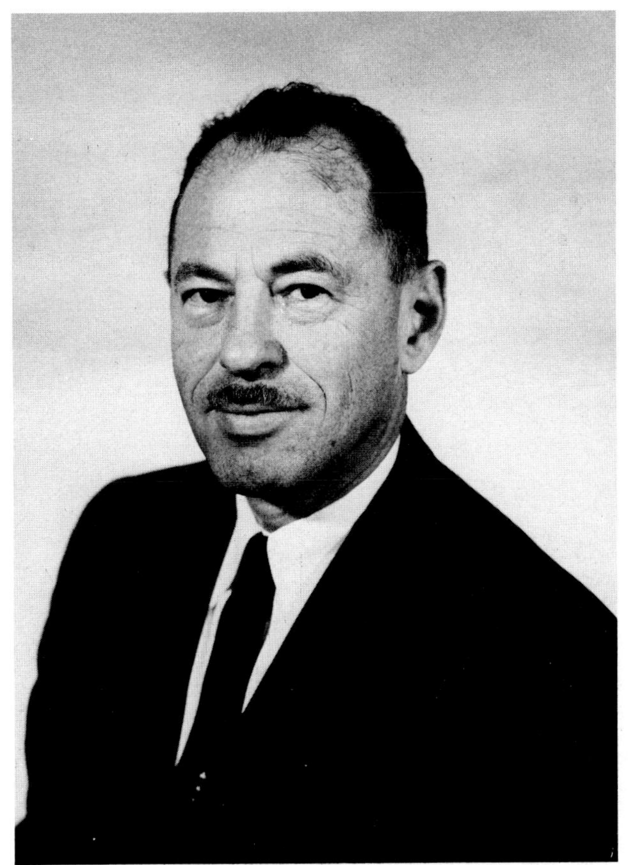

Preface to the First Edition

In the past twenty years the face of dentistry has changed, reflecting significant new attitudes about research, clinical practice, and education. For one thing, the focus of clinical attention has been placed more and more upon the *dentition* rather than upon the individual tooth. Dentistry has become more concerned with maintaining the integrity of the masticatory system than with the treatment of an isolated tooth. The rapidly increasing influx of basic scientists into the field of dental education and research has broadened the biological foundation of teaching and training, and has widened the scope of dental inquiry. The pressures of expanding knowledge have forced dental educators to modify and to broaden the traditional dental curriculum.

This book attempts to fulfill a vital need in dental education. There is a definite requirement early in the dental curriculum for a single text that combines the anatomy of the individual teeth with an exposition of the total dental complex acting as a component of the masticatory system. The function of the masticatory system is now taught as the science of occlusion, a word that once referred simply to the act of closure of the teeth (from the Latin *ob* + *claudo* = *occludo*, to shut against). The concept of combining dental anatomy with occlusion in a single book is not unique, but the manner in which it has been done in this text may represent something new in dentistry. To provide a broad basis for understanding tooth anatomy and occlusion, an entire chapter has been devoted to the tissues of the teeth and investing structures. The information has been brought up to date and includes data at all levels, from the histological to the cellular. Finally, an often neglected area of dental education has been strongly emphasized—the significance of the dentition in the non-dental biological sciences. This integration of interrelated data and subject material with its special emphasis upon occlusion represents the central theme in the modern dental curriculum. It is precisely in the study of occlusion that all clinical fields of dentistry converge.

Because of the changing character of dental practice and new concepts of oral health, it is necessary that the clinician today reevaluate the academic foundation upon which his clinical philosophy rests. It is the intent of the authors that this text will serve to provide him with the basis for his reevaluation. The book has been divided into four chapters, each subdivided into several sections. The first chapter, "The Anatomy of the Individual Teeth," is organized in a way that classifies the various teeth into families on the basis of morphological characteristics held in common. Thus, there are traits which separate the teeth of the upper from the lower arches, the permanent from the primary teeth, the molars from the incisors, and the first molar from the second molar. This introduces a more orderly arrangement into descriptive anatomy, sorting out the key, or *diagnostic*, traits that make each type of tooth distinctive in the dental arch. At the same time it permits the exposition of a central theme in biology, that of variability, which is applicable to the teeth as truly as to any other trait of the human organism. Thus two important concepts are stressed practically simultaneously: (1) there is an "average" or "stereotypic" tooth in the sense that all permanent mandibular first molars, for example, have a number of basic traits in common which easily identify them as such; and (2) there is almost an infinite number of ways in which permanent mandibular first molars can vary (and still be identified on the basis of these traits) so that no two will be identical. These two concepts must be thoroughly appreciated. They are complementary, not mutually exclusive.

Great care has been taken to collect and photograph unworn, intact, non-restored teeth, both permanent and primary. They have been photographed using large film size to minimize distortion and permit maximum detail. Because the enamel is translucent and presents optical difficulties in obtaining satisfactory photographs, casts of the crowns were made, using precise dental impression techniques. Photographs of the casts reveal minute details of the crown that have hitherto not been consistently observable. These are presented side-by-side with the occlusal photographs of the actual crowns.

The second chapter is entitled "The Histology of the Teeth and Their Investing Structures," and contains sections on enamel, dentin, pulp, and the periodontium. Special attention has been devoted to the biochemistry, histology, and ultrastructure of the enamel, since it is in this area that the newest contributions to knowledge have been made.

Chapter III is devoted to a detailed account of the

masticatory system under the headings of "The Temperomandibular Joint and Mandibular Function," "The Dentition: Its Alignment and Articulation," and "The Self-Protective Features of the Dentition." A new nomenclature has been adopted for the occlusal landmarks of teeth, simplifying discussion of the articulation of teeth in both static and dynamic function. The treatment of occlusion is accompanied by a large series of illustrations, presented in an animated, step-by-step fashion. The relationship of tooth structure to periodontal health is closely integrated with the subject matter of the previous chapter.

The final chapter, "The Human Dentition in Biological Perspective," reintroduces to the dental student the once traditionally taught subject of comparative vertebrate odontology and dental evolution. This material, once found in most of the old dental anatomy books, has been almost completely neglected in modern dental education. In reviving the subject it has been updated in the light of neo-Darwinism, modern genetics, and the latest fossil finds. Important new understanding of the human dentition is gained when it is viewed against the background of evolution and the living vertebrates. Armed with this kind of knowledge, the dental student will no longer fall prey to the oft-repeated and quite unfounded statements about "nature's intent" in evolutionary processes with respect to human dental occlusion. The role of heredity in the determination of dental structure is discussed in considerable detail. This is followed by sections devoted to variation and its genetic and embryological bases.

The section on normal and abnormal crown structure is based upon new research showing the effect upon tooth crown anatomy of prenatal and postnatal disturbances. The possible role of the dentition in disclosing the action and time of onset of teratogenic agents is pointed out. Abnormal tooth crowns found in association with cleft lip and/or palate and Mongolism are illustrated.

We are heavily indebted to the contributions of the authorities listed on the cover. It must be pointed out that their material has not been presented herein in its original form. We have taken the liberty of editing and rewriting their texts in order to achieve maximum conformity and continuity with the concepts we have tried to put forth. It must, therefore, be clearly understood that any errors of fact or interpretation are solely our own.

B.S.K.
R.E.J.
L.A.

Contributors to the First Edition

Morton Amsterdam, D.D.S.
Professor and Chairman
Department of Prosthodontics
School of Dental Medicine
University of Pennsylvania.

Percy M. Butler, Ph.D.
Professor and Chairman
Department of Zoology
Royal Holloway College, University of London
Englefield Green, Surrey, England.

D. Walter Cohen, D.D.S.
Professor and Chairman
Department of Periodontology
School of Dental Medicine
University of Pennsylvania.

W. Krogh-Poulsen, L.D.S.
Dr. med. dent., Odont. Dr. hc.
Department of Occlusion and Stomatognathic Dysfunction
The Royal Dental College
Copen-Hagen, Denmark.

Edmundo B. Nery, D.M.D.
Research Associate in Dental Anatomy
Cleft Palate Research Center
School of Dental Medicine
University of Pittsburgh.

Sidney I. Rosen, M.S.
Research Associate in Histochemistry and Electronmicroscopy
Cleft Palate Research Center
School of Dental Medicine
University of Pittsburgh.

Sam Weinstein, D.D.S., M.S.
Professor and Chairman
Department of Orthodontics
College of Dentistry
University of Nebraska.

Preface to the Second Edition

The objectives stated in the preface to the first edition remain unchanged. In order to serve our original purpose, the second edition contains an update of the previous knowledge. This includes new contributors and consultants on the pulp, calcified tissues of the teeth, periodontium, temporomandibular joint, and human evolution.

In addition to the above, a new section on neuromuscular mechanisms in the masticatory system has been added.

The chapters devoted to morphology have been totally rearranged to make them easier to read. In addition, a large number of clinical color illustrations have been added to exemplify a wide range of clinical applications of morphological details.

The portions denoted to comparative dental anatomy and evolution of the masticatory system have been amplified to better fill a void that exists in standard dental anatomy books.

The chapter devoted to enamel and dentin has been enhanced by the addition of relevant material on enamel and dentin bonding.

To increase the readability of the text, in some chapters material has been reorganized into what we hope will be a more usable form. Color has been added to many of the figures to enhance their presentation.

We would again like to pay tribute to the contributors to the second edition who have enabled us to bring the state of information to its most current level.

R.E.J.
L.A.

Contributors to the Second Edition

Percy Butler, M.A., Ph.D., B.S.C.
Former Professor of Zoology
University of London
Comparative Dental Anatomy and Evolution

Frank Celenza, D.D.S.
Diplomate
American Board of Prosthodontists
Neuromuscular Physiology

Alan Hannum, B.D.S., Ph.D., F.D.S., R.C.S.
Professor of Oral Biology
Faculty of Dentistry
The University of British Columbia
TMJ and Neuromuscular Physiology

Edwin S. Rosenberg, B.D.S., H. Dip. Dent., D.M.D.
Professor of Periodontics
School of Dental Medicine
University of Pennsylvania
Anatomy of the Periodontium

Louis Rossman, D.M.D.
Chairman of Postdoctoral Endodontics
The I.B. Bender Division of Endodontics
Albert Einstein Medical Center
Director, American Board of Endodontics
Pulpal Anatomy

Farshid Sanavi, D.M.D.
Assistant Professor of Periodontics and Periodontal Research
School of Dental Medicine
University of Pennsylvania
Anatomy of the Periodontium

Geoffrey Sperber, B.S.C., B.D.S., M.Sc., Ph.D.
Professor of Oral Biology
University of Alberta
Comparative Dental Anatomy and Evolution/ Dental Anthropology

John G. Winnett, B.D.S., Ph.D., L.D.S., R.C.S., F.A.D.M.
Professor of Oral Biology and Pathology
School of Dental Medicine
State University of New York/Stonybrook
Anatomy of the Enamel

D. Walter Cohen, D.D.S.
President
Medical College of Pennsylvania
Anatomy of the Periodontium

Contents

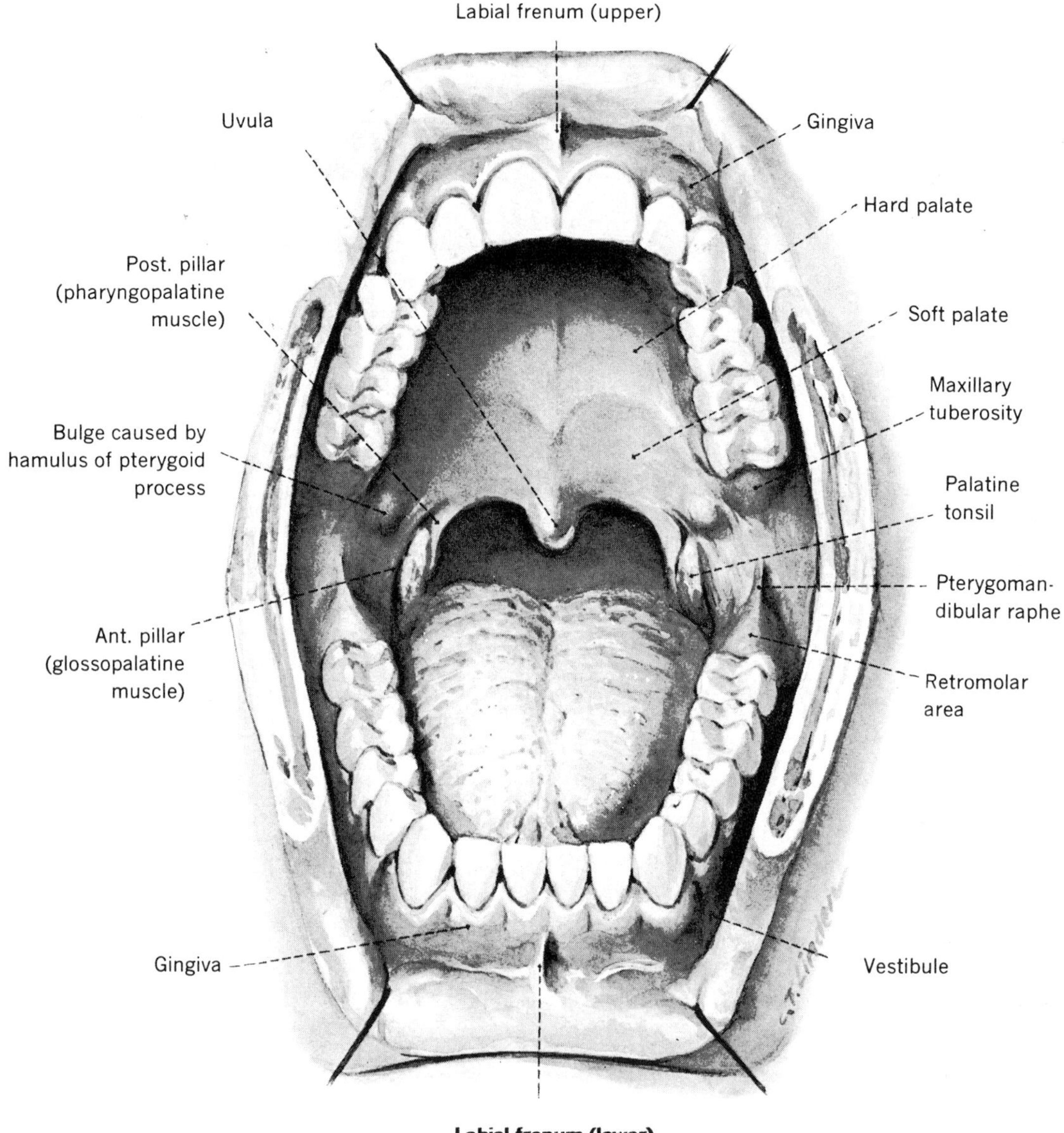

Plate I

The oral cavity. Reproduced from M. Massler and I. Schour, 1958, *Atlas of the Mouth,* by permission of the American Dental Association, Chicago.

Glossary

Terms of Orientation

Angle the junction of two or more surfaces
Apex the terminal end or tip of a root
Apical toward the apex of a root
Axial pertaining to the longitudinal (long) axis of the tooth, *i.e.*, labial, buccal, lingual, mesial, and distal surfaces
Axial root center an imaginary line passing through the geometric center of a tooth root parallel to its long axis
Buccal next to or toward the cheek
Buccal surface that surface of a posterior tooth positioned immediately adjacent to the cheek
Distal away from the median line
Distal surface the surface of a tooth facing away from the median line following the curve of the dental arch
Facial surfaces refers to labial and buccal surfaces collectively
Labial next to or toward the lips
Labial surface that surface of an anterior tooth positioned immediately adjacent to the lip
Lingual next to or toward the tongue
Lingual surface the surface of a tooth that faces towards the tongue
Line angle that angle formed by the junction of two surfaces *along a line, e.g.*, the mesiobuccal angle
Mesial toward the median line
Mesial surface the surface of a tooth facing toward the median line following the curve of the dental arch
Occlusal toward the biting surface of a posterior tooth
Occlusal surface the surface of a premolar or molar within the marginal ridges which contacts the corresponding surfaces of antagonists during closure of the posterior teeth
Point angle that angle formed by the junction of three surfaces *at a point, e.g.*, the mesiolabioincisal angle
Proximal surface the surface of a tooth which faces toward an adjoining tooth in the same arch, *i.e.*, both mesial and distal surfaces are proximal surfaces

Anatomical Terms

Cementoenamel junction junction of enamel and cementum, *i.e.*, cervical line
Cervix (neck) a narrow or constricted portion of a tooth in the region of the junction of crown and root
Cervical line a curved line formed by the junction of enamel and cementum of a tooth, *i.e.*, cementoenamel junction
Cingulum a bulbous convexity on the cervical third of the lingual surface of an anterior tooth
Contact area that region of the mesial or distal surface of a tooth that touches the adjacent tooth in the same arch
Crown that portion of a tooth, covered with enamel, which is normally visible in the oral cavity
Cusp 1) A pronounced elevation on the occlusal surface of a tooth terminating in a conical, rounded, or flat surface
2) Any crown elevation which begins calcification as an independent center
Embrasure a V-shaped space between the proximal surfaces of two adjoining teeth in contact
Fissure a cleft or crevice in a tooth surface thought to result from the imperfect fusion of the enamel of adjoining cusps or lobes
Fossa a rounded or angular depression on the surface of a tooth. There are three common types:
1) Lingual fossa—a broad shallow depression on the lingual surface of an incisor or canine
2) Central fossa—a relatively broad deep angular valley in the central portion of the occlusal surface of a molar
3) Triangular fossa—a comparatively shallow pyramid-shaped depression on the occlusal surfaces of posterior teeth located just within the confines of the mesial and/or distal marginal ridges
Groove a shallow linear depression on the surface of a tooth. There are two common types:
1) Developmental groove—marks the boundaries between adjacent cusps and other major divisional parts of a tooth
2) Supplemental groove—an indistinct linear depression, irregular in extent and direction, which does not demarcate major divisional portions of a tooth
Lobe a major division of a tooth erroneously believed to be formed during development from a separate center of calcification
Mamelon a rounded or conical prominence on the incisal ridge of a newly erupted incisor
Proximal root concavity a depression extending longitudinally on the mesial or distal surface of an anterior or posterior tooth
Pit a sharp, pointed depression usually located at the junction of two or more intersecting developmental grooves or at the termination of a single developmental groove

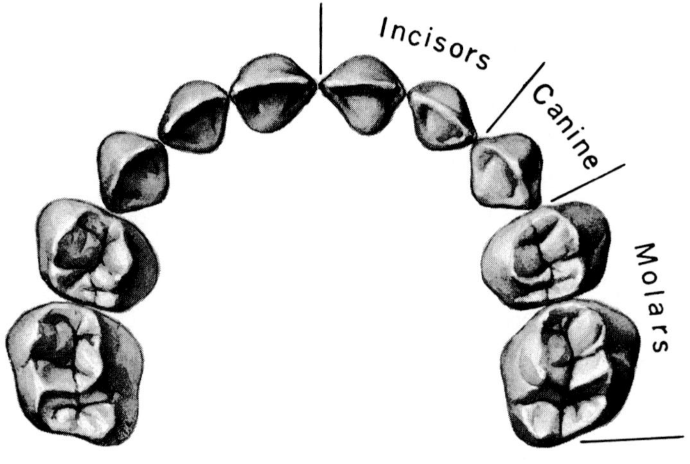

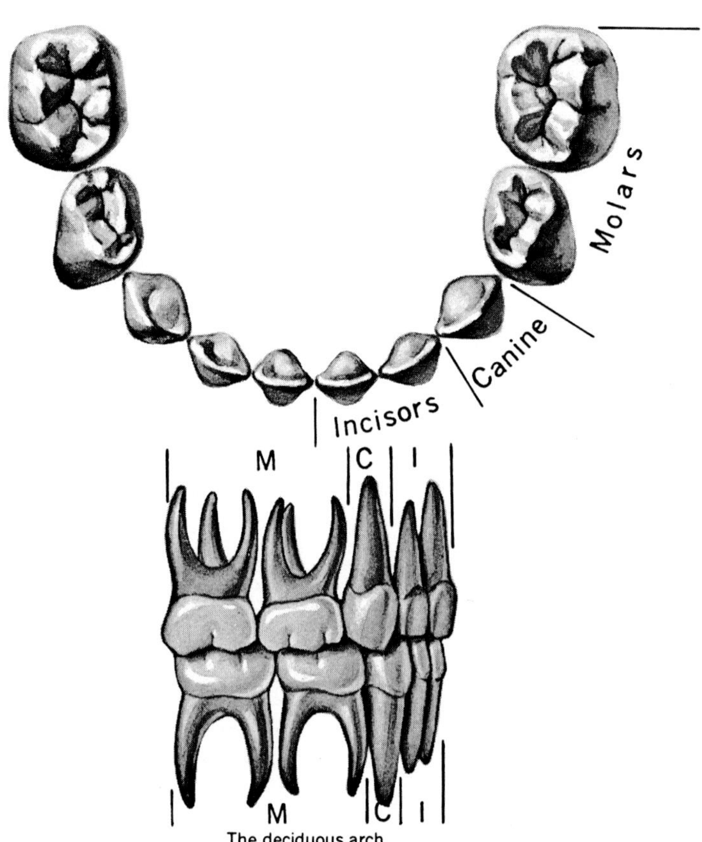

Plate II

The deciduous arch. Reproduced with modification from M. Massler and I. Schour, 1958, *Atlas of the Mouth,* by permission of the American Dental Association, Chicago.

Ridge a linear elevation on the surface of a tooth. There are several common types:
1) Marginal ridges—elevated crests which form the mesial and distal margins of a) the occlusal surfaces of posterior teeth, and b) the lingual surfaces of anterior teeth
2) Triangular ridges—prominent elevations, triangular in cross-section, which extend from the tip of a cusp towards the central portion of the occlusal surface of a tooth
3) Cusp ridges—elevations which extend in a mesial and distal direction from cusp tips. Cusp ridges form the buccal and lingual margins of the occlusal surfaces of posterior teeth
4) Incisal ridge—the incisal portion of a newly erupted anterior tooth
5) Oblique ridge—an elevated prominence on the occlusal surfaces of a maxillary molar extending obliquely between the tips of the distobuccal and mesiolingual cusps
6) Transverse ridge—made up of the triangular ridges of a buccal and a lingual cusp which join to form a more or less continuous elevation extending transversely across the occlusal surface of a posterior tooth

Root that portion of a tooth normally embedded in the alveolar process and covered with cementum

Root bifurcation that point at which a root trunk divides into two separate branches

Root trifurcation that point at which a root trunk divides into three separate branches

Root trunk (base) that portion of a multirooted tooth between the cervical line and bifurcation or trifurcation of the separate roots

Sulcus an elongated valley in the surface of a tooth formed by the inclines of adjacent cusps or ridges which meet at an angle

Thirds imaginary divisions of a tooth crown or root as to length (*i.e.*, occlusal, middle, and gingival thirds) or mesiodistal breadth (*i.e.*, mesial, middle, and distal thirds)

Tubercle a slightly rounded elevation on the surface of a tooth, *e.g.*, the lingual tubercle of the maxillary anterior teeth

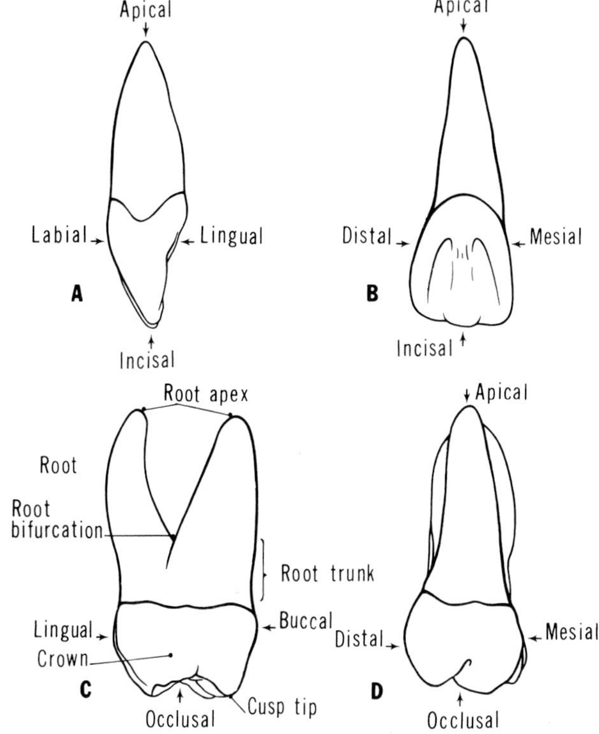

Plate III

A, maxillary left central incisor, distal view; *B*, maxillary left central incisor, lingual view; *C*, maxillary left first molar, mesial view; *D*, maxillary left first molar, lingual view.

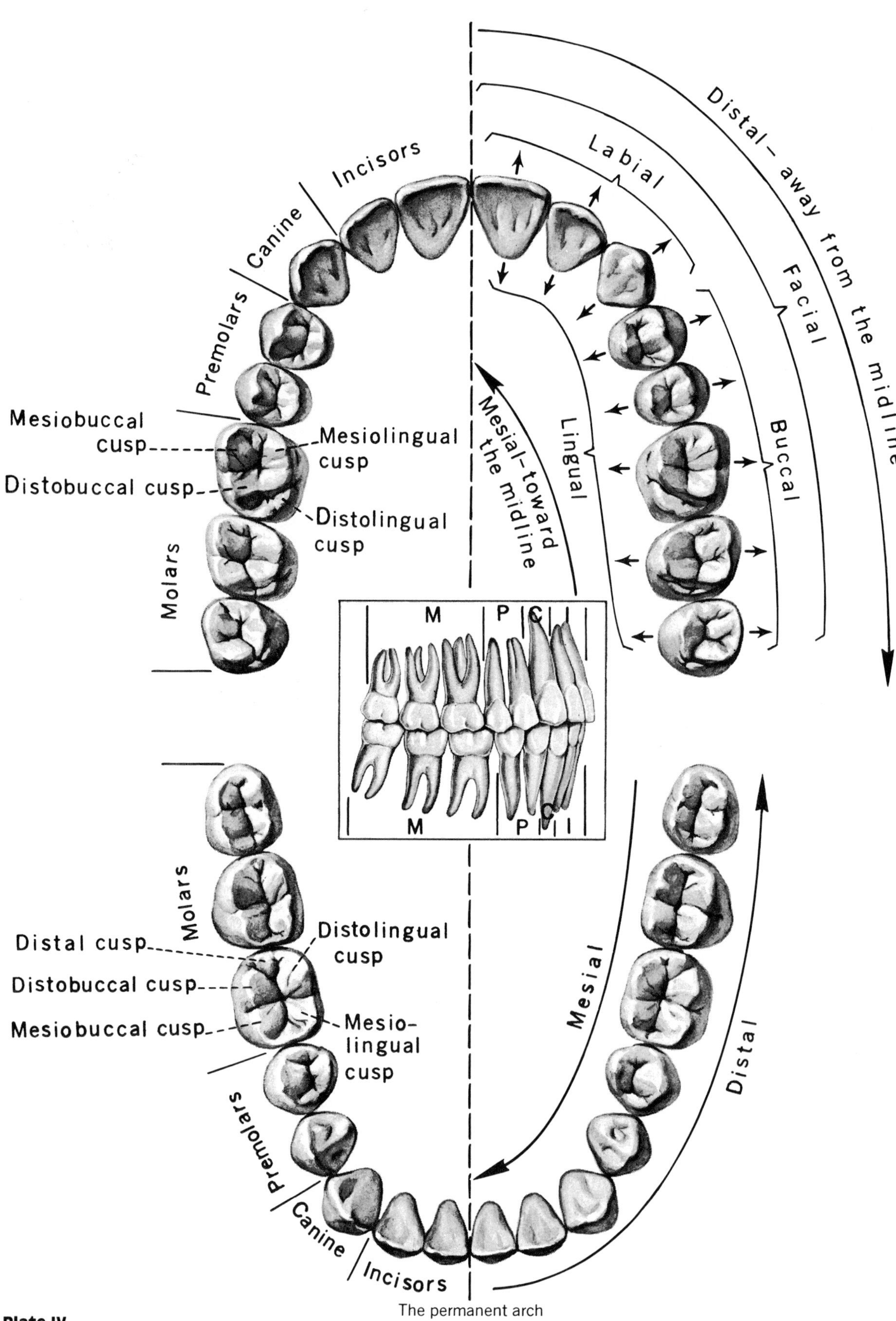

Plate IV

The permanent arch (terms of orientation). Reproduced with modification from M. Massler and I. Schour, 1958, *Atlas of the Mouth*, by permission of the American Dental Association, Chicago.

Kraus' Dental Anatomy and Occlusion

Part One

Anatomy of the Individual Teeth

1

Introduction

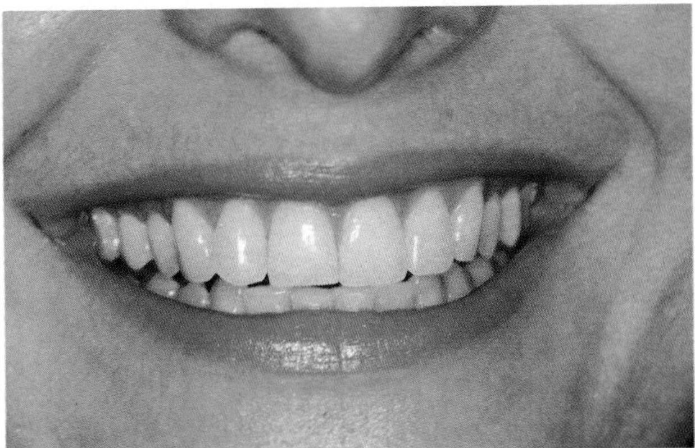

Figure 1.1
Frontal view of the human dentition.

Man, like all mammals, has two *sets* of teeth. The first set, comprising 20 teeth in all, is called the *primary* or *deciduous* dentition. These teeth first begin to appear in the oral cavity at a mean age of 6 months and the last one erupts into the mouth at about 28 ± 4 months. For approximately the next 4 years (from 2 to 6 years of age) the child must function with his 20 primary teeth. Then, commencing at 6 years, the first of the *permanent* teeth appears. From 6 until 12 years of age the primary teeth are replaced, in rather definite succession, by the permanent teeth (Fig. 1.1). Additional teeth appear until, by the age of 18 (or even as late as 25), the full complement of 32 permanent teeth is present in the mouth. There are, then, three periods of dentition in man: (1) the primary dentition (6 months to 6 years), (2) the mixed dentition (6 to 12 years), and (3) the permanent dentition (12+ years). If man is assigned an average life span of 70 years, it is obvious that he spends only 6 percent of this time chewing with his primary teeth but 91 percent, if he is fortunate, masticating with his permanent dentition. For this reason it has been the practice in most dental anatomy texts to describe first the permanent dentition, and this practice is followed here.

Just as the student in zoology first becomes acquainted with the taxonomic (or classification) system, so the dental student must first acquire a knowledge of dental systematics. In this way he is introduced to dentistry in an orderly, progressive manner. There is system and order in the dentition and its arrangement, and it greatly facilitates learning and remembering if the student is oriented to his subject in a scientific way. As in gross anatomy, there are special terms of orientation, movement, structure, and location that are part of the professional jargon language of dentistry. Furthermore, the peculiar kinds and arrangement of the dentition lend themselves to a special kind of taxonomical system that may be new to dentistry but is old hat to other fields such as archeology, from which we have borrowed the classification to be used in describing the permanent and primary dentitions.

To begin with there are two dental *arches:* the maxillary, which is part of the cranium and is immovable apart from it, and the mandibular, which is part of the lower jaw and is the movable part of the skull. In man the units of the primary and the permanent dentition are equally divided between the two arches. Thus, in the primary dentition there are 10 maxillary and 10 mandibular teeth, and in the permanent dentition there are 16 maxillary and 16 permanent units. Looking at the two arches face-on, we can divide the total tooth-bearing apparatus into four quadrants: a right maxillary, a left maxillary, a right mandibular, and a left mandibular. In the permanent dentition there are eight teeth in each quadrant. The vertical line dividing the arches into right and left halves denotes the *midsagittal plane.* A horizontal line between the arches separates the upper from the lower dentitions.

On the basis of form and function the human teeth fall into three or four *classes.* In the primary dentition there are three classes of teeth: incisors, canines, and molars. In the permanent dentition there are four classes: incisors, canines, premolars (or bicuspids), and molars. Canines, for example, differ in form from the molars in that they possess a single rather pointed cusp, whereas molars have three to five somewhat flattened cusps. The form predicts the function in both cases. Canines are primarily piercing teeth while molars are grinders. Class traits, then, are basically those characteristics that place teeth into functional categories. The labiolingually compressed crowns of incisors make them cutting teeth as opposed to the cone-shaped cusps of the canines, which limit them to piercing functions.

The number of teeth in each class constitutes the *dental formula,* and is usually stated in terms of one

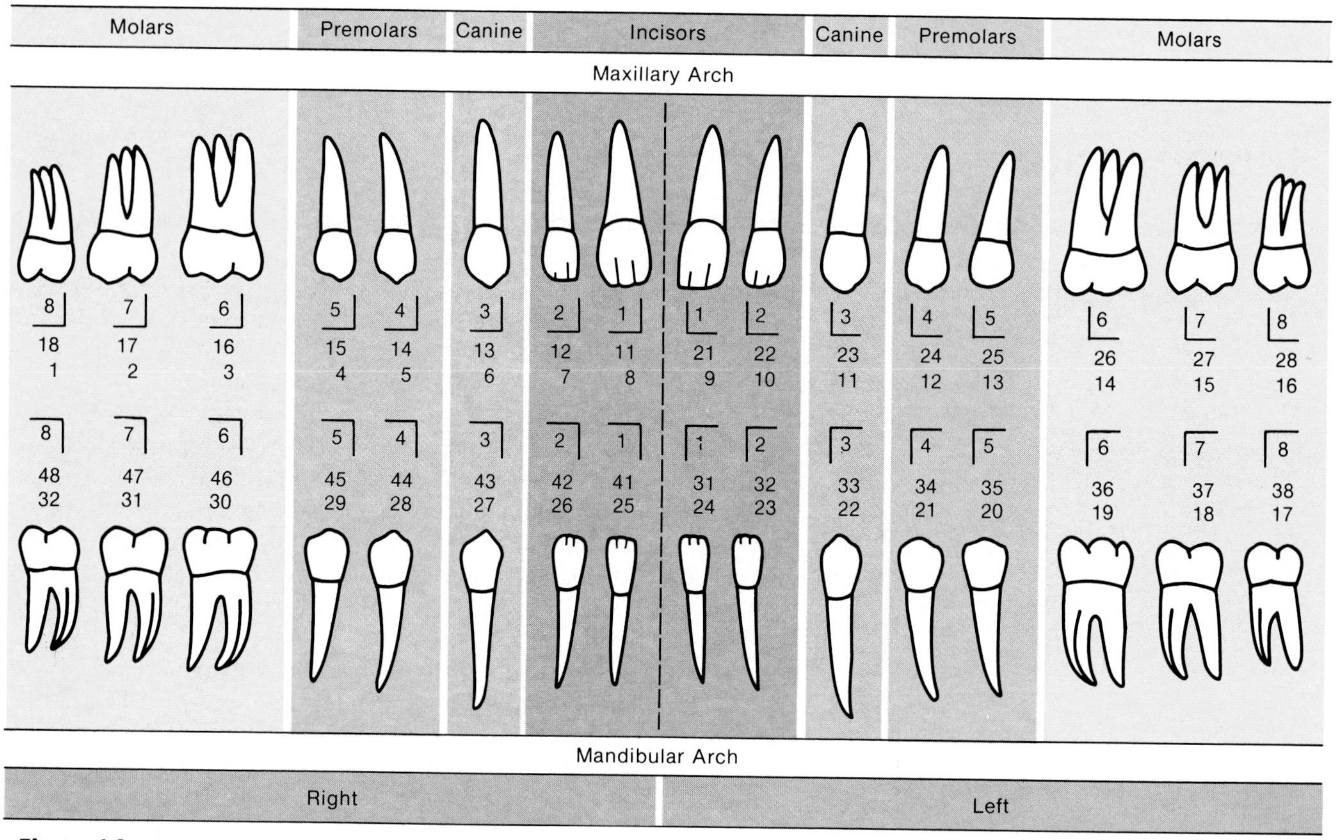

Molars			Premolars		Canine	Incisors				Canine	Premolars		Molars		
Maxillary Arch															
8┘	7┘	6┘	5┘	4┘	3┘	2┘	1┘	└1	└2	└3	└4	└5	└6	└7	└8
18	17	16	15	14	13	12	11	21	22	23	24	25	26	27	28
1	2	3	4	5	6	7	8	9	10	11	12	13	14	15	16
8┐	7┐	6┐	5┐	4┐	3┐	2┐	1┐	┌1	┌2	┌3	┌4	┌5	┌6	┌7	┌8
48	47	46	45	44	43	42	41	31	32	33	34	35	36	37	38
32	31	30	29	28	27	26	25	24	23	22	21	20	19	18	17
Mandibular Arch															
Right								Left							

Figure 1.2
A classification of the permanent dentition.

quadrant, the upper left. For example, in the permanent dentition there are two incisors, one canine, two premolars, and three molars in each quadrant. They are written as follows: 2-1-2-3. In each quadrant the teeth closest to the midline are the incisors, followed distally by the canine, the two premolars, and finally the three molars. The entire dental formula would be written

$$\frac{3\text{-}2\text{-}1\text{-}2 \mid 2\text{-}1\text{-}2\text{-}3}{3\text{-}2\text{-}1\text{-}2 \mid 2\text{-}1\text{-}2\text{-}3}.$$

Since in man each quadrant contains the same number and classes of teeth, the formula need be written for only one quadrant. In other mammals, however, there are differences between maxillary and mandibular arches, so that upper and lower left quadrants are designated (see Figs. 1.2 and 1.3).

Not only are there differences within each class between the upper and lower arches (these differences being called *arch traits*), but there are differences between the arch components of each class which render them easily identifiable. For example, in the incisor class there are two components in each quadrant. The most mesial of the two is the *central incisor,* so designated for its proximity to the midsagittal plane. Distal to it is the *lateral incisor.* Although both incisors possess distinctive class traits and arch traits, they also have individual characteristics that differentiate them from each other. The latter are termed *type traits.** In addition to these three kinds of traits, a fourth is the *set* trait, which differentiates the permanent tooth from its analogue (or counterpart) in the primary dentition. In other words, those features that enable the dental anatomist to differentiate between a permanent maxillary central incisor and a primary maxillary central incisor are called *set traits.*

Several shorthand notation methods have been devised for designating the type of tooth and the quadrant in which it is found. There are three systems of numerical designation. The most common and perhaps most convenient notation is the *Palmer System,* which employs cursive upper case letters for the primary teeth and arabic numerals for the permanent teeth. Thus, for the primary teeth the designation is as follows:

*There are arch traits and set traits for canines, but no type traits.

A = central incisor
B = lateral incisor
C = canine
D = first molar
E = second molar

For the permanent dentition it is:

1 = central incisor
2 = lateral incisor
3 = canine
4 = first premolar
5 = second premolar
6 = first molar
7 = second molar
8 = third molar (wisdom tooth)

To indicate a particular quadrant the following symbols are used:

⌊ = maxillary left
⌋ = maxillary right
⌈ = mandibular left
⌉ = mandibular right

In this way it is a simple matter to designate any one of the 52 units of the dentition; ⌊5, for example, denotes a maxillary permanent left second premolar, and E⌉ signifies a mandibular right primary first molar.

A second frequently used numerical designation system is the *International System*, in which the quadrants are designated as follows:

maxillary permanent right = 1
maxillary permanent left = 2
mandibular permanent left = 3
mandibular permanent right = 4

The individual teeth in each quadrant have the same numerical designation as in the Palmer System, namely,

11 = maxillary right central incisor
12 = maxillary right lateral incisor
13 = maxillary right canine incisor
14 = maxillary right first premolar

21 = maxillary left central incisor
22 = maxillary left lateral incisor
23 = maxillary left canine incisor
24 = maxillary left first premolar

The primary quadrants in the International System are numbered as follows:

maxillary primary right = 5
maxillary primary left = 6
mandibular primary left = 7
mandibular primary right = 8

The individual primary teeth are numerically designated as follows:

51 to 55 = maxillary right central incisor to maxillary right second molar

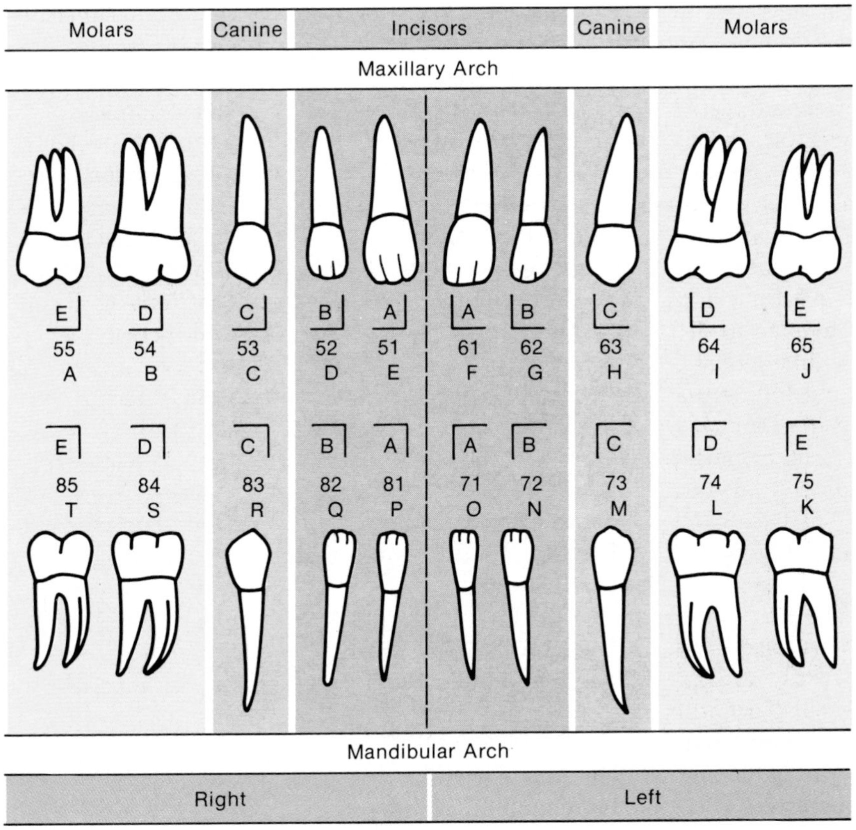

Molars		Canine	Incisors				Canine	Molars	
Maxillary Arch									
E⌋	D⌋	C⌋	B⌋	A⌋	⌊A	⌊B	⌊C	⌊D	⌊E
55	54	53	52	51	61	62	63	64	65
A	B	C	D	E	F	G	H	I	J
E⌉	D⌉	C⌉	B⌉	A⌉	⌈A	⌈B	⌈C	⌈D	⌈E
85	84	83	82	81	71	72	73	74	75
T	S	R	Q	P	O	N	M	L	K
Mandibular Arch									
Right					Left				

Figure 1.3
A classification of the primary dentition.

61 to 65 = maxillary left central incisor to maxillary left second molar
71 to 75 = mandibular left central incisor to mandibular left second molar
81 to 85 = mandibular right central incisor to mandibular right second molar

There is a third system of numerical designation, the *American* or *Universal System*, which numerically designates the teeth in sequential order beginning with the most posterior tooth in the maxillary right permanent arch on the maxillary right third molar as #1, thence proceeding sequentially to the maxillary right central incisor, #8, to the maxillary left central incisor, #9, sequentially to the maxillary left third molar, #16, thence to the mandibular left third molar, #17, sequentially to the mandibular left central incisor, #24, to the mandibular right central incisor, #25, sequentially to the mandibular right third molar, #32.

The primary dentition is designated from A to T in sequential order in the same manner. Thus:

A = maxillary right second primary molar
E = maxillary right primary central incisor
F = maxillary left primary central incisor
J = maxillary left primary second molar
K = mandibular left primary second molar
O = mandibular left primary central incisor
P = mandibular right primary central incisor
T = mandibular right primary second molar

If, out of the totality of 52 teeth, a single tooth were to be selected at random, how would one proceed to identify it? Generally one would follow this order. (1) Is it one of the primary or permanent teeth? (2) Is it an incisor, canine, premolar, or molar? (3) Is it a maxillary or mandibular tooth? (4) If it is an incisor, is it a central or lateral; if a premolar or molar, which specific one is it? Therefore, we might say that the usual order of classification is first to identify the *set* trait, next the *class* trait, then the *arch* trait, and finally the *type* trait. Since it is unsystematic to describe primary and permanent teeth simultaneously, we omit the set traits in this chapter but follow the remaining sequence. If we were to consider the various groups or populations of mankind, and even the other kinds of Primates, then we would be forced to use additional diagnostic categories, such as *racial traits* and *species traits.* Indeed, in a later chapter we do just that.

The arrangement of this chapter differs from the standard dental texts in that the teeth are discussed by class rather than by type. In other words, we deal with the incisors (central and lateral, maxillary and mandibular) as a group rather than as individual units. This not only facilitates description and analysis of basic features held in common, but also emphasizes arch and type differences. In addition, it eliminates unnecessary repetition.

With each class the same order of treatment is followed. The maxillary units are discussed first, then the mandibular. Since each tooth can be described from five different views, the maxillary and mandibular teeth are treated in the following order: labial (or buccal), lingual, mesial, distal, and incisal (or occlusal) aspects. Under each aspect the types of teeth in that class are considered, always in the same order; thus, for the maxillary incisors, the labial aspect of the central incisor is discussed first, followed by the lingual aspect, and so on. In addition, for each aspect the tooth may best be divided into three areas for purposes of systematic description: *crown profile, crown surface,* and *root.* Following the description of the five aspects, the pulp and the normal variations in structure of the crown and root are discussed. The same order is followed for the description of the lateral incisors. The chapters end with summary charts that show in abbreviated form the diagnostic arch and type traits for the particular class and arch.

Since this arrangement is deemed to be of particular use to the student in making various kinds of comparisons, the following outline of the above arrangement is presented, with the outline for the permanent incisors expanded as an example:

The Permanent Incisors

The Maxillary Incisors
- Size and Eruption
- Central Incisor
  - Labial Aspect
  - Lingual Aspect
  - Mesial Aspect
  - Distal Aspect
  - Incisal Aspect
  - Pulp
  - Variations
- Lateral Incisor
- Summary
  - Arch Traits
  - Type Traits

The Mandibular Incisors
- Size and Eruption
- Central Incisor
  - Labial Aspect
  - Lingual Aspect
  - Mesial Aspect
  - Distal Aspect
  - Incisal Aspect
  - Pulp
  - Variations
- Lateral Incisor
- Summary
  - Arch Traits
  - Type Traits

The Permanent Canines

The Maxillary Canines
The Mandibular Canines

The Permanent Premolars

The Maxillary Premolars
The Mandibular Premolars

The Permanent Molars

The Maxillary Molars
The Mandibular Molars

2

The Permanent Incisors

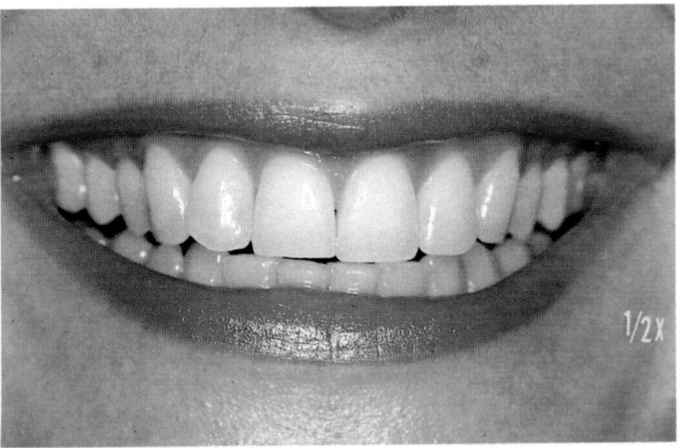

Figure 2.1
The permanent incisors appear prominently in a smile.

There are two incisors on each side of the midline of both maxillary and mandibular arches (Fig. 2.1). The *central* or *first* incisor is that member of the class closest to the midline, whereas the *lateral* or *second* incisor is farther removed from (or more distal to) the midline (Fig. 2.2).

The mandibular central incisor is generally the first of its class to erupt, at approximately 7 years of age. It is soon followed by the maxillary central incisors. The maxillary and mandibular lateral incisors are usually the last members of the class to appear, generally during the eighth year.

Incisors, as a class, constitute the "cutting blades" of the human grinding mill. In the animal kingdom, they may have a variety of functions, such as fur combing in the insectivores, tree chopping in certain rodents, and meat stripping in the carnivora. In man, however, their chief function is that of cutting or shearing food in preparation for grinding.

The incisors, together with the canines, form a particular group referred to as the *anterior teeth.* The anterior teeth are highly important esthetically, since they are readily seen during eating, speech, and facial gesticulation. In addition they play an important role in the formulation of many speech sounds, particularly in the Romance, Anglo-Saxon and Germanic languages. For example, a 6-year-old child who has lost the deciduous maxillary central incisors is unable to produce such sounds as "v," "f," or "th" until the permanent maxillary incisors erupt.

The incisors, then, as a class provide a significant contribution: (1) functionally, as cutting instruments; (2) esthetically in that their presence, proper form, and arrangement are important adjuncts to pleasing facial configuration; (3) phonetically, in that they play a major role in the proper enunciation of certain speech sounds.

Certain class traits distinguish all incisors: (1) the incisal two-thirds of the crown appears flattened or compressed labiolingually, providing a long horizon-

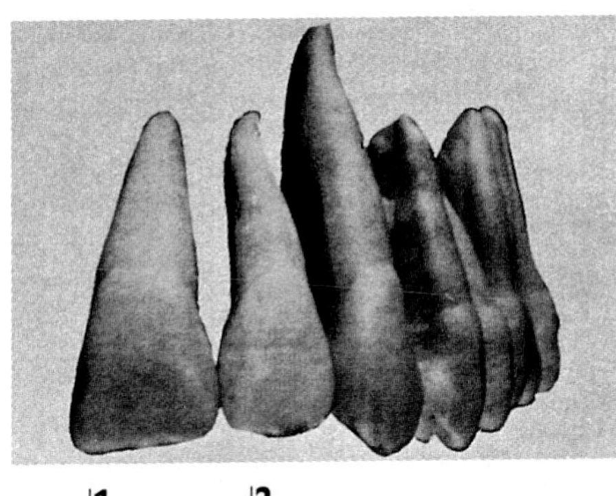

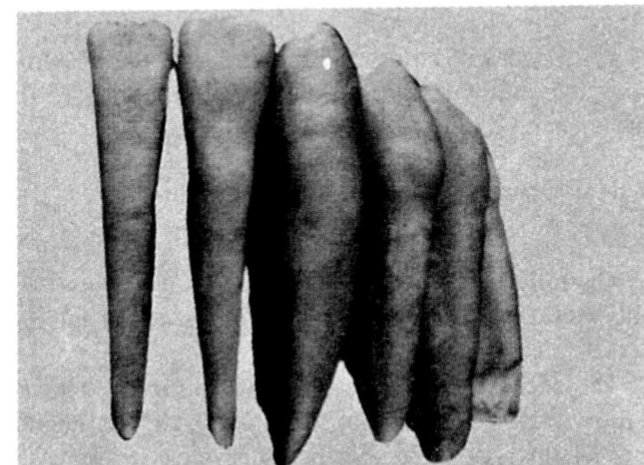

Figure 2.2
Labial view of the left quadrants.

tal "biting" edge or margin; (2) two or more distinct and rounded protuberances (or *mamelons*) surmount the incisal margins of all newly erupted incisors (the form, distribution, and number of these mamelons may differ in each type of incisor); (3) the marginal ridges of all incisors are located on the mesial and distal borders of the lingual surfaces and are roughly parallel to the long axis of each tooth.

All incisors, maxillary and mandibular, as well as central and lateral, show these features in common (class traits). As is seen in the following sections, however, maxillary incisors present distinctive features (i.e., arch traits) that differentiate them from their mandibular counterparts; in addition, lateral incisors may be distinguished from central incisors in a number of morphological characteristics (type traits).

The Maxillary Incisors

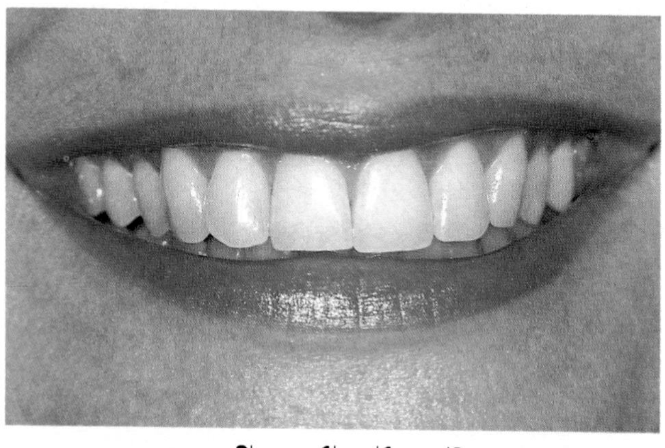

Figure 2.3
Maxillary incisors.

Size and Eruption

Maxillary Incisors	Crown Height (mm)	Mesiodistal Crown Diameter (mm)	Labiolingual Crown Diameter (mm)	Tooth Length (mm)	Age at Eruption (yr)
Central incisors	10.5	8.5	7.0	23.5	7
Lateral incisors	9.0	6.5	6.0	22.0	8

The maxillary incisors are chisel-shaped cutting teeth. Viewed labially or lingually they are the widest teeth of the incisor class (arch trait). In addition, in the maxillary arch the central incisor is larger in crown area than the lateral (arch trait, since the reverse is true in the mandibular arch). Apart from size the two incisors are basically similar in form. As is discussed later, the lateral incisor morphologically has a diminutive modification of the basic form exhibited by the central incisor.

Central Incisor

Labial Aspect (Fig. 2.4)

The crown of the maxillary central incisor is by far the widest (mesiodistally) of the four types of incisors (type trait).

The incisal margin of the newly erupted, unworn tooth reveals three minor elevations representing the tips of three or more so-called mamelons. Generally there are three such elevations, of which the central is the smallest in terms of breadth. The mesial and distal mamelons are of approximately equal width. The former often has a slightly raised "shoulder" on the mesial portion of the incisal profile, and it joins

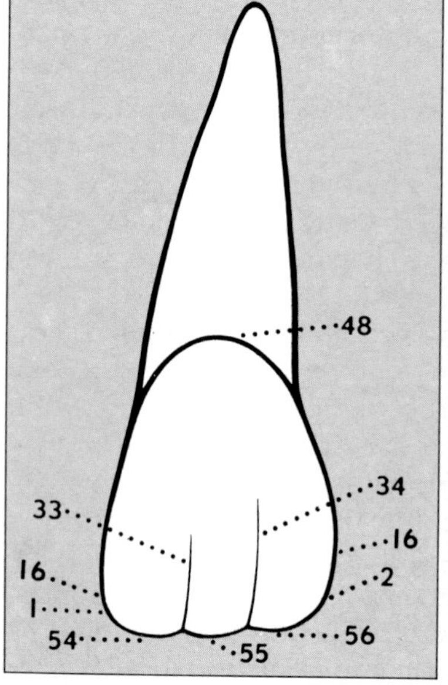

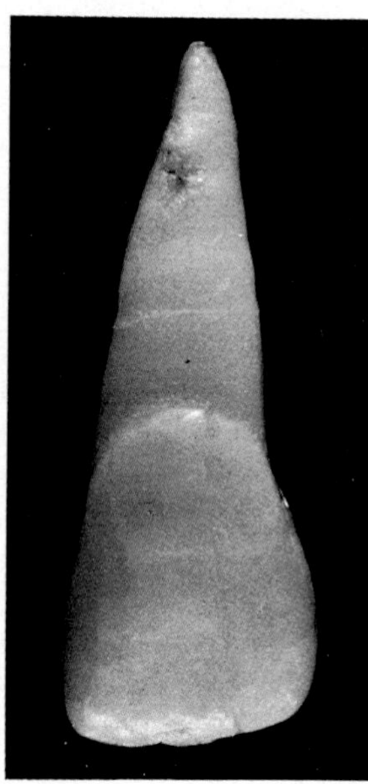

Figure 2.4
Maxillary left central incisor (labial aspect). For Numerical Nomenclature Code, see page 9 (also inside front and back covers).

Numerical Nomenclature Code

1. Mesioincisal Angle
2. Distoincisal Angle
3. Mesiolabial Line Angle
4. Distolabial Line Angle
5. Mesiobuccal Angle
6. Distobuccal Angle
7. Mesiolingual Angle
8. Distolingual Angle
9. Root Apex
10. Cusp Apex
11. Axial Root Center
12. Cervix
13. Cingulum
14. Proximal Root Concavity
15. Mesial Concavity
16. Contact Area
17. Buccal Cusp
18. Lingual Cusp
19. Mesiobuccal Cusp
20. Mesiolingual Cusp
21. Distobuccal Cusp
22. Distolingual Cusp
23. Distal Cusp
24. Carabelli Cusp
25. Mesial Marginal Ridge Cusp
26. Lingual Fossa
27. Mesiolingual Fossa
28. Distolingual Fossa
29. Mesial Triangular Fossa
30. Distal Triangular Fossa
31. Central Fossa
32. Distal Fossa
33. Mesiolabial Groove
34. Distolabial Groove
35. Mesial Marginal Groove
36. Supplemental Groove
37. Mesial Groove
38. Distal Groove
39. Central Groove
40. Mesiobuccal Groove
41. Distobuccal Groove
42. Mesiolingual Groove
43. Distolingual Groove
44. Lingual Groove
45. Buccal Groove
46. Carabelli Groove
47. Height of Contour
48. Cervical Line
49. Buccal Verticle Apex Line
50. Lingual Verticle Apex Line
51. Mesial Lobe
52. Middle Lobe
53. Distal Lobe
54. Mesial Mamelon
55. Middle Mamelon
56. Distal Mamelon
57. Median Longitudinal Axis
58. Lingual Pit
59. Mesial Pit
60. Distal Pit
61. Buccal Pit
62. Central Pit
63. Carabelli Pit
64. Incisal Ridge
65. Mesial Marginal Ridge
66. Distal Marginal Ridge
67. Mesial Cusp Ridge
68. Distal Cusp Ridge
69. Distal Transverse Ridge
70. Transverse Ridge
71. Buccal Ridge
72. Lingual Ridge
73. Oblique Ridge
74. Anterior Transverse Ridge
75. Triangular Ridge
76. Buccal Root
77. Lingual Root
78. Mesiobuccal Root
79. Distobuccal Root
80. Mesial Root
81. Distal Root
82. Root Bifurcation
83. Root Trunk (base)
84. Lingual Tubercle

the mesial margin of the crown at right angles, the so-called mesioincisal angle (type trait). The distal mamelon, on the other hand, presents a relatively low shoulder, which slopes cervically to meet the distal profile margin of the crown in a more or less rounded "distoincisal" angle.

The mesial margin of the crown forms a more or less straight line. The height of contour (i.e., the contact area with the adjacent tooth) of the mesial margin is located relatively close to the incisal edge (within the incisal third). The distal margin, on the other hand, is somewhat rounded with the height of contour located further away from the incisal edge at the junction of the middle and incisal thirds.

Both mesial and distal margins converge cervically and end in the cervical line (cementoenamel junction, or CEJ). The CEJ is a smoothly curved arc that is convex cervically.

From the incisal margin two or more grooves may extend toward the cervical line. These mark the borders of the lobes that culminate in mamelons at the incisal margin. They are of variable length and prominence. We will call them *labial lobe grooves.*

The root is conical in outline and is inclined distally from cervix to apex.

Lingual Aspect (Fig. 2.5)

The crown profile in lingual aspect is the same as in labial aspect.

The lingual surface of the crown is "scoop-like" in form. It is marked by a broad depression in its central portion (the *lingual fossa*), which is bordered by three distinct elevations: namely, the *mesial* and *distal marginal ridges* respectively, and the *cingulum*, a bulbous protuberance just below the cervical line. Marginal ridges and cinguli are prominent features of the

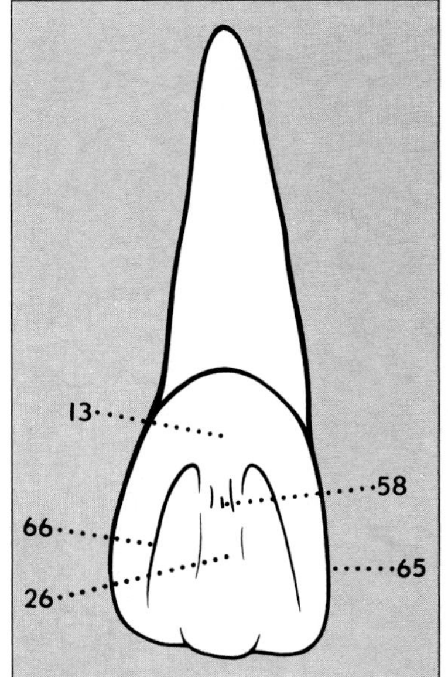

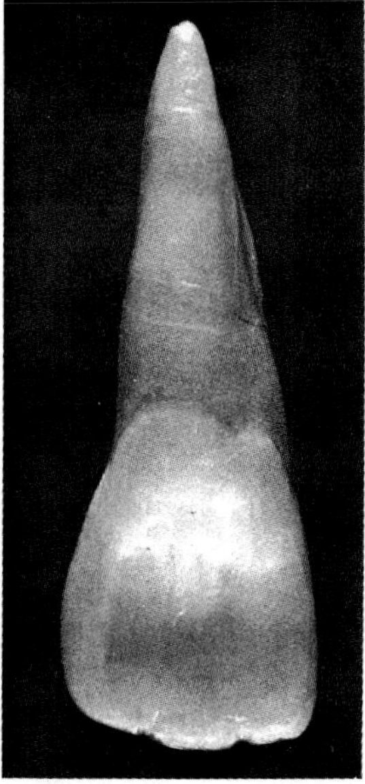

Figure 2.5

Maxillary left central incisor (lingual aspect).

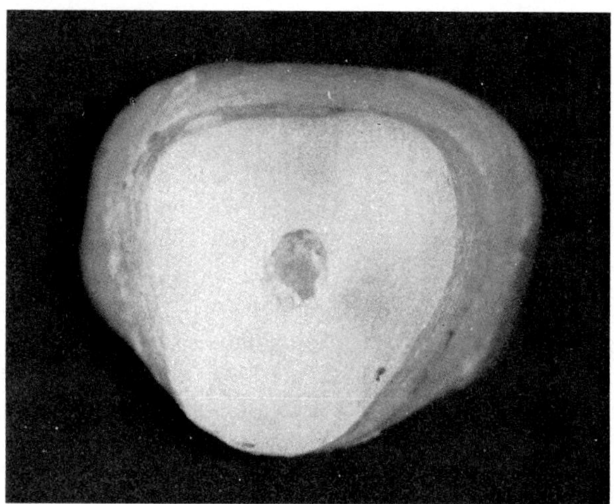

Figure 2.6

Root of the maxillary left central incisor in transverse section.

lingual surfaces of all maxillary incisors (arch trait); as a result, the lingual fossa is invariably a well-defined depression (arch trait).

Faint grooves mark the inner borders of the marginal ridges, and a small pit (the lingual pit) is often found just below the central portion of the cingulum.

The CEJ of the lingual surface forms a distinctly curved arc that differs from that of the labial surface in two respects: (1) the lingual CEJ forms an arc with a much smaller radius than that of the labial; (2) the point of maximum convexity of the lingual CEJ is situated near the distal margin of the root.

The root is narrower seen from the lingual than from the labial aspect. This is because in horizontal cross-section the root converges lingually (Fig. 2.6). From this view the more labially placed portion of the root, both mesial and distal, can be seen. This feature is characteristic of all maxillary incisors; hence it is an arch trait.

Mesial Aspect (Fig. 2.7)

The crown appears chisel-shaped in outline because of an incisal convergence of the labial and lingual margins. The labial margin is smoothly curved from its height of contour in the cervical third up to the incisal edge. The lingual margin is S-shaped, being convex in the region of the cingulum and concave thence to the incisal edge.

The mesial surface of the maxillary central incisor is unique in that the CEJ shows the most pronounced curvature of any tooth in the dentition (type trait).

The root is conical in outline and tapers to a pointed apex.

Distal Aspect (Fig. 2.8)

The crown profile in distal aspect is not different from the mesial view.

The crown surface has two features that characterize its distal aspect; the cervical line is less sharply curved on the distal aspect, and the distal contact area is located further from the incisal margin than is the mesial contact area.

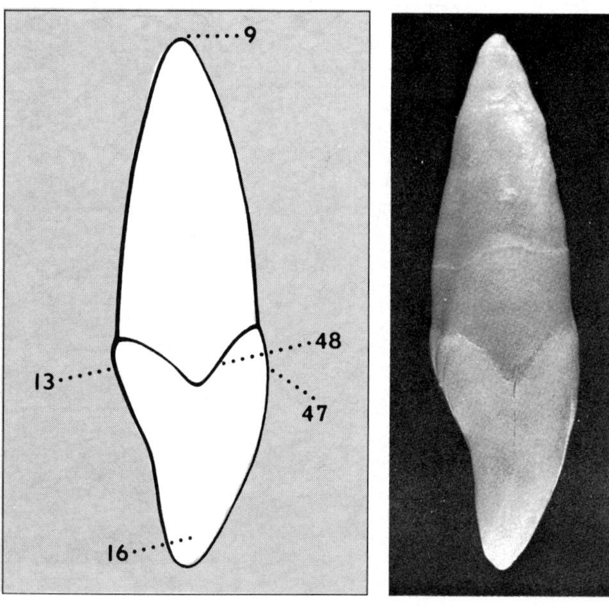

Figure 2.7

Maxillary left central incisor (mesial aspect).

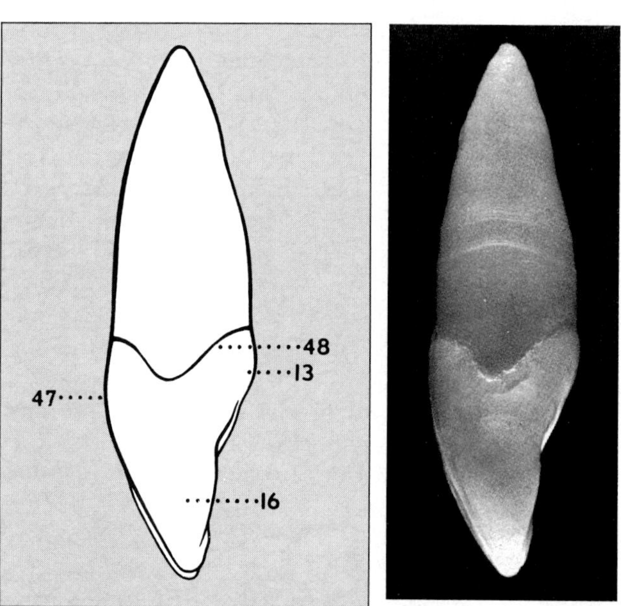

Figure 2.8

Maxillary left central incisor (distal aspect).

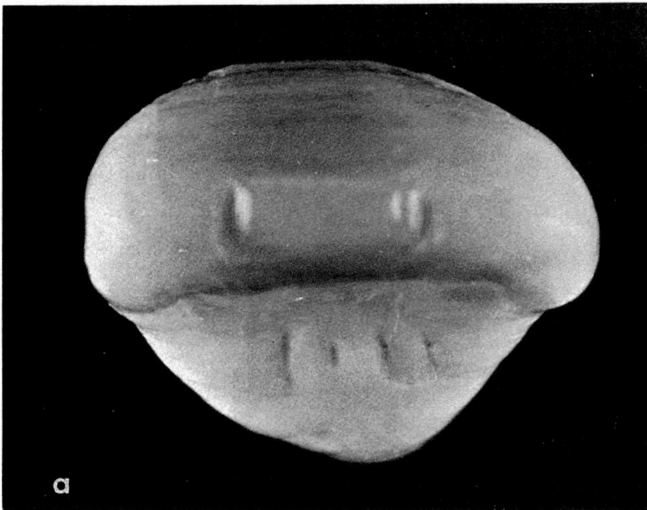

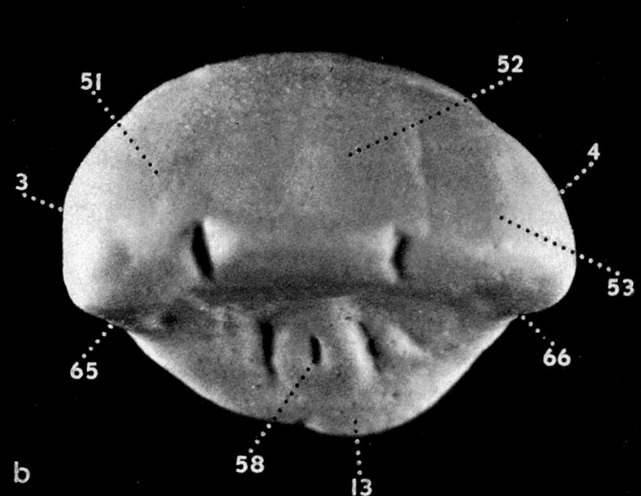

Figure 2.9

Maxillary left central incisor (incisal aspect): *a,* actual crown; *b,* cast.

Incisal Aspect (Fig. 2.9)

The crown is roughly triangular in outline from the incisal aspect (type trait). The labial profile forms the "base" of the triangle, the mesial and distal profiles its "sides," and the "apex" is located lingually.

The labial profile, which is in general bilaterally symmetrical and only slightly convex from the mesial to distal (type trait), meets the mesial and distal profiles to form relatively sharp, distinct line angles, i.e., the mesiolabial and distolabial line angles respectively (type trait). The mesial and distal profiles, which converge lingually, are unequal in length, the mesial being the longer of the two. As a result the apex is located distal to the midline of the tooth.

The labial surface as seen from the incisal aspect often shows three or more faint depressions, the labial lobe grooves, extending gingivally from the incisal edge. These demark the lobes of the crown. They are important esthetically because their presence causes light to be reflected laterally, thereby giving a "textured" appearance to the labial surface (see Figs. 2.10, 2.11).

The details of the lingual surface, which include the prominent cingulum and distinct mesial and distal marginal ridges, are clearly seen from the incisal aspect. The pit (or pits) on the cingulum, when present, are clearly visible.

Pulp (Fig. 2.12)

The structure of the pulp cavity roughly mirrors the external configuration of the crown and root as seen in both labiolingual and mesiodistal sections. The wid-

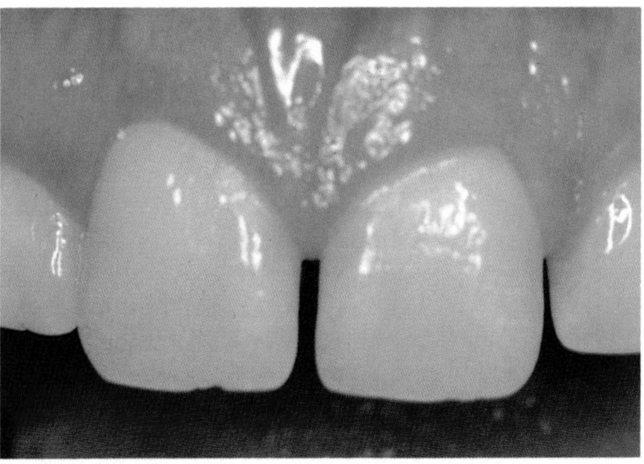

Figure 2.10

Unsightly spacing (diastema) between maxillary anterior teeth—a disfigurement observed in over 20 percent of patients.

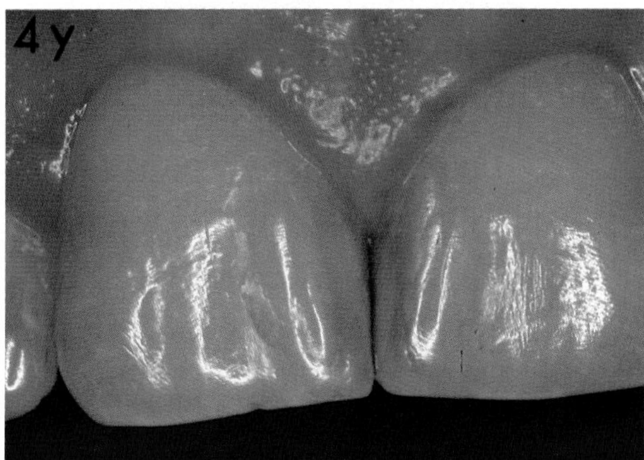

Figure 2.11

The same anterior dentition as shown in Figure 2.10 four years after space closure using bonded composite material.

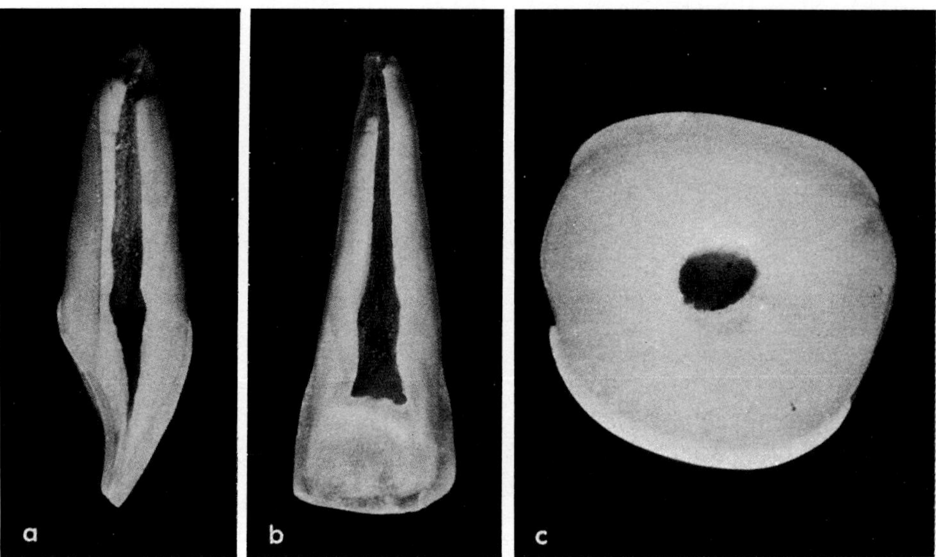

Figure 2.12

Pulp cavity of the maxillary left central incisors: *a*, labiolingual section; *b*, mesiodistal section; *c*, transverse section at the cervix.

est diameter of the cavity labiolingually occurs at the level of the cervix, where in horizontal cross-section the pulp cavity is almost rounded (Fig. 2.12*a–c*). In the incisal two-thirds of the crown the pulp cavity flattens out labiolingually in keeping with the external structure. In other words, an endocast of the pulp cavity would very much resemble a cigar holder, flat at the lip portion and rounded where the cigar is inserted.

Variations

The maxillary central incisor may show a wide range of variability, particularly with regard to (1) labial outline; (2) labial lobe grooves; (3) labial profile curvature; (4) the mammelons; (5) the cingulum; (6) root size.

Labial Outline The mesial and distal borders of the maxillary central incisor crown as seen from the labial

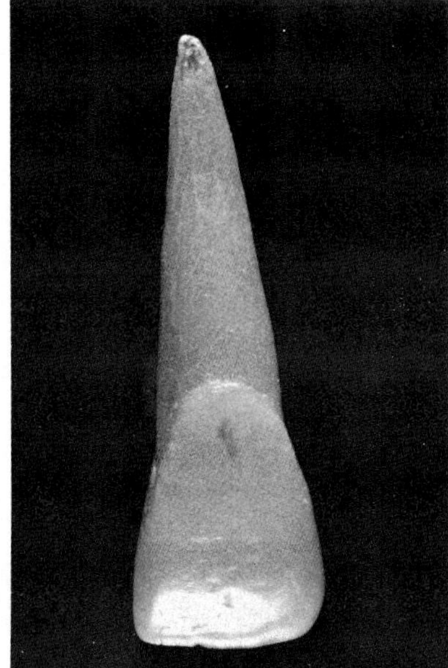

Figure 2.13

Labial aspect of the maxillary left central incisor showing tapered crown outline.

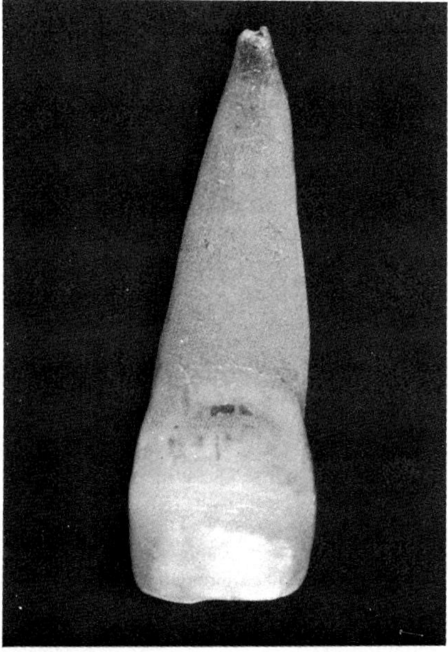

Figure 2.14

Labial aspect of the maxillary left central incisor showing square crown outline.

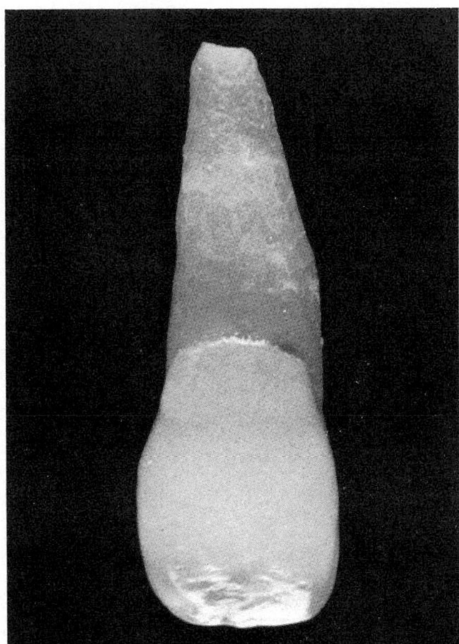

Figure 2.15
Labial aspect of the maxillary right central incisor showing ovoid crown outline.

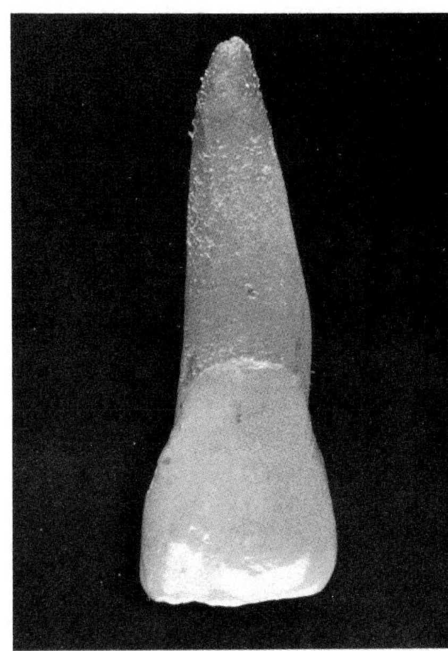

Figure 2.16
Labial aspect of the maxillary left central incisor showing square-tapered crown outline.

aspect usually converge toward the cervix. In other words, the narrowest portion of the crown from this aspect is located in the cervical area. Central incisor crowns characteristically show a high degree of variation with regard to this outline, and in this respect may be classified into three basic types: (1) *tapering,* where the mesial and distal borders show a pronounced convergence toward the cervix (Fig. 2.13); (2) *square,* where mesial and distal borders show only slight cervical convergence, imparting to the crown a square outline (Fig. 2.14); (3) *ovoid,* where the widest dimension is found in the middle third of the crown, and the mesial and distal borders converge cervically as well as slightly incisally (Fig. 2.15).

In addition, there may be many combinations of the three basic types. For example, the central incisor shown on Figure 2.16 might be classified as a square-tapered type.

Labial Lobe Grooves As we have already seen, labial lobe grooves or depressions extend from the incisal edge cervically to demarcate three distinct lobes on the labial surface (Fig. 2.17*a* and *b*). The grooves are highly variable with regard to their degree of expres-

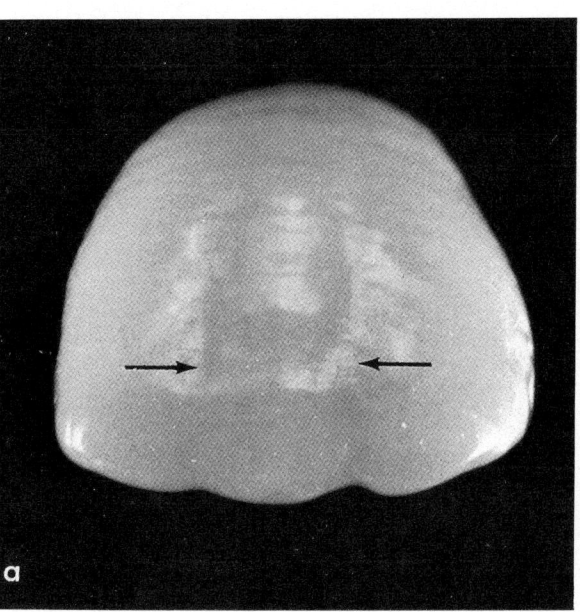

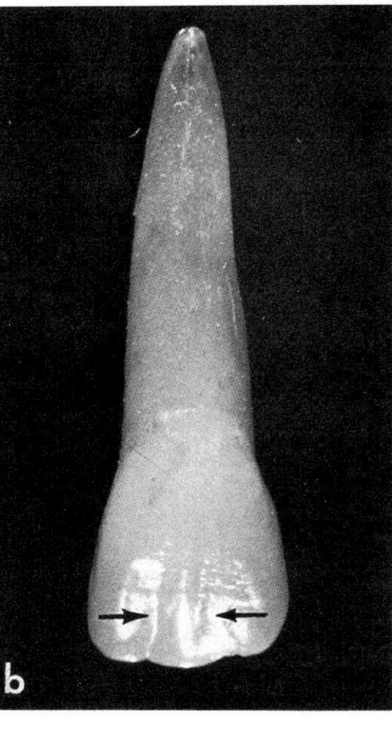

Figure 2.17
Labial grooves (*arrows*) of the maxillary left central incisor: *a,* incisal aspect; *b,* labial aspect.

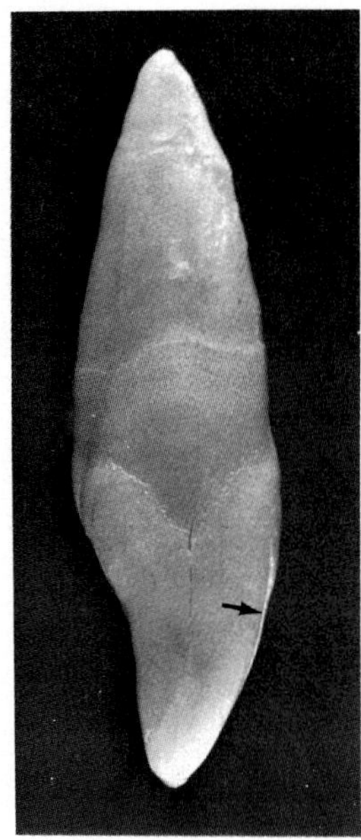

Figure 2.18
Mesial aspect of the maxillary left central incisor showing slight convexity of the labial profile of the crown.

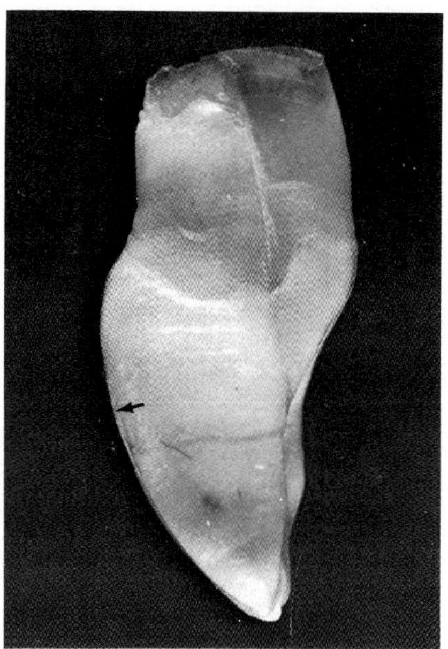

Figure 2.19
Mesial aspect of the maxillary right central incisor showing marked convexity of the labial profile of the crown.

sion. They may take the form of only slight "dips" of the labial surface, in which case the lobes are only faintly outlined, or they may be relatively deep depressions which clearly demarcate the trilobed form of the labial surface.

Labial Profile Curvature Usually the labial profile of a maxillary central incisor seen from the mesial aspect shows only a slight convexity from its height of contour (located just below the cervix) to the incisal edge (Fig. 2.18). Occasionally the labial surface presents a more marked convexity, as shown in Figure 2.19.

Mamelons Usually three mamelons surmount the incisal edges of newly erupted central incisors. Their form and distribution have already been described. Mamelons may vary with regard to number and regularity. Figure 2.20*a* and *b* show central incisors exhibiting an increased number and irregular distribution of mamelons respectively.

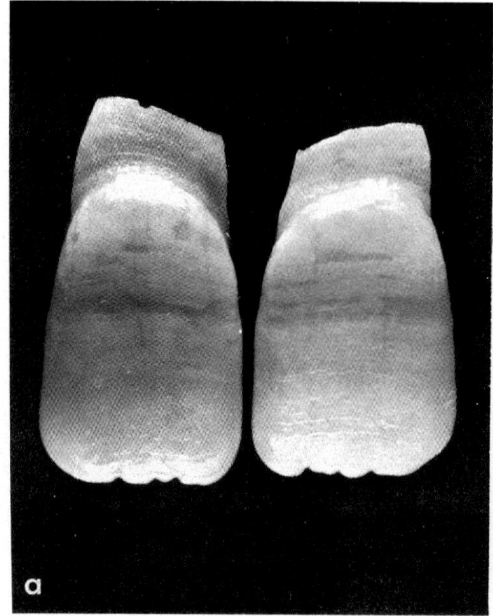

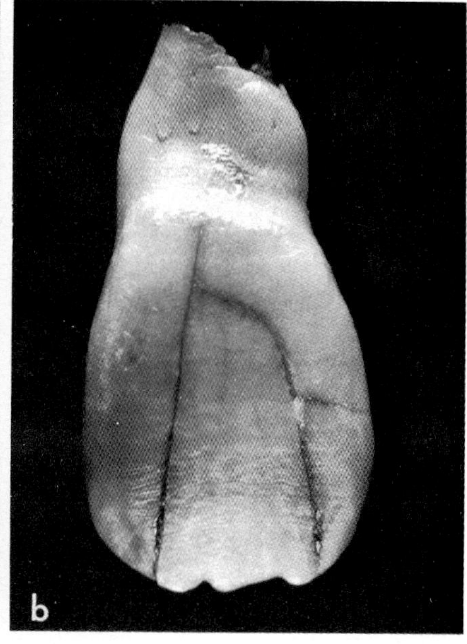

Figure 2.20
Variations in the incisal margins of the maxillary central incisors: *a*, increased number of mamelons; *b*, irregular distribution of mamelons.

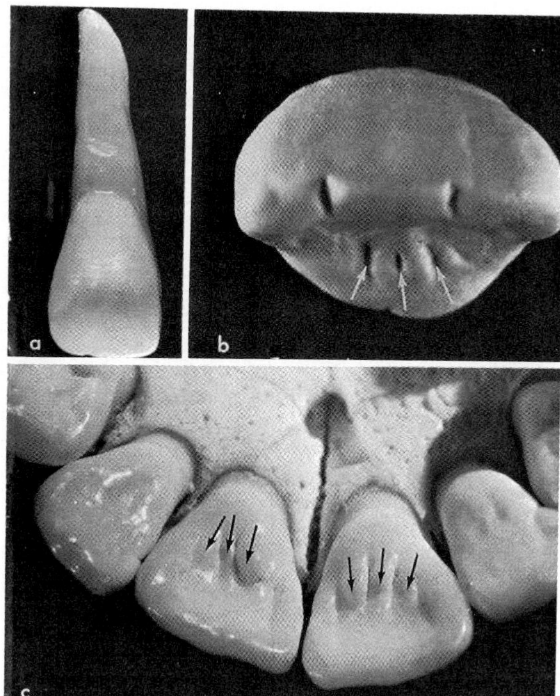

Figure 2.21
Variations of the cingulum in maxillary incisors: *a,* smooth cingulum, left central incisor, lingual aspect; *b,* cingulum marked by grooves or pits (*arrows*)—cast of right central incisor, incisal aspect; *c,* multiple tubercles (*arrows*) right and left central incisors, lingual aspect.

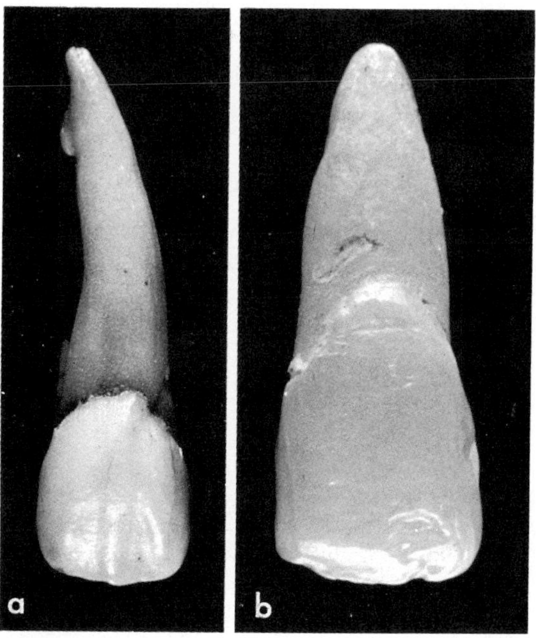

Figure 2.22
Extremes of root lengths in maxillary central incisors: *a,* unusually long root, right central incisor, labial aspect; *b,* unusually short root, left central incisor, labial aspect.

The Cingulum The cingulum has previously been described as a bulbous protuberance of the lingual surface located just above the cervical line. The incisal portion of the cingulum varies widely. It may be completely smooth (Fig. 2.21*a*), or, not uncommonly, it may be marked by single or multiple grooves and pits (Fig. 2.21*b*) with one or more distinct tubercles (Fig. 2.21*c*).

Root Size Central incisors are highly variable with regard to root length. Figure 2.22*a* and *b* show extremes in the form of uncommonly long and short roots respectively.

Lateral Incisor

Labial Aspect (Fig. 2.23)

The lateral incisor crown is noticeably narrower (mesiodistally) and shorter (incisocervically) than the central (type trait). The root, however, is of approximately the same length. Roundness is a characteristic feature of the lateral incisor. The mesioincisal angle is slightly more rounded and the distoincisal angle is distinctly more rounded than the corresponding features of the central incisor (type trait). In addition, both mesial and distal crown margins are more rounded in the lateral incisor than in the central (type trait). This places the heights of contour relatively farther from the incisal margin than is the case in the central incisor. The mesial height of contour is located at the junction of the incisal and middle thirds,

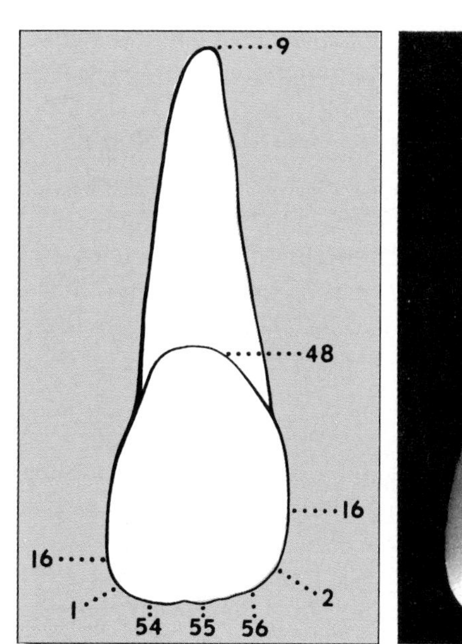

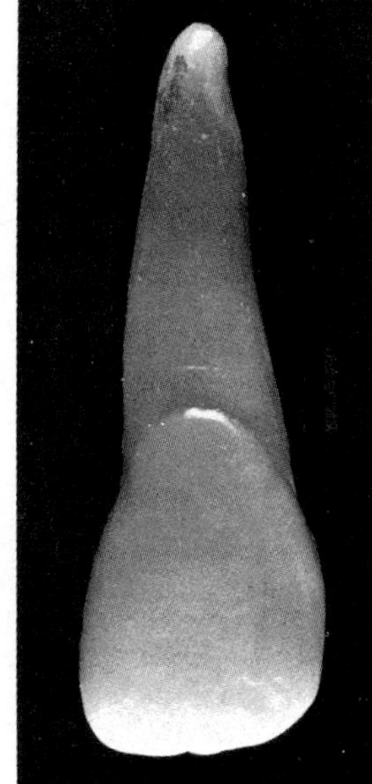

Figure 2.23
Maxillary left central lateral incisor (labial aspect).

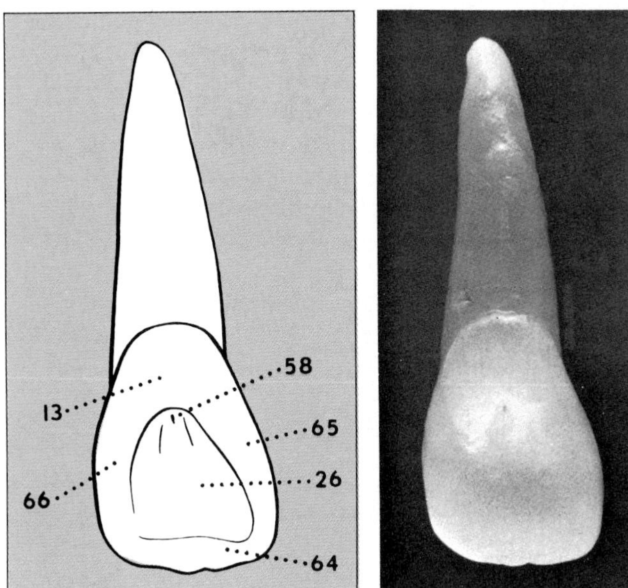

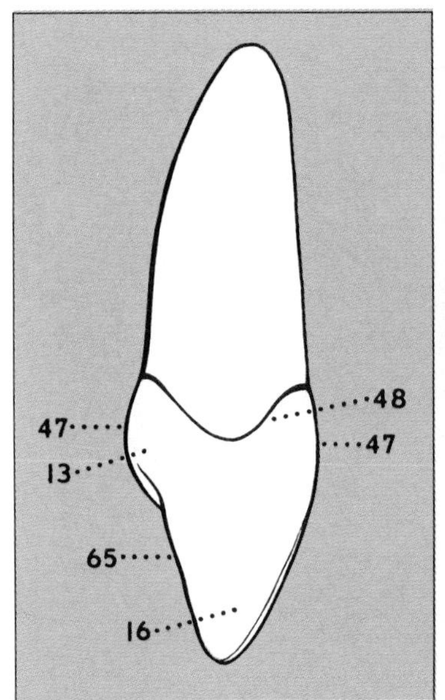

Figure 2.24
Maxillary left lateral incisor (lingual aspect).

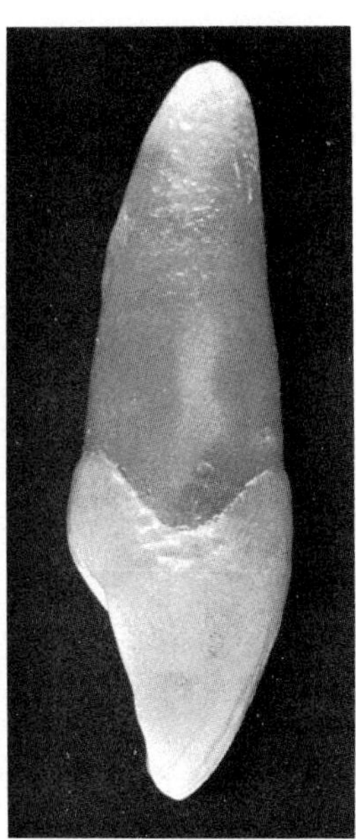

Figure 2.25
Maxillary left lateral incisor (mesial aspect).

whereas the distal height of contour is positioned in the center of the middle third (type trait).

The root of the lateral incisor, like that of the central, is conical and shows the same distal inclination.

Lingual Aspect (Fig. 2.24)

Apart from the size differential and generally rounded profile already described, the lingual aspect of the lateral incisor bears a strong resemblance to that of the central incisor. However, the marginal ridges and cingulum are often more prominent in the lateral incisor, and the lingual fossa is deeper than in the corresponding features of the central incisor (type trait).

Mesial Aspect (Fig. 2.25)

In addition to size, the crown of the lateral incisor differs from that of the central incisor in the following respects (type traits): (1) the cingulum often appears more convex in outline than that of the central incisor; (2) the CEJ is less curved than that of the central incisor.

Distal Aspect (Fig. 2.26)

The distal aspect reveals the same relationship to the mesial noted for the central incisor, namely that the cervical line is less sharply curved on the distal aspect and the distal contact area is located farther from the incisal margin as compared with the mesial contact area.

Incisal Aspect (Fig. 2.27)

The terms "small" and "round" might once again be used to describe the lateral incisor as related to the central incisor. From the incisal aspect the lateral incisor is noticeably smaller (mesiodistally) than the central incisor. In addition, the labial profile of the lateral incisor is distinctly rounded (type trait) in contrast to the relatively flat labial profile of the central

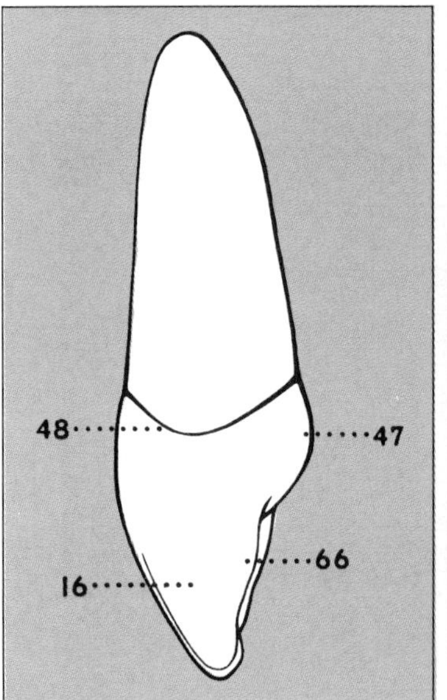

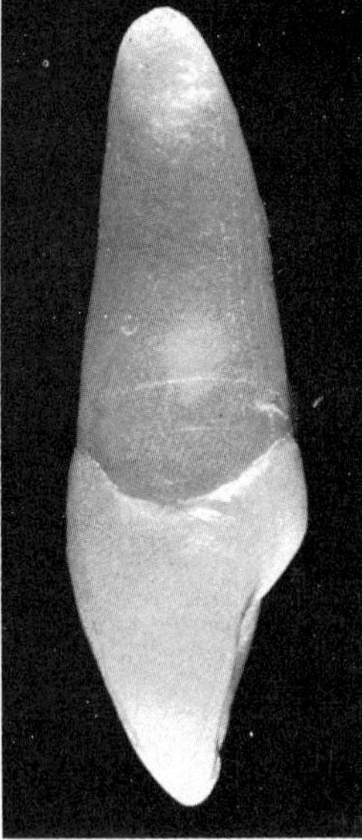

Figure 2.26
Maxillary left lateral incisor (distal aspect).

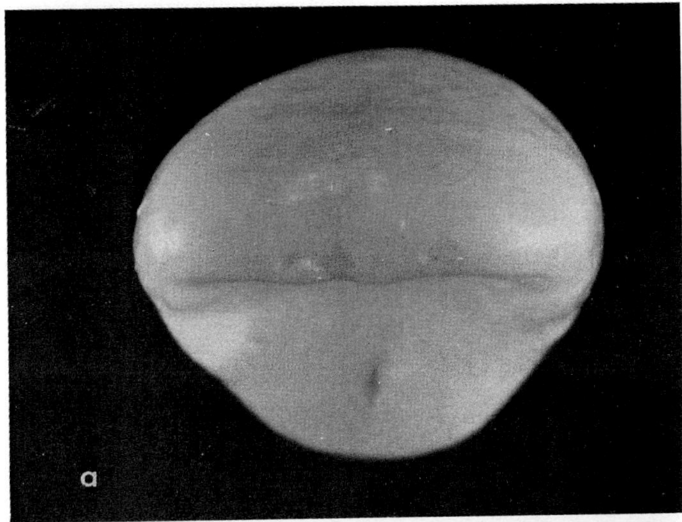

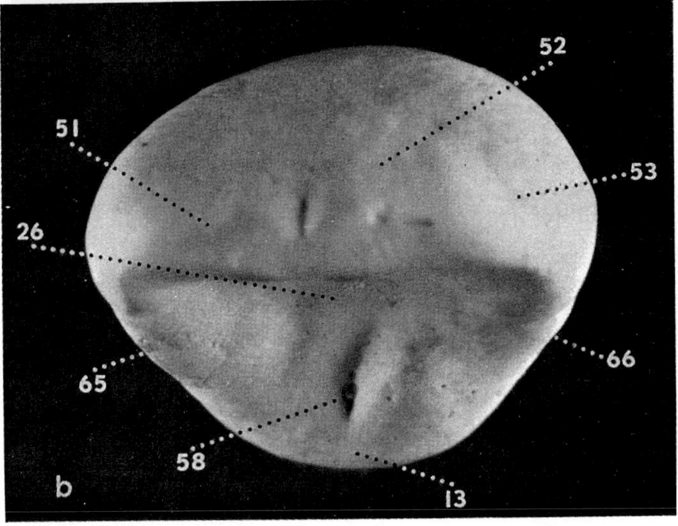

Figure 2.27
Maxillary left lateral incisor (incisal aspect): *a*, actual crown; *b*, cast.

incisor. Further, because of the high degree of convexity of the labial surface, the mesiolabial and distolabial line angles in the lateral incisor are much more rounded (type trait) and the lobes of the labial surface are less clearly demarcated in the lateral incisor. As a result of the rounding of the labial surface, the total profile of the lateral incisor from the incisal aspect is more or less ovoid in form (type trait) in contrast to the triangular outline of the central incisor.

Pulp

There are no diagnostic differences between the pulp cavities of the central and lateral maxillary incisors (Fig. 2.28).

Variations

The maxillary lateral incisor is perhaps the most variable tooth in the mouth with the exception of the third molar. It is not uncommonly missing entirely from the dental arch. On the other hand, supernumerary lateral incisors are by no means rare (Fig. 2.29). Maxillary lateral incisors also show a wide range of morphological variation with respect to (1) labial outline, (2) cingulum, (3) mesial and distal surfaces, (4) root curvature.

Labial Outline Like the central incisor, the lateral incisor commonly shows a wide range of variation with regard to its outline as viewed from the labial aspect. The variability centers around the degree of prominence of the distal lobe. Figure 2.30*a*, *b*, and *c* shows three different degrees of prominence of the lobe: slight, moderate, and pronounced. The latter strongly resembles the maxillary central incisor because of the prominence of its distal lobe.

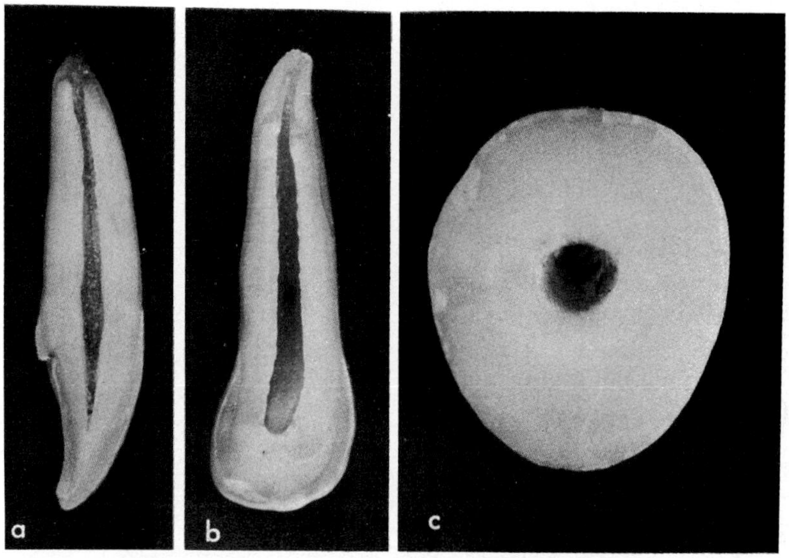

Figure 2.28

Pulp cavity of the maxillary left lateral incisor: *a*, labiolingual section; *b*, mesiodistal section; *c*, transverse section at the cervix.

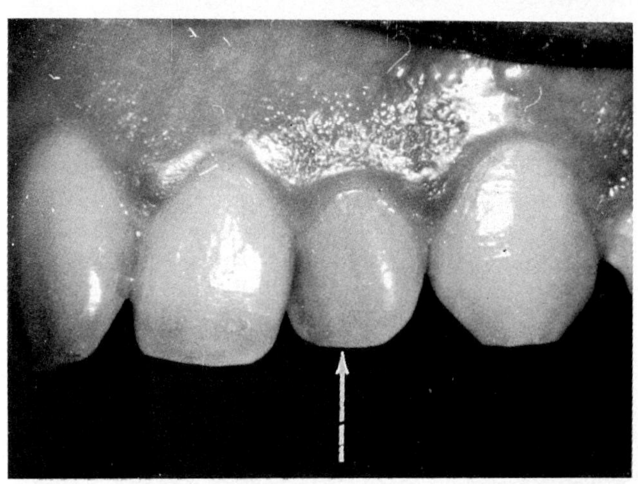

Figure 2.29

Maxillary left anterior dentition (labial aspect) showing a supernumerary lateral incisor.

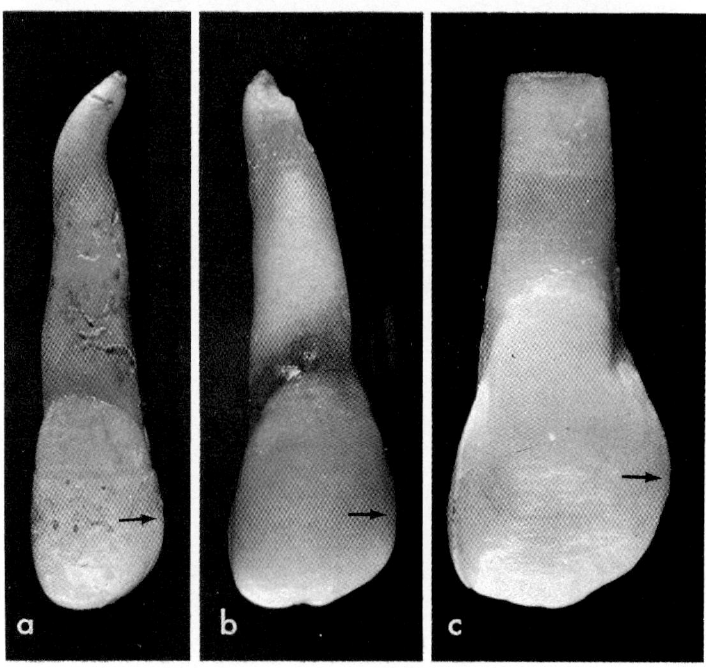

Figure 2.30

Variations in prominence in the distal lobe (*arrows*) of the maxillary left lateral incisor (labial aspect): *a*, slight prominence; *b*, moderate prominence; *c*, pronounced prominence.

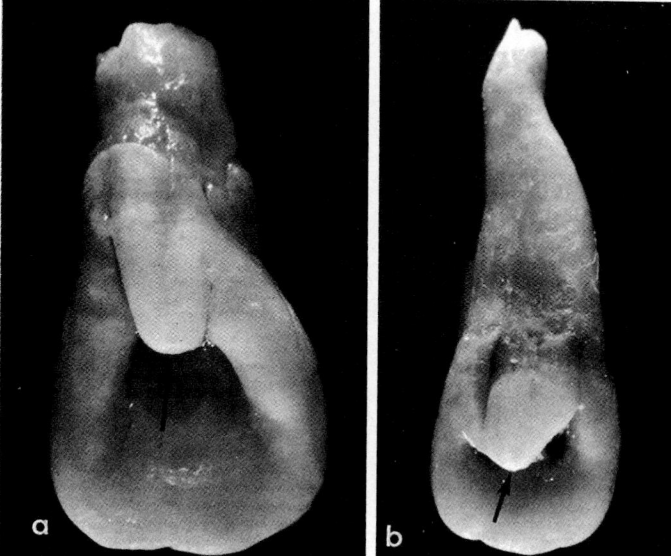

Figure 2.31

Variations in the tubercle (*arrows*), maxillary right lateral incisor (lingual aspect): *a*, slight tubercle; *b*, pronounced tubercle.

Cingulum As in the central incisor, the cingulum of the lateral incisor may be surmounted by one or more small cusps or tubercles. These may vary in prominence from a slightly rounded bulge (Fig. 2.31*a*) to a pronounced conical eminence (Fig. 2.31*b*). Instead of tubercles, one or more pits may be found at the same site. The latter may in turn show a variety of expressions from slight concavity to deep indentation.

Mesial and Distal Surfaces A groove may cross from the lingual cingulum over the mesial or distal margin onto the mesial or distal surface of the crown, and continue onto the root surface. The groove may vary in depth (Fig. 2.32*a* and *b*).

Root Curvature Maxillary lateral incisors commonly show a pronounced distal curvature of the apical portions of their roots (Fig. 2.33). This type of variation often complicates treatment in the fields of surgery and endodontics.

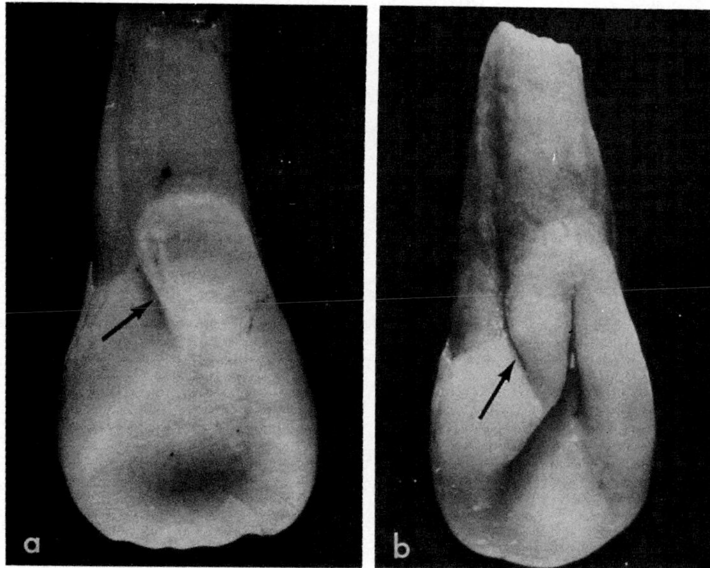

Figure 2.32

Variations in depth of the lingual marginal groove (*arrows*) in maxillary lateral incisors (lingual aspect): *a*, shallow distal groove, left lateral incisor; *b*, deep mesial groove, right lateral incisor.

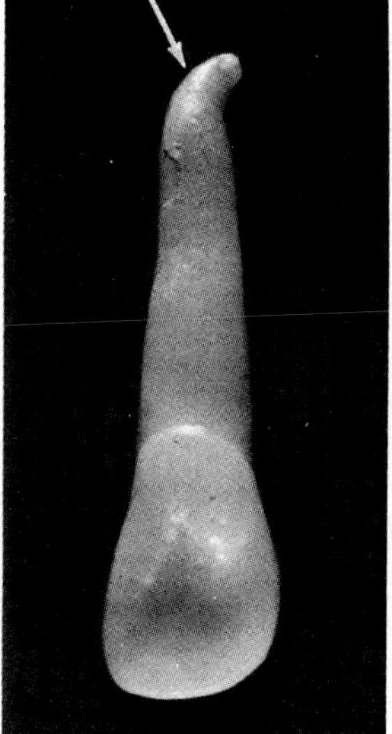

Figure 2.33

Distal apical curvature of root (*arrow*), maxillary right lateral incisor (lingual aspect).

Summary

Maxillary Incisors—Arch Traits

1. Wider than the corresponding mandibular incisors
2. Central incisor larger than lateral incisor

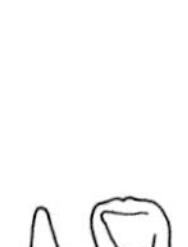

3. Marginal ridges and cinguli relatively more prominent than in the mandibular incisors
4. Lingual fossae deeper than in mandibular incisors
5. Roots rounded or triangular in cross-section, with equal labiolingual and mesiodistal widths

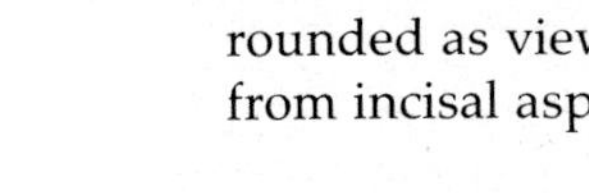

6. Labial surfaces more rounded as viewed from incisal aspect

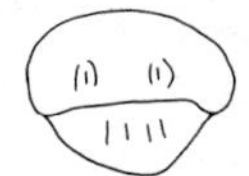

7. Crown wider mesiodistally than labiolingually

Maxillary Incisors—Type Traits

Crown	Central Incisor	Lateral Incisor
Labial Aspect		
Mesiodistally	Wide	Narrow
Mesioincisal angle	Sharp (90 degrees)	Slightly rounded
Distoincisal angle	Slightly rounded	Distinctly rounded
Mesial profile	Straight	Slightly rounded
Distal profile	Round	Highly rounded
Mesial contact	Incisal third	Junction of incisal and middle thirds
Distal contact	Junction of incisal and middle thirds	Middle third
Labial surface	Relatively flat	Rounded
Lingual Aspect		
Marginal ridges and cingulum	Moderately pronounced	More prominent
Lingual fossa	Moderately deep	Deep
Mesial Aspect		
CEJ	Moderately curved within incisal third	Less curved
Contact area		Junction of incisal and middle thirds
Cingulum	Moderately convex	Convex
Incisal Aspect		
Outline	Triangular	Ovoid
Labial surface	Slightly convex	Highly convex
Lobes	Visible labially	Slightly visible to absent
Mesio- and distolabial angles	Prominent	Rounded

The Mandibular Incisors

Size and Eruption

Mandibular Incisors	Crown Height (mm)	Mesiodistal Crown Diameter (mm)	Labiolingual Crown Diameter (mm)	Tooth Length (mm)	Age at Eruption (yr)
Central incisors	9.0	5.0	6.0	21.5	7
Lateral incisors	9.5	5.5	6.5	23.5	8

The mandibular incisors are generally the first permanent teeth to appear in the oral cavity. The central incisor usually erupts during the seventh year of life and is followed within 1 year by the lateral incisor.

Mandibular incisors might be referred to as the "moving cutting blades" of the dentition; that is, the incisal thirds of the labial surfaces of mandibular incisors glide over the incisal thirds of the lingual surfaces of the maxillary incisors during the protrusive and closing movements of the mandible, thereby providing the shearing or cutting function of the masticatory apparatus.

In general the mandibular incisors are much narrower mesiodistally than their maxillary antagonists (arch trait). In addition, no marked difference in size exists between the mandibular central and lateral incisors, although the latter is almost invariably slightly wider than the former (arch trait). Partly as a result of their near equality in size, mandibular incisors tend to resemble one another to a greater extent than do the maxillary incisors.

Central Incisor

Labial Aspect (Fig. 2.34)

The central incisor is the narrowest mesiodistally of all incisor crowns (type trait). It is unique in that it is the only member of its class that is bilaterally symmetrical when viewed from the labial aspect (type trait).

The incisal margin of the unworn crown is made up of three definite elevations (i.e., mesial, central, and distal) representing the tips of the mamelons. In contrast to all other members of the incisor class, the mesial and distal mamelons of the mandibular central incisor are of approximately equal prominence (type trait). They form almost 90-degree angles (the mesioincisal and distoincisal) with the adjacent mesial and distal margins of the crown (type trait). The mandibular central incisor is the only member of its class in which the distoincisal angle is as sharp and distinct as the mesioincisal angle. All other incisors show a more or less rounded distoincisal angle.

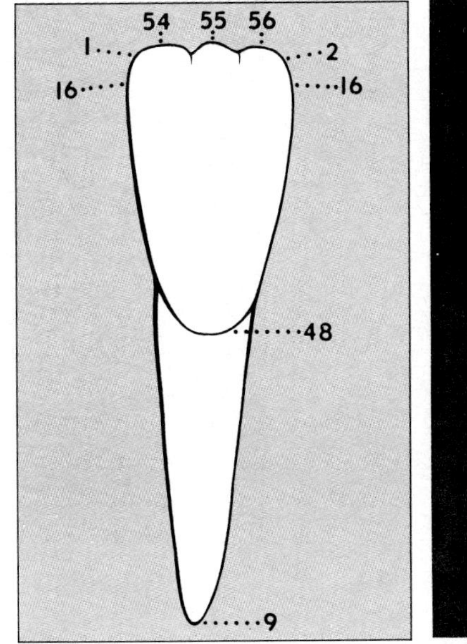

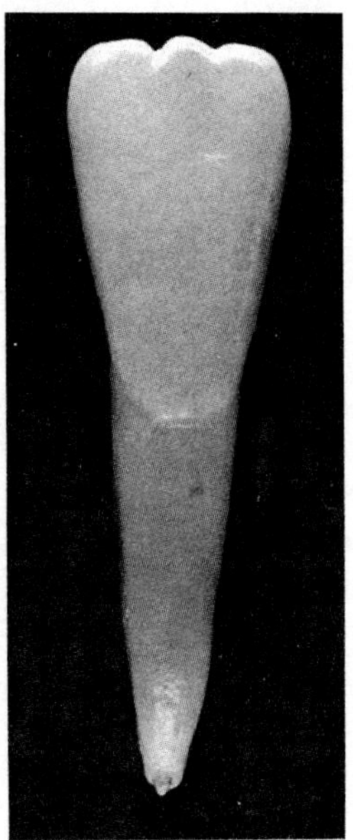

Figure 2.34
Mandibular left central incisor (labial aspect).

The contact areas of the mesial and distal borders are at the same relative crown height, well within the incisal third (type trait). In all other members of the incisor class the distal contact area is located cervical to the mesial contact area.

Both mesial and distal margins of the crown form relatively straight lines (type trait) and converge equally toward the CEJ. In this respect, the mandibular central incisor is unique, since in all other members of the class the distal margin is more or less convex.

The maximum convexity of the CEJ occurs midway between the mesial and distal borders of the root.

Occasionally the incisal third of the labial surface is divided into three lobes by shallow depressions that extend cervically from the incisal edge.

The root is narrow and conical when viewed from the labial aspect.

Lingual Aspect (Fig. 2.35)

The profile of the crown corresponds in outline to that already described for the labial aspect.

The lingual surface of the crown presents the same elevations that mark the lingual surfaces of maxillary

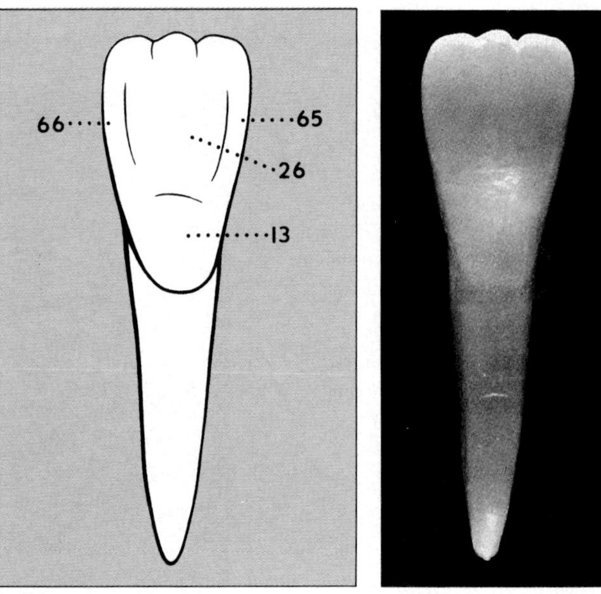

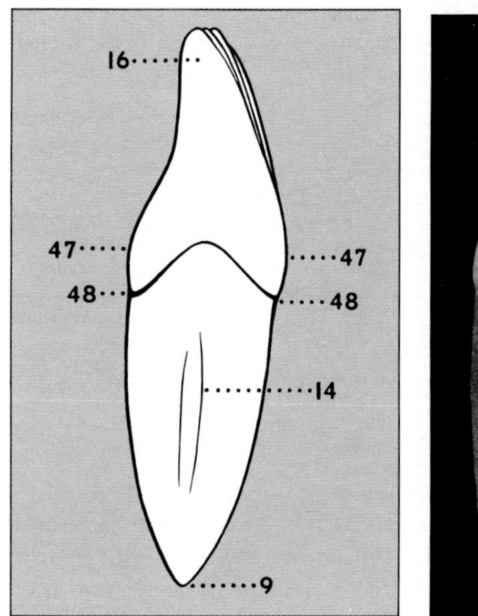

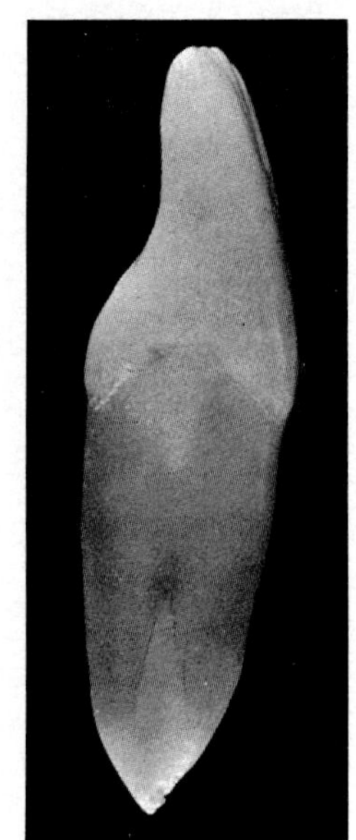

Figure 2.35
Mandibular left central incisor (lingual aspect).

Figure 2.36
Mandibular left central incisor (mesial aspect).

incisors, namely, *mesial and distal marginal ridges* and *lingual cingulum* respectively. The marginal ridges and cingulum enclose a shallow depression in the middle of the lingual surface, the *lingual fossa.* In the mandibular incisors, however, the marginal ridges and cinguli are far less prominent than the corresponding features of the maxillary incisors (arch trait). In addition, the lingual fossa of the mandibular incisor is more shallow than that of the maxillary incisor (arch trait). Accordingly, the scoop-like form characteristic of the lingual surfaces of maxillary incisors is barely noticeable in mandibular incisors.

The lingual CEJ presents approximately the same degree of curvature as that of the labial aspect.

The root is narrow and conical in outline.

Mesial Aspect (Fig. 2.36)

As is characteristic of all incisors, the crown is chisel-shaped in outline because of incisal convergence of both labial and lingual margins. The labial margin forms almost a straight line from its height of contour up to the incisal ridge. The lingual margin, on the other hand, is S-shaped, being convex in the region of the cingulum and concave up to the incisal ridge.

The mesial surface of the crown is convex and prominent in its incisal third, i.e., contact area, whereas the middle and cervical thirds are relatively flat.

The root is broad and flat (arch trait) and tapers more or less abruptly in the apical third to a relatively blunt apex. A shallow depression (proximal root concavity) extends longitudinally down the midportion of the root. In cross-section (Fig. 2.37) the root is ovoid in outline, being much broader labiolingually than mesiodistally (arch trait).

Distal Aspect (Fig. 2.38)

Because of the bilateral symmetry of the mandibular central incisor, the distal aspect is nearly the exact mirror image of the mesial aspect. The distal CEJ, however, is slightly less curved than the mesial CEJ.

Incisal Aspect (Fig. 2.39)

Like the maxillary central incisor, the crown presents a roughly triangular outline, the labial profile forming the base of the triangle and the mesial and distal pro-

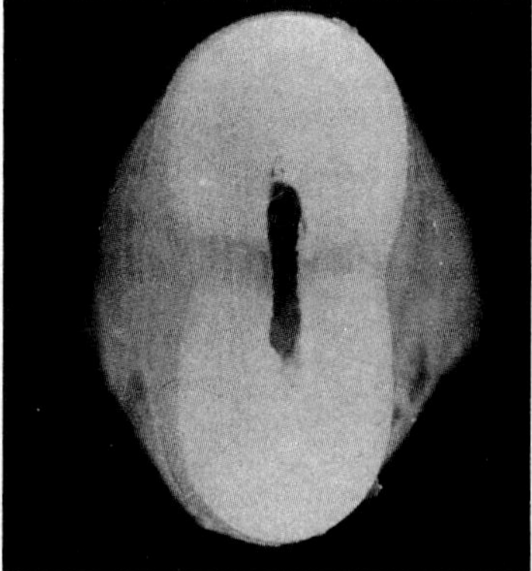

Figure 2.37
Transverse section of the root, mandibular left central incisor.

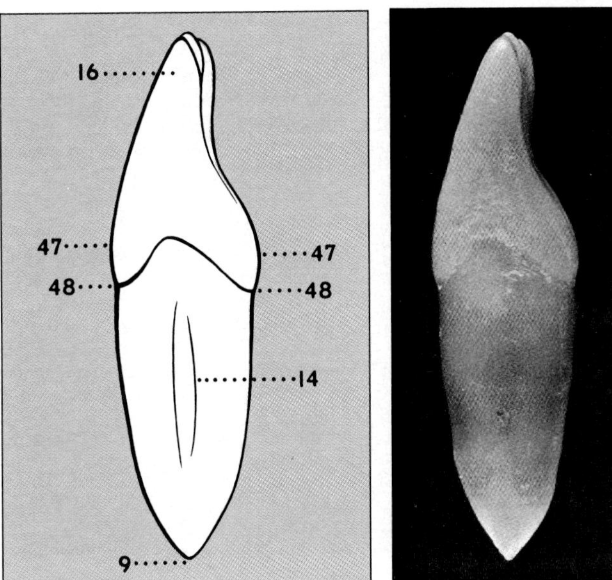

Figure 2.38
Mandibular left central incisor (distal aspect).

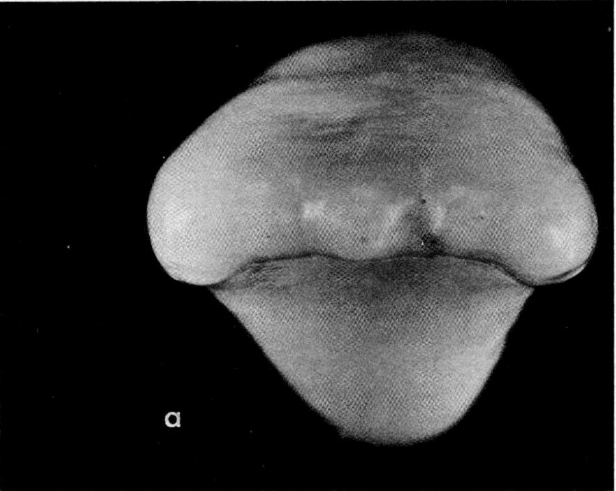

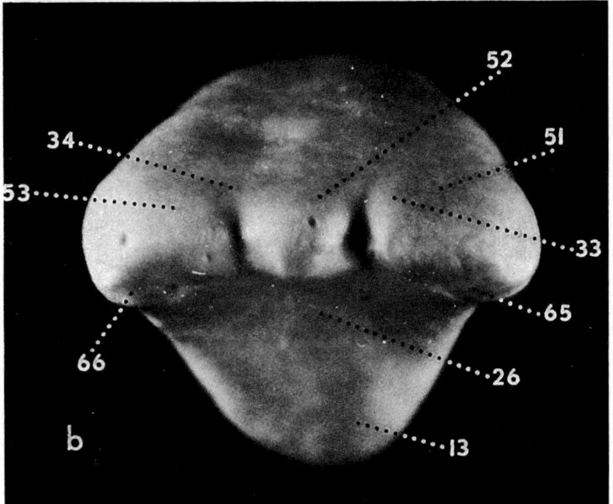

Figure 2.39
Mandibular left central incisor (incisal aspect): *a,* actual crown; *b,* cast.

files its sides. The latter converge lingually to form an apex.

The labial surface of the mandibular incisor is flat compared with that of the maxillary (arch trait), and seldom are the labial lobe grooves visible. The long axis of the incisal ridge is at right angles to a line bisecting the crown labiolingually (type trait). This feature serves to differentiate the central from the lateral mandibular incisor.

The lingual fossa, mesial and distal marginal ridges, and lingual cingulum are all clearly visible from the incisal aspect.

Pulp

The pulp cavity of the mandibular central incisor can easily be distinguished from that of the maxillary incisor. It is flattened mesiodistally, in conformity with the root shape. In the coronal portion it is very similar to its maxillary counterpart (Fig. 2.40).

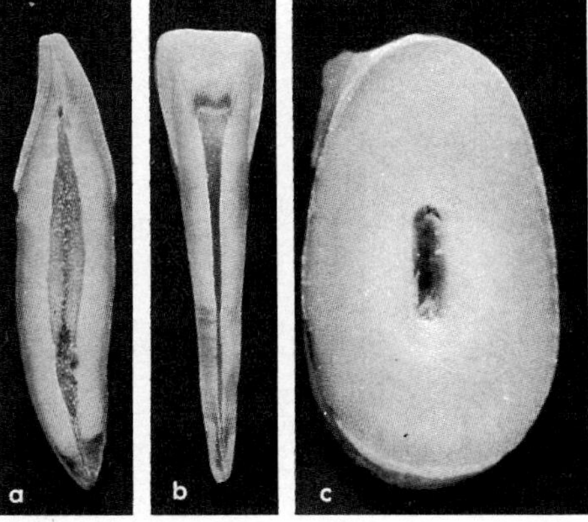

Figure 2.40
Pulp cavity of the left central incisor: *a,* labiolingual section; *b,* mesiodistal section; *c,* transverse section at the cervix.

Variations

Mandibular incisors do not show the wide range of variability exhibited by the maxillary incisors. However, there is variation involving (1) labial surface inclination; (2) mamelons; (3) root.

Labial Surface Inclination Characteristically, the labial profile of mandibular incisors, as viewed from the mesial aspect, is inclined lingually from the cervix to the incisal edge. There is variability in the degree of inclination of the labial profile. The specimens shown

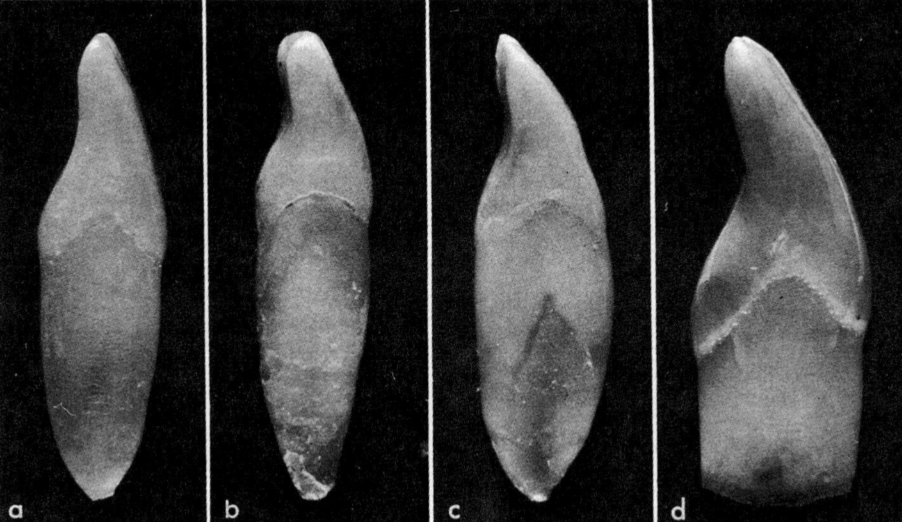

Figure 2.41

Variations in degree of inclination of the labial profile, mandibular left central incisor (mesial aspect): *a*, slight inclination; *b*, moderate inclination; *c*, pronounced inclination; *d*, very marked inclination.

in Figure 2.41*a* to *d* show a progressively increasing degree of inclination of the labial profile.

Mamelons Newly erupted mandibular incisors characteristically have three small mamelons (Fig. 2.42*a*). With regard to size they may show a great deal of variation. Figure 2.42*b* shows a central incisor with exaggerated cusplike mammelons separated by distinct grooves.

Root Mandibular incisor roots are usually straight, converging gradually to the apex. They are more labiolingually than mesiodistally inclined. Occasionally, however, the root may bend abruptly, or have an irregular curvature as shown in Figure 2.43. In addition, the proximal grooves that are commonly found on the root surface may be unusually deep, imparting to it a double-rooted appearance (Fig. 2.44).

Lateral Incisor

Labial Aspect (Fig. 2.45)

Two features of the mandibular lateral incisor when viewed from this aspect serve to distinguish it from

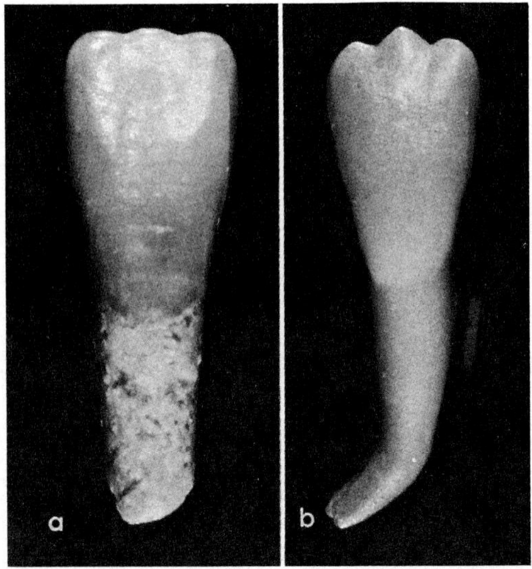

Figure 2.42

Variations in the size of mammelons, mandibular left central incisor (labial aspect): *a*, small mammelons; *b*, large mammelons.

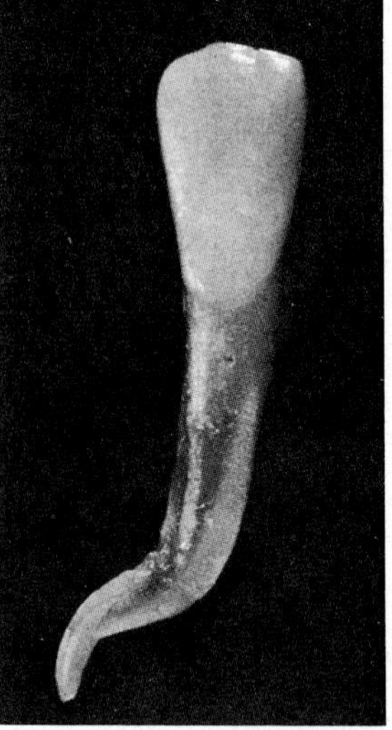

Figure 2.43

Irregular curvature in root of mandibular right lateral incisor.

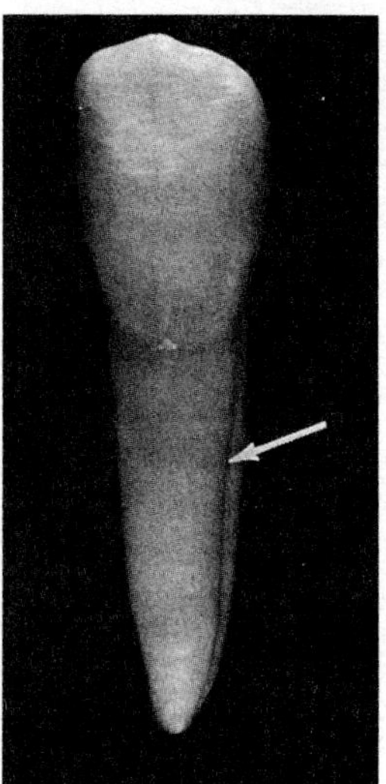

Figure 2.44
Deep proximal grooves (*arrow*) on root of mandibular left lateral incisor (labial aspect).

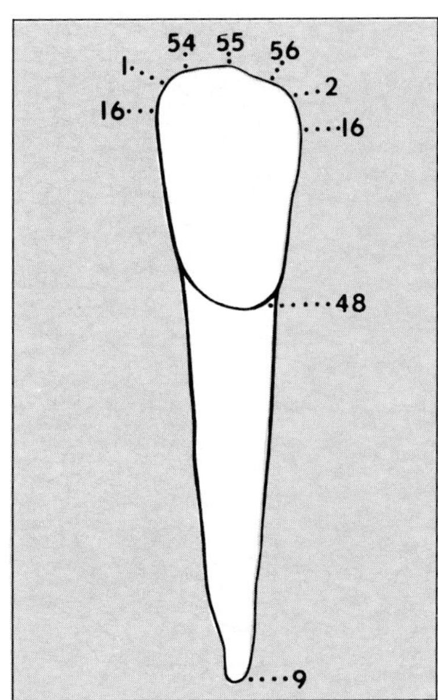

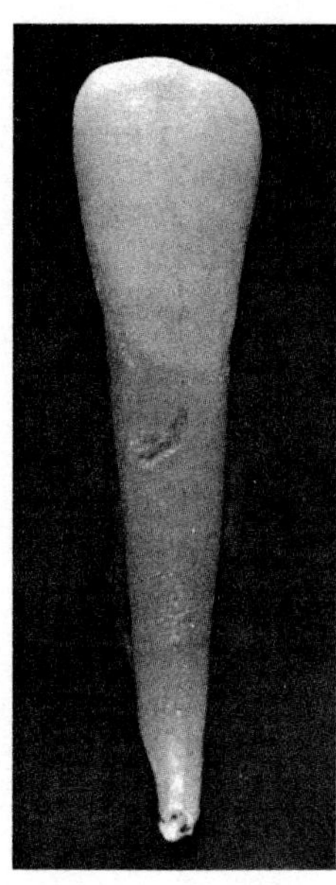

Figure 2.45
Mandibular left lateral incisor (labial aspect).

the central incisor, namely *size* and *lack of bilateral symmetry.* In the mandibular arch the lateral incisor is usually slightly wider than the central incisor (arch trait). The mesioincisal angle is sharp and distinct, whereas the distoincisal angle is rounded and more cervically situated.

The distal half of the crown provides a distinctive profile that gives the lateral incisor its characteristic appearance.

Lingual Aspect (Fig. 2.46)

Apart from the difference in size and lack of bilateral symmetry already noted, the lateral incisor from the lingual aspect is nearly identical to the central incisor.

Mesial Aspect (Fig. 2.47)

Except for a slightly less curved CEJ, the mesial aspect of the mandibular lateral incisor is very nearly identical to that of the central incisor.

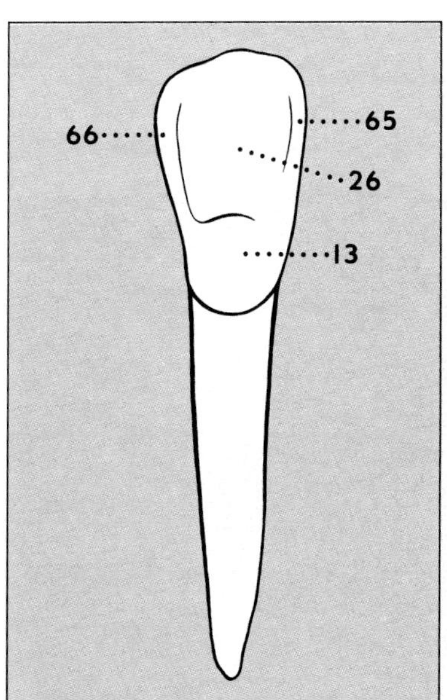

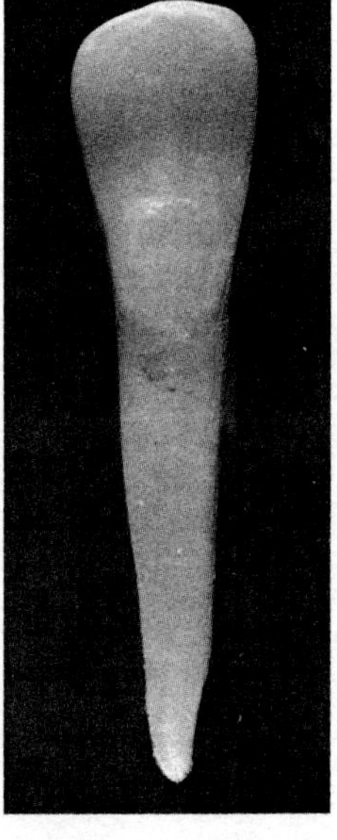

Figure 2.46
Mandibular left lateral incisor (lingual aspect).

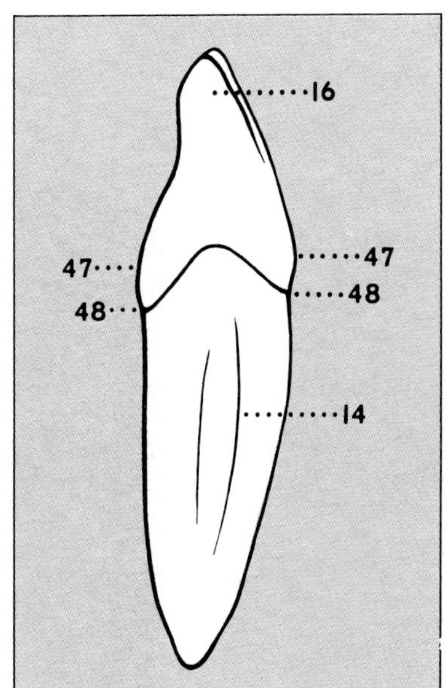

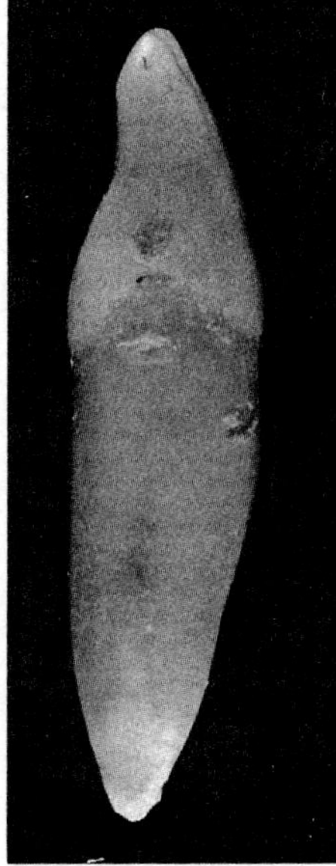

Figure 2.47
Mandibular left lateral incisor (mesial aspect).

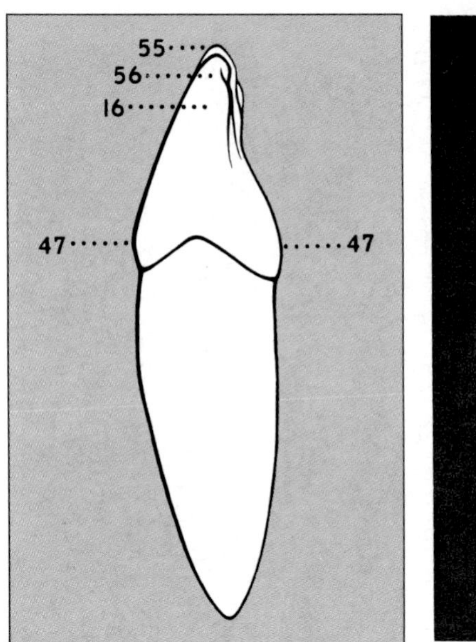

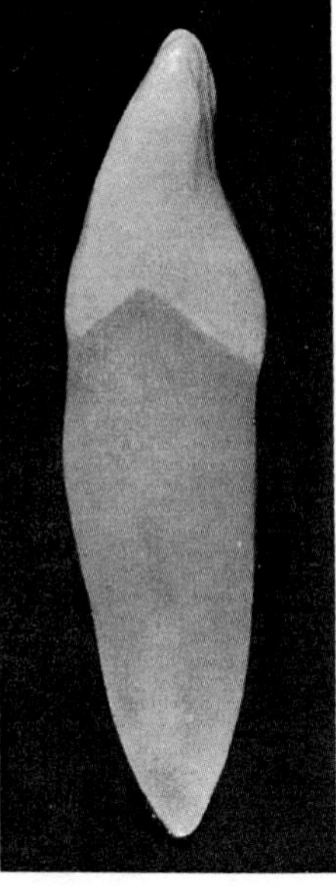

Figure 2.48
Mandibular left lateral incisor (distal aspect).

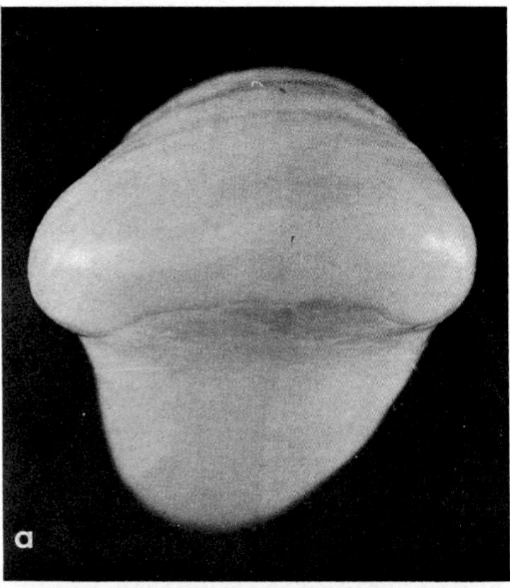

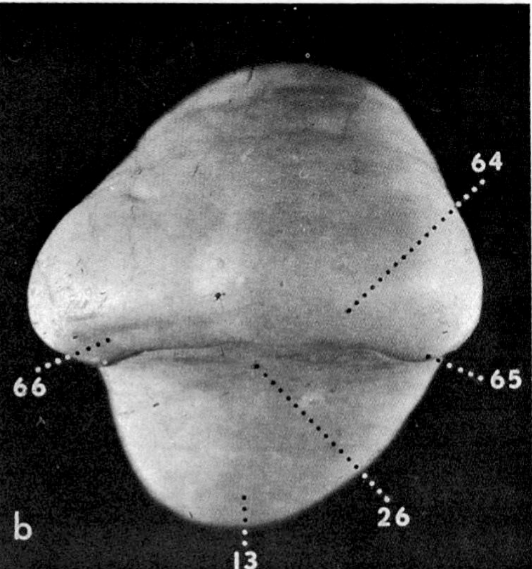

Figure 2.49
Mandibular left lateral incisor (incisal aspect): *a*, actual crown; *b*, cast.

Distal Aspect (Fig. 2.48)

Two relatively minor features distinguish the lateral mandibular incisor from the central incisor as viewed from the distal aspect: (1) more of the incisal ridge is visible when the lateral incisor is viewed from its distal aspect; (2) the curvature of the CEJ is less pronounced.

Incisal Aspect (Fig. 2.49)

A single feature distinguishes the lateral from the central incisor in incisal view. The incisal edge of the lateral incisor does not form a right angle with a line bisecting the crown labiolingually. Instead, it takes an oblique course, appearing as if twisted around the long axis of the root.

Figure 2.50
Pulp cavity of the mandibular left lateral incisor: *a*, labiolingual section; *b*, mesiodistal section; *c*, transverse section at the cervix.

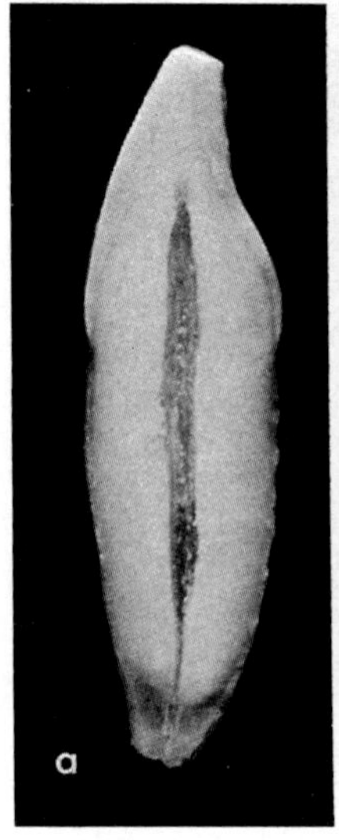

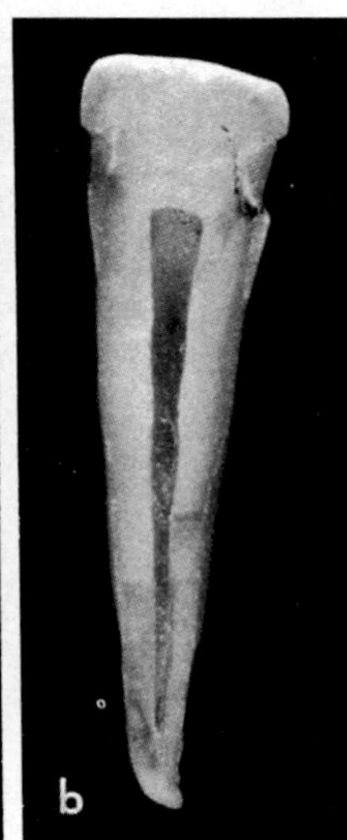

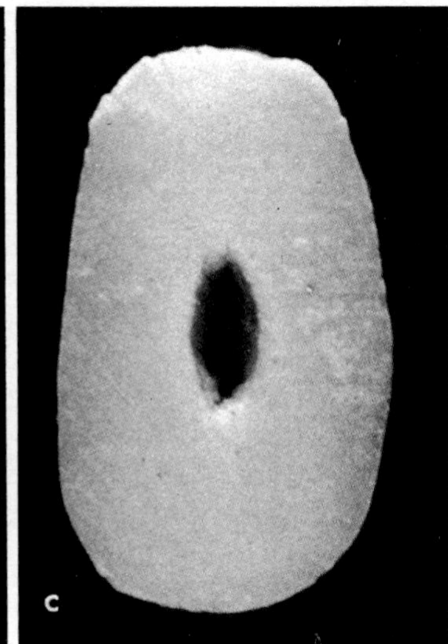

Pulp

The pulp cavity of the mandibular lateral incisor is almost identical to that of the central incisor. In the root it is flattened mesiodistally in conformity with the root shape (Fig. 2.50*c*). Coronally it is wide mesiodistally and narrow labiolingually, conforming to the crown shape (Fig. 2.50*a* and *b*).

Summary

Mandibular Incisors—Arch Traits

1. Narrowest teeth of incisor class
2. Lateral incisor wider than central

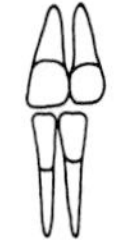

3. Marginal ridges and cinguli not prominent
4. Lingual fossa shallow
5. Roots oval in cross-section, much wider labiolingually than mesiodistally

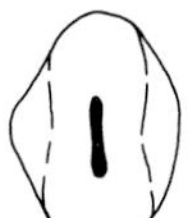

6. Labial surfaces flat

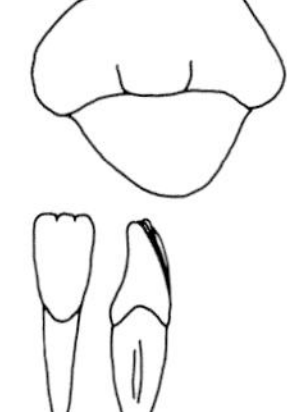

7. Crown wider labiolingually than mesiodistally

Mandibular Incisors—Type Traits

	Central Incisor	Lateral Incisor
Labial aspect	Narrow mesiodistally Bilaterally symmetrical Mesial and distal mammelons equally prominent Mesioincisal and distoincisal angles sharp 90 degrees	Slightly wider than central mesiodistally Asymmetrical Distal mammelon not prominent Distoincisal angle rounded
Incisal aspect	Incisal ridge forms right angle with labiolingual bisecting line	Incisal ridge twisted on crown

3

The Permanent Canines

Canines are the "single" members of the dental arches. Only one member of this class is present in each of the four quadrants (Fig. 3.1).

Canines are important throughout the animal kingdom since they may be used as seizing, digging, slashing, piercing, and fighting tools. Accordingly, in many orders of mammals the canines are indispensable to the survival of the animal. In man, who has devised many other means of defense and access to food, this important function has been lost. Nevertheless the canines are considered to be among the most strategic teeth in the mouth for a variety of reasons.

Canines are the most stable teeth in the dental arches. Their roots are almost invariably the longest and thickest (labiolingually) of any teeth, and hence are extremely well anchored in the alveolar bone. Clinically, therefore, they are usually among the last teeth to be lost. Canines occupy significant positions at the four corners of the dental arches. Indeed, they are commonly referred to as the "cornerstones" of the dental arches. They help support the facial musculature, and their loss often results in a flattening of the face in this region that is difficult to restore to normality. Further, because of their firm anchorage and strategic position in the dental arches, canines are thought to be important as "guideposts" in occlusion. They are well able to withstand masticatory stress and therefore serve as "buffers" that tend to relieve the posterior teeth of excessive, potentially damaging horizontal forces engendered during excursive movements of the mandible.

Certain class traits characterize all canines: (1) they are the only teeth in the dentition possessing a single conical cusp; (2) they possess the largest *single* roots of all the dental units; (3) they are the only cusped teeth that feature a functional lingual surface rather than an occlusal surface.

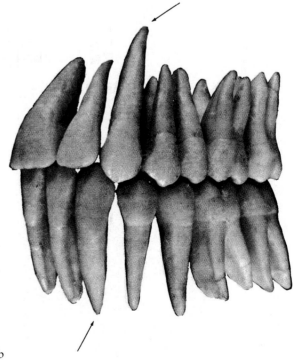

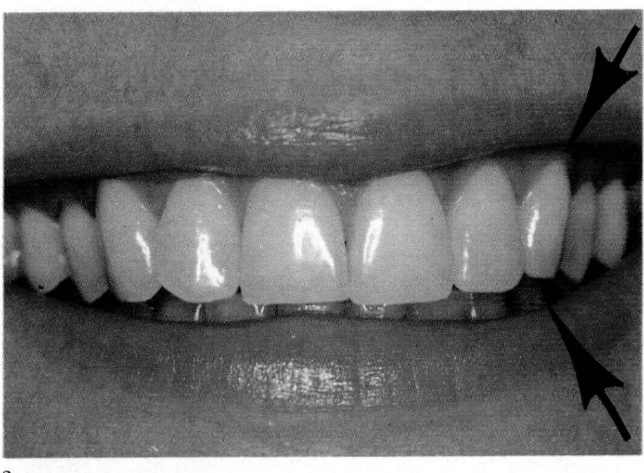

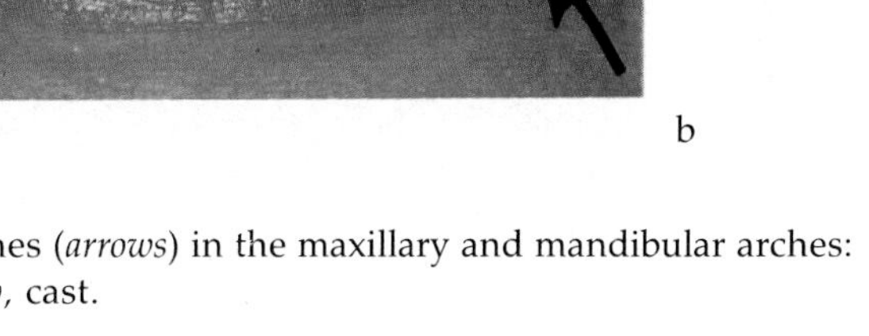

a b

Figure 3.1

Position of the canines (*arrows*) in the maxillary and mandibular arches: *a,* actual dentition; *b,* cast.

The Maxillary Canine

Size and Eruption

Arch	Crown Height (mm)	Mesiodistal Crown Diameter (mm)	Labiolingual Crown Diameter (mm)	Tooth Length (mm)	Age at Eruption (yr)
Maxillary	10.0	7.5	8.0	27.0	11

The maxillary canine, one of the last teeth to appear in the oral cavity (with the exception of the second and third molars), erupts toward the end of the 11th year of age. It is larger than the mandibular canines (arch trait) and morphologically it presents certain features that mark it as more or less a transitional form between incisors and premolars.

Labial Aspect (Fig. 3.2)

The incisal margin, unlike that in the incisors, is not flat but has two sloping sides that rise to a point approximately midway between the mesial and distal margins of the crown. Generally the mesial ridge slopes less markedly than the distal and is shorter, resulting in a high "shoulder" (mesioincisal angle). The distal ridge meets the distal margin to form a more rounded distoincisal angle. The entire incisal margin constitutes at least one-third of the total crown height and often as much as one-half (arch trait).

The mesial profile of the crown is only slightly convex, with its height of contour relatively close to the incisal margin. The distal profile is strongly convex with its height of contour in the middle portion of the crown, so that part of the crown appears to "overhang" the root. This results in a marked convergence of the mesial and distal margins toward the cervix (arch trait).

The CEJ forms a slightly convex arc.

The labial surface of the crown is marked by a pronounced ridge that extends cervically from the cusp tip. Slight depressions located on either side of the ridge delineate three distinct lobes of the labial surface. The incisal view in Figure 3.6 illustrates these features more clearly.

The root is relatively long and narrow from the labial aspect.

Lingual Aspect (Fig. 3.3)

Since both crown and root are narrower lingually than labially, almost the entire labial profile can be seen from the lingual aspect.

The mesial and distal crown margins, seen from the lingual aspect, present the same outline as those already described for the labial aspect.

The following features of the lingual surface, however, are highly distinctive and serve to distinguish the maxillary from the mandibular canine:

1. Two distinct, well-elevated ridges, the *mesial*

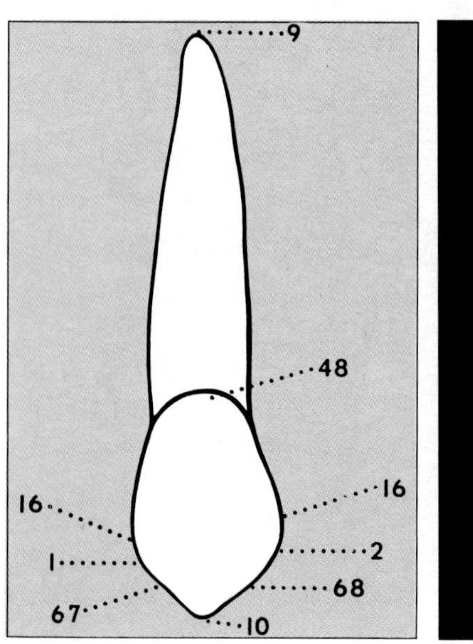

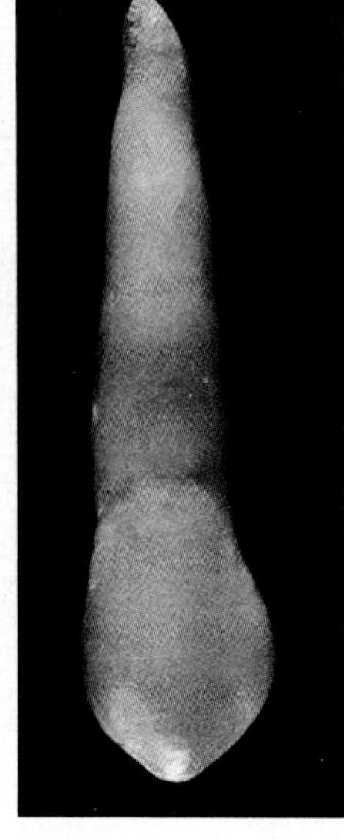

Figure 3.2
Maxillary left canine (labial aspect).

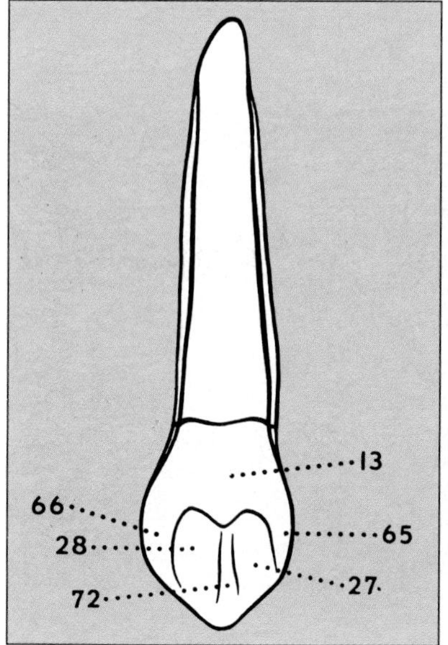

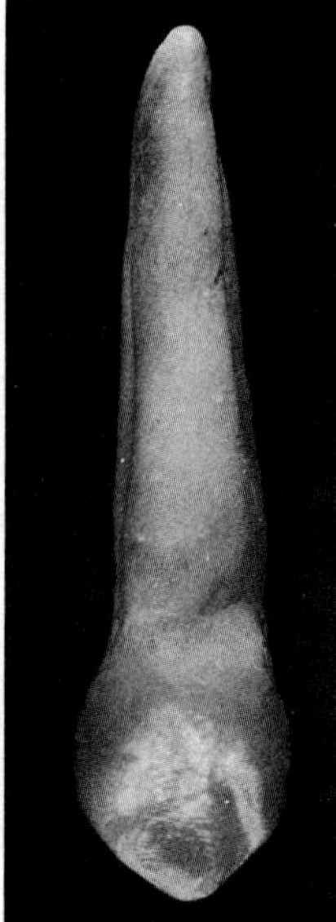

Figure 3.3
Maxillary left canine (lingual aspect).

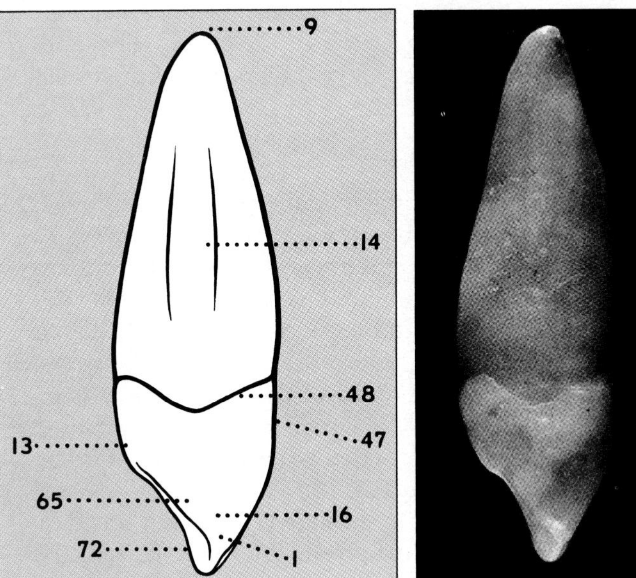

Figure 3.4
Maxillary left canine (mesial aspect).

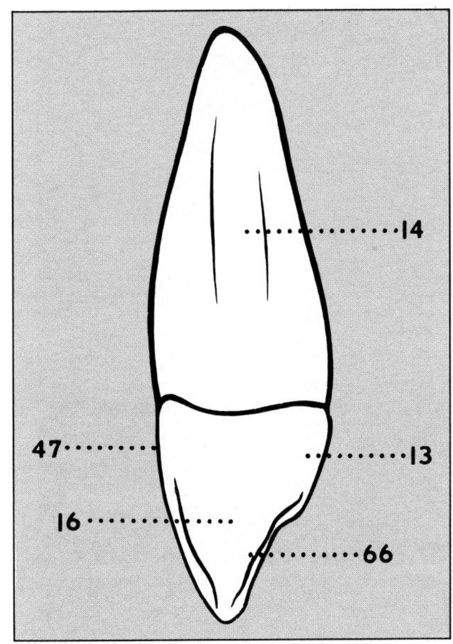

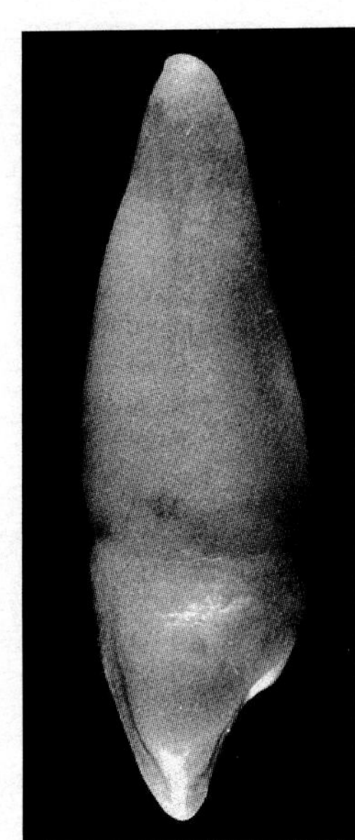

Figure 3.5
Maxillary left canine (distal aspect).

and *distal marginal ridges* respectively, make up the proximal boundaries of the lingual surface. Accentuated marginal ridges can be considered an arch trait for the maxillary canine.

2. A bulbous convexity, the lingual cingulum, makes up the cervical portion of the lingual surface. An accentuated lingual cingulum can be considered an arch trait for the maxillary canine. The incisal portion of the lingual cingulum may support one or more lingual tubercles.

3. A prominent elevation extends from the incisal portion of the cingulum to the cusp tip in the form of a more or less continuous ridge or crest. This elevation is referred to as the lingual ridge. At its midpoint it is interrupted by a slight concavity. Although the mandibular canine also exhibits a lingual ridge, it is usually more pronounced in the maxillary canine (arch trait).

4. The mesial and distal marginal ridges, together with the lingual ridge, form the boundaries of two shallow concavities of the lingual surface, the *mesiolingual* and *distolingual* fossae respectively.

5. A lingual pit and/or developmental grooves are common features of the lingual surface (arch trait). The lingual pit is usually located near the incisal portion of the lingual cingulum, and the mesial and distal developmental grooves mark the inner boundaries of their respective marginal ridges.

Mesial Aspect (Fig. 3.4)

The most striking feature of the mesial aspect is the extreme thickness of the cervical third of both crown and root. The labial margin is relatively straight from the middle of the root to the junction of the cervical and middle thirds of the crown, where the height of contour is located (arch trait). From this point the labial margin slopes downward and incisally in a straight line to the apex of the crown.

The lingual profile, on the other hand, is more irregular. It exhibits a pronounced convexity (i.e., the lingual cingulum) from the cervical line to the midpoint of the crown, then a slight concavity (i.e., the midpoint of the lingual ridge) followed by a marked convexity (i.e., the incisal portion of the lingual ridge) extending up to the cusp apex. The height of contour of the lingual profile is situated close to the cervical line. The labial and lingual profiles, in general, converge incisally from their respective heights of contour toward the cusp apex.

The incisal ridge is relatively thick labiolingually (arch trait).

The mesial marginal ridge is prominent, as viewed from the mesial aspect, and the junction of the mesioincisal ridge and mesial surface is marked by a distinct angle (i.e., the mesioincisal).

In the mesial aspect, the root is extremely broad from the cervix up to roughly one-half to two-thirds of its length, from which point it tapers to a more or less blunt apex. A slight longitudinal concavity may mark the root surface for a variable portion of its length.

Distal Aspect (Fig. 3.5)

The profiles from the distal aspect of the crown and root in general resemble those already described for the mesial aspect. The longitudinal concavity of the

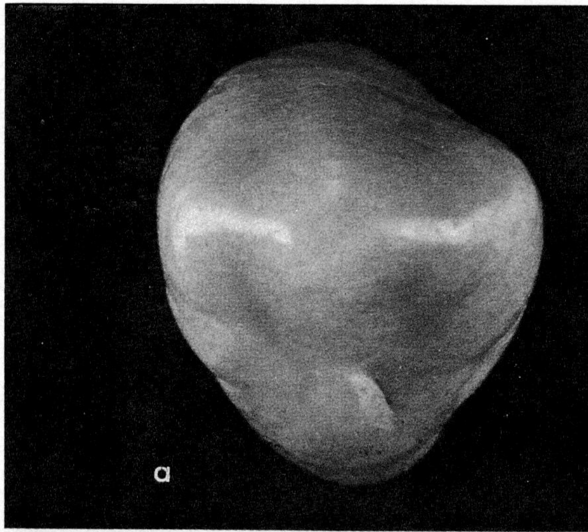

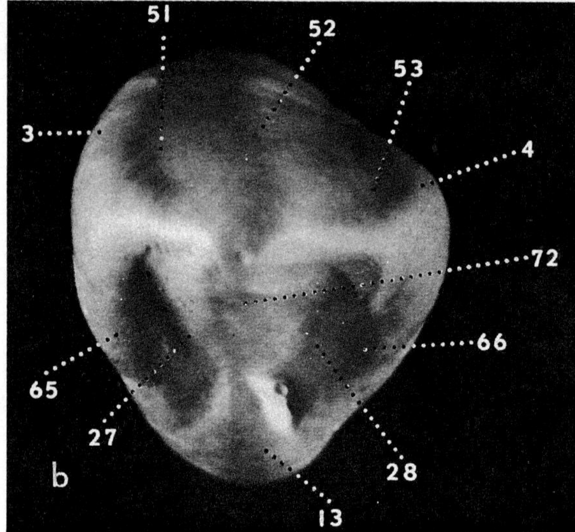

Figure 3.6
Maxillary left canine (incisal aspect): *a*, actual crown; *b*, cast.

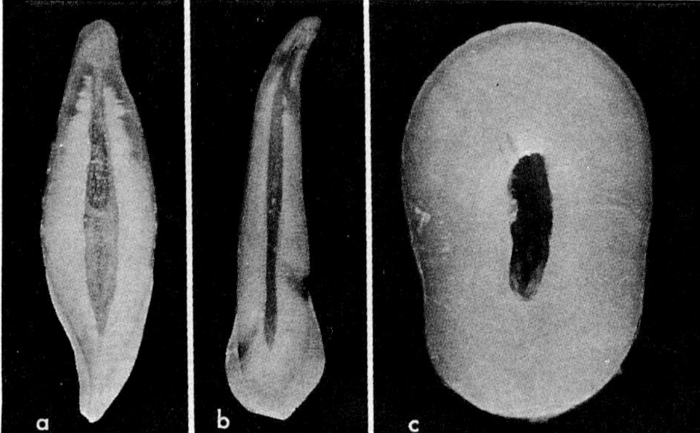

Figure 3.7
Pulp cavity of the maxillary left canine: *a*, labiolingual section; *b*, mesiolingual section; *c*, transverse section at the cervix.

root on the distal surface is usually deeper and longer than that of the mesial surface. The cervical line tends to be flatter (i.e., less convex) than that of the mesial surface.

Incisal Aspect (Fig. 3.6)

A striking feature of the incisal aspect of the canine is the asymmetry of the crown. If a line is drawn bisecting the lingual cingulum and passing through the cusp apex, that portion of the crown distal to the line is noticeably wider and more concave labially than is the mesial portion.

The height of contour of the labial profile is directly in line with the cusp apex. The mesial half of the labial profile is rounded whereas the distal is flattened or even a little concave.

The mesial profile is relatively flat and broad labiolingually. The distal profile, on the other hand, is highly convex and narrow labiolingually. The mesial and distal borders converge lingually more or less abruptly from their respective heights of contour to form the convex outline of the lingual cingulum.

There are three distinct lobes (i.e., the mesial, middle, and distal) marked by depressions on the labial surface. The middle lobe is by far the most prominent. The mesial and distal cusp ridges are relatively thick labiolingually (arch trait) and incline slightly lingually from the cusp apex to become confluent with the respective marginal ridges of the lingual surface.

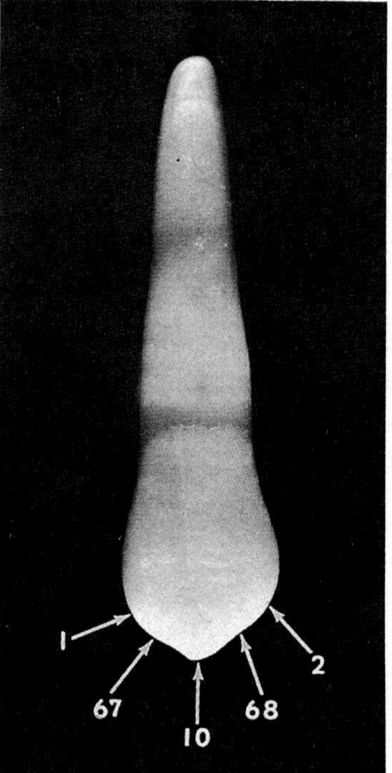

Figure 3.8
Typical topography of the maxillary left canine crown (labial aspect).

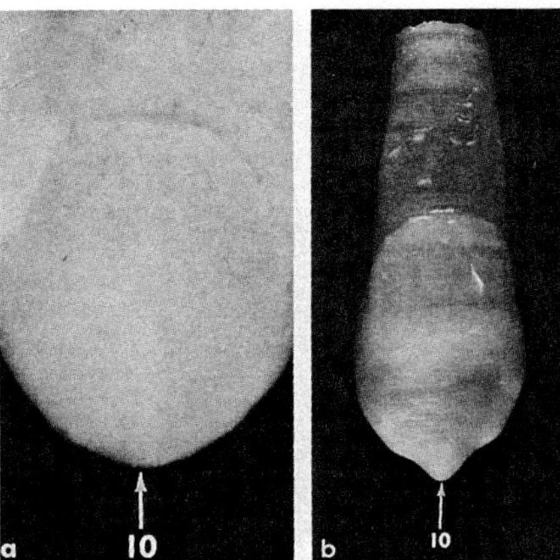

Figure 3.9
Variations in the cusp tip, maxillary left canine (labial aspect): *a*, blunted apex; *b*, "nippled" apex.

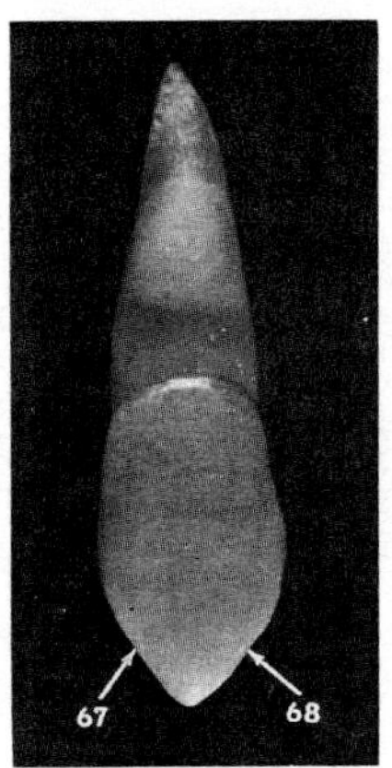

Figure 3.10
Almost vertical pitch of maxillary left canine cusp ridges (labial aspect).

The prominent lingual ridge and two adjacent lingual fossae are clearly visible from the incisal aspect, as are the lingual tubercle and mesial and distal grooves.

Pulp

A labiolingual section of the canine reveals a double-convex, lens-shaped pulp cavity, with the widest diameter situated well below the cervix near the middle of the tooth. In mesiodistal section the cavity is very narrow from top to bottom. In its entire length the cavity is constricted mesiodistally (Fig. 3.7*a*, *b*, and *c*).

Variations

In order to understand the wide range of variation found in the maxillary canine, one must keep in mind the essential topography of the crown as seen in labial aspect. There is a single cusp tip, a mesial and a distal sloping cusp ridge, and a mesial and distal "shoulder" (mesioincisal and distoincisal angle) (Fig. 3.8). Each of these features may vary. The cusp tip may be more or less accentuated, ranging from a barely perceptible blunted apex to a sharply conical or "nippled" point (Fig. 3.9*a* and *b*). Each ridge may vary in its degree of slope from practically no slope at all to an almost vertical pitch (Fig. 3.10); however, the two slopes are not necessarily symmetrical in this respect but may be present in any number of combinations (Fig. 3.11). The so-called shoulders of the canine are actually more or less accentuated "styles" that develop on either or both slopes of the central cusp during the ontogeny of the tooth. At one extreme of the range of variation, both styles may be absent or obscured so that the canine takes on a peg-shaped or fang-like appearance (see Fig. 3.10). On the other hand one or both styles may be present in varying degrees of development (Fig. 3.12*a* and *b*). Rarely, both styles may be so strongly uplifted as to give an incisor-like appearance to the crown (Fig. 3.13*a*). A

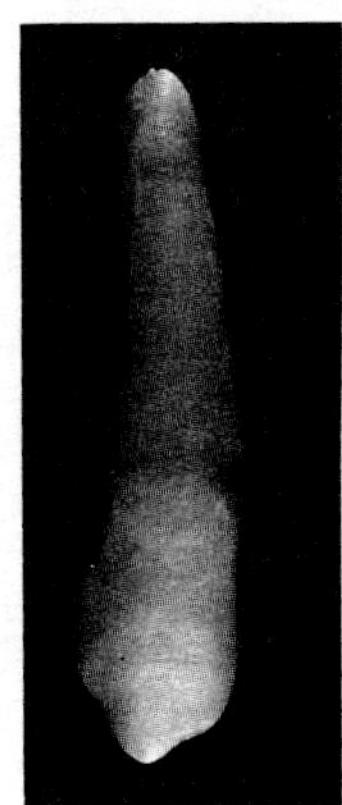

Figure 3.11
Asymmetrical slopes of maxillary right canine cusp ridges (labial aspect).

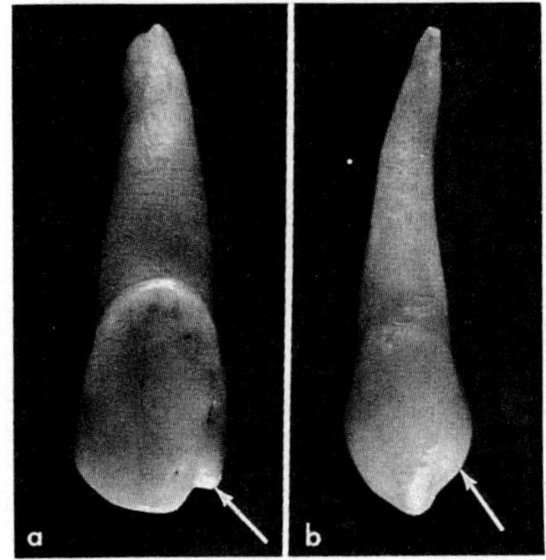

Figure 3.12
Variation in appearance of styles on the cusp ridges of the maxillary right canine (labial aspect); *a*, pronounced mesial shoulder or style (*arrow*); *b*, slight mesial shoulder or style (*arrow*).

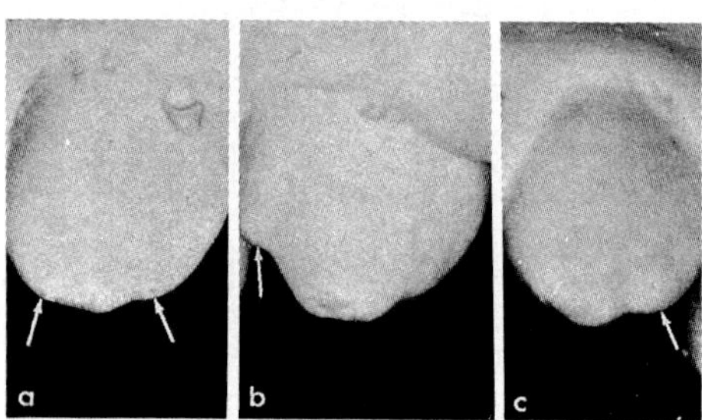

Figure 3.13

Further variations in styles, maxillary left canine (labial view, casts): *a*, strongly uplifted styles, giving incisor-like appearance to the crown (*arrows*); *b*, mesial style situated close to cervix (*arrow*); *c*, distal style situated close to cusp apex (*arrow*).

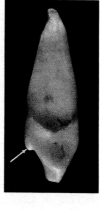

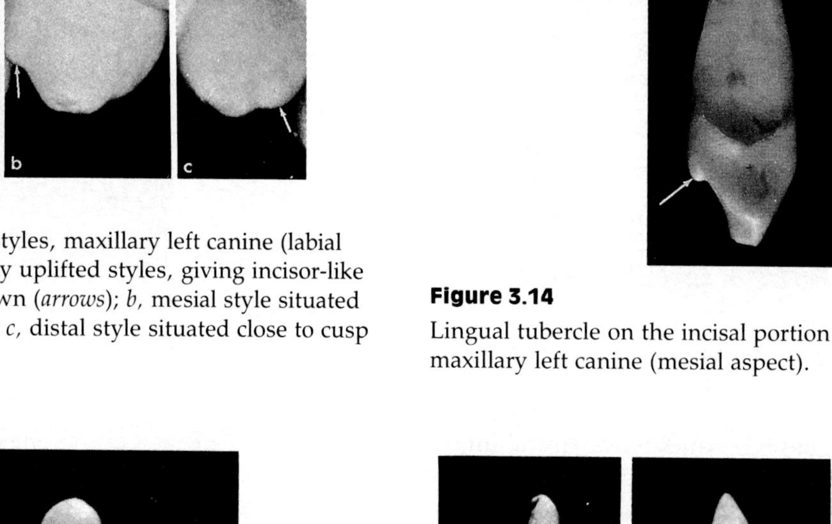

Figure 3.14

Lingual tubercle on the incisal portion of the cingulum, maxillary left canine (mesial aspect).

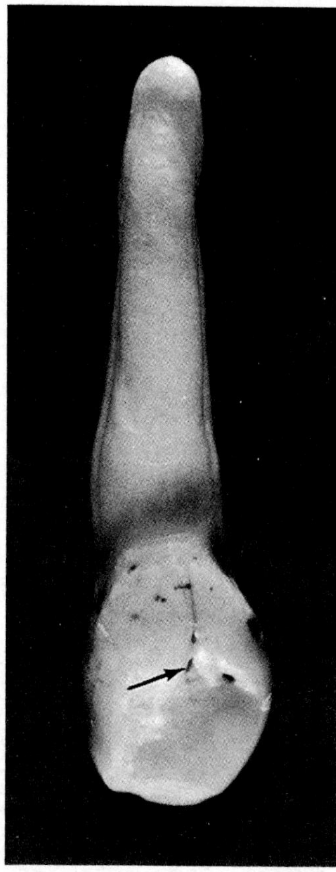

Figure 3.15

Pit (*arrow*) associatd with tubercle, maxillary right canine (lingual aspect).

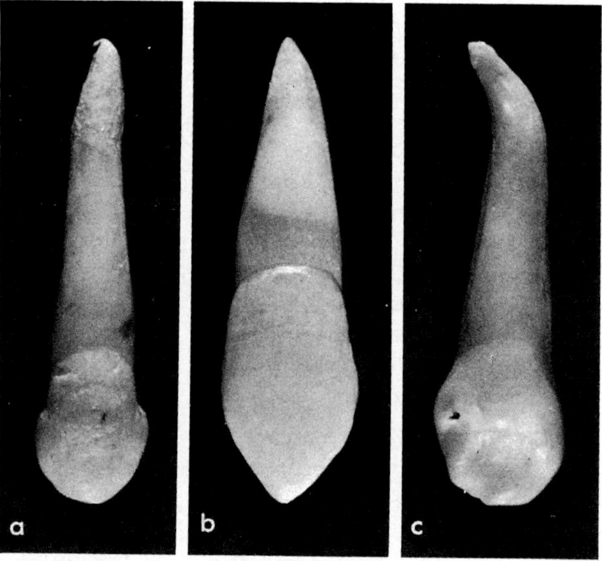

Figure 3.16

Variations in the root of the maxillary left canine: *a*, unusually long root (labial aspect); *b*, unusually short root (labial aspect); *c*, hooked root (lingual aspect).

further aspect of variation lies in the positioning of the styles; they may be situated quite close to the cervix or may occupy a position very high on the crown (Fig. 3.13*b* and *c*).

As noted previously, the lingual cingulum in the maxillary canines is more strongly developed than in the mandibular canines. Quite commonly the incisal portion of the cingulum is elevated in the form of a small cusp—the "lingual tubercle" (Fig. 3.14). As in the maxillary incisors, a pit may be found associated with the tubercle (Fig. 3.15).

The maxillary canine root may be unusually long (Fig. 3.16*a*), abnormally short (Fig. 3.16*b*), distally inclined throughout its length, or abruptly curved or "hooked" in its apical portion (Fig. 3.16*c*).

Summary

Maxillary Canine—Arch Traits

1. The crown is larger than the mandibular canine in the same dentition.

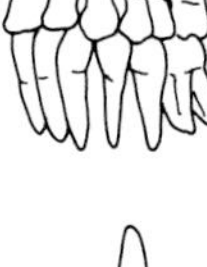

2. The mesial and distal margins as seen from the labial aspect tend to converge markedly toward the cervix.

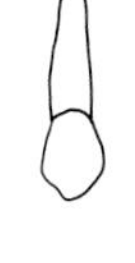

3. The incisal margin of the crown occupies at least one-third of the crown height and often as much as one-half.

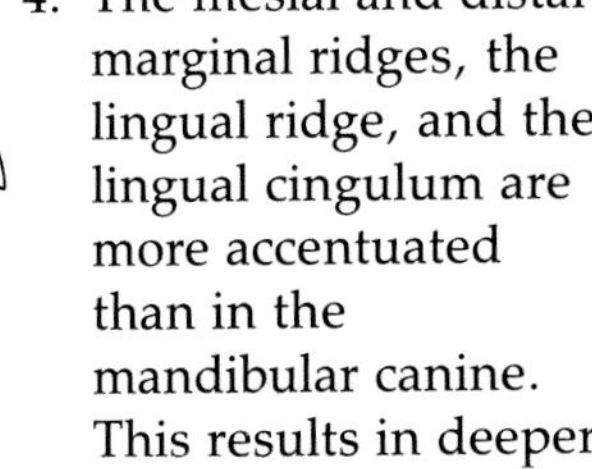

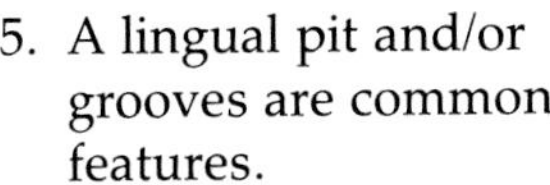

4. The mesial and distal marginal ridges, the lingual ridge, and the lingual cingulum are more accentuated than in the mandibular canine. This results in deeper lingual fossae.

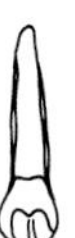

5. A lingual pit and/or grooves are common features.

6. The labiolingual diameter of the crown near the cervix is greater than in the mandibular canine.

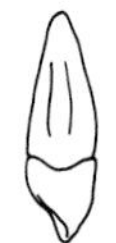

7. There is marked asymmetry of the mesial and distal halves of the crown when viewed from the incisal aspect.

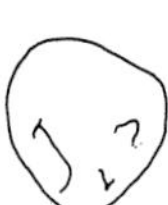

The Mandibular Canine

Size and Eruption

Arch	Crown Height (mm)	Mesiodistal Crown Diameter (mm)	Labiolingual Crown Diameter (mm)	Tooth Length (mm)	Age at Eruption (yr)
Mandibular	11.0	7.0	7.5	26.0	11

The mandibular canine is the first member of its class to appear in the oral cavity. Relative to the maxillary canine, it is noticeably narrower mesiodistally (arch trait) and hence appears longer incisocervically. In addition, the mandibular canine is slightly narrower in the labiolingual dimension. Along with the mandibular incisors, the canine is generally the last tooth to be lost through dental disease (i.e., caries, periodontal disease).

Labial Aspect (Fig. 3.17)

The cusp does not appear as long and pointed as that of its maxillary counterpart (arch trait). This is because the mesial cusp ridge forms a high shoulder adjacent to the cusp apex and the distal cusp ridge forms a low shoulder—this is sometimes referred to as the "scoliosed" appearance of the mandibular canine. The incisal margin of the crown is confined to the incisal one-fourth or one-fifth of the crown, giving the tooth a long, narrow appearance (arch trait). The mesial profile of the crown is relatively straight and is almost directly in line with the mesial root profile. The distal crown profile, on the other hand, is highly convex and "overhangs" the corresponding root profile in the form of a bulbous protuberance. The mesial and distal margins tend to parallel each other or to converge only slightly toward the cervix (arch trait).

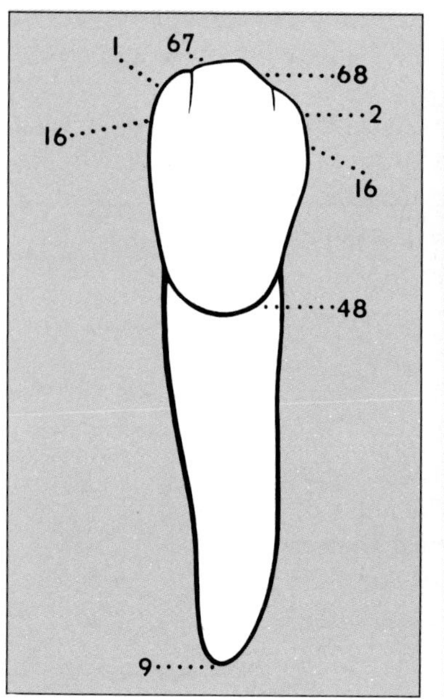

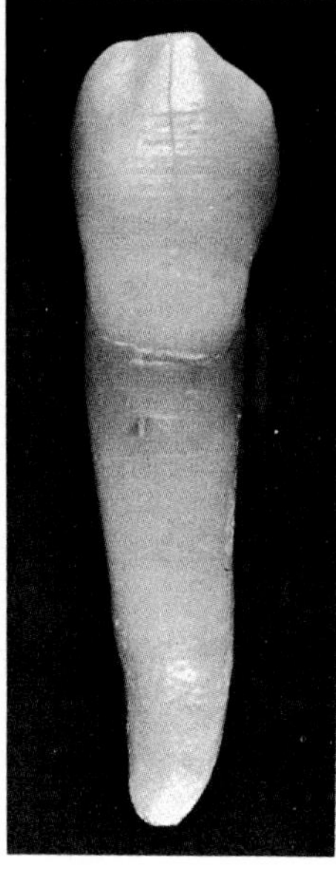

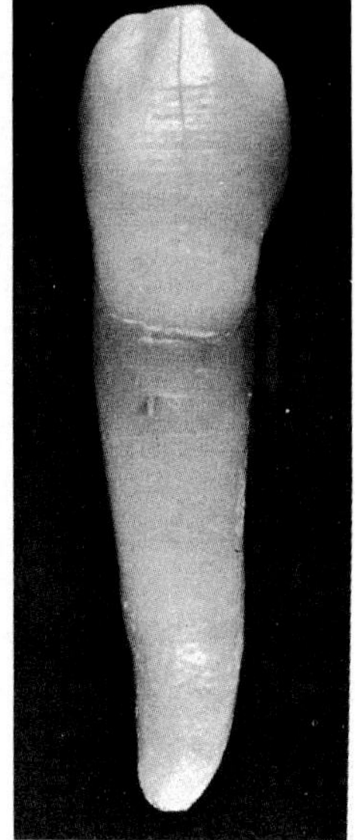

Figure 3.17
Mandibular left canine (labial aspect).

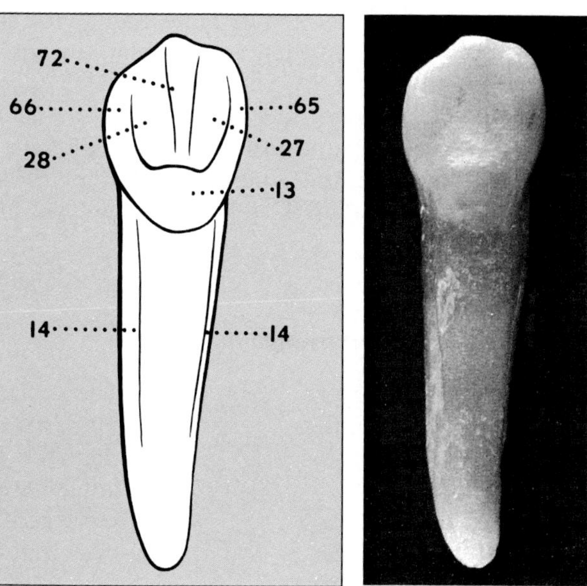

Figure 3.18
Mandibular left canine (lingual aspect).

The mesial contact area is located high on the crown just below the mesioincisal angle. The distal contact area is more cervical, and is located at the junction of the incisal and middle thirds.

The labial CEJ is slightly convex toward the root apex.

As in the maxillary canines, three lobes are visible from the labial aspect, marked off by two shallow depressions or grooves.

The root is conical in form, tapering from the cervix to a more or less blunted apex. There is generally a slight mesial inclination from cervix to apex. The crown-root orientation is distinctive in this tooth; the crown often appears to be tilted distally in relation to the long axis of the root (arch trait).

Lingual Aspect (Fig. 3.18)

The profile of the lingual aspect corresponds to that of the labial aspect.

The lingual surface presents essentially the same features as that of the maxillary canine, namely, mesial and distal marginal ridges, lingual cingulum, lingual ridge, and mesio- and distolingual fossae. Nevertheless, there are certain distinct differences: (1) the two marginal ridges, the lingual ridge, and the lingual cingulum are much less prominent in the mandibular canine (arch trait); (2) the mesio- and distolingual fossae are shallow and barely discernible in the mandibular canine (arch trait); (3) pits or grooves of the lingual surface are rarely if ever present (arch trait); (4) the root is narrower lingually than labially, and distinct longitudinal depressions or grooves extend down the proximal surfaces.

Mesial Aspect (Fig. 3.19)

The cervical third of the mandibular canine is narrower than that of the maxillary canine (arch trait). The height of contour on the labial profile is just above

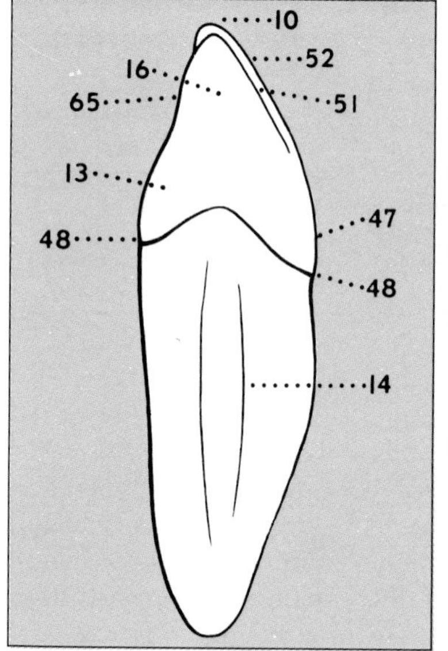

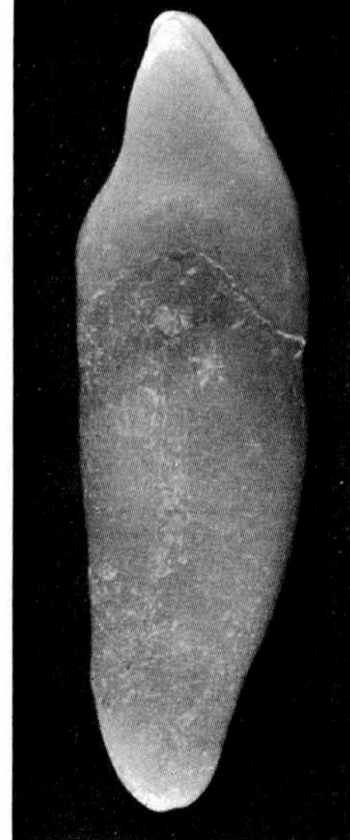

Figure 3.19
Mandibular left canine (mesial aspect).

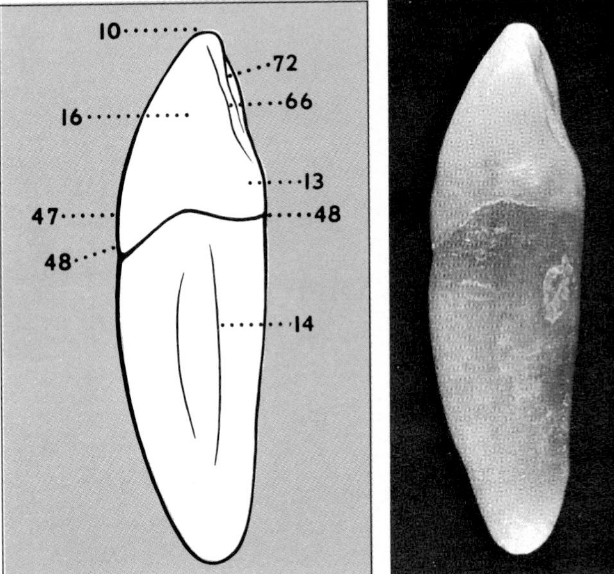

Figure 3.20
Mandibular left canine (distal aspect).

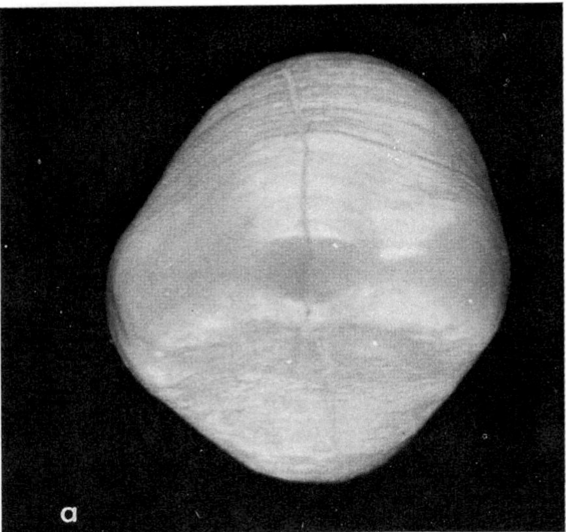

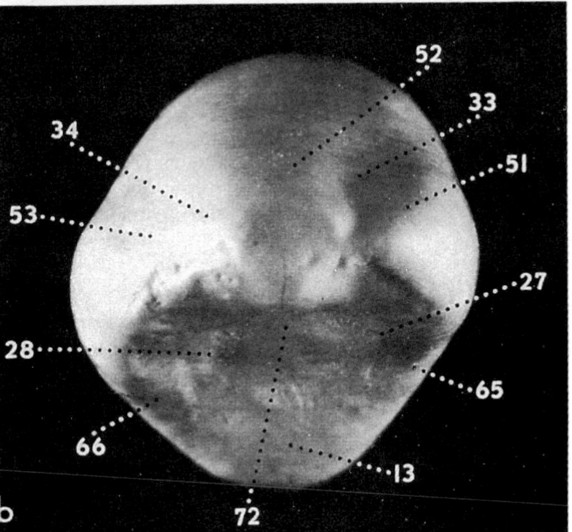

Figure 3.21
Mandibular left canine (incisal aspect): *a*, actual crown; *b*, cast.

the cervical line (arch trait). The entire labial profile is strongly convex, so that much of the labial surface can be seen from the incisal view. The lingual cingulum is generally less prominent on the mandibular than on the maxillary canine (arch trait).

Unlike the maxillary canine, the mesial marginal ridge is confluent with the lingual profile and cannot be distinguished as such.

The root of the mandibular canine is narrower than that of the maxillary.

Distal Aspect (Fig. 3.20)

The crown profile and surface are the same in distal as in mesial aspect. The same applies to the root.

Incisal Aspect (Fig. 3.21)

If a line were drawn perpendicular to the incisal axis and passing through the apex of the cusp, the mesial and distal halves of the crown would be more nearly symmetrical than in the maxillary canine (arch trait). The lingual profile is usually less round (or more blunt) than in the maxillary canine.

Several features of the crown surface distinguish the mandibular from the maxillary canine. The mesial and distal marginal ridges are less strongly developed. The diminution of the lingual ridge gives a less bulky appearance to the central portion of the incisal edge. There is only a slight lingual tubercle at best, and rarely, if ever, does a lingual pit occur. Finally, the vertical grooves separating the three lobes on the labial surface are less marked than on the maxillary canine.

Pulp

The pulp cavity is morphologically similar to that of the maxillary canine (Fig. 3.22*a*, *b*, and *c*).

Variations

All of the basic structural characteristics of the mandibular canine display a range of variations about the mean described above. For example, in some cases the lingual ridge may be quite marked (Fig. 3.23). Likewise, the marginal ridges may be relatively prominent. As in the maxillary canine, the mesial and distal styles run through a gamut of expressions, both in position and prominence (Fig. 3.24*a*, *b*, and *c*). The "bending" of the crown relative to the longitudinal root axis may be strongly emphasized or barely perceptible (Fig. 3.25*a* and *b*).

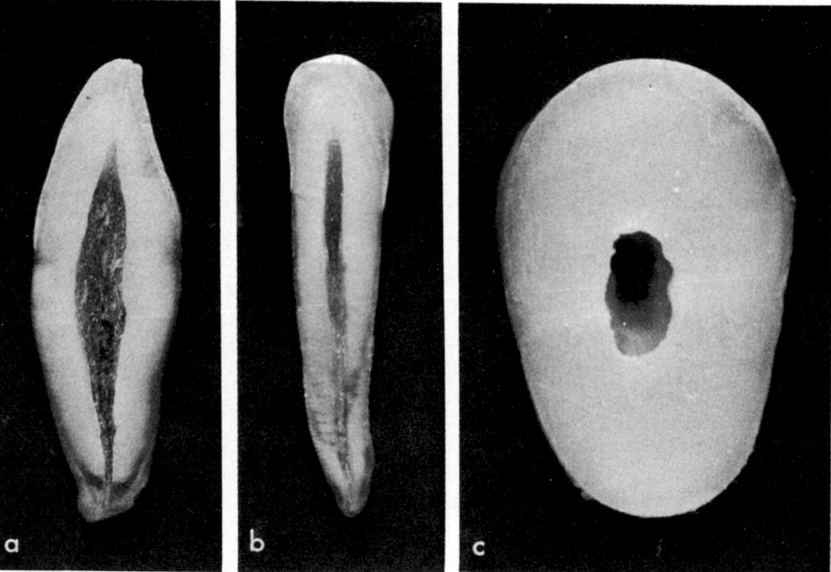

Figure 3.22

Pulp cavity of the mandibular left canine: *a*, labiolingual section; *b*, mesiodistal section; *c*, transverse section at the cervix.

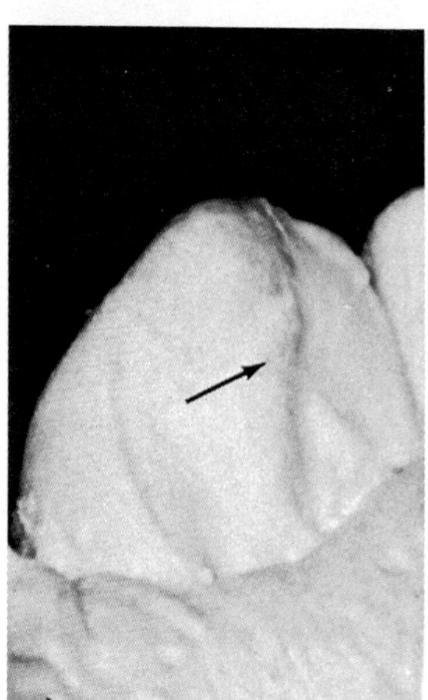

Figure 3.23

Prominent lingual ridge (*arrow*) on mandibular left canine crown (lingual aspect, cast).

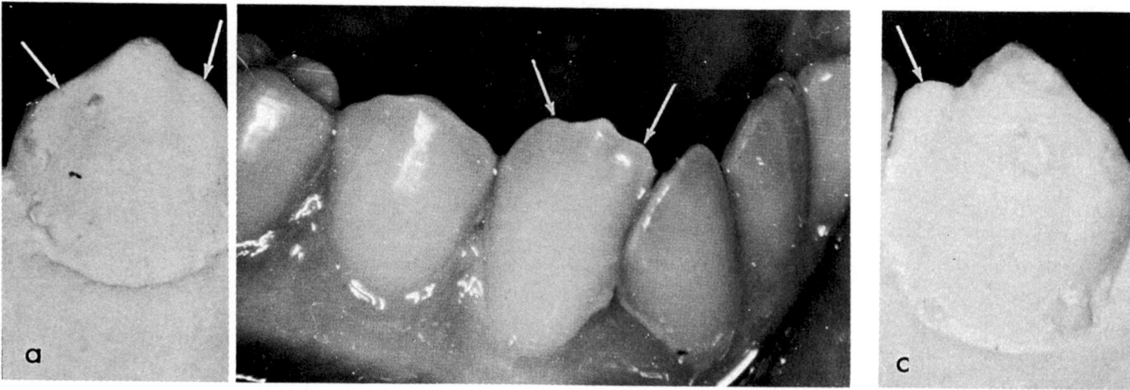

Figure 3.24

Variations in the expressions of style (*arrows*) on the mandibular right canine crowns (labial aspect): *a*, slight styles (cast); *b*, pronounced mesial and distal styles; *c*, exaggerated mesial style (left canine, cast).

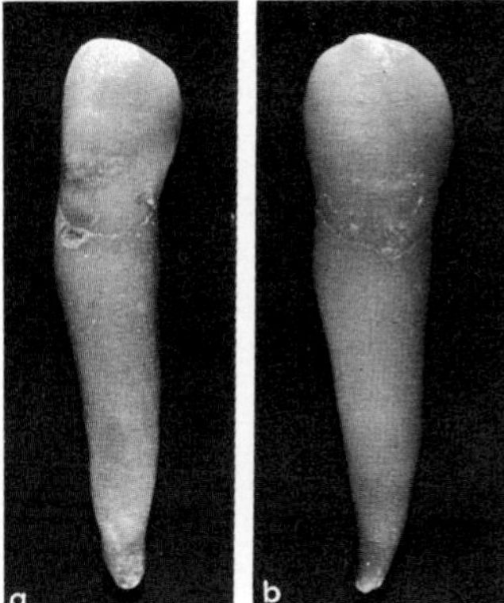

Figure 3.25

Degrees of "bending" of the crown, mandibular left canine (labial aspect): *a,* pronounced "bending"; *b,* slight "bending."

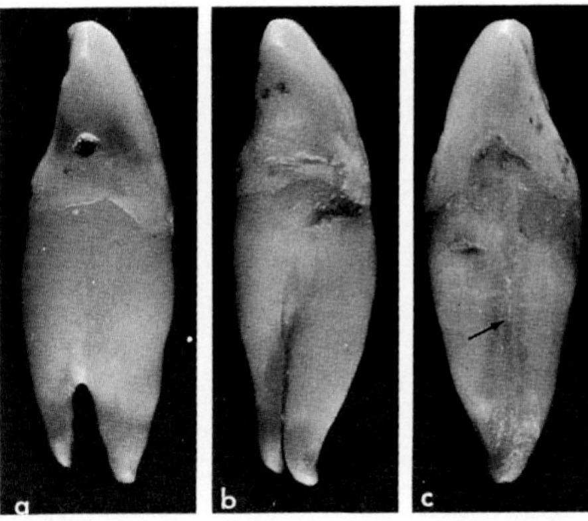

Figure 3.26

Variations in double root expressions of mandibular left canines: *a,* clearly separated roots; *b,* roots juxtapositioned; *c,* deep groove (*arrow*) on the proximal root surface.

The mandibular canine occasionally has a double root situated labiolingually. The two roots may be in juxtaposition or clearly separated. On the other hand, this tendency for doubling may take the expression of unusually deep grooves on the proximal root surfaces which divide the single root into a buccal and lingual component (Fig. 3.26).

Summary

Mandibular Canine—Arch Traits

1. The crown is smaller than the maxillary canine in the same dentition.

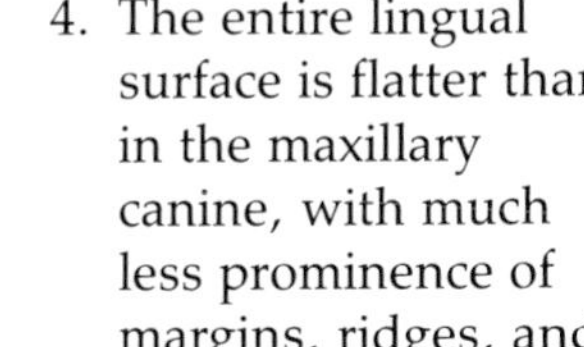

2. The mesial and distal margins as seen from the labial aspect tend to be parallel or only slightly convergent toward the cervix.

3. The incisal margin of the crown is confined to the incisal one-fourth or one-fifth of the crown, giving the tooth a long, narrow appearance as compared with the maxillary canine.

4. The entire lingual surface is flatter than in the maxillary canine, with much less prominence of margins, ridges, and cingulum.

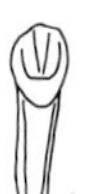

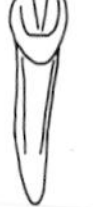

5. There are no lingual pits or grooves.

6. The mesial and distal halves of the crown when viewed from the incisal aspect are more symmetrical.

7. The labiolingual diameter of the crown near the cervix is less than in the maxillary canine.

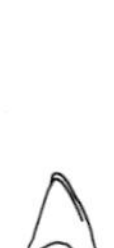

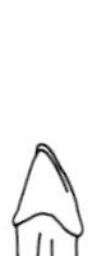

Clinical Applications

The incisor and canine teeth are critically important clinically not only from a standpoint of function but also for esthetic reasons. They may be involved in a wide variety of abnormalities in the form of discoloration, fracture, malformation and malalignment to mention only a few. Accordingly an intimate knowledge of precise morphological detail is highly important to the student of dentistry.

Examples of successful restorations for a wide variety of common clinical problems, including crown fracture, discoloration, malformation and malalignment are shown in Figures 3.27, 3.28, 3.29, and 3.30.

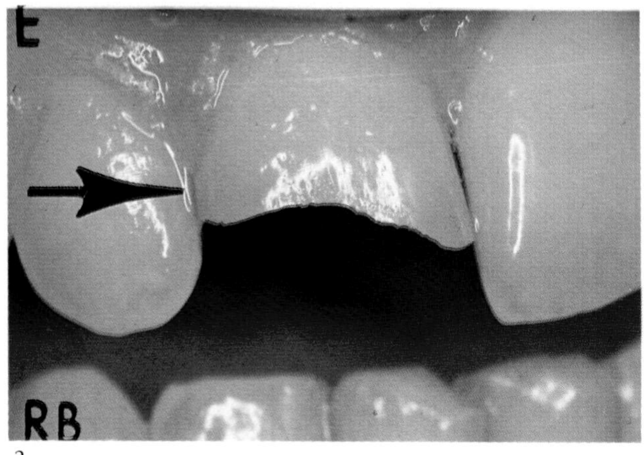

a

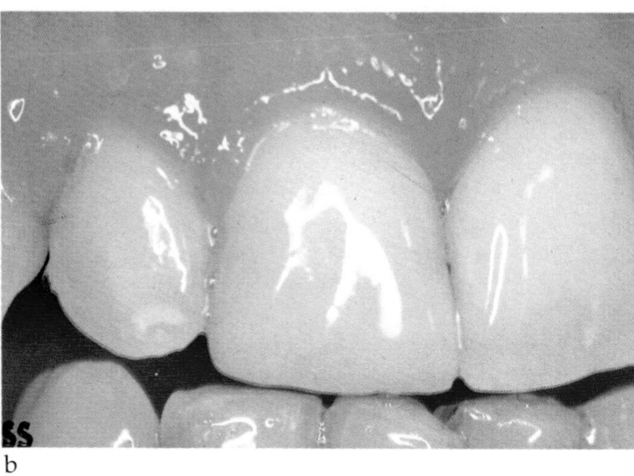

b

Figure 3.27

a, An extensively fractured central incisor crown in a 17-year-old patient; *b*, the same crown anatomically restored with a composite resin restorative material. Note the anatomic details of the labial surface of the restoration.

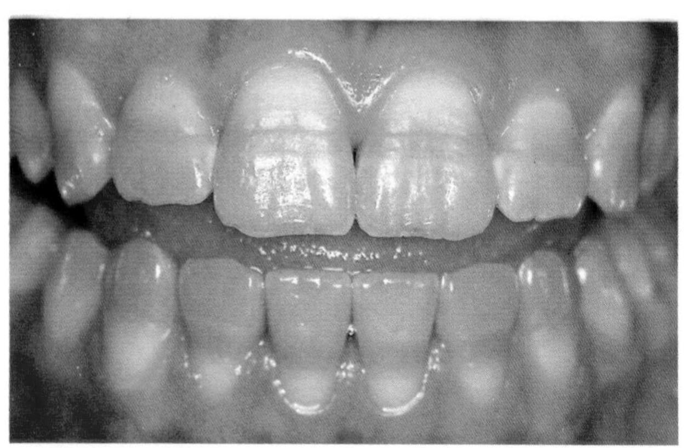

a

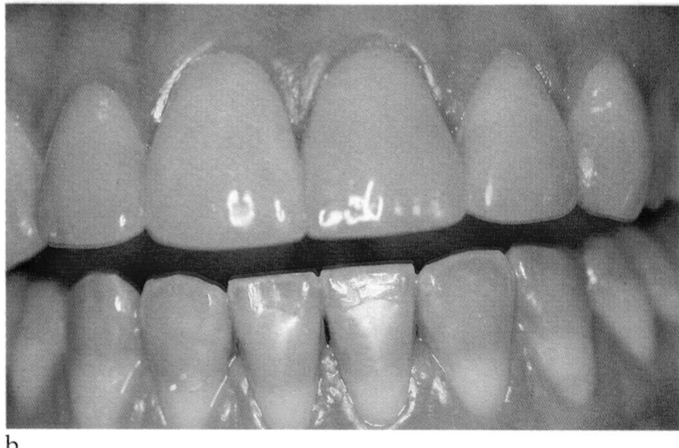

b

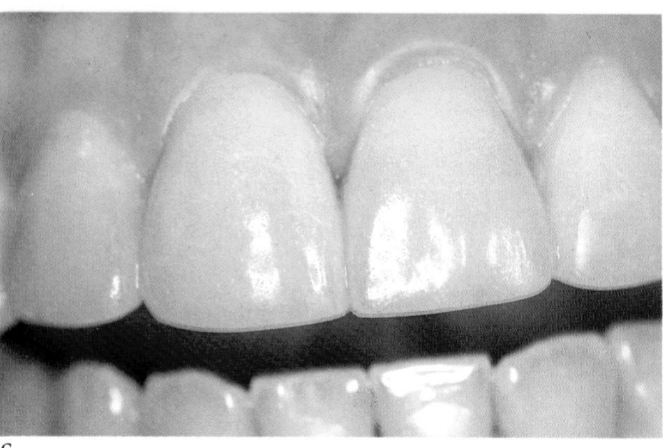

c

Figure 3.28

a, Tetracycline discoloration in a 24-year-old patient; *b*, *c*, the same dentition 4 years after treatment using bonded porcelain veneer restorations.

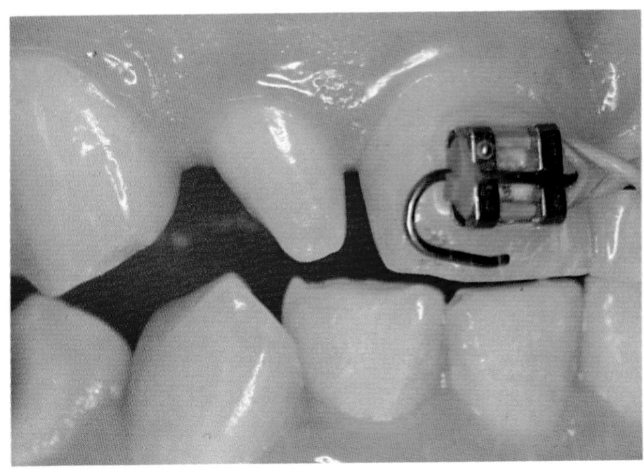

a

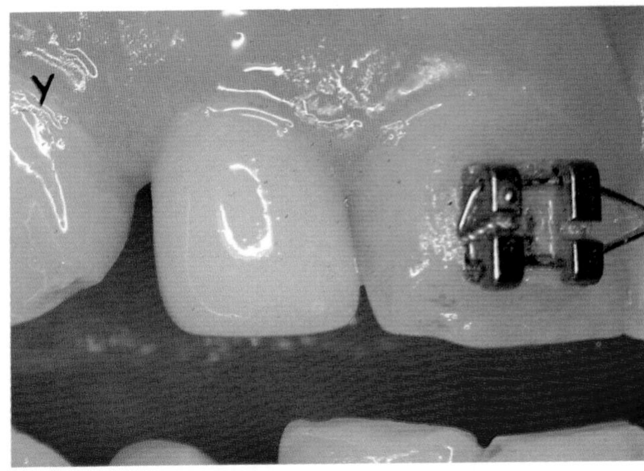

b

Figure 3.29

a, A "peg" lateral incisor in a mid-adolescent patient; *b,* the same incisor restored with a direct bonded composite restoration.

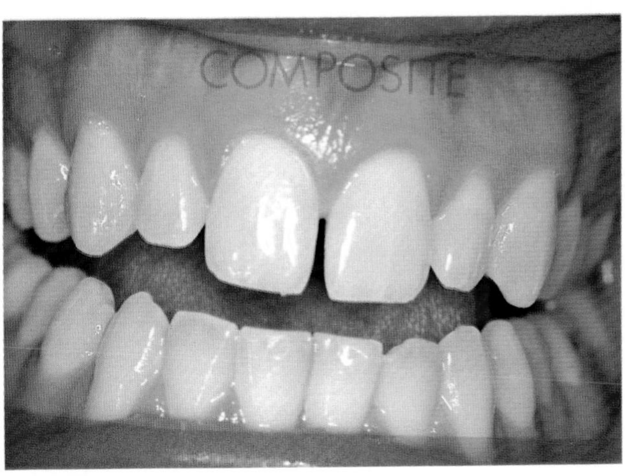

a

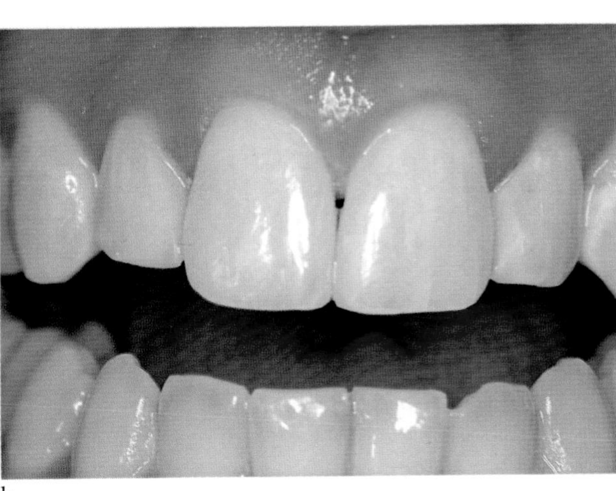

b

Figure 3.30

a, A midline diastema space in the dentition of a young adolescent; *b,* the same dentition after space closure using bonded composite restorative materials.

The Premolars

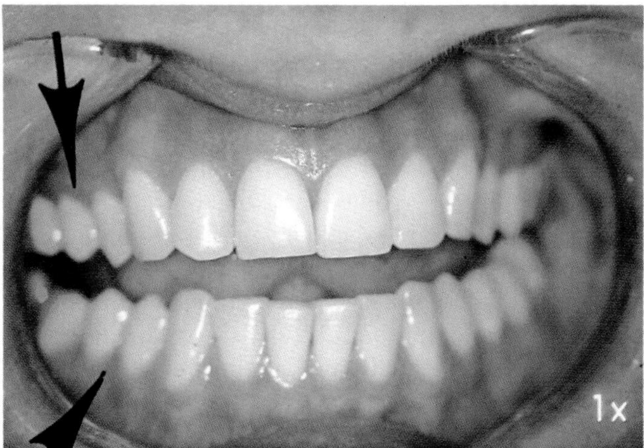

Figure 4.1
Fronto-lateral view of the right premolar dentition.

There are eight premolars in the human permanent dentition, two in each quadrant of the maxillary and mandibular arches (Fig. 4.1).

The premolars succeed the primary molars and erupt between the ages of 10 and 12 years, i.e., just before the appearance of the canines and second molars. The maxillary and mandibular first premolars erupt more or less contemporaneously, and are followed by the maxillary and mandibular second premolars in that order.

The premolars are often referred to as "bicuspids." The latter term, however, is misleading since it connotes two cusps. As is seen later, some members of this class do not necessarily exhibit a "two-cusp" structure.

Premolars occupy a position in the dental arch between the canines and molars. Morphologically they may be regarded as "intermediate" or "transitional" forms between canines and molars. We have already seen that the single-cusp, wedge-shaped form of canines lends itself nicely to a piercing or tearing function. Molars, on the other hand, are multicusped with broad occlusal surfaces that render them particularly suited for a grinding function. Premolars, as "intermediate" members of the dental arch, invariably possess at least one sharp projecting major cusp, the buccal, in addition to a somewhat restricted occlusal surface that participates in the grinding function.

Just as the incisors and canines constitute a special group called the "anterior teeth," the premolars and molars together are referred to as the "posterior teeth."

There are certain class traits diagnostic for all premolars: (1) premolars generally have at least two cusps, but may have additional cusps or cusplets; (2) premolars alone have a single buccal cusp with one or more lingual cusps.

The human premolars, although designated as the "first" and "second," are considered to be the "third" and "fourth" premolars by paleontologists, since it is believed that in the course of evolution the original first and second premolars were lost, leaving only the last two (the third and fourth).

Maxillary Premolars

Size and Eruption

Maxillary Premolars (mm)	Crown Height (mm)	Mesiodistal Crown Diameter (mm)	Bucco-lingual Crown Diameter (mm)	Tooth Length (mm)	Age at Eruption (yr)
First	8.5	7.0	9.0	23.5	9
Second	8.5	7.0	9.0	22.5	10

Maxillary first and second premolars are much more alike than are the mandibular first and second premolars (arch trait). Certain other arch traits clearly distinguish them from their mandibular antagonists. (1) All maxillary premolars have two major cusps that are approximately equal in size and prominence. The same is not true of mandibular premolars. (2) All maxillary premolar crowns, as viewed from the occlusal aspect, are distinctly wider buccolingually than

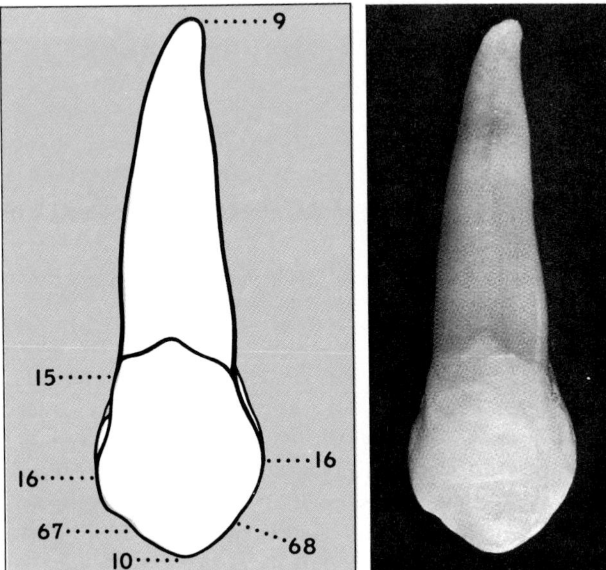

Figure 4.2
Maxillary left first premolar (buccal aspect).

mesiodistally. The mesiodistal and buccolingual dimensions of mandibular premolars more closely approximate one another. (3) The buccal profiles of all maxillary premolars (as viewed from the proximal aspects) show only a slight lingual inclination from the height of contour to the cusp apex. The buccal profiles of mandibular premolars are strongly inclined lingually. (4) The height of contour of the lingual profiles of all maxillary premolars is located approximately at the midportion of the crown. The corresponding crest of curvature in mandibular premolars is closer to the cusp apex, i.e., in the occlusal third of the crown.

First Premolar (Fig. 4.2)

Buccal Aspect

When viewed from the buccal aspect the maxillary first premolar bears a distinct resemblance to the adjoining canine although it is somewhat smaller. It is very similar to the second premolar in form but is slightly larger.

The mesial and distal cuspal ridges incline at about a 30-degree slope to form a rather rounded apex. At the margins of the crown they form prominent bulging shoulders (the mesio- and disto-occlusal angles), which overhang the cervical portion (type trait). The appearance of the crown from this aspect is somewhat ovoid. Near the cervix the two margins (mesial and distal) become rather parallel and confluent with the root. From the buccal aspect a small portion of the mesial profile of the lingual cusp can occasionally be seen. In between lies the *mesial concavity,* a depression between the lingual and buccal cervical thirds of the crown and root on the mesial side.

Occasionally two lobes or "styles" are visible on either side of the cusp apex. They may be demarcated by slight depressions running partway up the crown from the cuspal margin.

There is little to distinguish the root from that of the maxillary canine. It is conical and converges gradually to a somewhat blunt apex.

Lingual Aspect (Fig. 4.3)

The buccal portion of the crown of the maxillary first premolar is larger in all dimensions than the lingual, so that from the lingual aspect almost the entire buccal profile is visible (type trait). The lingual cusp is almost always slightly mesial to the midline of the crown. The bulging shoulders found on the buccal portion of the crown are not seen on the lingual portion, nor are lobes or styles visible on the marginal ridge of the lingual cusp. The two halves of the lingual profile are quite symmetrical.

There are no protuberances, ridges, or depressions to be seen on the lingual surface.

The two root apices are visible from the lingual aspect. The mesial concavity observed only in the crown portion of the tooth from the buccal aspect can now be observed along most of the root length.

Mesial Aspect (Fig. 4.4)

Two cusps of unequal prominence (i.e., the buccal and the lingual) make up the occlusal profile of the

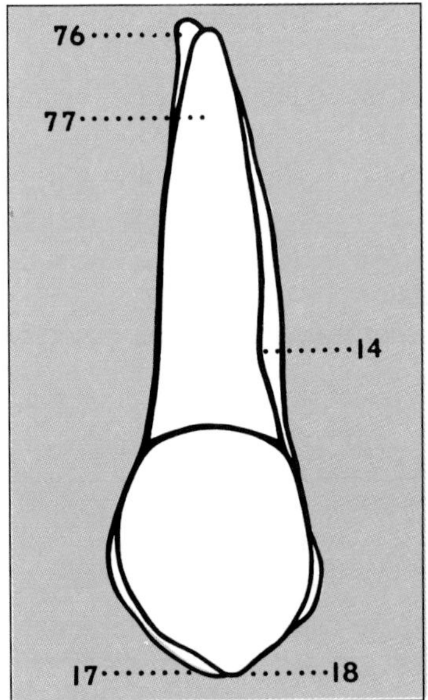

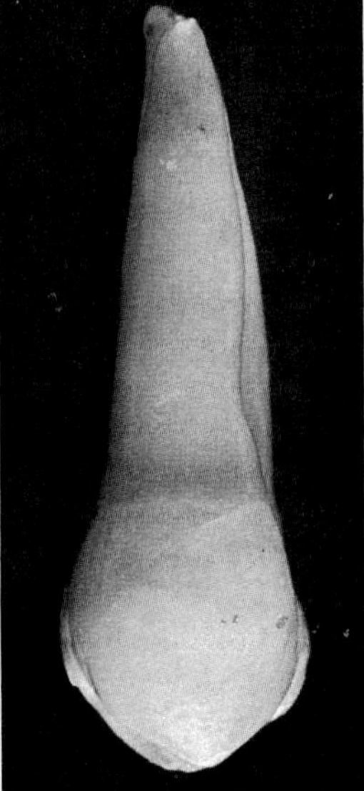

Figure 4.3
Maxillary left first premolar (lingual aspect).

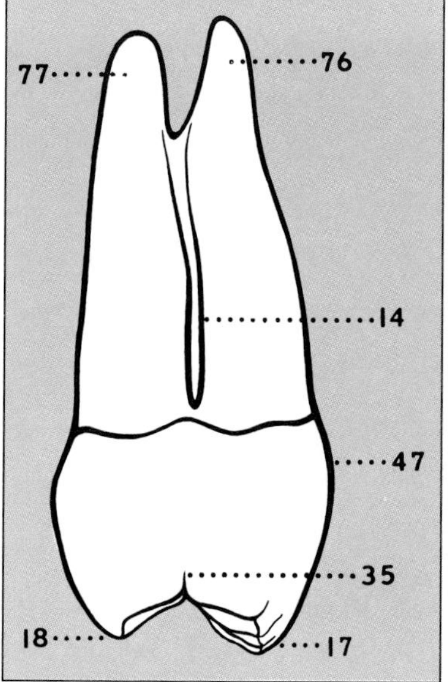

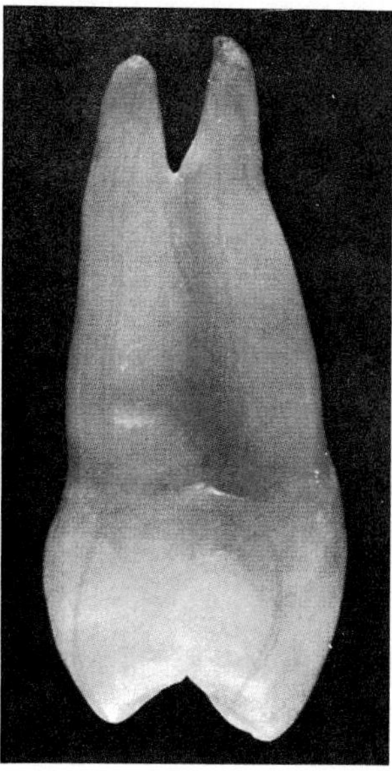

Figure 4.4
Maxillary left first premolar (mesial aspect).

mesial aspect of the maxillary first premolar. The buccal cusp is distinctly more prominent in terms of height than the lingual cusp. "Triangular ridges" incline from both cusp apices with a slope of roughly 45 degrees toward the center of the occlusal surface. The mesial marginal ridge is seen as a prominent elevation from this aspect. It is interrupted just lingual to its midpoint by the *mesial-marginal groove* (type trait), which crosses the marginal ridge from the occlusal surface, forming a distinct notch. Such marginal ridge depressions are called "spillways," and it is claimed that they permit the escape of food from the occlusal surface during mastication.

The buccal profile of the crown is marked by a slight convexity in its cervical third. From the height of contour (which is located well within the cervical third) to the cusp apex, the buccal profile shows only a slight inclination toward the lingual. This is also a feature that distinguishes maxillary from mandibular premolars.

The lingual profile of the crown shows a more or less uniform convexity from the cervical line to the cusp apex, and the height of contour is located at approximately the midpoint of the crown. The cervical line is irregularly convex toward the occlusal. At its midpoint it may extend apically in the form of a small V-shaped "incipient enamel extension."*

The cervical third exhibits a deep depression, the *mesial concavity*, which extends down the crown onto the root surface in the form of a deep groove (the *mesial interradicular groove*), which divides the root trunk into buccal and lingual moieties. The mesial interradicular groove lies directly in line with the mesial marginal groove. Accordingly, the entire mesial surface of the maxillary first premolar appears to be divided into two segments (i.e., buccal and lingual). The mesiobuccal and mesiolingual cusp ridges extend mesially from their respective cusp apices and become confluent with the mesial marginal ridge. The point of junction of the mesiobuccal cusp ridge with the mesial marginal ridge is marked by a distinct angle measuring roughly 90 degrees (type trait). The corresponding junction between the mesiolingual cusp ridge and the mesial marginal ridge is, on the other hand, ill defined, since the two ridges join in the form of a rounded arc.

The occlusal table, as viewed from the mesial aspect, is clearly centered over the root trunk. This is an important feature since it clearly differentiates maxillary from mandibular posterior teeth.

Two roots (i.e., buccal and lingual) are seen from the mesial aspect (type trait). They are joined from the cervix to about two-thirds of the length where they bifurcate in the apical third. As is seen later, the bifurcation point is variable, but the mesial surface of the entire root is almost always divided into two components by a deep groove extending vertically from the cervix.

*This may be found in the bifurcational area of any multirooted tooth and is a frequent characteristic of Eskimo teeth.

Distal Aspect (Fig. 4.5)

The distal aspect of the maxillary first premolar resembles the mesial aspect except for the following

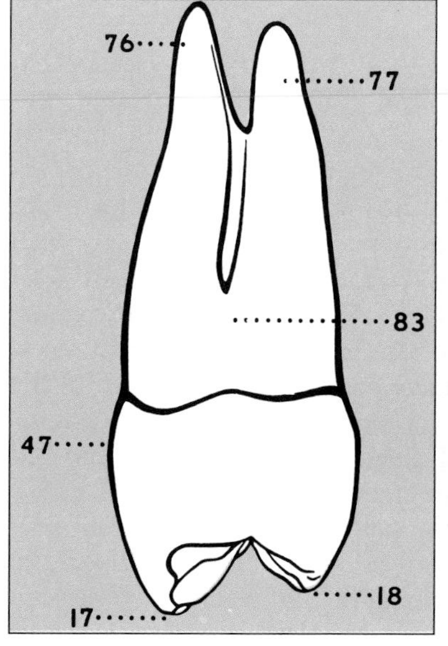

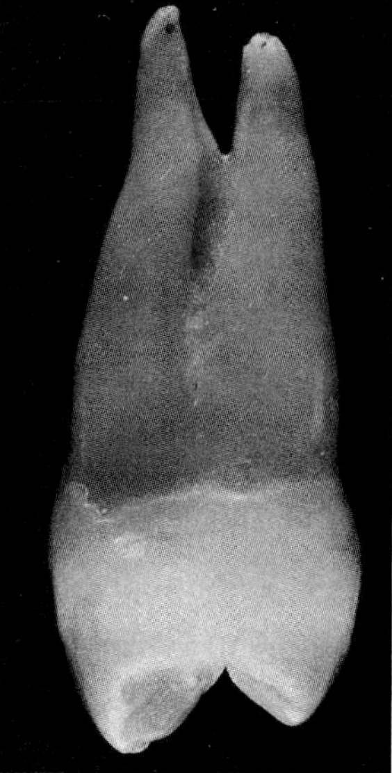

Figure 4.5
Maxillary left first premolar (distal aspect).

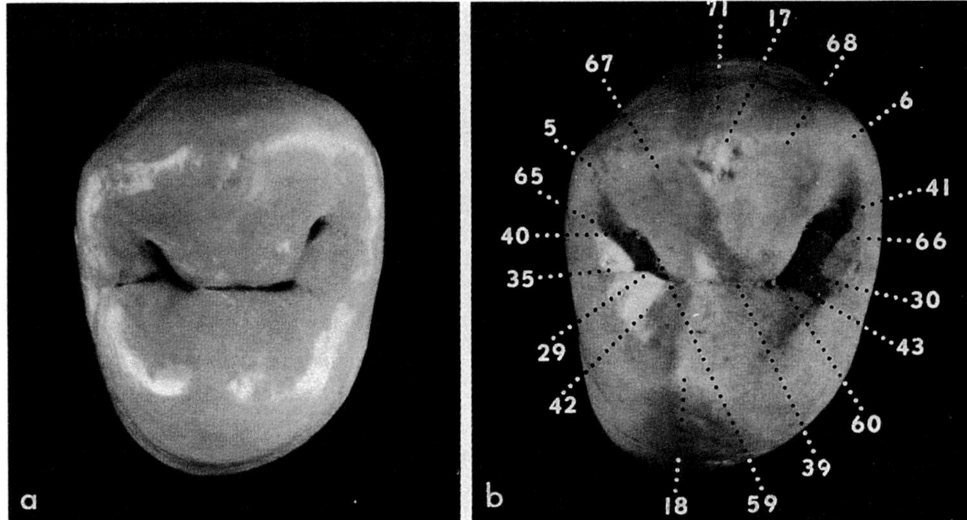

Figure 4.6
Maxillary left first premolar (occlusal aspect): *a*, actual crown; *b*, cast.

features: (1) more of the occlusal surface may be seen from the distal aspect; (2) the continuity of the distal marginal ridge is not broken by a marginal groove; (3) a concavity is not present in the cervical third of the distal surface of the crown; (4) the distal interradicular groove is much less pronounced than the mesial interradicular groove; (5) the distobuccal cusp ridge meets the distal marginal ridge in a more looping curve.

Occlusal Aspect (Fig. 4.6)

The crown profile is roughly hexagonal (type trait) in the first premolar of the maxillary dentition. The buccal profile takes the form of an inverted V. A central prominence (corresponding to the apex of the V) is directly in line with the tip of the buccal cusp. On either side of the central prominence the buccal profile inclines slightly toward the lingual in a more or less straight line to meet the mesial and distal profiles. The buccal profile curves sharply to form the mesial and distal borders. The points of maximum flexure are known as the mesiobuccal and distobuccal angles (type trait). This feature is characteristic of the maxillary first premolar. The mesio- and distobuccal angles mark the widest mesiodistal dimension of the crown.

The mesial and distal profiles show a slight but definite lingual convergence (type trait). The proximal profiles become confluent with the lingual profile, which is uniformly strongly convex. The occlusal halves of both buccal and lingual *surfaces* may be seen from the occlusal aspect. The buccal surface is marked by a central prominence, the *buccal ridge,* which extends cervically from the apex of the buccal cusp for more than one-half of the length of the crown. Distinct concavities or depressions on either side of the ridge divide the buccal surface into three lobes. The lingual surface, on the other hand, being uniformly convex, shows no evidence of lobes or styles.

The mesial and distal marginal ridges, together with the cusp ridges, mark the boundaries of the *occlusal table.*

If straight lines are drawn along the crests of the marginal ridges and connected with similar lines drawn through the apices and ridges of both cusps, the resultant figure will approximate a trapezoid (type trait). The buccal and lingual cusp ridges form the parallel sides of the trapezoid and the mesial and distal marginal ridges form the converging sides of the figure. The buccal is the wider of the two parallel sides and the distal is the longer of the two converging sides.

Two cusps, buccal and lingual, constitute the most conspicuous features of the occlusal surface. The buccal cusp is relatively wide compared with the lingual. The buccal cusp ridge is oriented mesiolingually (type trait) giving the buccal cusp a "twisted" appearance.

The apex of the lingual cusp is located slightly mesial to the midline of the crown. Accordingly the mesiolingual cusp ridge is shorter than the distolingual cusp ridge (just the reverse of the buccal cusp).

Prominent triangular ridges (i.e., the buccal and lingual triangular ridges) extend from the respective cusp apices toward the center of the occlusal surface.

The triangular ridges (particularly the buccal) are often flanked on either side by shallow trough-like supplemental grooves.

The mesial and distal marginal ridges form strongly marked elevated platforms. The mesial marginal ridge contrasts with the distal marginal ridge in that it is shorter in length and is interrupted by a groove at its midpoint.

The buccal and lingual triangular ridges are separated by the *central groove,* which extends mesiodistally across the center of the occlusal surface. The central groove, which is longer in the first premolar (type trait), terminates mesially and distally in the *mesial* and *distal triangular fossae* respectively. The mesial triangular fossa is bounded by the mesial marginal ridge and by the buccal and lingual triangular ridges. The distal triangular fossa occupies a similar position in the distal moiety of the occlusal table. The former is definitely greater in area and in depth than the distal triangular fossa. Each fossa contains the following markings: (1) a pit (the *mesial* and *distal pits* respectively) located in the depths of the fossae and marking the proximal terminations of the central groove; (2) a buccal groove (the *mesiobuccal* and *distobuccal grooves* respectively), which extends from each pit toward the respective buccal corners of the crown; (3) a lingual groove (the *mesiolingual* and *distolingual grooves* respectively), which is a faint depression of short length extending from each pit toward the respective lingual corners of the crown.

The mesial triangular fossa contains an additional groove, the *mesial marginal groove,* which extends in a mesial direction from the mesial pit and crosses the marginal ridge to end on the proximal surface (type trait).

Pulp

In transverse cross section at the cervix the pulp cavity of the maxillary first premolar is kidney shaped, being broad buccolingually and extremely narrow mesiodistally. There are two pulp horns; the buccal is larger and reaches farther apically than the lingual. Almost invariably there are two pulp canals, whether or not there are two separate roots. In mesiodistal section the pulp cavity resembles that of the maxillary canine very closely (Fig. 4.7).

Variations

When viewed from the occlusal aspect, the mesial and distal profiles of the maxillary first premolar generally converge lingually. There is considerable variation, however, with regard to their *degree of convergence* as illustrated in Figure 4.8. The proximal borders of one specimen (*a*) show only a slight degree of lingual convergence, whereas those of a second specimen (*b*) show a moderate and a third (*c*) a marked degree of convergence.

The intercuspal width (i.e., the distance between the apices of buccal and lingual cusps) in the maxillary first premolar, as in all posterior teeth, may vary greatly between individuals. Figure 4.9*a* and *b* shows two extremes in this regard, from a limited or restricted interapical diameter (*a*) to maximum dimension (*b*).

The cusps of maxillary first premolars (like canines and all posterior teeth) may show a high degree of variability with regard to the inclination of their mesial and distal cusp ridges. Figure 4.10 shows buccal views of two first premolars, one with a sharp, highly conical cusp form (*a*) and the other with a blunted cusp form (*b*).

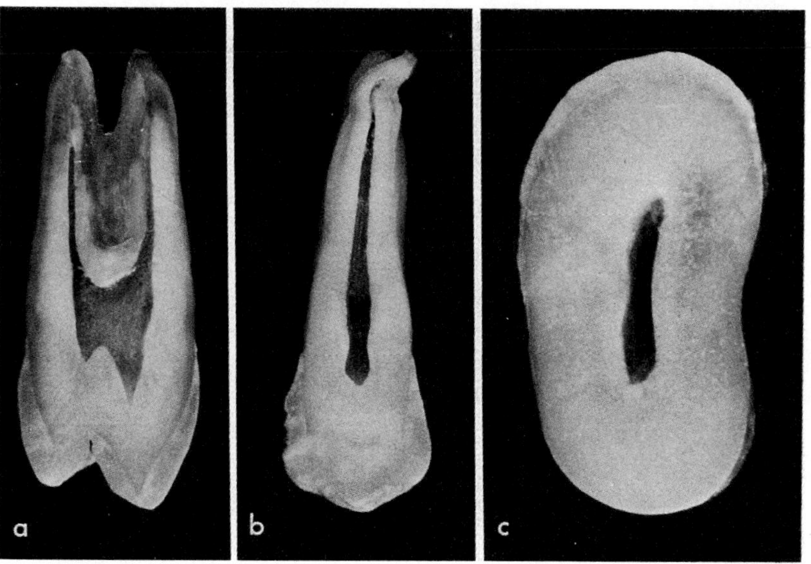

Figure 4.7
Pulp cavity of the maxillary first premolar: *a,* buccolingual section; *b,* mesiodistal section; *c,* transverse section at the cervix.

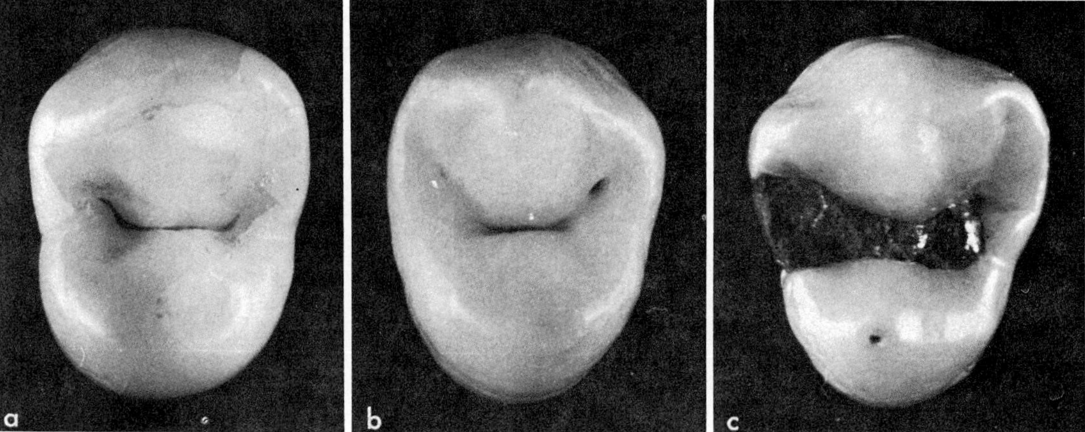

Figure 4.8

Variations in degree of conversions of the proximal borders, maxillary first premolars (occlusal aspect): *a*, slight lingual convergence; *b*, moderate lingual convergence; *c*, marked lingual convergence.

The widest mesiodistal diameter of the maxillary premolars (and all posterior teeth) occurs close to the occlusal surface, just cervical to the marginal ridges. The proximal profiles converge cervically from their maximum mesiodistal diameter, imparting a more or less bell-shaped appearance to the crown (Fig. 4.11). This bell-shaped outline may vary among individuals from slight (*a*), to moderate (*b*), to pronounced (*c*).

The buccal ridge of a maxillary first premolar is bordered on each side (i.e., mesial and distal) by a shallow groove or depression that extends cervically from the cusp ridge and outlines three buccal lobes (Fig. 4.12*a*). The mesial groove is almost invariably the most distinct of the two depressions (Fig. 4.12*b*). Not infrequently a deep pit or fissure of the buccal surface may mark the usual position of the mesial groove (Fig. 4.12*c*).

Maxillary first premolar roots show a particularly wide range of variability. Although two roots are usually present on this tooth, a single root is by no means

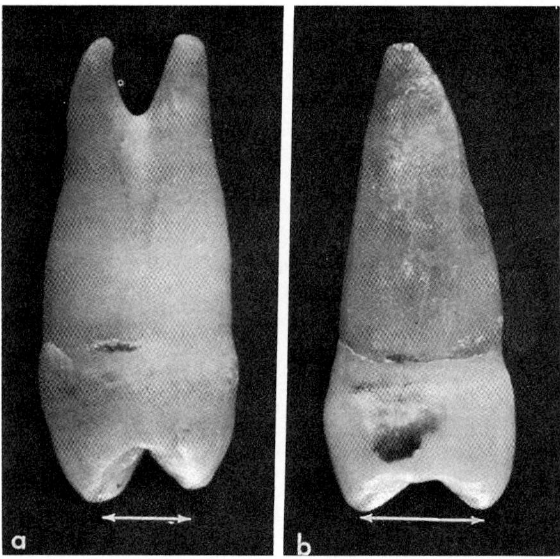

Figure 4.9

Variations in intercuspal diameter, maxillary first premolars (mesial aspect): *a*, short interapical diameter (*arrows*); *b*, maximal interapical diameter.

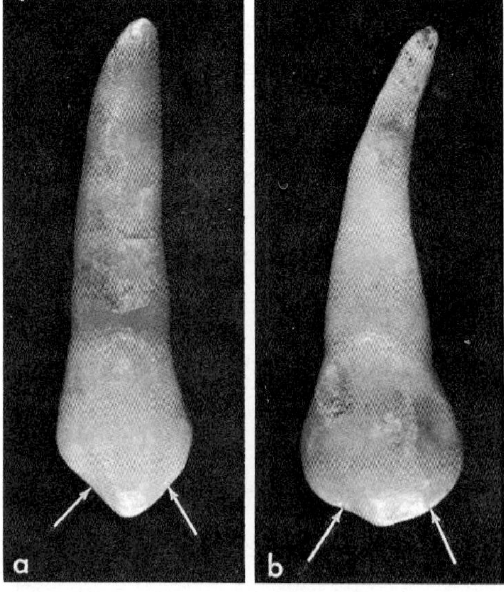

Figure 4.10

Variations in the inclination of cusp ridges (*arrows*) in maxillary first premolars (buccal aspect): *a*, highly conical cusp form; *b*, blunted cusp form.

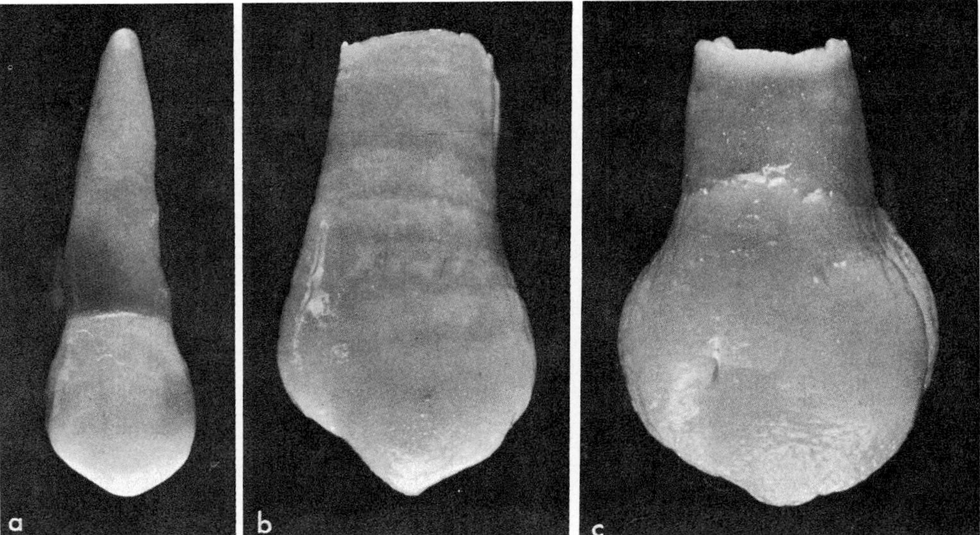

Figure 4.11
Variations in the crown outline of maxillary first premolars (buccal aspect): *a*, slight bell-shaped outline; *b*, moderate bell-shaped outline; *c*, pronounced bell-shaped outline.

an uncommon feature (Fig. 4.9*b*). In the case of a single root there may be considerable variation in the outline when it is viewed from the proximal. Both sides may converge toward the apex in an even, regular, and almost straight line (Fig. 4.13*a*) or they may take a somewhat parallel course until quite near the apex where they converge sharply, the result being a broad root with a sharp or pointed apex (Fig. 4.13*b*).

In the usual two-rooted first premolar the pointed bifurcation varies greatly. It may be relatively close to the cervical line at the junction of the cervical and middle thirds (Fig. 4.14*a*) or it may be located in the apical third (Fig. 4.14*b*).

The maxillary first premolar root(s) may be irregularly curved (Fig. 4.15) or be distally inclined in the apical third.

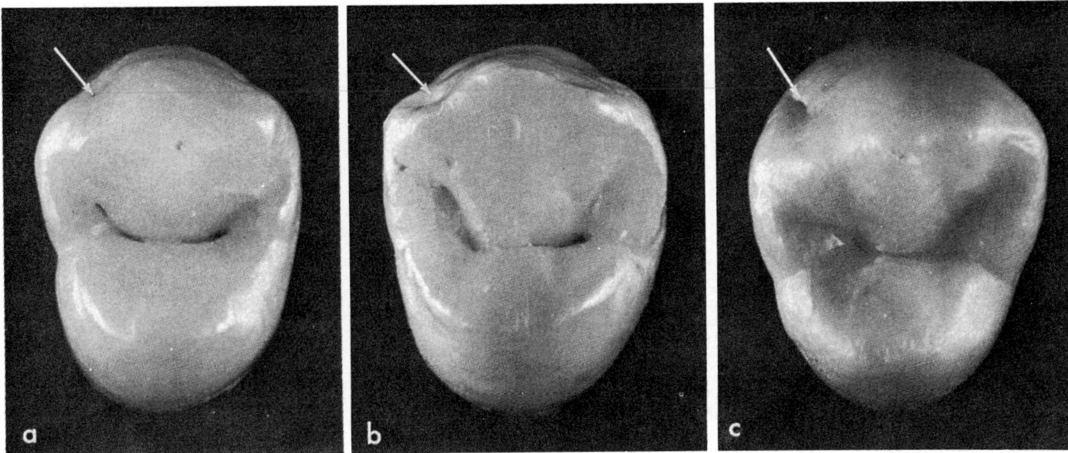

Figure 4.12
Variations in the buccal groove (*arrows*), maxillary first premolar (occlusal aspect): *a*, shallow buccal groove; *b*, deep buccal groove; *c*, fissure in buccal groove.

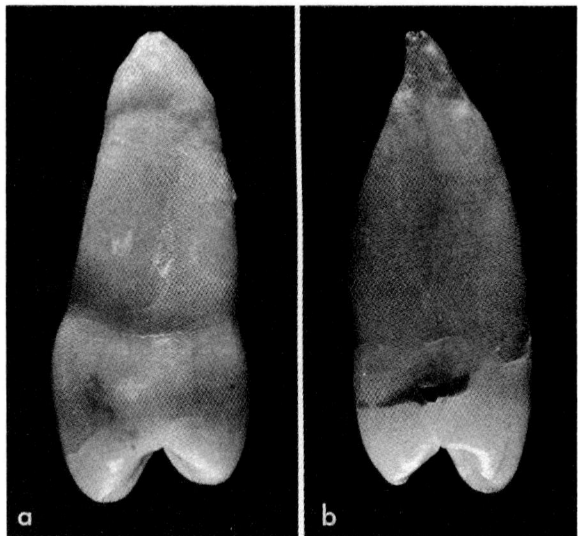

Figure 4.13

Variation in convergence of root profile, maxillary first premolars (mesial aspect): *a,* slight regular convergence; *b,* sharp convergence to apex.

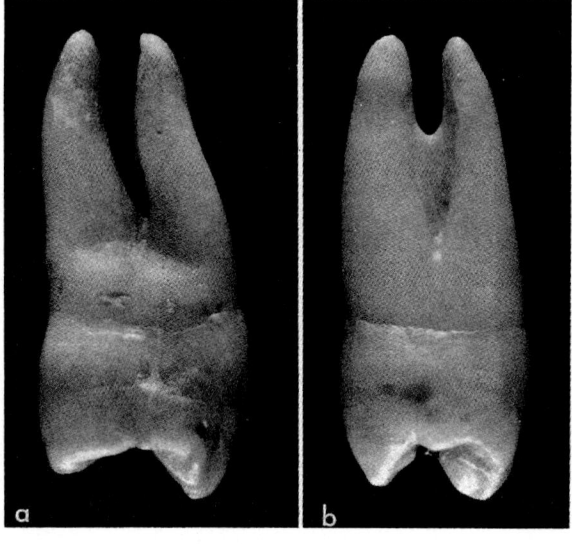

Figure 4.14

Variation in the point of bifurcation of double-rooted maxillary first premolars (mesial aspect): *a,* bifurcation at the junction of the cervical and middle thirds; *b,* bifurcation in the apical third.

Second Premolar

Buccal Aspect (Fig. 4.16)

Although basically similar in form to the first, the maxillary second premolar possesses a few type traits that distinguish it from the other premolars. The crown is smaller in breadth and in height. The mesio- and disto-occlusal angles are much less prominent, giving the crown a "narrow-shouldered" rather than an ovoid appearance. The mesial concavity is much less pronounced than in the first premolar. Lobes or styles are seldom seen, and the vertical depressions are generally absent.

Lingual Aspect (Fig. 4.17)

Seldom can any of the buccal profile be observed (type trait) in the maxillary second premolar. This is

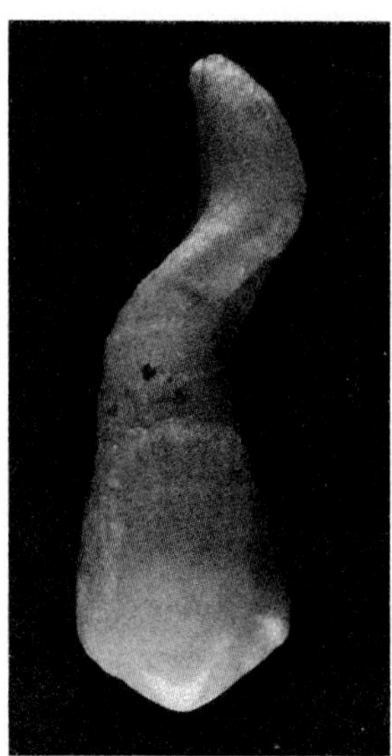

Figure 4.15

Irregular curvature of the root, maxillary first premolar (buccal aspect).

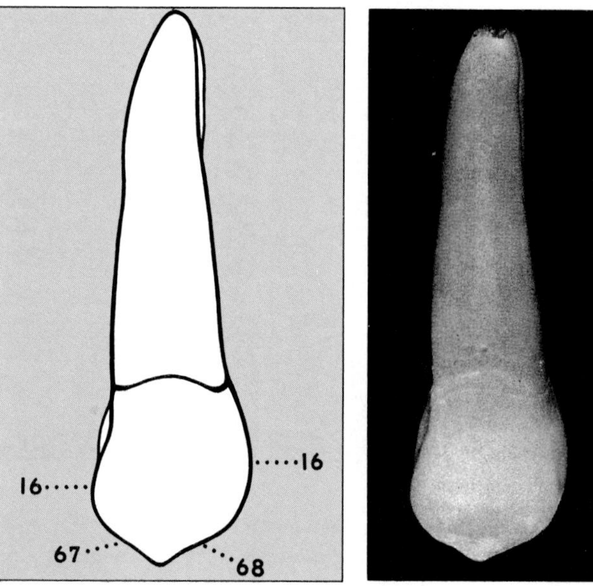

Figure 4.16

Maxillary left second premolar (buccal aspect).

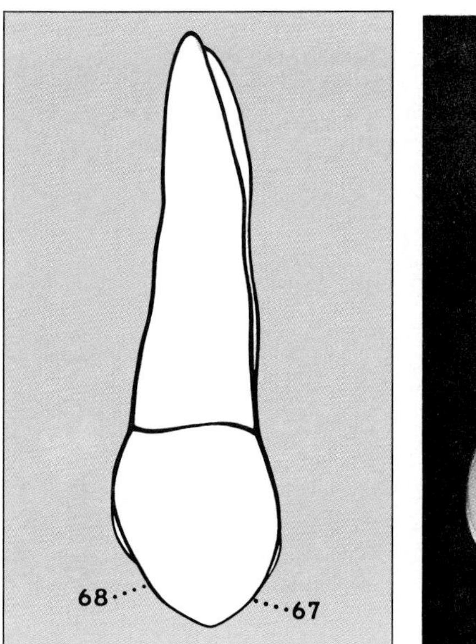

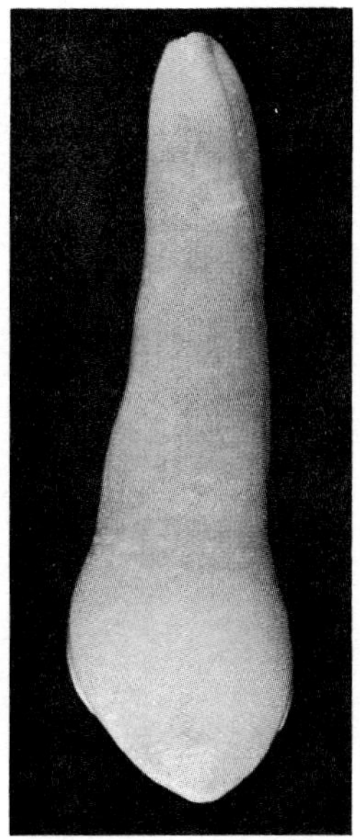

Figure 4.17
Maxillary left second premolar (lingual aspect).

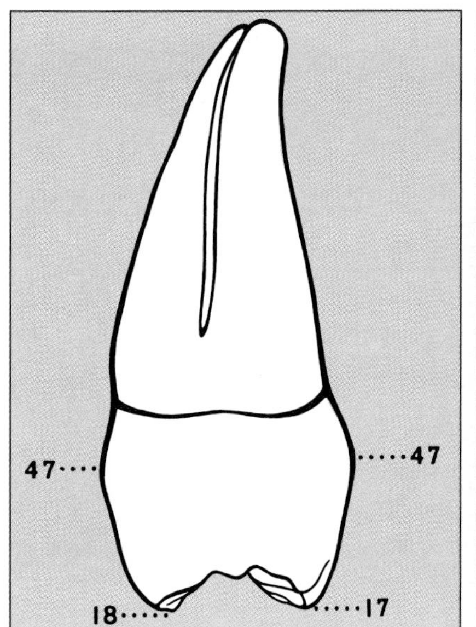

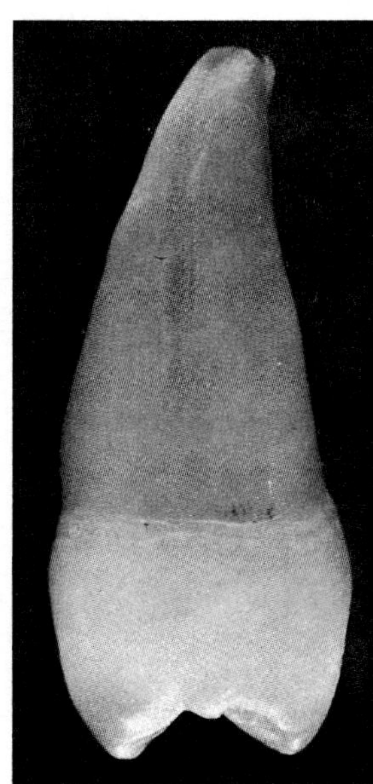

Figure 4.18
Maxillary left second premolar (mesial aspect).

because the lingual and buccal cusps are practically identical in dimensions. There is only one root, but a portion of the mesial concavity can be seen in the apical area.

Mesial Aspect (Fig. 4.18)

From the mesial aspect the type traits of the maxillary second premolar are: (1) the buccal and lingual cusps are more nearly equal in height (the buccal cusp is only slightly more prominent than the lingual cusp); (2) the mesial marginal ridge is not interrupted by a groove; (3) the mesial surface of the crown is not marked by a concavity but is evenly convex from marginal ridge to cervical line; (4) a single root is seen from the mesial aspect.

Distal Aspect (Fig. 4.19)

The distal aspect of the maxillary second premolar presents essentially the same features as that of the first premolar. However, the lingual cusp of the second premolar more nearly equals the buccal cusp in height, and only a single root is present on the second premolar.

Occlusal Aspect (Fig. 4.20)

The occlusal aspect of the maxillary second premolar differs in many ways from the first. In profile it is *ovoid* rather than hexagonal (type trait). The mesio- and distobuccal corners are more rounded (type trait) and the mesial and distal borders show little if any lingual convergence (type trait).

The buccal surface is evenly convex from mesial to distal (type trait). The buccal ridge and lobes are barely discernible (type trait). The occlusal table outline is rectangular rather than trapezoidal in form (type trait). The lingual cusp very nearly equals the buccal cusp in width (mesiodistally). The marginal ridges of the second premolar extend buccolingually with little if any convergence (type trait). This trait,

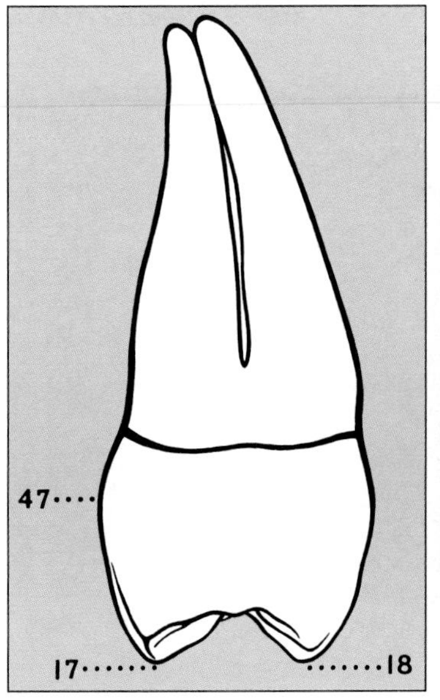

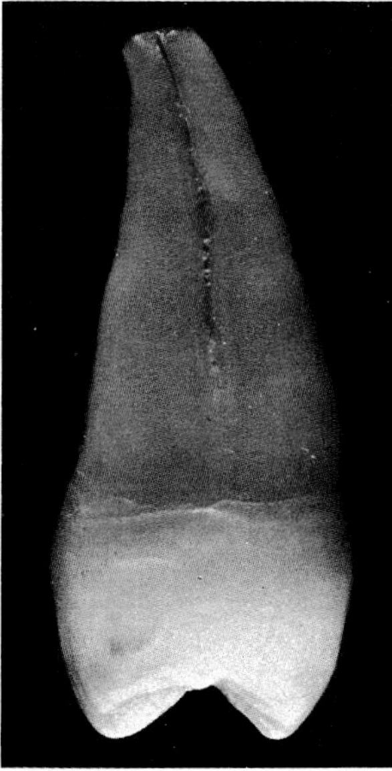

Figure 4.19
Maxillary left second premolar (distal aspect).

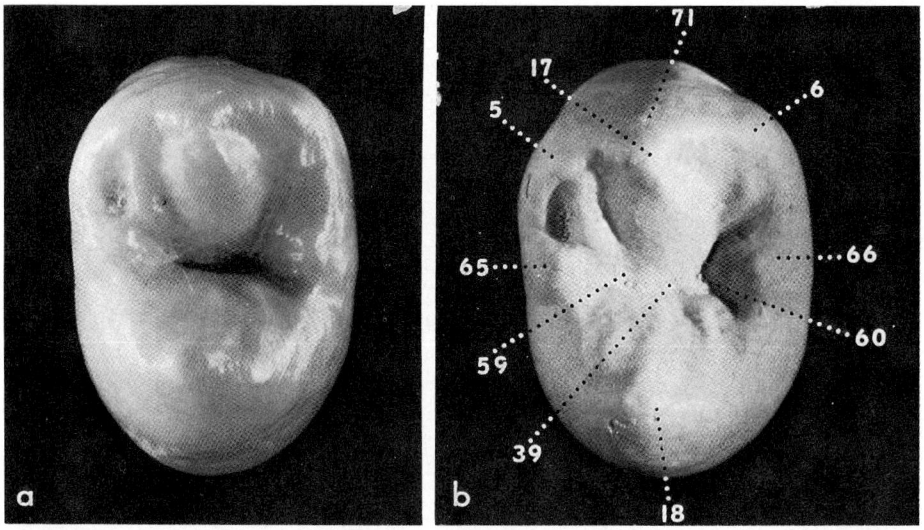

Figure 4.20
Maxillary second premolar (occlusal aspect): *a*, actual crown; *b*, cast.

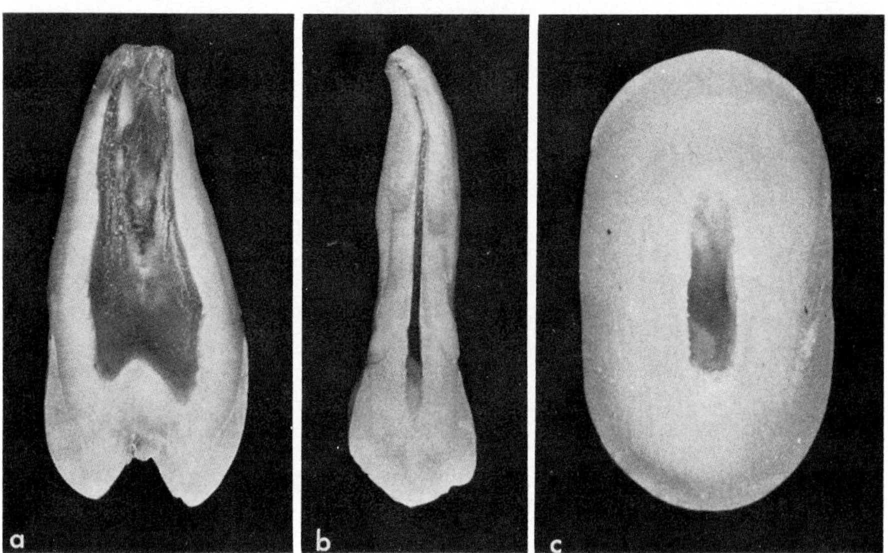

Figure 4.21
Pulp cavity of the maxillary second premolar: *a*, buccolingual section; *b*, mesiodistal section; *c*, transverse section at the cervix.

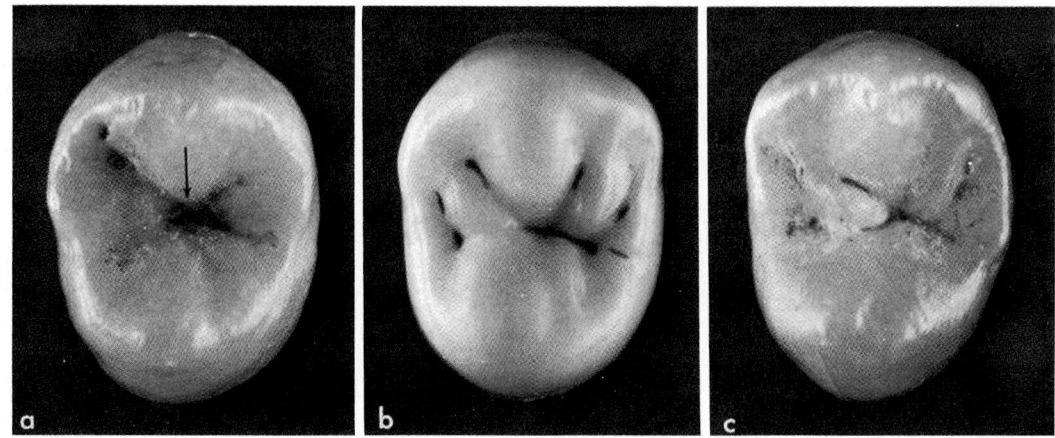

Figure 4.22
Variations in the pit-groove pattern, maxillary second premolars (occlusal aspect): *a*, absence of central groove and mesial and distal pits, with deep pit (*arrow*) in middle of occlusal surface; *b* and *c*, irregular patterns of supplemental grooves.

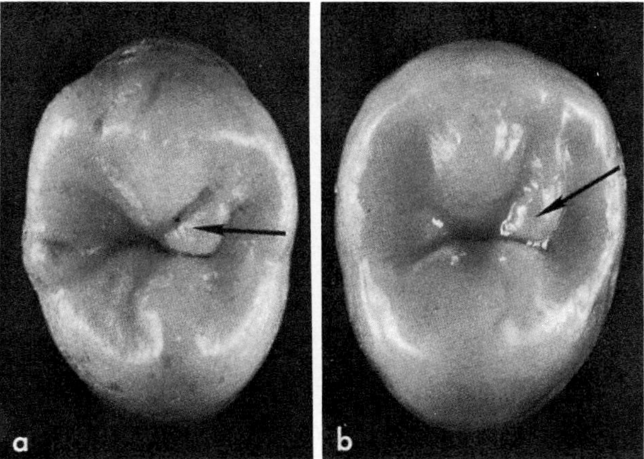

Figure 4.23
a and *b*, examples of the distal and transverse ridge (*arrows*), maxillary second premolars (occlusal aspect).

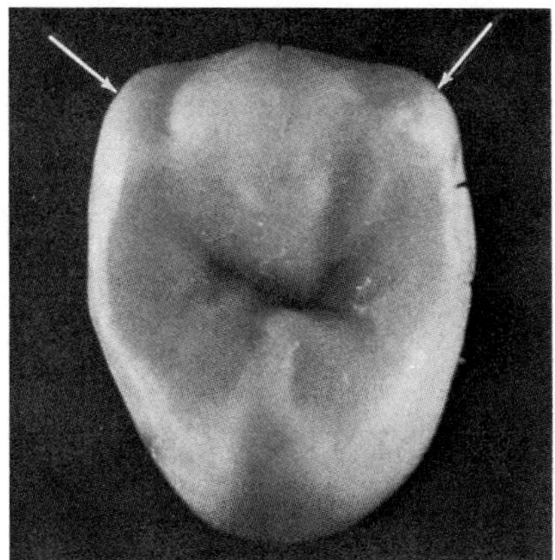

Figure 4.24
Strongly developed styles (*arrows*), maxillary second premolar (occlusal aspect).

along with the similarity in width of the two cusps, results in the rectangularly shaped occlusal table outline.

The occlusal surface pit-groove pattern differs from that of the first premolar in the following ways: (1) the central groove is shorter in length, so that the mesial and distal pits are closer to the middle of the occlusal surface (type trait); (2) there is no mesial marginal groove (type trait); (3) supplemental grooves, which radiates in a buccal and lingual direction from the central groove, are more numerous (type trait); (4) either one or both lingual grooves may be more deeply etched into the surface, so that a variety of groove patterns are produced.

Pulp

In the maxillary second premolar a transverse section shows the pulp cavity to be cigar shaped at the cervix. In buccolingual section there are two pulp horns of almost equal height with a relatively greater width at the cervix than is the case with the first premolar. There is usually a single pulp canal. The two premolars in mesiodistal section show no significant difference in structure of the pulp cavity (Fig. 4.21).

Variations

The central groove of the maxillary second premolar may vary in form from a deep fissure to a shallow depression in the occlusal surface. Occasionally the central groove and mesial and distal pits are absent and a single deep pit marks the middle of the occlusal surface (Fig. 4.22*a*). Commonly, in this type of variation, supplemental grooves may be seen radiating from the central pit in the form of an X. Other supplemental grooves, irregular in their distribution and course, frequently complicate the pit-groove pattern of the occlusal surface (Fig. 4.22*b* and *c*).

Occasionally an additional ridge is found lying between the buccal triangular ridge and the distal marginal ridge. It is bounded by a mesial and distal groove (Fig. 4.23). This might be termed the *distal transverse ridge*.

The buccal cusp shows a considerable range of variations with regard to the mesial and distal styles. As indicated above, the styles may be imperceptible or one or both may be strongly developed (Fig. 4.24).

The buccal cusp is generally rounded (Fig. 4.25*a*). Occasionally, however, the mesial and distal cusp ridges may incline steeply from the apex, resulting in a sharply conical cusp tip (Fig. 4.25*b*). The mesial

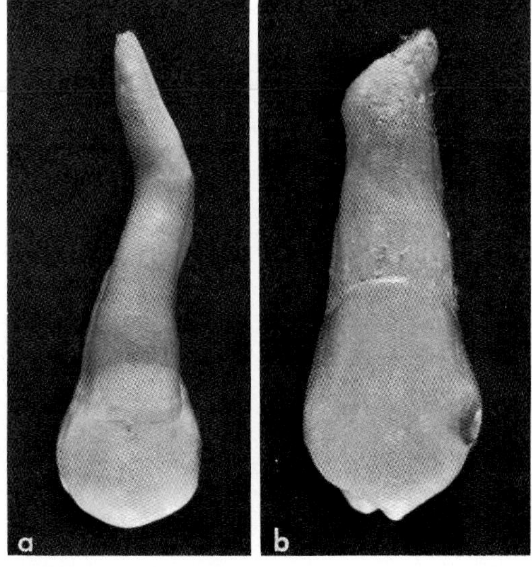

Figure 4.25
Variations in form of buccal cusps, maxillary second premolars (buccal aspect): *a*, rounded buccal cusp; *b*, sharply conical buccal cusp.

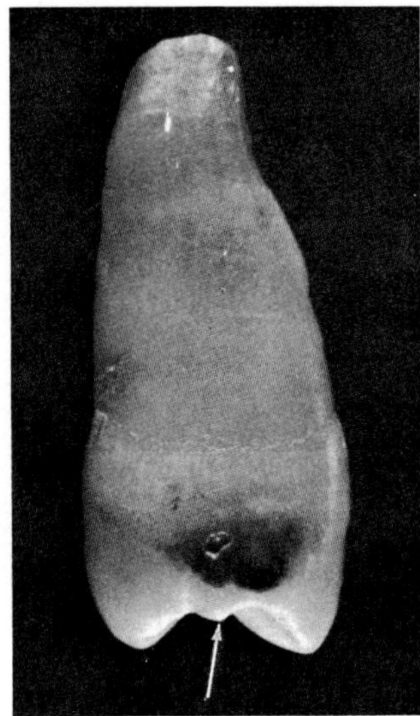

Figure 4.26
Presence of a cusplet (*arrow*) on the mesial marginal ridge, maxillary left second premolar (mesial aspect).

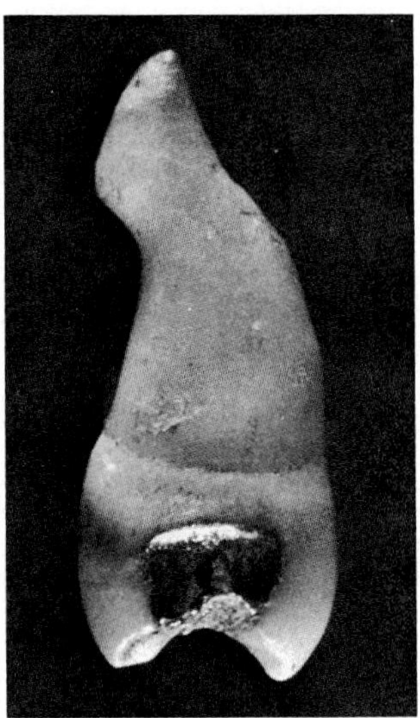

Figure 4.27
Irregular curvature of the root, maxillary right second premolar (mesial aspect).

marginal ridge of the maxillary second premolar is usually a prominent uninterrupted crest connecting the mesial ridges of the buccal and lingual cusps. Occasionally a small but distinct cusplet occupies the approximate midpoint of the mesial marginal ridge (Fig. 4.26).

Like all the other dental units, this tooth has a wide range of variability with respect to root size, curvature, and form. The root may be unusually short (Fig. 4.25*b*) or abnormally long (Fig. 4.25*a*). In addition, it may be curved in a variety of ways (Figs. 4.25*a* and 4.27).

Summary

Maxillary Premolars—Arch Traits

1. There are two major cusps, buccal and lingual, which are approximately equal in size and prominence.

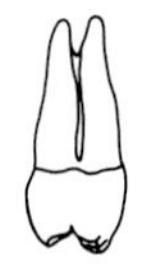

2. The crowns, from the occlusal aspect, are wider buccolingually than mesiodistally.

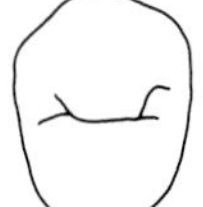

3. Buccal profiles, viewed from the proximal aspect, are only slightly inclined lingually from height of contour to cusp apex.

4. The lingual height of contour is situated approximately midway between cervix and apex.

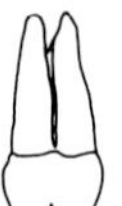

5. There is, overall, a much greater morphological similarity between the two maxillary than between the two mandibular premolars.

Maxillary Premolars—Type Traits

	First Premolar	Second Premolar
Buccal aspect	Prominent bulging shoulders	Narrow shoulders
Lingual aspect	Entire buccal profile of crown visible	None of buccal profile visible

	First Premolar	Second Premolar
Mesial aspect	Mesial marginal groove interrupts mesial marginal ridge Generally two roots, buccal and lingual	No mesial marginal groove Single root
Occlusal aspect	Crown profile hexagonal Mesiobuccal and distobuccal corners sharp Mesial and distal profiles converge lingually Occlusal table outline trapezoidal Buccal cusp ridge oriented mesiolingually, giving crown a twisted appearance Buccal cusp wider than lingual cusp Central groove long Supplemental grooves rare Buccal, central, and mesial marginal grooves form characteristic pattern Buccal ridge and lobes visible	Crown profile ovoid Mesiobuccal and distobuccal corners more rounded No lingual convergence; mesial and distal profiles are parallel Occlusal table outline rectangular Crown not twisted in appearance Buccal and lingual cusps similar in width Central groove short Frequent and numerous supplemental grooves Accentuation of one or both lingual grooves provides different patterns Buccal ridge and lobes not present

Mandibular Premolars

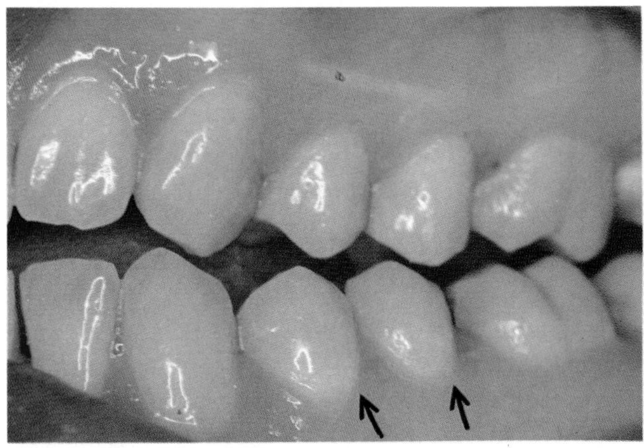
a

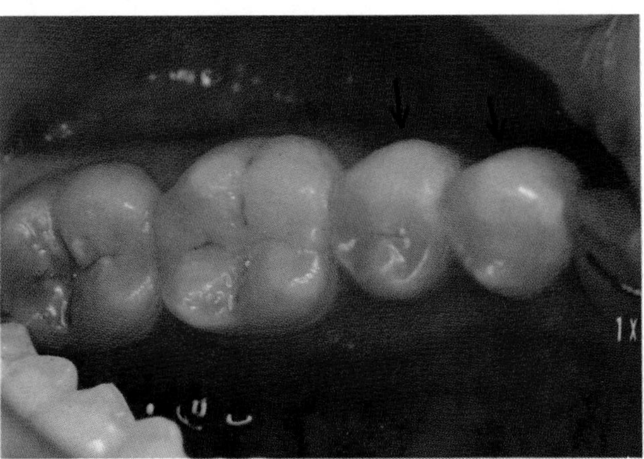
b

Figure 4.28
a, Lateral view of mandibular left premolars; *b*, occlusal view of mandibular left premolars.

Size and Eruption

Mandibular Premolars (mm)	Crown Height (mm)	Mesiodistal Crown Diameter (mm)	Bucco-lingual Crown Diameter (mm)	Tooth Length (mm)	Age at Eruption (yr)
First	8.5	7.0	7.5	22.5	9
Second	8.0	7.0	8.0	22.5	10

The mandibular first premolar, from a purely functional standpoint, may be regarded as a canine. The second premolar, on the other hand, resembles in some respects a small molar. Accordingly the two do not resemble each other nearly as much as do the maxillary premolars (arch trait).

First Premolar

Buccal Aspect (Fig. 4.29)

A long, pointed buccal cusp constitutes the occlusal profile of the mandibular first premolar. The mesial cusp ridge is shorter in length than the distal. Both cusp ridges incline cervically from the cusp apex with a slope of approximately 30 degrees to the horizontal and meet the respective proximal crown profiles to form angulated margins.

The crown is not bilaterally symmetrical since the mesial and distal profiles present differing degrees of curvature (type trait). Both converge cervically from their heights of contour to meet their respective root profiles. The cervical line is relatively flat mesiodistally in comparison to that of the canine.

The buccal aspect of the root is conical in outline and its proximal borders converge to form a relatively sharp apex.

Lingual Aspect (Fig. 4.30)

The entire extent of the buccal profile of the mandibular first premolar is visible from the lingual aspect (type trait). From this view the greatest mesiodistal diameter lies across the buccal moiety of the crown near the buccal surface. What is more, the mandibular first premolar is the only member of its class in which almost the entire occlusal surface can be seen from the lingual aspect (type trait). The occlusal plane in all other premolars (and molars) lies perpendicular to the longitudinal axis of the tooth. In the mandibular first premolar, on the other hand, it tilts lingually in relationship to the long axis.

A prominent ridge (i.e., the *buccal triangular ridge*) inclines lingually and cervically from the apex of the buccal cusp on its occlusal surface with a slope of roughly 45 degrees and crosses the midportion of the occlusal surface to the apex of the lingual cusp. In addition, the mesial and distal marginal ridges (which are visible throughout their entire extent from the lingual aspect) incline lingually and cervically at a slope of 45 degrees to join the corresponding ridges of the lingual cusp.

The lingual cusp is a minor elevation in terms of height (type trait) and presents a highly conical, sharply pointed apex. The apex of the lingual cusp may lie directly in line with the apex and triangular

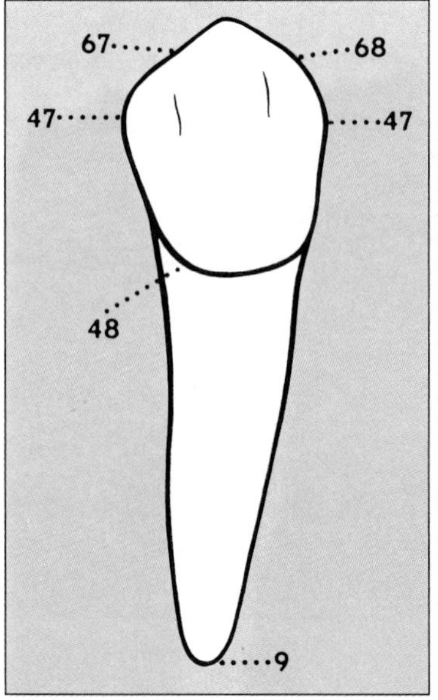

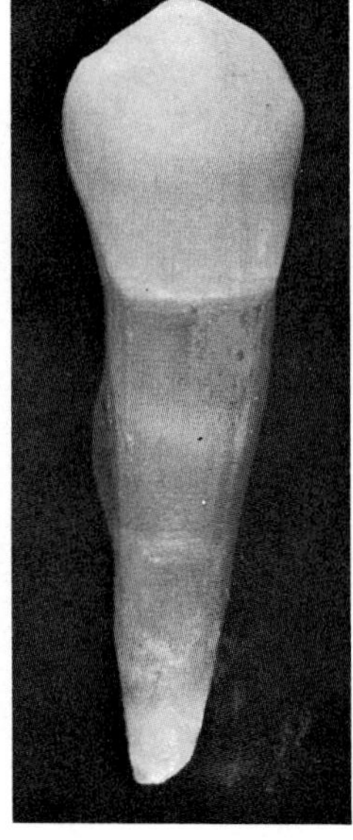

Figure 4.29
Mandibular left first premolar (buccal aspect).

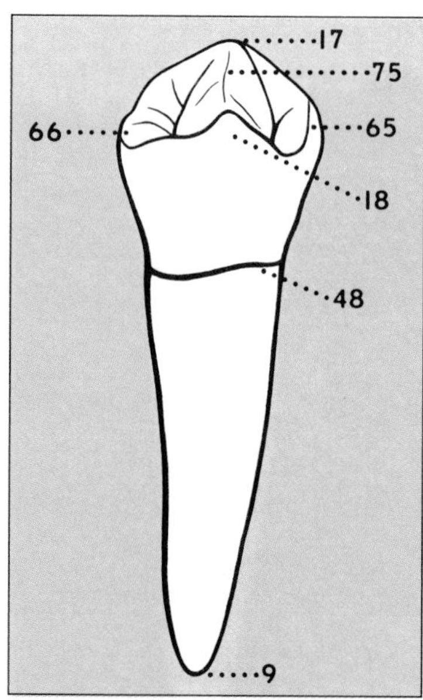

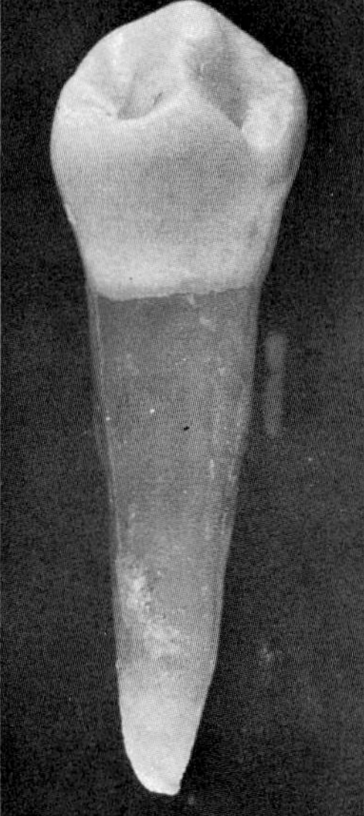

Figure 4.30
Mandibular left first premolar (lingual aspect).

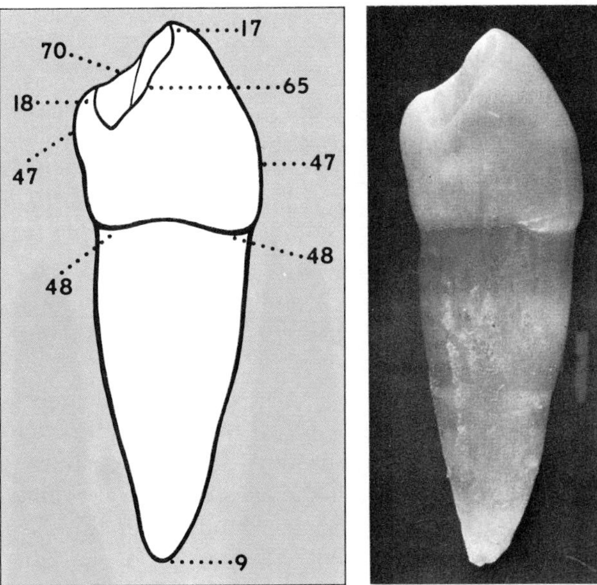

Figure 4.31
Mandibular left first premolar (mesial aspect).

ridge of the buccal cusp, or may be situated either mesial or distal to the midline of the crown.

The lingual surface, which is distinctly narrower mesiodistally than the buccal surface (type trait), is uniformly convex and unmarked by lobes or ridges. The cervical line presents only a slight degree of curvature.

The lingual aspect of the root is narrower than its buccal aspect and tapers to a relatively blunt apex.

Mesial Aspect (Fig. 4.31)

The mandibular first premolar is the only posterior tooth in which the occlusal plane is tilted lingually in relation to the horizontal plane (type trait). This unique feature is more clearly seen from the mesial aspect.

The occlusal profile is made up, for the most part, of the *transverse ridge*, a pronounced elevation that extends buccolingually across the occlusal surface to link the apices of the buccal and lingual cusps (type trait). The transverse ridge is made up of two moieties, the triangular ridge of the buccal and that of the lingual cusp. The two components may be separated by a *central groove* that extends mesiodistally across the center of the occlusal surface. On the other hand, the groove may be ill defined or entirely absent, and the transverse ridge, accordingly, is seen as a continuous uninterrupted crest.

The mesial marginal ridge inclines in a cervical direction (from buccal to lingual) at about 45 degrees (type trait). The point of junction between the mesial marginal ridge and the mesiolingual cusp ridge is marked by a deep V-shaped cleft, the *mesiolingual groove* (type trait).

The buccal profile, which is prominent and highly convex in its cervical third, shows a pronounced lingual inclination from the height of contour to the apex of the buccal cusp.

The lingual profile is relatively straight from the cervical line to the junction of the middle and occlusal thirds. It then shows a distinct convexity up to the lingual cusp apex. The latter is almost in line with the lingual profile of the root. This feature is generally true of all mandibular posterior teeth and serves to distinguish them from their maxillary counterparts. Apices of the lingual cusps in all maxillary posterior teeth are located well *within* the root profiles. The lingual height of contour is located well within the occlusal third of the crown.

The mesial contact area, which is directly in line with the apex of the buccal cusp, forms a highly prominent convexity of the mesial surface of the crown. Below (i.e., cervical to) the contact area the crown surface is relatively flat or concave, and immediately lingual to the contact area the mesial surface is marked by the mesiolingual groove (type trait).

The root is very broad buccolingually at the cervix and tapers sharply to the apex. Its surface may be marked by deep longitudinal depressions.

Distal Aspect (Fig. 4.32)

In the mandibular first premolar the distal crown profile corresponds almost exactly to that of the mesial aspect. However, certain surface features of the crown differ. For instance, the distal marginal ridge is more prominent than the mesial marginal ridge and does not show as marked an inclination relative

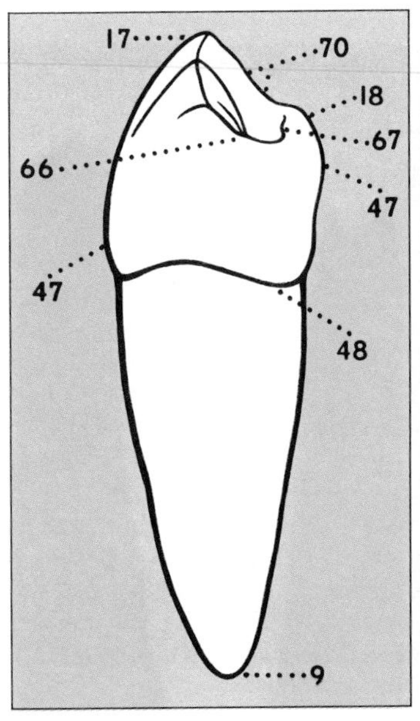

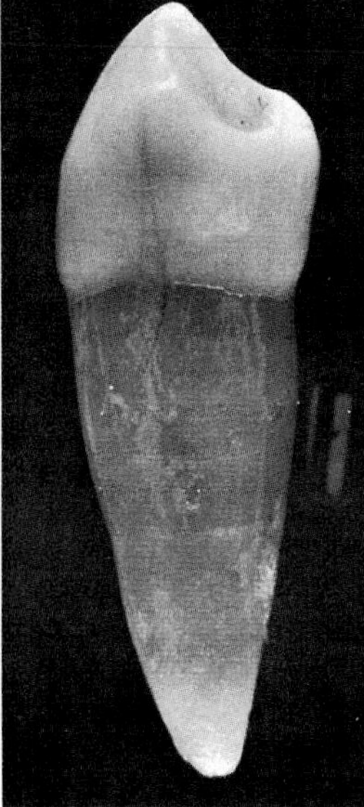

Figure 4.32
Mandibular left first premolar (distal aspect).

to the longitudinal root axis. The distal marginal ridge meets the lingual cusp ridge in an unbroken line and the distal surface is unmarked by the presence of a developmental groove. The distal surface, in general, is broader buccolingually than the mesial surface and its contact area is more extensive.

Occlusal Aspect (Fig. 4.33)

The occlusal outline of the mandibular first premolar is diamond shaped (type trait). The buccal profile takes the form of an inverted V. A central prominence (corresponding to the apex of the V) is directly in line with the tip of the buccal cusp. On either side of the central prominence the buccal profile inclines more or less abruptly toward the lingual to join the mesial and distal profiles to form the mesiobuccal and distobuccal angles respectively. The mesio- and distobuccal angles mark the widest mesiodistal diameter of the crown. The mesial and distal profiles converge lingually (type trait); the mesial profile is in the form of a slightly curved margin interrupted by the mesiolingual groove (type trait); the distal profile is considerably more convex. The lingual profile forms a narrow, irregularly convex arc measuring roughly one-half of the width of the buccal profile (type trait).

More than two-thirds of the buccal surface is visible from the occlusal aspect. A prominent elevation, the *buccal ridge,* extends cervically from the apex of the buccal cusp for more than half the length of the buccal surface of the crown. Shallow depressions on either side of the buccal ridge divide the buccal surface into three more or less distinct lobes.

Only a small portion of the lingual surface (i.e., the occlusal third) is visible from the occlusal aspect. The lingual surface is convex and unmarked by lobes or depressions.

The occlusal table, as outlined by the cusp and marginal ridges, is distinctly triangular in form (type trait). The base of the triangle corresponds to the buccal cusp ridge, and the apex to the tip of the lingual cusp.

Two cusps, quite opposite in size, constitute the predominant features of the occlusal surface (type trait). The buccal cusp, a broad, sharp elevation, occupies the widest mesiodistal diameter of the crown. The apex of the buccal cusp is generally near the midline of the crown.

The lingual cusp, a small elevation, is merely a fraction of the size of the buccal cusp (type trait). The mesiolingual cusp ridge extends from the cusp apex in a straight line to join the mesial marginal ridge. The distolingual cusp ridge extends from the cusp apex to become confluent with the distal marginal ridge, forming a highly convex crest.

The triangular ridges of the buccal and lingual cusps often form a continuous crest, the *transverse ridge,* which extends buccolingually across the center of the occlusal surface to link the apices of the two cusps (type trait). The transverse ridge appears to divide the occlusal surface into two moieties, mesial and distal.

The mesial marginal ridge is distinctly shorter in length and less prominent in height than the distal marginal ridge (type trait). It is clearly demarcated from the mesiolingual cusp ridge by a deep V-shaped depression, the mesiolingual groove (type trait).

The distal marginal ridge forms a prominent elevation on the distal portion of the crown and measures nearly twice the length of the mesial marginal ridge.

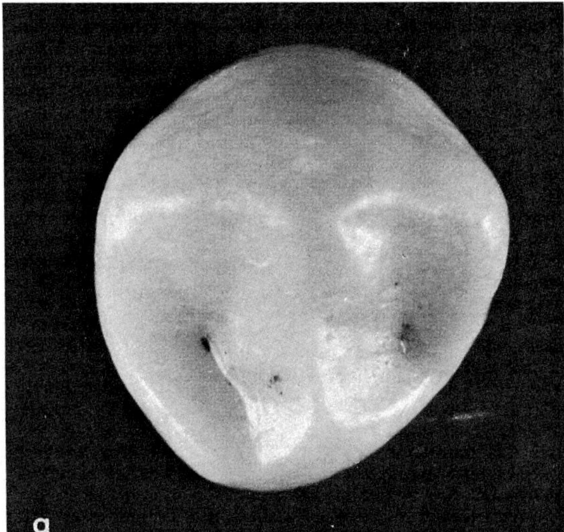

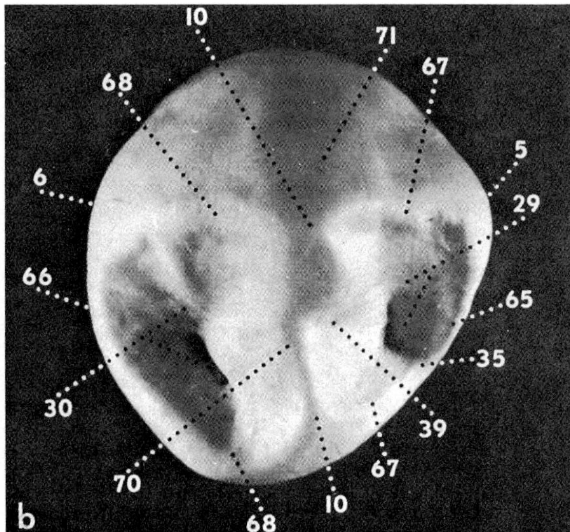

Figure 4.33
Mandibular left first premolar (occlusal aspect): *a,* actual crown; *b,* cast.

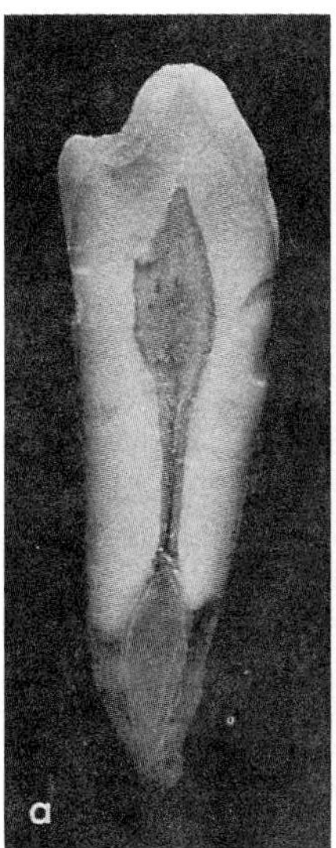
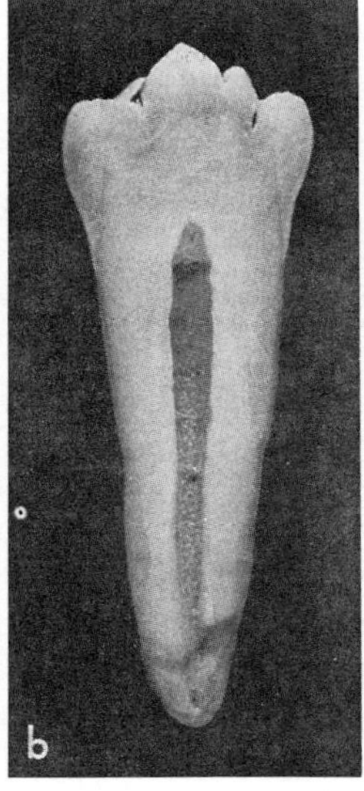
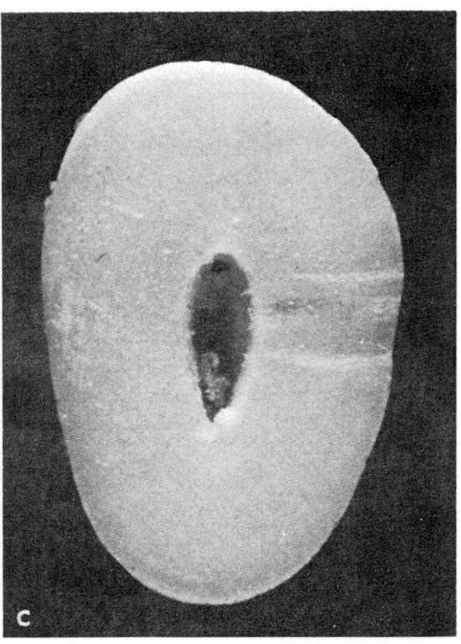

Figure 4.34

Pulp cavity of the mandibular first premolar: *a*, buccolingual section; *b*, mesiodistal section; *c*, transverse section at the cervix.

Two relatively deep valleys cross the occlusal surface. They are on either side of the transverse ridge just within the confines of the marginal ridges, and are called the *mesial* and *distal fossae* respectively. Each fossa contains in its depths (1) a pit, (the *mesial* or *distal*); (2) a groove, (the *mesial* or *distal*), extending buccolingually and roughly paralleling the marginal ridges; (3) a supplemental depression at the buccal termination of each groove. A *mesiolingual groove* is found in the mesial fossa only. It extends in a mesiolingual direction from the mesial pit and crosses the marginal ridge onto the proximal surface. It may be highly variable in extent.

Pulp (Fig. 4.34)

A mesiodistal section of the mandibular first premolar shows the pulp cavity to be very similar to that of the canine. It is rounded at the occlusal end and is quite narrow. In buccolingual section two pulpal horns are seen—a large buccal horn, corresponding to the buccal cusp, and a much smaller lingual horn. The pulp chamber is bulbous and tapers to a narrow canal, which may be bifurcated in the apical third. In transverse section the canal outline is ovoid, being compressed mesiodistally.

Variations

The mandibular first premolar is one of the most variable in the entire dentition. In practically every trait of the crown and root it shows a wide range of variation.

1. The transverse ridge may extend uninterrupted from buccal to lingual cusp apices (Fig. 4.35*a*). On the other hand, it may be divided into a buccal and

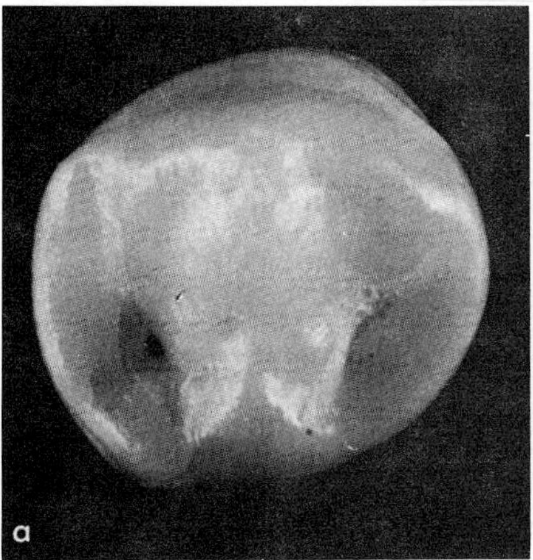
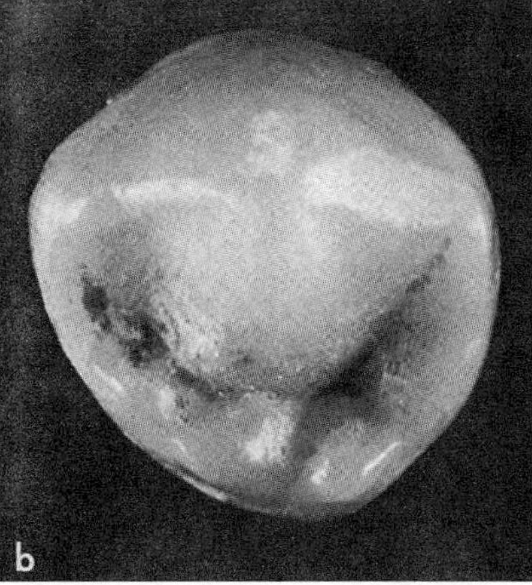
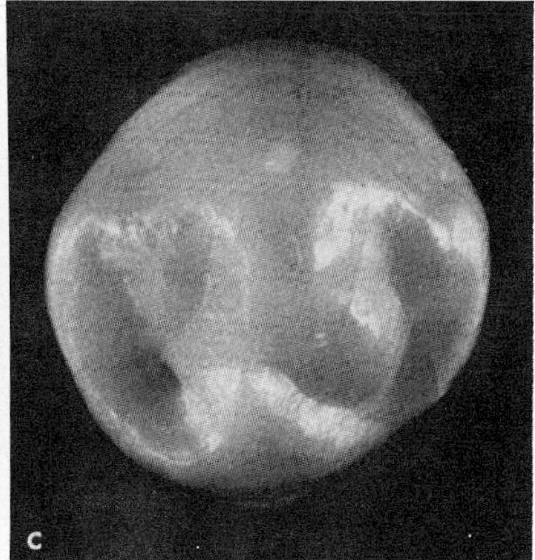

Figure 4.35

Variations in the transverse ridge, mandibular first premolars (occlusal aspect): *a*, uninterrupted ridge; *b*, division into two moieties by a central groove; *c*, shallow central groove crossing the transverse ridge.

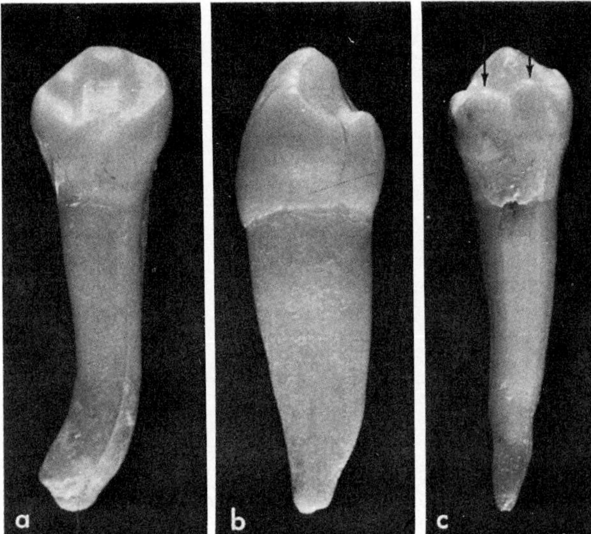

Figure 4.36

Variations in number of lingual cusps, mandibular first premolar (lingual aspect): *a*, absence of lingual cusps; *b*, a single lingual cusp; *c*, two lingual cusps (*arrows*).

lingual moiety by a deep central groove extending from the deepest portions of the mesial and distal fossae (Fig. 4.35*b*). A third variation consists of a shallow groove that runs across the transverse ridge and splits it into a large buccal portion and a relatively slight lingual tubercle (Fig. 4.35*c*). In the latter instance the lingual cusp cannot be distinguished as such but appears very much like a Carabelli tubercle.

2. Although most frequently there is but a single lingual cusp or tubercle there may be as many as four and rarely there may be a complete absence of a lingual cusp (Fig. 4.36).

3. The position of the lingual cusp relative to the midline of the crown, as determined by the position of the buccal cusp apex, may be mesial, distal, or exactly in the midline.

4. Although it is more common to find a single mesiolingual groove it is not unusual for two grooves, one mesial and one distal, to extend down the lingual surface of the crown (Fig. 4.37). They may be shallow and short, or fairly deep and of moderate length. Frequently the lingual margin appears to be devoid of any groove, but close inspection will reveal the presence of a notch at the site.

5. There may be one or more accessory transverse ridges located on the occlusal aspect of the buccal cusp. As many as five, including the main ridge, have been observed. In addition, there may be a bifurcating ridge running obliquely from the center of the transverse ridge to the central groove.

6. The size and prominence of the transverse ridge varies greatly, from low and narrow to high and broad.

7. The mesial and distal marginal ridges may be strongly accentuated along their entire lengths and even up to the apex of the buccal cusp. On the other hand, they may be so attenuated as to be difficult to see.

8. A distal lobe or style is occasionally seen on the buccal cusp margin. It may be very slight or so marked as to resemble a cusplet (Fig. 4.38).

9. Occasionally there may be two roots, a buccal and a lingual. There may also be unusually deep longitudinal grooves on the proximal root surfaces (Fig. 4.39).

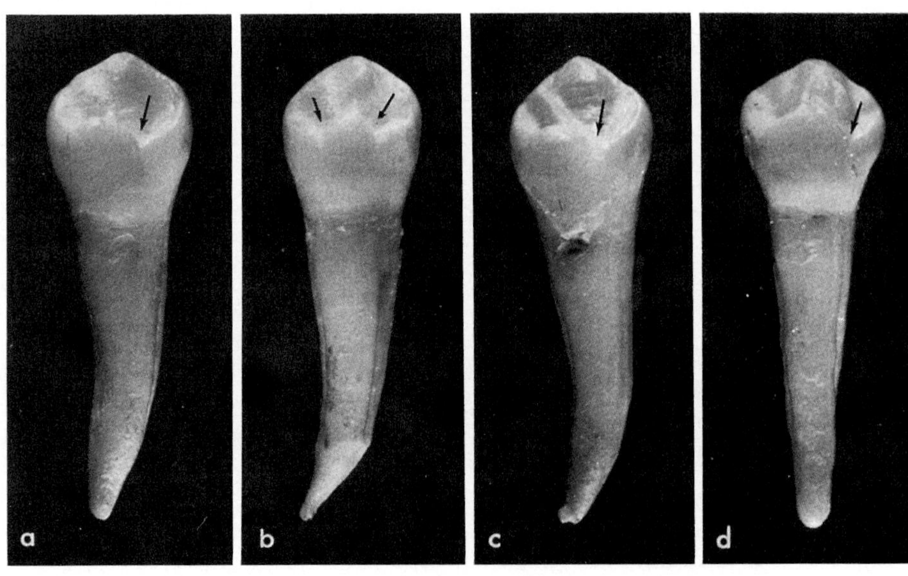

Figure 4.37

Variations in the mesiolingual groove (*arrows*), mandibular first premolars (lingual aspect): *a*, a single mesiolingual groove; *b*, two lingual grooves; *c*, cleft-like mesiolingual groove; *d*, slight notch at the site of the mesiolingual groove.

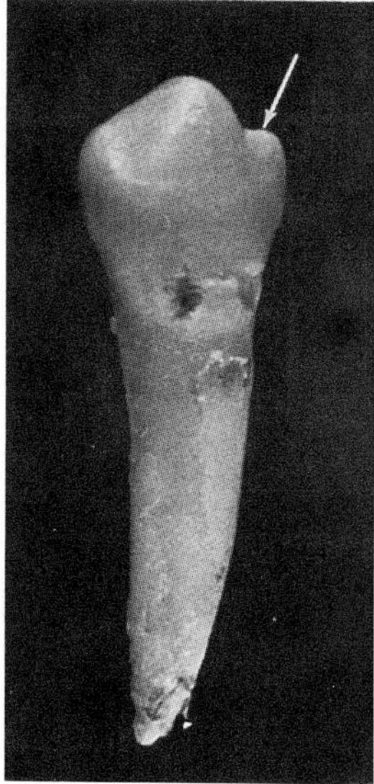

Figure 4.38
Distal style on buccal cusp margin (*arrow*), mandibular left first premolar (buccal aspect).

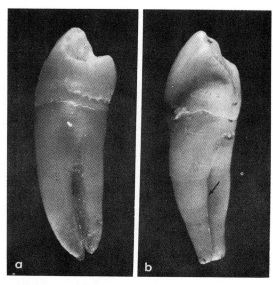

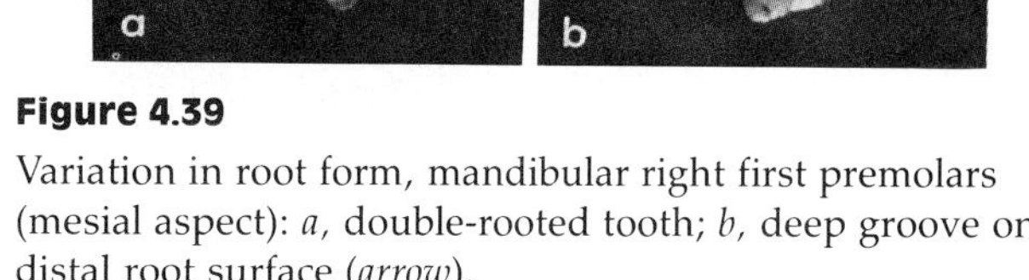

Figure 4.39
Variation in root form, mandibular right first premolars (mesial aspect): *a*, double-rooted tooth; *b*, deep groove on distal root surface (*arrow*).

Second Premolar

Buccal Aspect (Fig. 4.40)

From the buccal aspect the mandibular premolars are difficult to tell apart. The features already described for the buccal aspect of the first premolar closely resemble those of the second premolar.

Lingual Aspect (Fig. 4.41)

The mesiodistal diameter of the lingual aspect of the second mandibular premolar is at least as wide as that of its buccal aspect (type trait). Accordingly, the only portion of the buccal profile visible is the outline of the buccal cusp, and little, if any, of the occlusal surface is visible from the lingual aspect (type trait). The

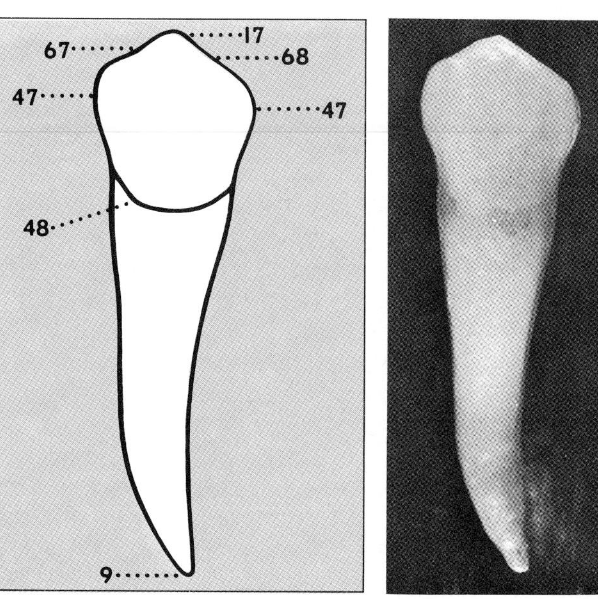

Figure 4.40
Mandibular left second premolar (buccal aspect).

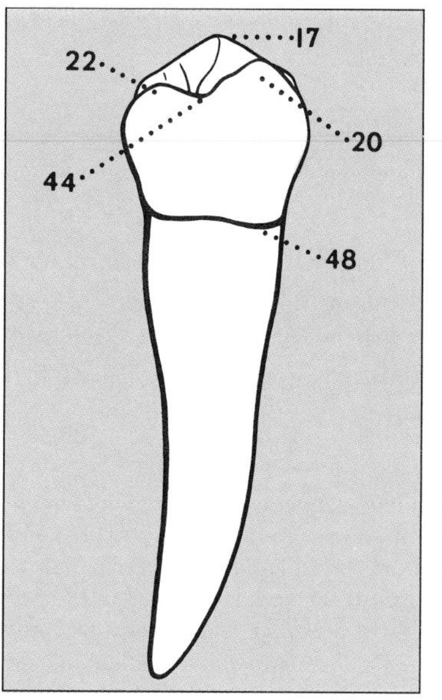

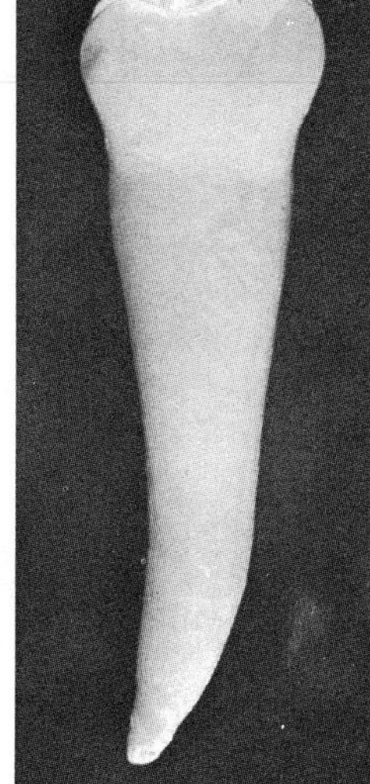

Figure 4.41
Mandibular left second premolar (lingual aspect).

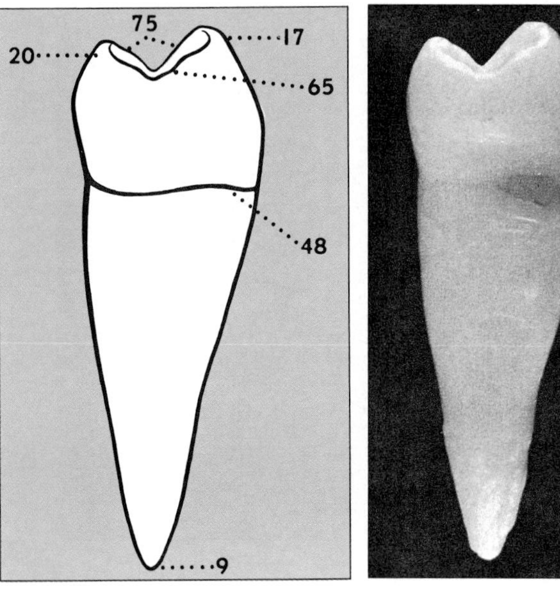

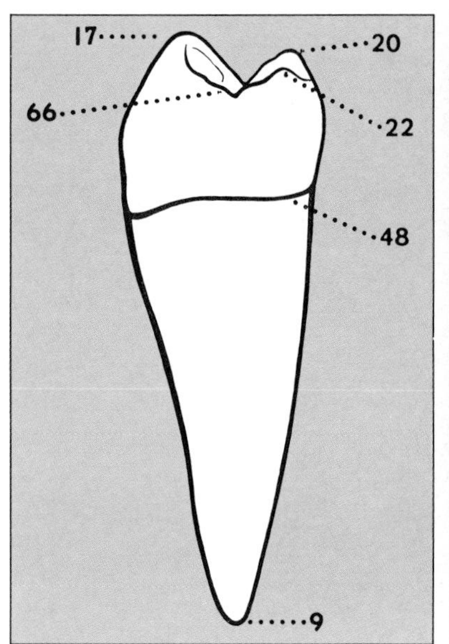

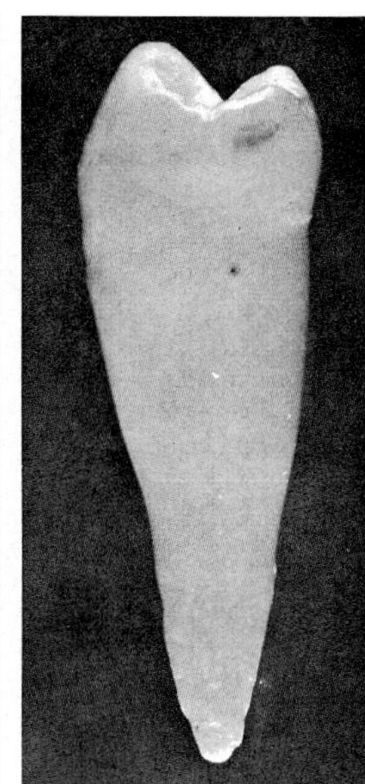

Figure 4.42
Mandibular left second premolar (mesial aspect).

Figure 4.43
Mandibular left second premolar (distal aspect).

occlusal plane of the second premolar is perpendicular to the longitudinal root axis.

There is invariably at least one major lingual cusp* present (i.e., the mesiolingual) which nearly equals the buccal cusp in terms of height (type trait) and occupies roughly two-thirds of the mesiodistal width of the lingual aspect of the crown. The distolingual cusp, a relatively minor elevation, measures less than half of the dimension of the mesiolingual cusp and is demarcated from the latter by a distinct notch (i.e., the termination of the lingual groove).

The mesial and distal crown profiles are strongly convex and converge cervically.

Mesial Aspect (Fig. 4.42)

The occlusal surface is not tilted lingually in the mandibular second premolar but is perpendicular to the longitudinal axis.

The occlusal profile consists of the triangular ridges of the buccal and mesiolingual cusps. The two ridges do not form a continuous crest, but end in a distinct groove at approximately the midpoint of the occlusal surface.

*The mandibular second premolar may exhibit either two cusps (i.e., one buccal and one lingual) nearly equal in size and prominence, or three cusps (i.e., one buccal and two lingual) of unequal size. Although the frequencies of occurrence in the human dentition of the two- and three-cusp crown patterns have not yet been determined, the three-cusp structure is apparently more common and will be considered more or less typical. The two-cusp form is described in a later section (Variations).

The mesiolingual cusp of the second premolar is a major elevation and nearly equals the buccal cusp in height (type trait).

Distal Aspect (Fig. 4.43)

The distal aspect reveals another distinguishing feature, namely, the presence of two lingual cusps. The distolingual cusp is clearly smaller in all dimensions than the mesiolingual cusp and often appears as a slight bulge on the distal corner of the crown.

Occlusal Aspect (Fig. 4.44)

In the mandibular second premolar the occlusal profile is more or less square (type trait). The mesial and distal profiles are straight and parallel to each other (type trait).

A little more than one-half of the buccal surface is visible from the occlusal aspect, and the buccal ridge is less prominent than that of the first premolar (type trait). The lingual moiety very nearly equals the buccal in width (type trait).

The occlusal table is much wider buccolingually in the second premolar (type trait) and is square or circular in form (type trait).

Generally three cusps occupy the occlusal surface. The buccal, the largest of the three, is followed in order of decreasing width and height by the mesiolingual and distolingual cusps. The mesial and distal marginal ridges are approximately equal in width (type trait).

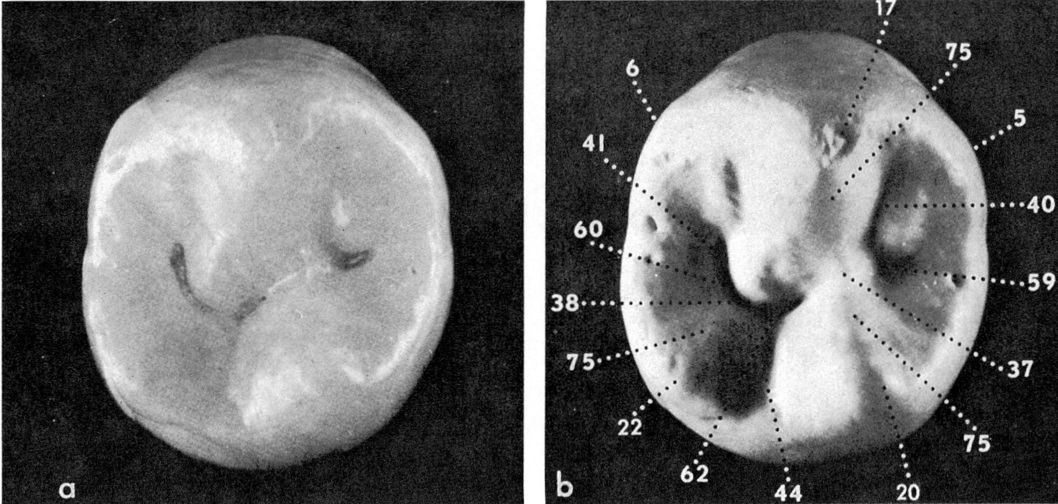

Figure 4.44

Mandibular left second premolar (occlusal aspect): *a,* actual crown; *b,* cast.

The three triangular ridges are demarcated by a distinctive pit-groove pattern. The mesial groove extends obliquely across the occlusal surface and separates the triangular ridges of the buccal and the mesiolingual cusps. The lingual groove separates the triangular ridges of the lingual cusps, and the distal groove (a relatively short depression) marks the boundary between the triangular ridges of the buccal and distolingual cusps. The mesial, distal, and lingual grooves intersect in the form of a Y at a point just distal to the midportion of the occlusal surface (type trait). The point of intersection is marked by the central pit (type trait).

Two shallow valleys (the *mesial* and *distal triangular fossae*) are located just within the confines of the respective marginal ridges. In each fossa there is (1) a pit (the *mesial* or *distal pit*), which marks the proximal termination of the mesial or distal groove; (2) a groove (the *mesiobuccal* or *distobuccal groove*), which extends from the pit toward the nearest corner of the crown; (3) one or more supplemental grooves that radiate from each pit toward the cusp apex.

Pulp (Fig. 4.45)

The pulp cavity of the mandibular second premolar is similar to that of the first premolar with minor exceptions. In buccolingual section the pulp chamber is wider and the two pulpal horns are more nearly equal in size. In transverse section, the canal is narrow me-

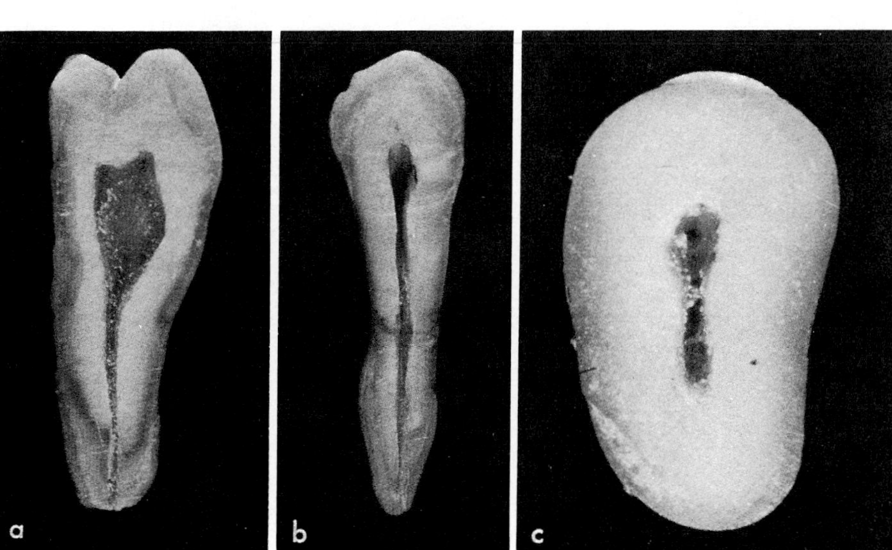

Figure 4.45

Pulp cavity of the mandibular second premolar: *a,* buccolingual section; *b,* mesiodistal section; *c,* transverse section at the cervix.

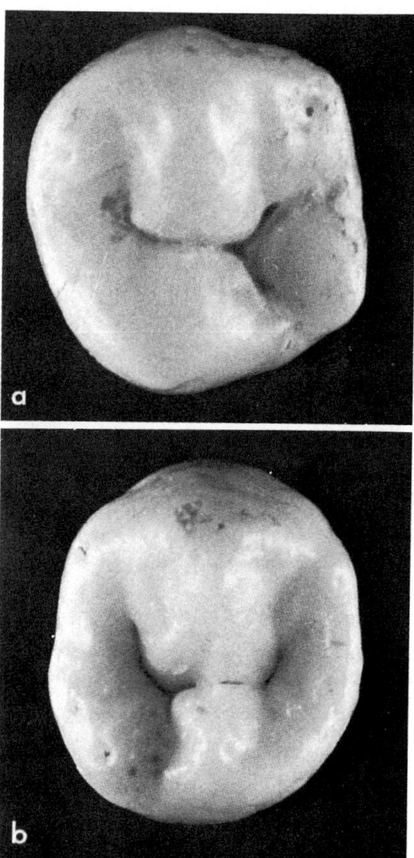

Figure 4.47
Types of pit-groove pattern, mandibular left second premolars (occlusal aspect): *a,* Y pattern; *b,* H pattern.

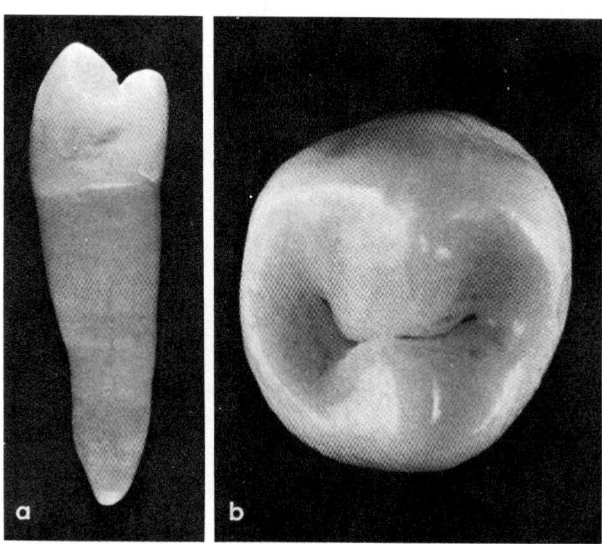

Figure 4.46
Two-cusped mandibular left second premolar: *a,* distal aspect; *b,* occlusal aspect.

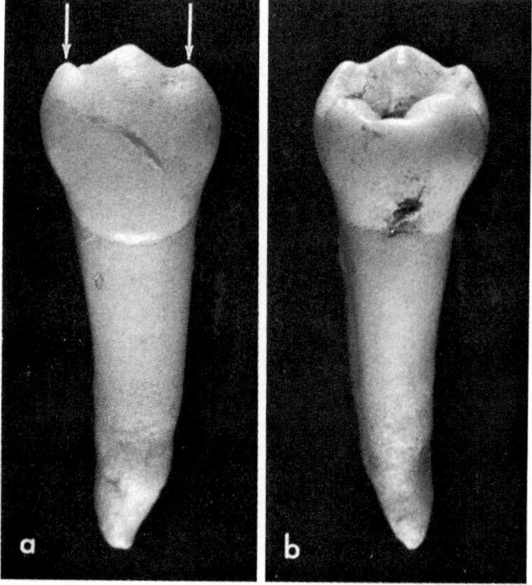

Figure 4.48
Mesial and distal styles (*arrows*) of the buccal cusp, mandibular left second premolar: *a,* buccal aspect; *b,* lingual aspect.

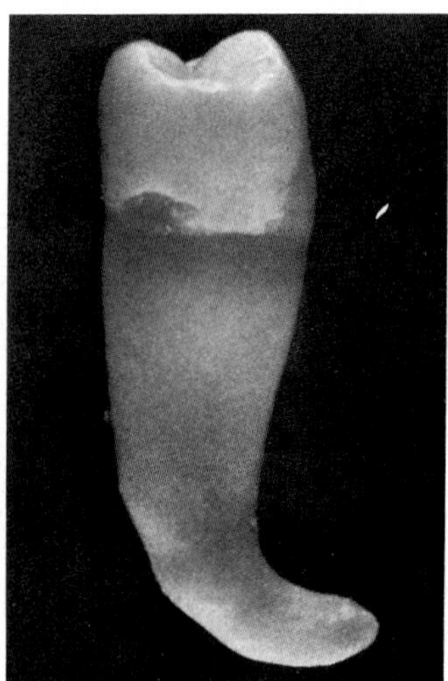

Figure 4.49
Marked root curvature, mandibular left second premolar (mesial aspect).

siodistally but is shaped somewhat like an hourglass, with a constricted area near the center.

Variations

The most common variation of the crown is the occurrence of two rather than three cusps (Fig. 4.46*a*). The single lingual cusp occupies the center of the lingual moiety of the tooth, and the distal marginal ridge, instead of supporting a distal lingual cusplet, is flat and smooth (Fig. 4.46*b*). The lingual groove and central pit are absent in this form; only a central groove occurs, extending mesiodistally across the occlusal surface between the triangular ridges of the two cusps.

The pit-groove pattern of the second premolar may take any one of three different forms, Y, H, or U. The Y pattern is found in the three-cusped premolar and is the result of the intersection of the mesial, distal, and lingual grooves in the middle of the occlusal surface (Fig. 4.47*a*). In the two-cusped premolar the central groove intersects the supplemental grooves in the mesial and distal fossae to form an H pattern (Fig. 4.47*b*). Occasionally the buccal triangular ridge projects sharply onto the lingual moiety of the occlusal surface so that the central groove takes a U-shaped course, with the base of the U on the lingual and the arms extending buccally. The H pattern is found on two-cusped premolars.

As in all other teeth thus far described the buccal cusp may have more or less prominent styles on either slope. In Figure 4.48*a* and *b* lingual and buccal views of a premolar with cusp-like styles on the distal and mesial slopes are presented.

Root variation consists mainly of differences in size and curvature (Fig. 4.49), with rare occurrences of double roots.

Summary

Mandibular Premolars—Arch Traits

1. The buccal cusp in each premolar is much larger than the lingual.
2. The mesiodistal and buccolingual dimensions of the crown are more nearly equal in the mandibular premolars.

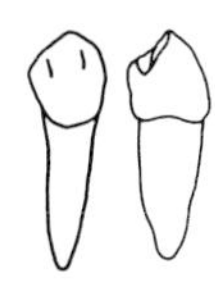

3. The buccal profiles of the mandibular premolars are strongly inclined lingually.

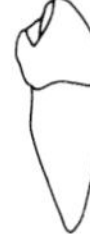

4. The lingual height of contour occurs in the occlusal third of the crown.

Mandibular Premolars—Type Traits

	First Premolar	Second Premolar
Buccal aspect	Crown bilaterally asymmetrical	Crown bilaterally symmetrical
Lingual aspect	Entire buccal profile visible	None of buccal profile visible
	Almost entire occlusal surface visible	Little if any of occlusal surface visible
	Lingual cusp much lower than buccal	Buccal and lingual cusps almost equal in height

continued

	First Premolar	Second Premolar
Mesial aspect	Occlusal plane tilted lingually	Occlusal plane horizontal
	Transverse ridge links apices of buccal and lingual cusps	No transverse ridge
	Mesial marginal ridge inclines cervically about 45 degrees	Mesial marginal ridge is horizontal
	Mesiolingual groove	No mesiolingual groove
Occlusal aspect	Occlusal outline diamond shaped	Occlusal outline square or round
	Mesial and distal profiles converge lingually	Mesial and distal profiles straight and parallel
	Occlusal table triangular in outline	Occlusal table square in outline
	Buccal cusp more than twice the size of lingual cusp	Buccal and lingual cusps nearly equal in size
	Mesial marginal ridge shorter and less prominent than distal marginal ridge	Mesial and distal marginal ridges about same length and prominence
	Absence of Y pattern formed by grooves	Main grooves form Y pattern
	No central pit	Central pit

The Premolars—Clinical Applications

Throughout the patient's lifetime the premolars may be subjected to a wide variety of clinical problems, including interproximal and occlusal caries, cervical demineralization, cervical erosion, and congenital absence. All of these require an intimate knowledge of anatomic tooth form for proper restoration (Figs. 4.50–4.59).

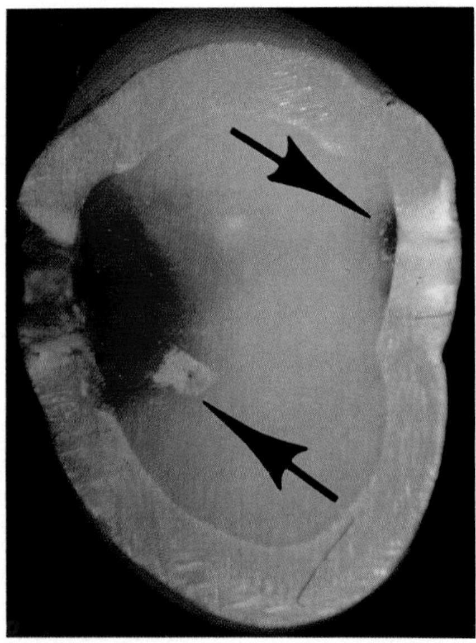

Figure 4.50

Cross section of crown showing proximal caries in a maxillary first premolar.

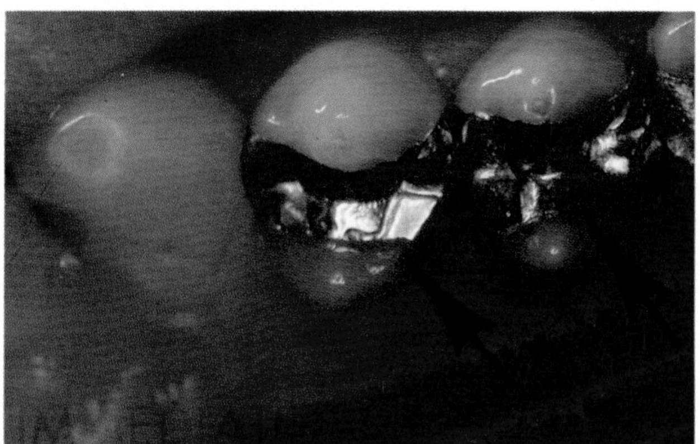

Figure 4.51

Resulting silver amalgam restorations in the maxillary premolars. Note the proper restoration of anatomic detail on marginal ridges; groove pattern.

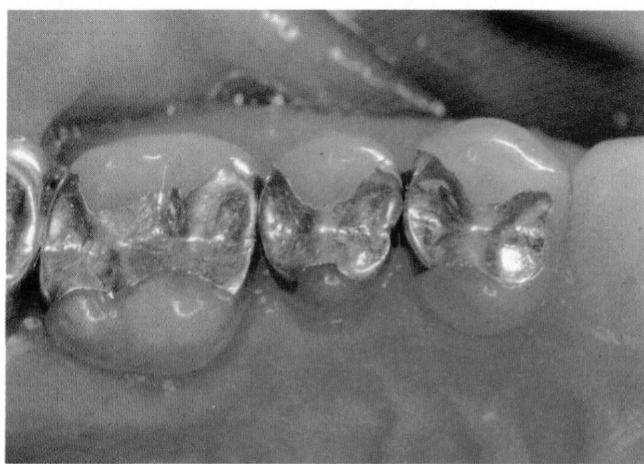

Figure 4.52

Class II gold inlays in the maxillary premolars at 18-year recall. Restored by a dental student.

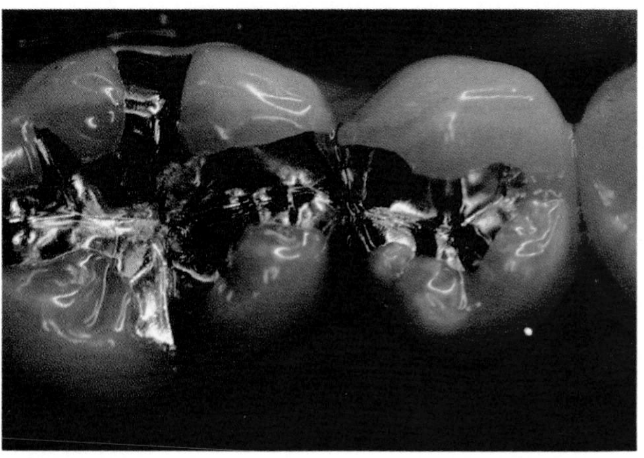

Figure 4.53

Class II silver amalgam restorations, mandibular left second premolar and first molar. Note anatomic detail of marginal and triangular ridges; groove pattern.

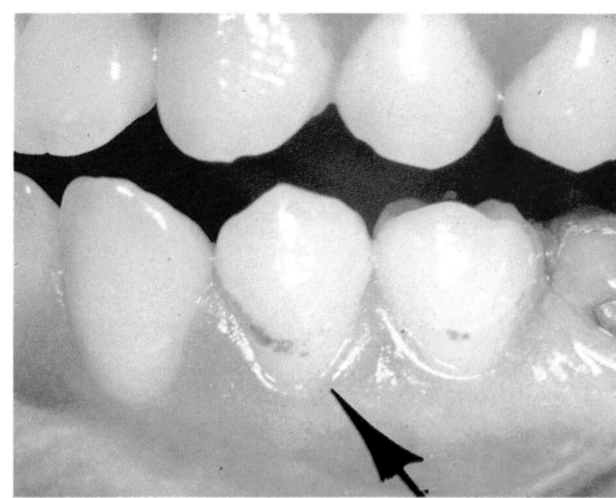

Figure 4.54

Cervical demineralization lesion, mandibular first premolar.

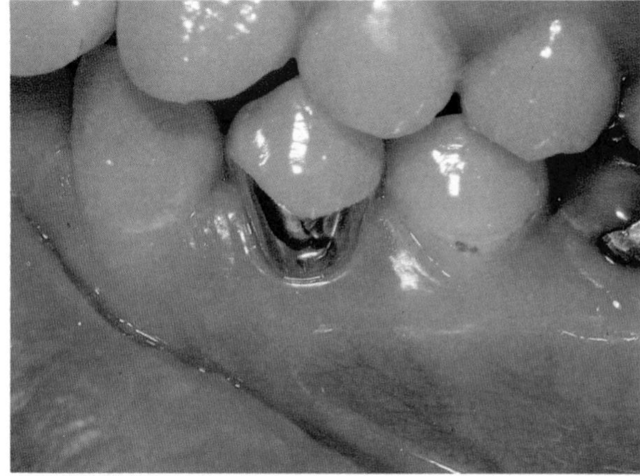

Figure 4.55

The same premolar as shown in Figure 4.54 after restoration with gold foil. Note excellent gingival tissue response.

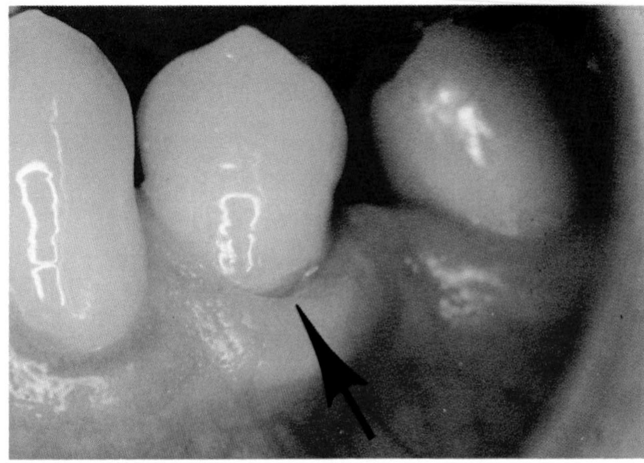

Figure 4.56

Cervical erosion lesion, mandibular first premolar.

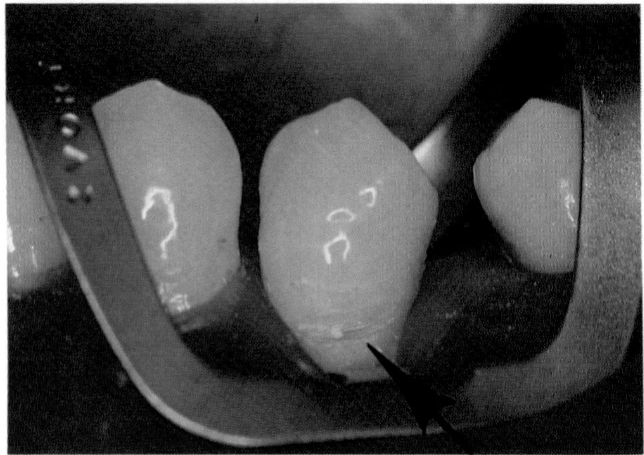

Figure 4.57

The same premolar as shown in Figure 4.56 after isolation and placement of retraction clamp.

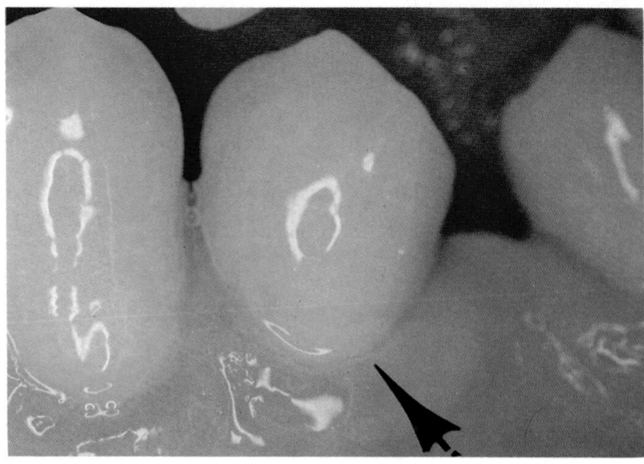

Figure 4.58

The same premolar as shown in Figures 4.56 and 4.57 after restoration with a bonded composite resin.

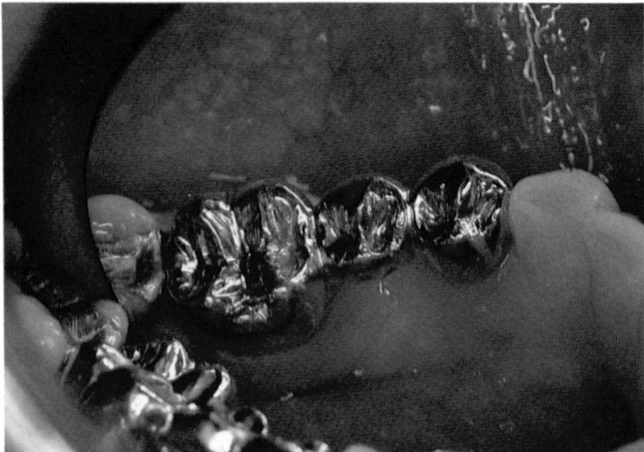

Figure 4.59

A three-unit fixed prosthesis replacing a congenitally missing mandibular second premolar. Note anatomic detail in the restoration.

5

The Molars

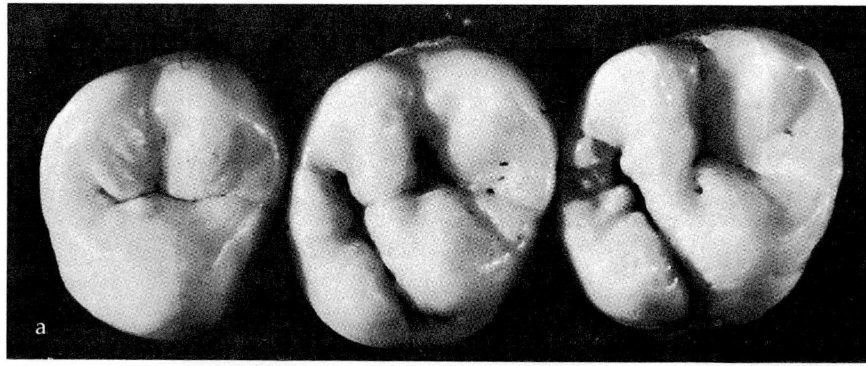

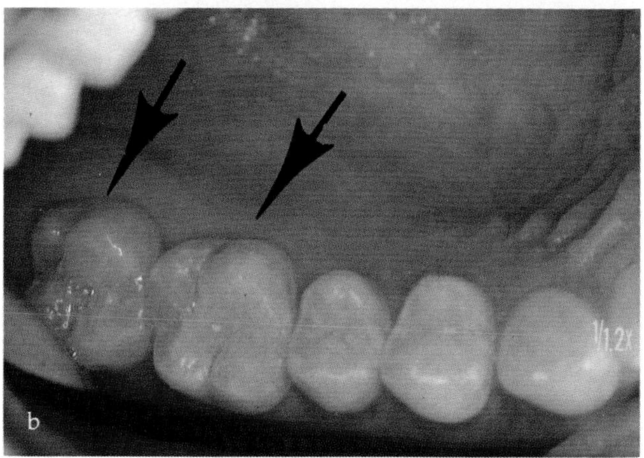

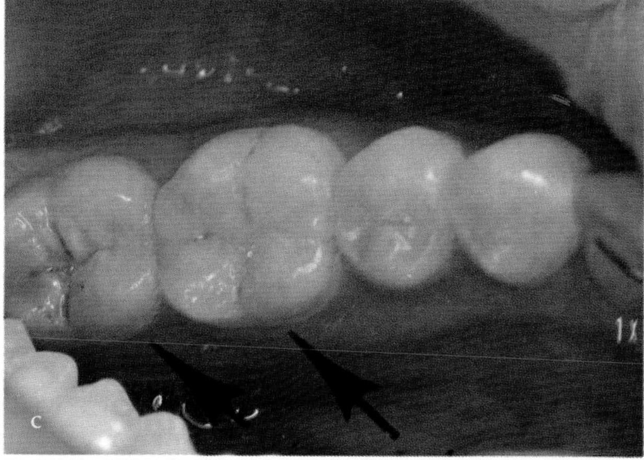

Figure 5.1
a, Maxillary right first, second, and third molars from the same arch; *b,* left maxillary molars, occlusal view; *c,* left mandibular molars, occlusal view.

Three molars occupy the posterior segments of each dental quadrant. Molars are the only units of the dentition that do not replace a primary predecessor.

The first permanent molar erupts into the oral cavity at approximately 6 years of age; hence it is sometimes referred to as the "6-year molar." The second molars erupt during the 12th year. The third molars, often called the "wisdom teeth," are quite irregular in their time of eruption, and, in fact, sometimes do not erupt at all, either because the tooth bud itself does not develop (*agenesis*), or because the tooth fails to erupt (*impaction*). Of the three permanent molars, the third is the most variable anatomically and developmentally.

Molars play a major role in the mastication of food. In addition they are highly important in supporting or sustaining the vertical dimension of the face.

There are several *class traits* that distinguish all molars: (1) molars have the largest occlusal surfaces of any teeth in the arch; (2) molars have three to five major cusps; (3) molars are the only teeth that have at least two buccal cusps; (4) molars have two or three large roots, the orientation and disposition of which are peculiar to these teeth and easily distinguish them from the premolars, the only other units of the dental arch that can possess two roots.

Their broad multicusped occlusal surfaces, strong root support, and positional relationship to the temporomandibular joints make the molars admirably suited for their grinding function.

Maxillary Molars

Size and Eruption

Maxillary Molars (mm)	Crown Height (mm)	Mesiodistal Crown Diameter (mm)	Bucco-lingual Crown Diameter (mm)	Tooth Length (mm)	Age at Eruption (yr)
First	7.5	10.0	11.0	19.5	6
Second	7.0	9.0	11.0	18.0	12
Third	6.5	8.5	10.0	17.5	18+

There are several *arch traits* that distinguish the maxillary molars as a group: (1) there are generally three roots, two buccal and one lingual; (2) generally there are three major cusps and the fourth is of lesser size; (3) the crowns are always broader buccolingually than mesiodistally; (4) the distobuccal and mesiolingual cusps are, with few exceptions, connected by a ridge, the *oblique ridge*; (5) the mesiobuccal, distobuccal, and mesiolingual cusps are arranged in a tricuspate-triangular pattern; (6) the two buccal cusps are of unequal size, the mesiobuccal (MB) cusp invariably being larger than the distobuccal (DB) cusp; (7) the distolingual (DL) cusp is at best a minor elevation and indeed may be greatly reduced or missing entirely.

There are numerous minor differences (*type traits*) that serve to identify each of the maxillary molars. For example, the DL cusp is generally most pronounced on the first molar and become progressively attenuated in second and third molars. Indeed, it may be missing entirely in the latter. The gradient in the degree of expression of the DL cusp is probably the most obvious type trait that distinguishes first from second and second from third maxillary molars (Fig. 5.1).

The first molar, by reason of its time of eruption (6 years) and position in the arch, is regarded as the anchor tooth of the maxillary dentition. Anatomically, it represents the *prototype* or *basic pattern* of the human permanent maxillary molars since, as will be seen later, the second and third molars differ from it morphologically only with regard to the proportionate interrelationships of their component parts. In addition, the first is the largest of the three permanent molars (type trait) and shows the least morphological variation.

First Molar

Buccal Aspect (Fig. 5.2)

Two cusps (MB and DB) make up the occlusal profile of the maxillary first molar. Although the buccal cusps are approximately equal in height (type trait) the MB cusp is slightly wider than the DB. The two are separated by a *buccal groove*, which terminates about halfway up the buccal surface. The slopes of the DB cusp are steeper relative to those of the MB cusp and, accordingly, the former appear sharper or more conical in outline. The apex of the mesiolingual

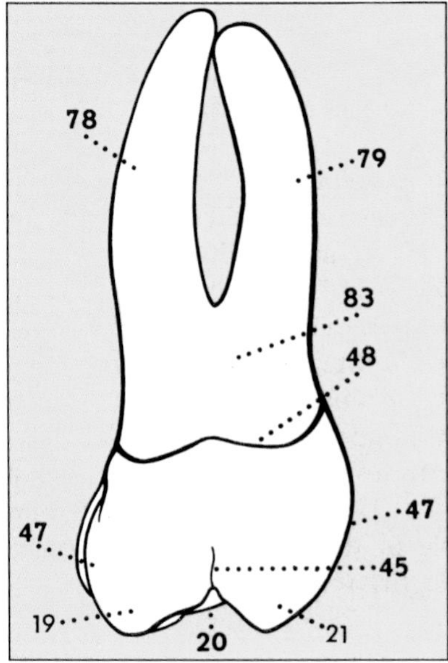

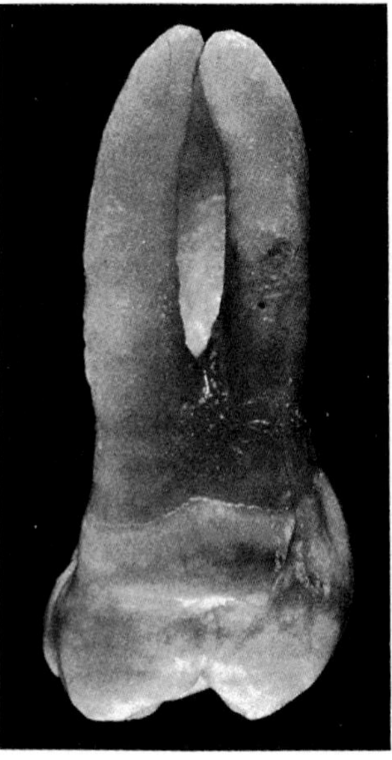

Figure 5.2
Maxillary left first molar (buccal aspect).

(ML) cusp is visible in the background approximately in line with the buccal groove.

The mesial and distal profiles are quite different. The mesial profile is highly convex in its occlusal and middle thirds. The contact area, which is located at the height of the convexity, is roughly three-fourths of the distance from the cervical line to the marginal ridge. The cervical third of the mesial profile is relatively flat or, in some cases, concave. The distal crown profile, on the other hand, is entirely convex from the cervical line to the marginal ridge. The height of contour is located closer to the cervix, approximately three-fifths of the distance from cervical line to marginal ridge.

The cervical line consists of two slightly curved segments separated by a sharp, apically directed peak at the midpoint of the buccal surface.

Both buccal and distal surfaces are visible when the first molar is viewed from its buccal aspect. The buccal surface has a prominent convexity in its cervical third and is relatively flat in the middle and occlusal thirds. The distal surface is uniformly convex occlusocervically. At the junction of the buccal and distal surfaces the crown shows a flattened or concave area in its cervical third.

Three roots are visible from the buccal aspect (the mesiobuccal, distobuccal, and lingual). The two buccal roots are joined in the form of a common root base for approximately one-third of the distance from the cervical line to the root apices. Just above the midpoint of the crown a shallow vertical groove marks the root base and marks the beginning of the buccal roots. The latter, which appear relatively narrow when viewed from the buccal aspect, often look like the handles of a pair of pliers, inclining toward each other in their apical thirds (type trait). The mesiobuccal root extends almost straight vertically from the cervical line and then curves distally in its apical third. Its apex is almost directly in line with the tip of the mesiobuccal cusp (type trait). The distobuccal root, on the other hand, shows a distal inclination from the cervical line and then curves mesially in its apical third. The lingual root, the longest of the three, is seen in the background between the two buccal roots.

Lingual Aspect (Fig. 5.3)

Two cusps of unequal size make up the occlusal profile of the maxillary first molar. The ML cusp, a relatively blunt, very prominent elevation, constitutes roughly three-fifths of the mesiodistal width of the crown. The DL cusp, noticeably shorter and narrower, has a rounded rather than a conical outline. The DL cusp of the first molar is invariably larger than that of the other two molars (type trait). The two lingual cusps are separated by the *lingual groove,* which terminates roughly halfway up the lingual surface.

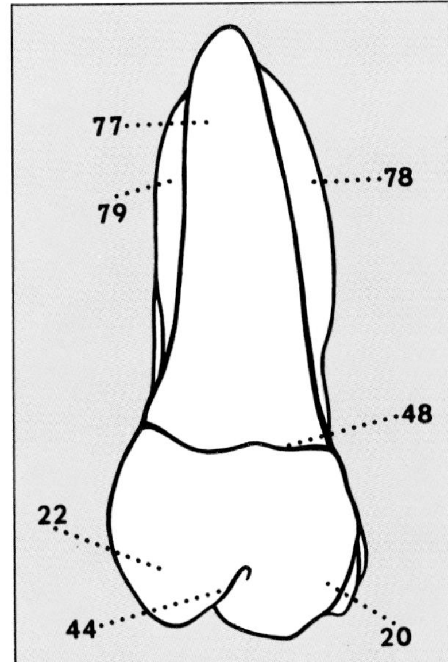

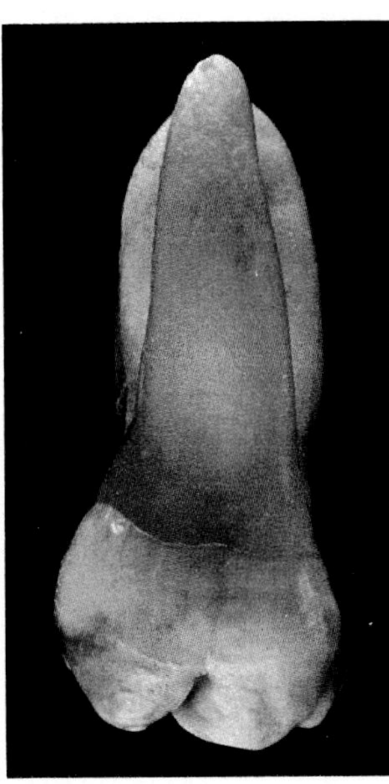

Figure 5.3
Maxillary left first molar (lingual aspect).

The mesial crown profile is convex except for a flattened area in its cervical third. The distal profile, on the other hand, is uniformly convex occlusocervically. The cervical line is very straight from mesial to distal.

The lingual surface is more or less evenly convex occlusocervically. It is divided into two distinct moieties by the lingual groove. The mesial moiety (the lingual aspect of the ML cusp) marks the site of the Carabelli (or fifth) cusp. This trait varies in both expression and frequency in the different races of mankind. Because of this, it cannot be considered a type trait, but is dealt with in a later chapter. The distal moiety (the lingual aspect of the DL cusp) is highly convex in all directions.

Three roots are observed from the lingual aspect. In the background the entire mesial profile of the mesiobuccal root is visible as well as a portion of the distal profile on the distobuccal root. In the foreground a single lingual root tapers evenly from a relatively broad base to a more or less blunted apex. The lingual root is the longest of the three roots and is marked by a shallow vertical depression that begins at the cervical line and extends about two-thirds of the distance to the root apex. The lingual root apex is almost directly in line with the midline of the crown (type trait).

Mesial Aspect (Fig. 5.4)

The maximum buccolingual diameter is at the cervix of the crown of the maxillary first molar. Both buccal

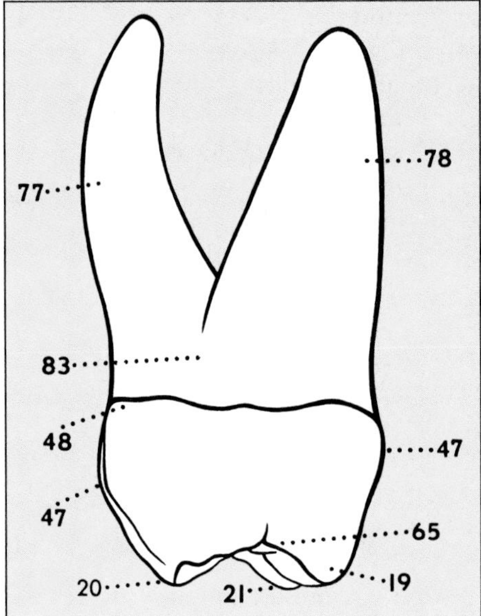

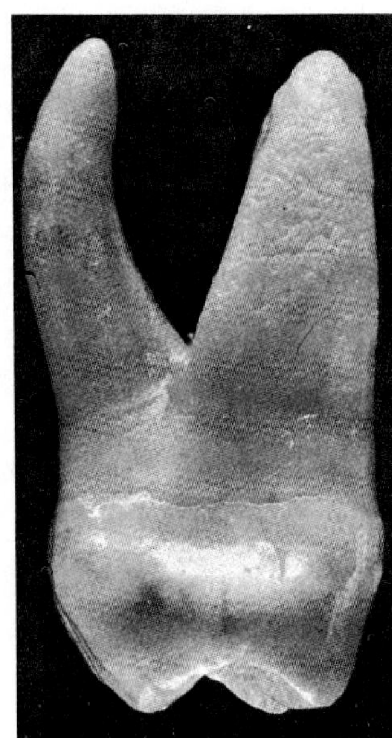

Figure 5.4
Maxillary left first molar (mesial aspect).

and lingual profiles converge occlusally, and the minimum crown diameter occurs between the apices of the MB and ML cusps. The crown is, therefore, roughly trapezoidal in outline.

The occlusal profile is made up of the apices of the MB and ML cusps and the triangular ridges. The ML cusp is higher than the MB. The buccal profile is strongly convex in its cervical third. It then inclines slightly toward the lingual in a more or less straight line and ends at the tip of the MB cusp. The lingual profile is more uniformly convex from the cervical line to the tip of the ML cusp. Its height of contour is approximately at the midpoint of the crown.

The cervical line, although irregular, is generally slightly convex toward the occlusal.

The mesial marginal ridge forms a prominent platform that extends buccolingually linking the mesial cusp ridges. It is marked by several distinct tubercles (type trait) that are faintly outlined by supplementary grooves (spillways) radiating from the occlusal surface.

The occlusal and middle thirds of the mesial surface are highly convex. The contact area is located at the most prominent portion of this convexity, i.e., at the junction of the occlusal and middle thirds just buccal to the center of the crown. The cervical third

Figure 5.5
Maxillary left first molar (distal aspect).

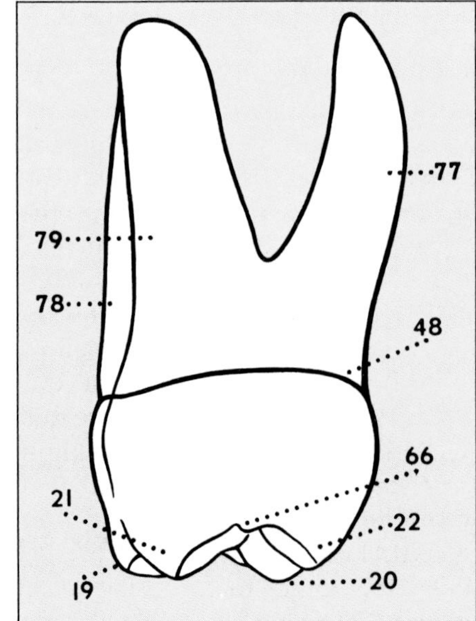

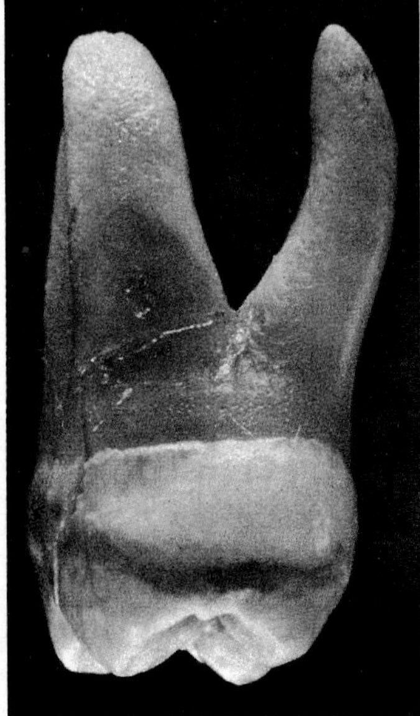

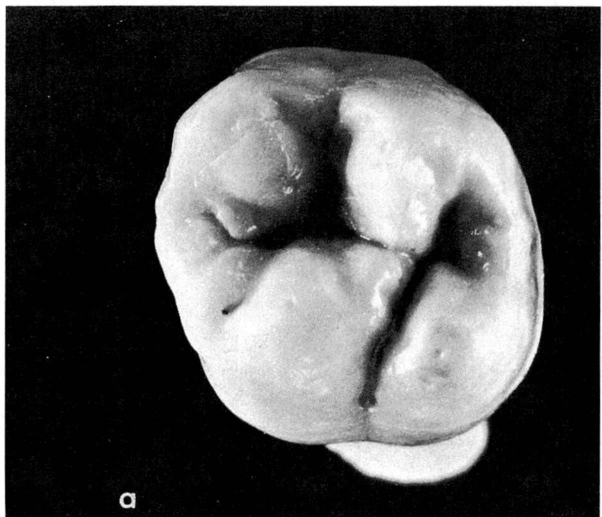

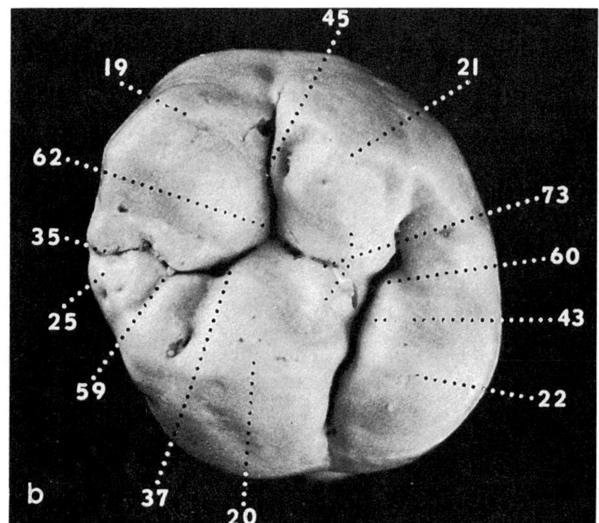

Figure 5.6
Maxillary left first molar (occlusal aspect): *a*, actual crown; *b*, cast.

of the crown is, on the other hand, either flat or concave.

Both mesiobuccal and lingual roots are seen from this aspect. The mesiobuccal root, which appeared narrow from the buccal aspect, now looks broad and flat buccolingually. The lingual root, which was relatively broad from the lingual aspect, now appears constricted buccolingually and looks somewhat banana shaped, curving lingually from the root base and then buccally toward the apex. The lingual profile of the entire tooth (crown and root) from the mesial aspect resembles the curvature of the human vertebral column (sigmoid).

A characteristic feature of the first molar is that both the mesiobuccal and lingual roots project beyond the adjacent crown profiles (type trait).

Distal Aspect (Fig. 5.5)

The DB cusp, the distal marginal ridge, and the DL cusp contribute to the occlusal profile of the crown of the maxillary first molar. The DB cusp is more prominent than the DL cusp. Since both DB and DL cusps are larger in the first molar, only a small portion of each mesial cusp is visible from the distal aspect. The distal marginal ridge is shorter buccolingually and far less prominent than the mesial marginal ridge. The crest of the distal marginal ridge is only rarely marked by the presence of accessory tubercles or cusplets.

The buccal and lingual crown profiles are identical in form to those already described for the mesial aspect. Since the distal moiety of the crown is relatively constricted buccolingually, almost the entire extent of the buccal surface is visible from the distal aspect. The distal cervical line is very nearly straight.

The distal surface is less extensive in area than the mesial surface. It is uniformly convex except for a slightly flattened area in the region of the distobuccal root. The contact area is located approximately at the midpoint of the crown buccolingually and occlusocervically.

Three roots are visible from the distal aspect. The entire buccal profile and apex of the mesiobuccal root form a background for the distobuccal root. The latter, shorter and narrower than the mesiobuccal, extends almost straight vertically with little if any projection beyond the buccal profile of the crown. The lingual root, the longest of the three, projects in a lingual direction for more of its length, then curves abruptly toward the buccal in its apical third.

Occlusal Aspect (Fig. 5.6)

The outline of the crown of the maxillary first molar is square to rhomboidal (Fig. 5.7). The MB and DL angles are acute and the DB and ML angles are obtuse.

Approximately one-third of the buccal surface and one-half of the lingual surface are visible. The buccal surface is relatively flat. Its distal portion is lingual to the mesial portion. The lingual surface is more convex than the buccal and is divided into two parts by the lingual groove.

The occlusal table consists of two separate and distinct components. The *trigon* (or mesial moiety of the tooth) bears three cusps, the MB, the ML, and the DB. The *talon* (or heel) consists of a single cusp, the DL, and the distal marginal ridge.

The three largest cusps (MB, DB, and ML) are arranged in a pattern typical of the maxillary molars.

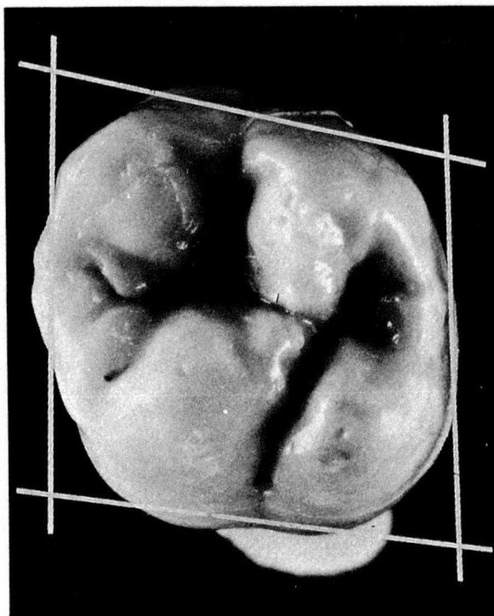

Figure 5.7

Rhomboidal crown outline, maxillary left first molar (occlusal aspect).

They are linked together in a tricuspate-triangular pattern by (1) the buccal cusp ridges that form the base of the triangle, (2) the mesial ridge that forms the mesial side of the triangle, and (3) the oblique ridge that courses diagonally across the occlusal surface (between DB and ML) to form the distal side of the triangle. If straight lines are drawn connecting the apices of the MB, DB, and ML cusps, in most cases the resultant figure will approximate an equilateral triangle. If we consider the apex to be the ML cusp, then the buccal ridge forms the base, and the mesial marginal and oblique ridges the sides of the triangle (Fig. 5.8).

This portion of the tooth represents the *trigon* or primitive cusp triangle which is both phylogenetically and ontogenetically the original molar crown. This is discussed in more detail in a later chapter.

The remaining portion of the occlusal table, namely the distal marginal ridge and the DL cusp, comprises the talon and projects distally and lingually from the tricuspate-triangle. The talon extends beyond the root base, and both ontogenetically and phylogenetically represents a more recent addition to the crown. The talon is relatively well developed in the first molar (type trait) but undergoes a progressive diminution in size in the second and third molars.

Four cusps make up the occlusal surface. In order of decreasing size they are ML, MB, DB, and DL.

The ML and MB cusps are quite broad and together make up almost two-thirds of the total area of the occlusal surface.

The mesial and distal marginal ridges are elevated crests that mark the proximal borders of the occlusal table. The mesial marginal ridge is longer and more prominent than the distal. The oblique ridge may be considered a marginal ridge in that it forms an elevated platform marking the distal border of the trigon. It is a prominent, more or less continuous crest, particularly in the first molar (type trait), and is made up of two structures, the triangular ridge of the DB cusp and the distal ridge of the ML cusp.

A broad, deep valley, the *central fossa,* marks the center of the trigon. The central fossa is itself roughly triangular in outline and contains (1) a *central pit,* located at a point in the middle of the triangle roughly equidistant from the apices of the three cusps; (2) a *buccal groove* that runs between the buccal cusps; (3) a *distal groove* that pursues a distolingual course toward the oblique ridge; (4) a *central groove* that radiates from the central pit in a mesial direction and terminates in the *mesial pit.*

A second fossa, running parallel and distal to the oblique ridge is known as the *distal fossa.* It contains (1) a *distal pit,* located just distal to the midpoint of the oblique ridge; (2) a *distolingual* (or distal oblique) *groove,* which runs parallel to the oblique ridge and

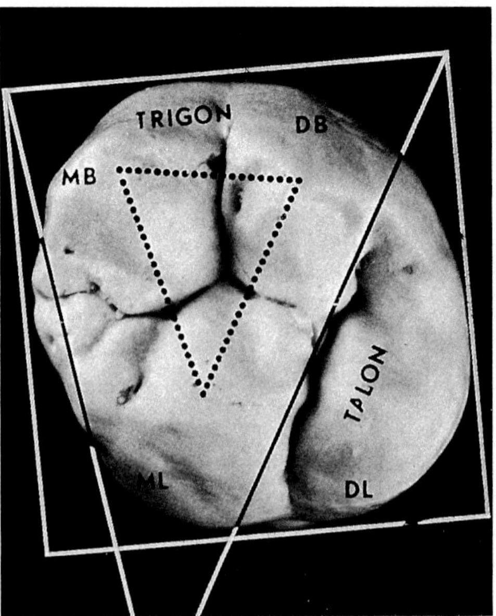

Figure 5.8

Triangular form of trigon and talon, maxillary left first molar (occlusal aspect): *MB,* mesiobuccal; *DB,* distobuccal; *ML,* mesiolingual; *DL,* distolingual.

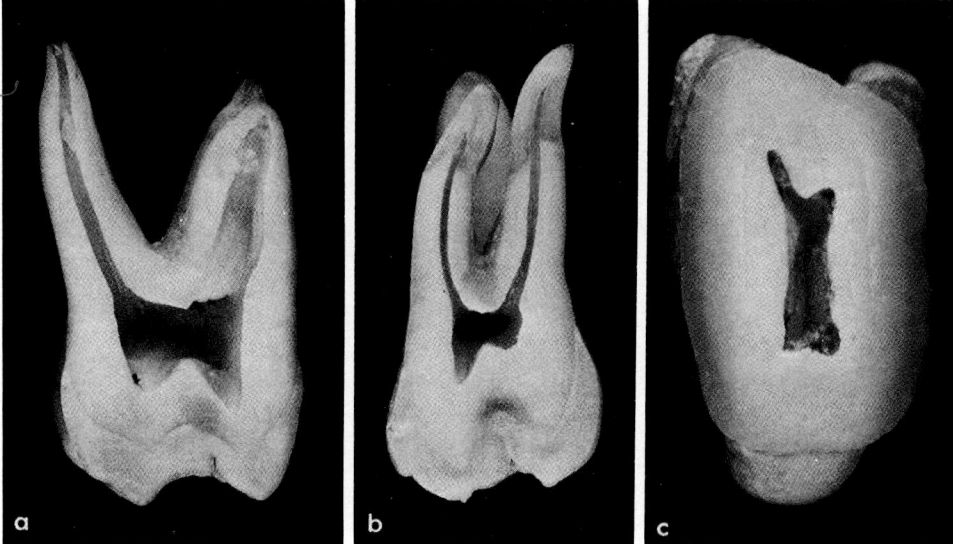

Figure 5.9
Pulp cavity of the maxillary left first molar: *a,* buccolingual section; *b,* mesiodistal section; *c,* transverse section at the cervix.

extends all the way to the lingual border. The distolingual groove continues onto the lingual surface as the *lingual groove.*

In addition to the two major fossae just described, two relatively minor depressions mark the occlusal surface: (1) the *mesial triangular fossa,* which is located just distal to the midpoint of the mesial marginal ridge, containing (a) the *mesial pit* and (b) two or more supplemental grooves, which radiate from the mesial pit toward the mesiobuccal and mesiolingual corners of the crown respectively; (2) the *distal triangular fossa,* which is situated just mesial to the midpoint of the distal marginal ridge, containing a small pit and two supplemental grooves radiating from it toward the corners of the crown.

Pulp (Fig. 5.9)

A mesiodistal section of the maxillary first molar shows a pulpal chamber with two horns, a mesiobuccal and a smaller distobuccal. The chamber itself is very small relative to the total crown area. The two canals are very narrow. In buccolingual section the pulpal chamber is wider and taller, but the two horns are more nearly equal in height. The mesiobuccal canal is broader and shorter than the lingual. In transverse section the pulp chamber at the cervical line shows the relative positions of the three canals. The mesiobuccal canal projects finger-like toward the mesiobuccal angle of the crown. The distobuccal canal is short and pointed toward the distobuccal corner of the crown. The two canals diverge at an angle of almost 90 degrees. The opening of the lingual canal is situated at the lingual extremity of the pulp chamber and cannot be distinguished at this level.

Variations

One of the most interesting features of the crown of the maxillary first molar from the point of view of evolution, race, and genetics is the so-called *Carabelli trait* (also known as Carabelli cusp or Carabelli tubercle). It includes a variety of expressions that manifest themselves on the mesiolingual surface of the ML cusp. These expressions range from complete absence to pits, grooves, tubercles, cusplets, or cusps. In some human populations, as among Melanesians, the Carabelli trait takes the form of a large fifth cusp, as large as any other on this molar. Other populations lack any expression of the trait other than a pit or groove. Among Caucasians the entire gamut of expressions may be found, as shown in Figures 5.10*a* to *d* and 5.11*a* to *c*. The Carabelli trait is discussed in greater detail in a later chapter.

The *anterior transverse ridge* (ATR) is a structure that may be encountered on the occlusal surface. It has received little mention in the dental literature. This elongated cusplike prominence extends diagonally from the mesiobuccal corner between the mesial marginal ridge and the triangle ridge of the MB cusp

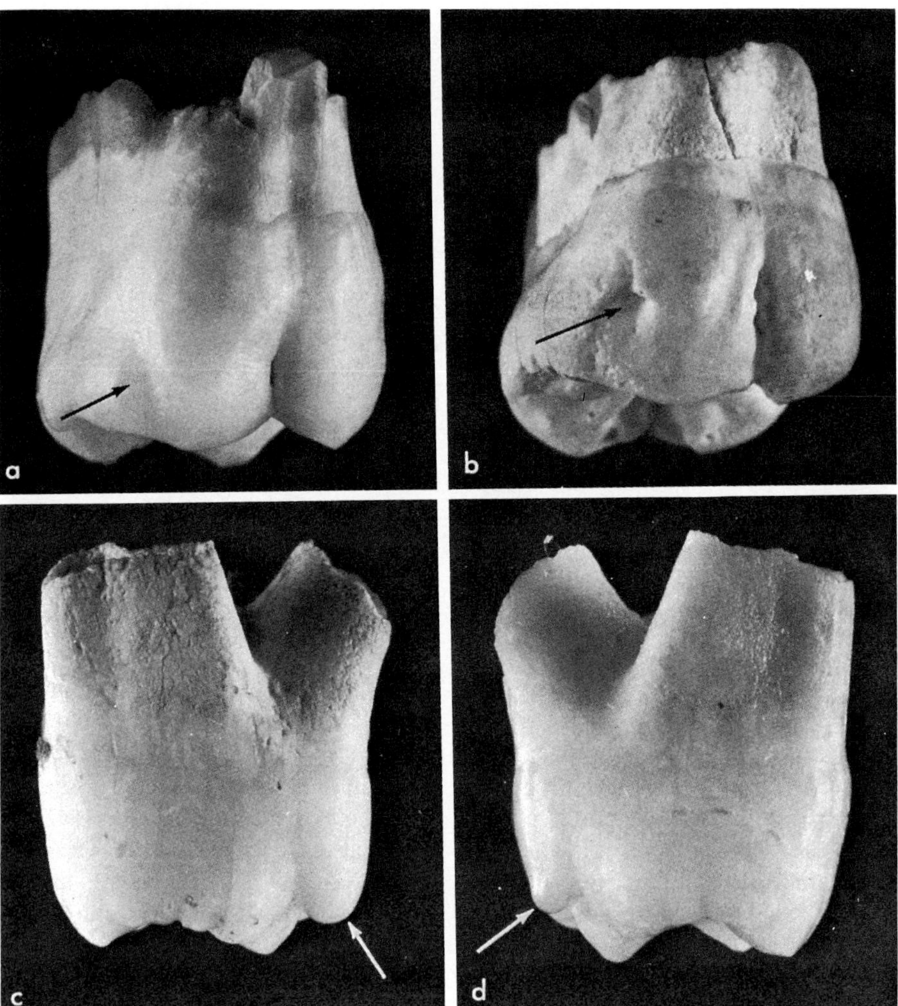

Figure 5.10

Variations of the Carabelli trait (*arrows*), maxillary first molar: *a*, Carabelli groove (lingual aspect); *b*, Carabelli pit (lingual aspect); *c*, pronounced Carabelli tubercle (mesial aspect); *d*, slight Carabelli tubercle (mesial aspect).

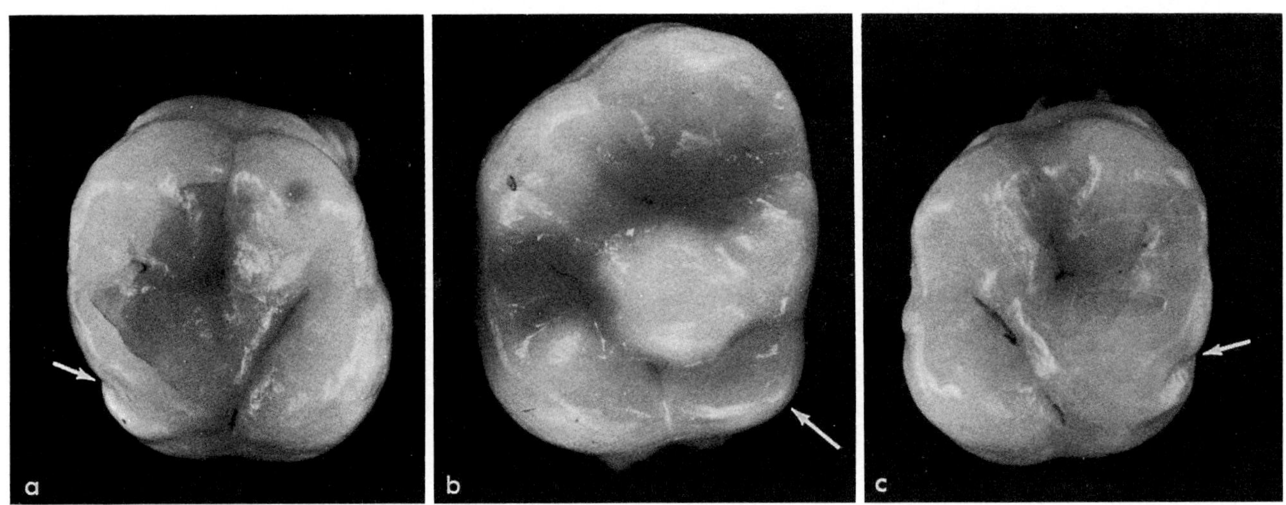

Figure 5.11

Variations of the Carabelli trait (*arrows*), maxillary first molar (occlusal aspect): *a*, slight tubercle; *b*, pronounced tubercle; *c*, groove.

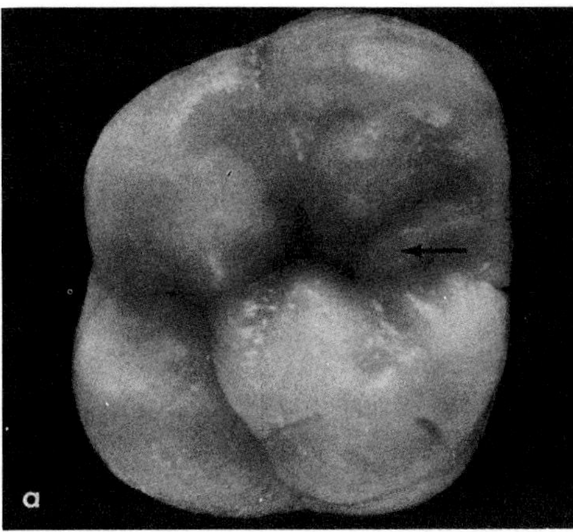

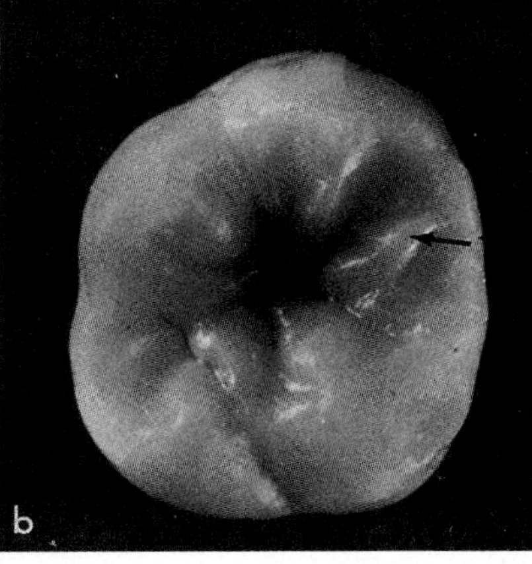

Figure 5.12

Anterior transverse ridge (*arrows*), maxillary right first molar (occlusal aspect): *a*, slightly developed; *b*, very prominent.

(Fig. 5.12*a*). It is highly variable with regard to degree of prominence, and when present in its most pronounced form (Fig. 5.12*b*) may almost completely obliterate the mesial triangular fossa.

Although the *oblique ridge* is one of the most constant features of the maxillary first permanent molar it may vary in size (Fig. 5.13*a* and *b*) and in continuity. The oblique ridge may be a continuous, uninterrupted crest (Fig. 5.14*a*) or be partially (Fig. 5.14*b*) or totally (Fig. 5.14*c*) interrupted at its approximate midpoint by the *distal groove.* The form and extent of the distal groove and its relationship to the oblique ridge are highly important considerations in restorative dentistry.

A common variation involves the number and prominence of *mesial marginal ridge tubercles* or cusps. Embryonically the mesial marginal ridge may show as many as five sharp conical eminences which often calcify as independent centers. The mesial marginal ridge of the completely calcified tooth may show one, two, or several rounded elevations along its length separated by distinct grooves (Fig. 5.15*a* and *b*) which provide "spillways" from the occlusal surface. The *distal marginal ridge,* on the other hand, rarely exhibits these tubercles, but commonly exhibits a single groove at its approximate midpoint (Fig. 5.16).

Supplemental grooves are highly variable features of the occlusal surface. A common type of supplementary groove is found in association with the triangular ridges of the main cusps. This type usually branches off from a main developmental groove and is found on either side of the triangular ridge. It roughly parallels the ridge in its course, and as it approaches the cusp ridge changes its direction and points toward the apex (Fig. 5.17).

The mesial and distal ridges of the MB cusp often slope evenly from the apex (see Fig. 5.2). Commonly, however, a small style may occur on either or both ridges (Fig. 5.18). These secondary elevations are not often seen clinically since they are obliterated by wear soon after eruption. They may be important considerations in understanding molar evolution.

A frequent variation occurs at the termination of the buccal groove in the form of a *buccal pit* (Fig. 5.19).

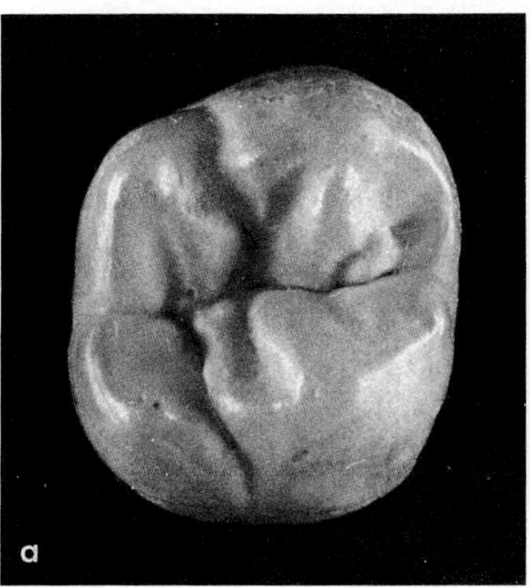

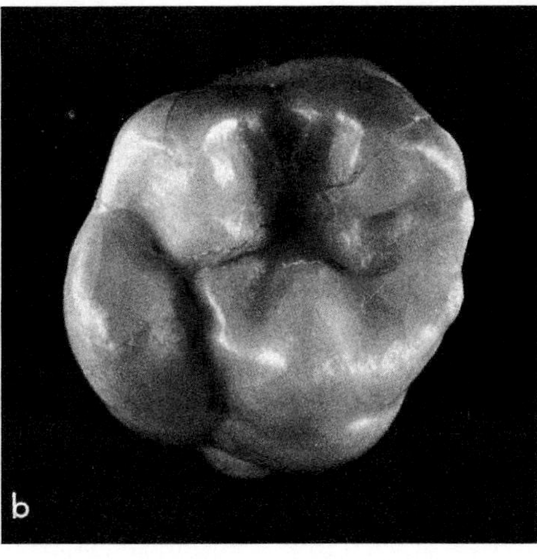

Figure 5.13

Variations in size of the oblique ridge, maxillary right first molar: *a*, small ridge; *b*, large ridge.

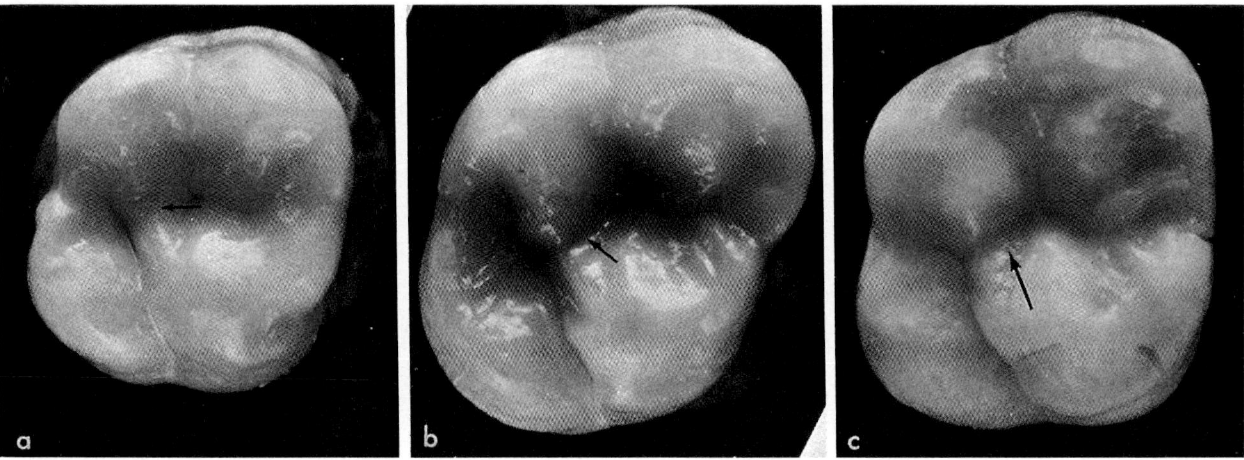

Figure 5.14

Variations in the form of the oblique ridge (*arrows*), maxillary right first molar (occlusal aspect): *a,* continuous ridge; *b,* partially interrupted; *c,* bisected by distal groove (totally interrupted).

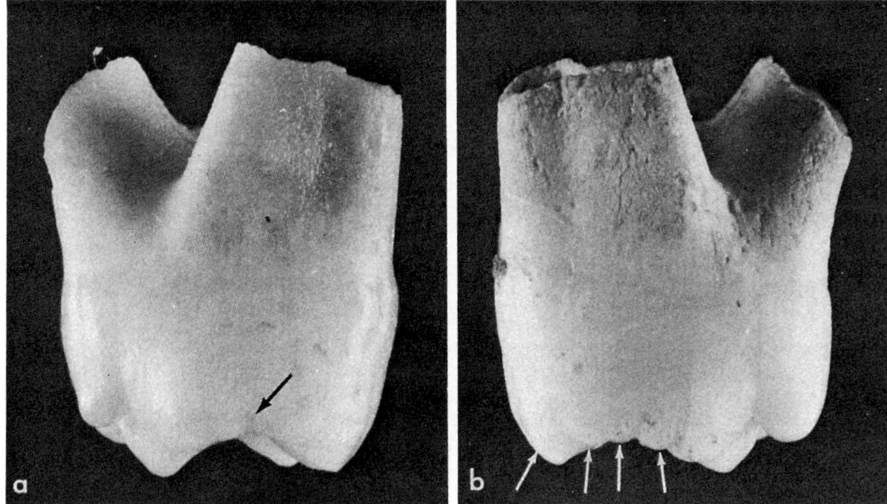

Figure 5.15

Mesial marginal ridge cusps (*arrows*), maxillary right first molar (mesial aspect): *a,* two mesial marginal ridge cusps; *b,* five mesial marginal ridge cusps.

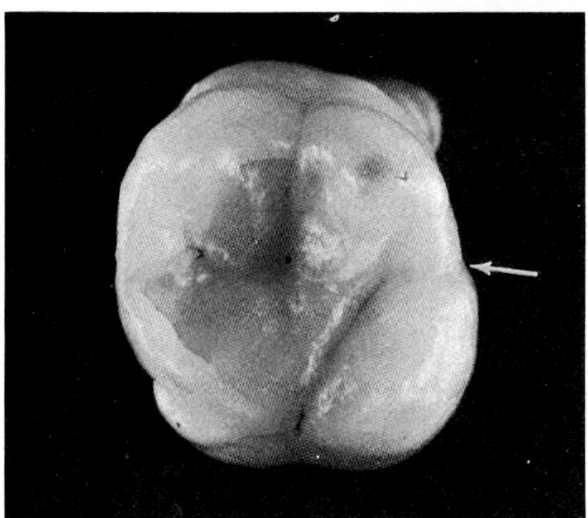

Figure 5.16

Groove on distal marginal ridge (*arrow*), maxillary left first molar (occlusal aspect).

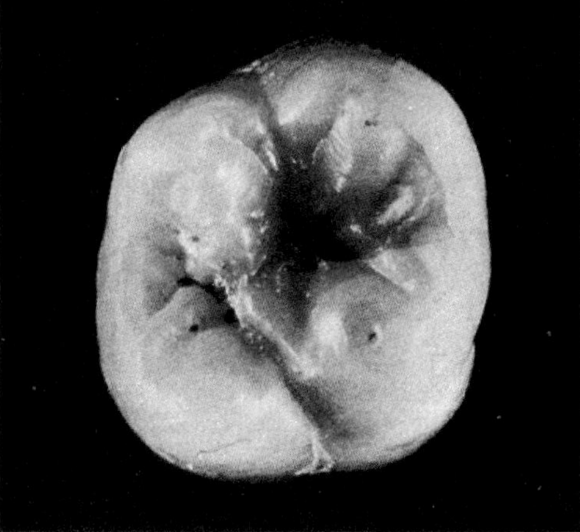

Figure 5.17

Supplemental groove pattern, maxillary right first molar (occlusal aspect).

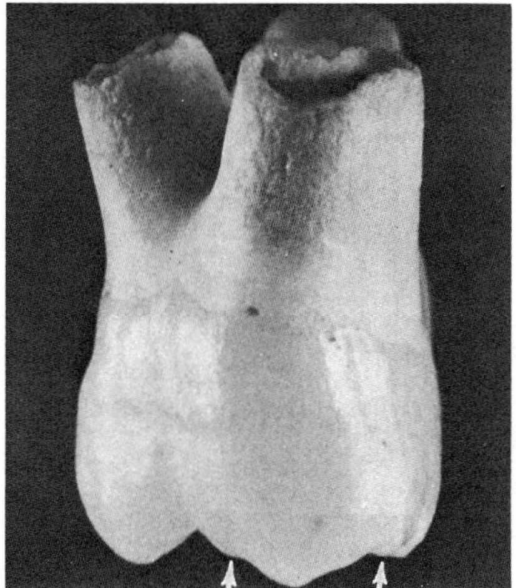

Figure 5.18
Styles on mesial buccal cusp ridge (*arrows*), maxillary right first molar (buccal aspect).

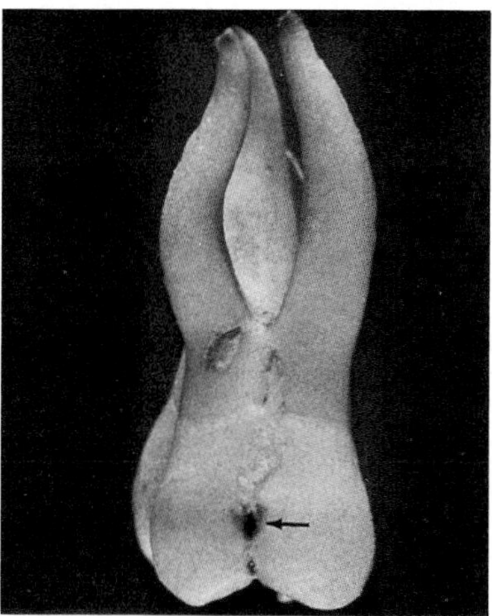

Figure 5.19
Buccal pit (*arrow*), maxillary right first molar (buccal aspect).

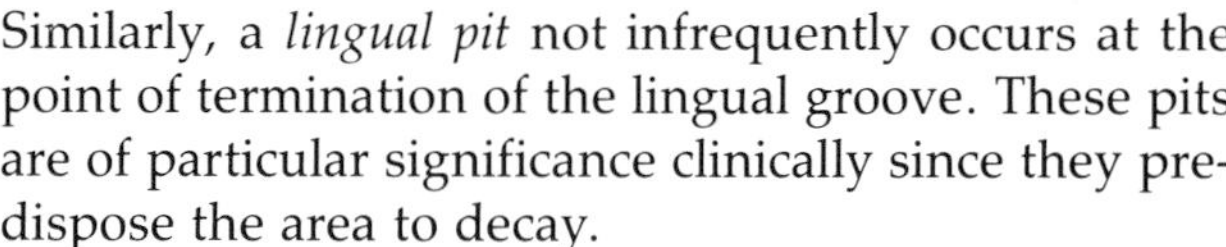

Similarly, a *lingual pit* not infrequently occurs at the point of termination of the lingual groove. These pits are of particular significance clinically since they predispose the area to decay.

The *buccal roots* may exhibit extreme curvature for their entire length (Fig. 5.20*a*), or they may curve abruptly only in their apical thirds (Fig. 5.20*b*). Both are occasionally abnormally short, or more often the distobuccal root alone is short relative to the mesiobuccal (Fig. 5.20*c*). The distobuccal root shows a particular tendency to distal inclination and/or irregular curvature (Fig. 5.20*d*).

The mesial aspect of both the mesiobuccal and lingual roots may show minor variations with regard to dimension and inclination. The mesiobuccal root may be unusually broad (Fig. 5.21*a*), and occasionally the lingual root, rather than showing the "plier handle" curvature referred to previously, is inclined lingually in a straight line (Fig. 5.21*b*). A relatively rare variation involves the fusion of distobuccal and lingual roots (Fig. 5.22).

Time and space do not permit a more exhaustive discussion of the seemingly limitless number of minor variations that may be encountered in the crown

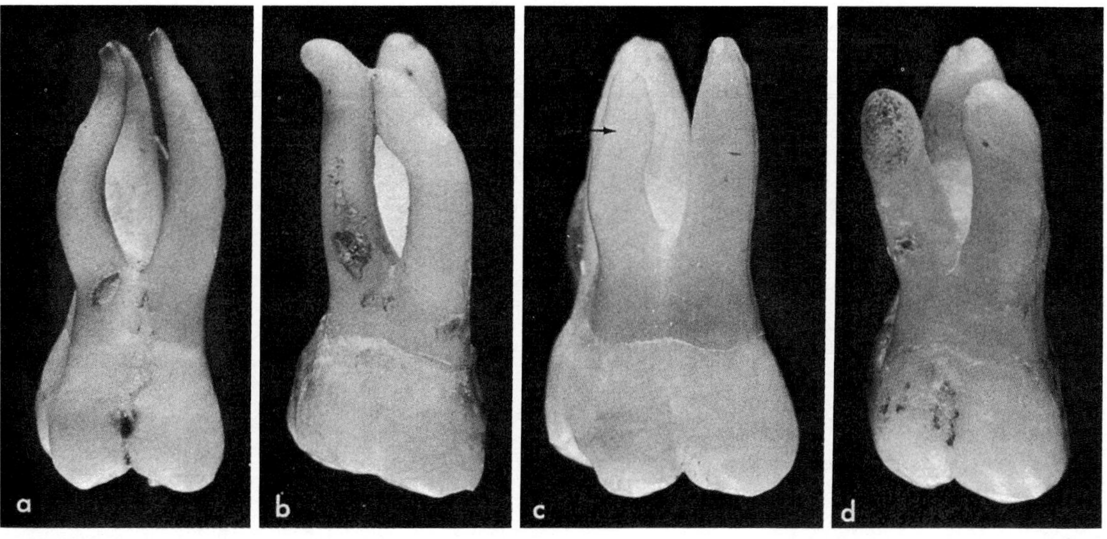

Figure 5.20
Variations in root configurations, maxillary right first molars (buccal aspect): *a*, extreme curvature of roots; *b*, abrupt curvature in apical thirds; *c*, short distobuccal root (*arrow*); *d*, distal inclination of distobuccal root.

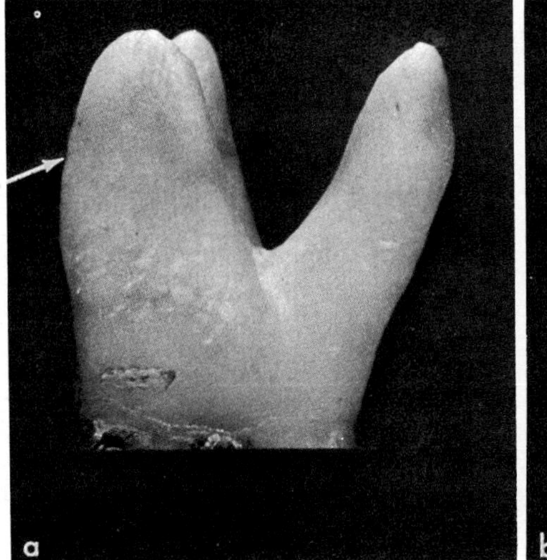

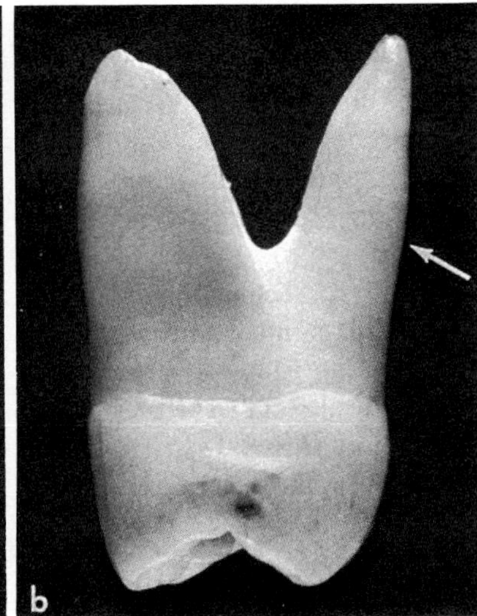

Figure 5.21
Root variations (*arrows*), maxillary first molar (mesial aspect): *a*, unusually broad mesial buccal root; *b*, straight lingual root.

and roots of the maxillary first permanent molar. We make no claims that the preceding discussion encompasses all the variable features of this tooth, for in fact we have illustrated only the more obvious. The student, throughout his clinical years, will encounter literally thousands of variations in tooth form, which often disguise or modify slightly the basic pattern. In addition, these seemingly minor morphological variations will, in many cases, alter the course of clinical treatment.

Second Molar

Buccal Aspect (Fig. 5.23)

Three features differentiate the maxillary second from the first molar: (1) crown size; (2) relative prominence of the DB cusp; (3) inclination of the buccal roots.

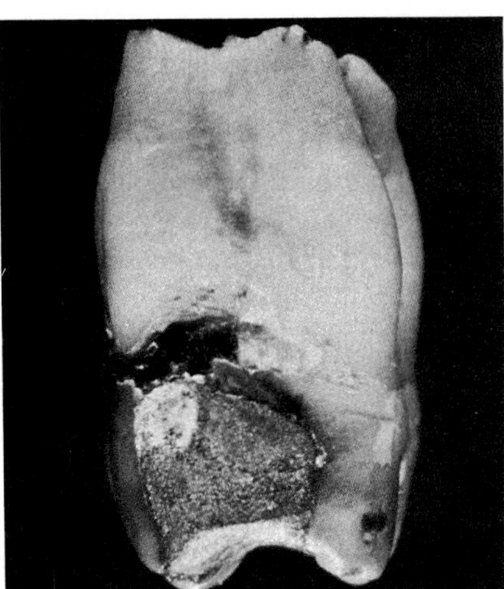

Figure 5.22
Fusion of distobuccal and lingual roots, maxillary left first molar (distal aspect).

The crown is smaller, both mesiodistally and cervico-occlusally, than in the first molar (type trait). The DB cusp is less prominent in terms of height and narrower mesiodistally in the second molar (type trait).

The buccal roots of the second molar show a distinct distal inclination. The apex of the MB root, for example, is directly in line with the midline of the crown. In addition, the roots are not "plier handled" in relation to each other but tend to be parallel throughout their lengths.

Lingual Aspect (Fig. 5.24)

Two features differentiate the lingual aspect of the maxillary second molar from that of the first: (1) the distolingual cusp is distinctly smaller in both width

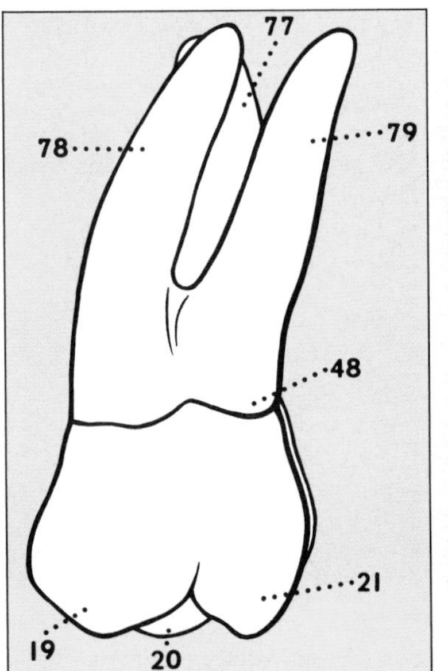

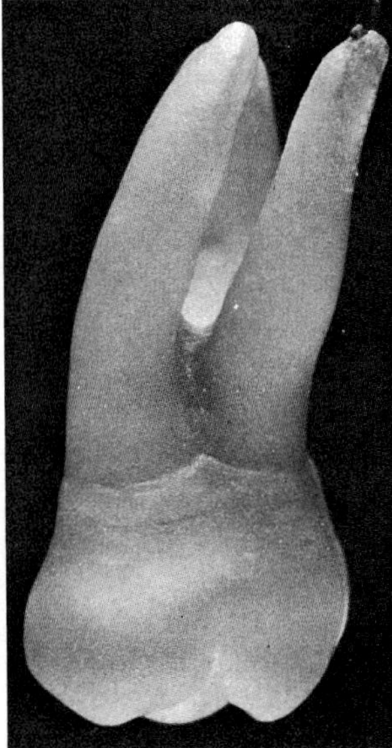

Figure 5.23
Maxillary left second molar (buccal aspect).

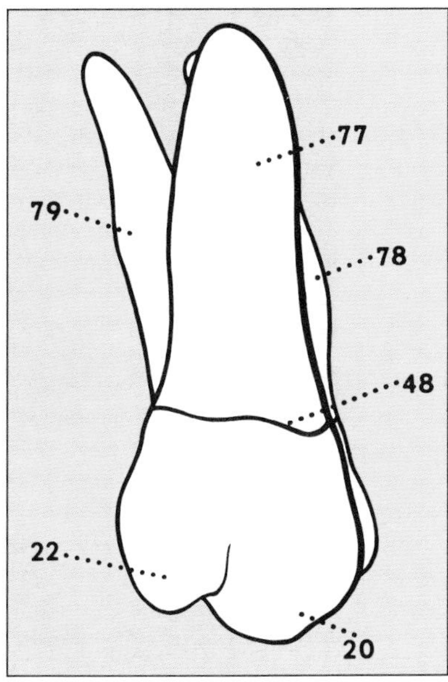

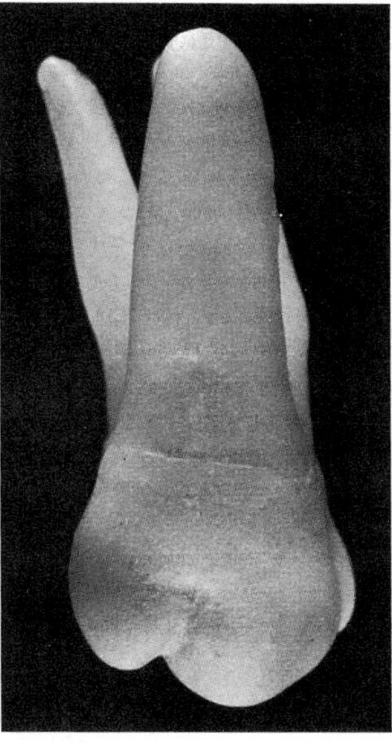

Figure 5.24
Maxillary left second molar (lingual aspect).

and height than in the first molar (type trait); (2) the lingual root is almost invariably narrower mesiodistally in the second molar (type trait) and may show a distinct distal inclination. The apex of the lingual root is often situated directly in line with the tip of the DL cusp (type trait).

Mesial Aspect (Fig. 5.25)

The maxillary second molar differs from the first in that the mesial marginal ridge tubercles are less numerous and less pronounced (type trait), and the mesiobuccal and lingual roots are much less divergent, being located well within the confines of the adjacent crown profiles (type trait).

Distal Aspect (Fig. 5.26)

Since both DB and DL cusps are less prominent in the second molar, a greater portion of the occlusal surface is visible from the distal aspect. In addition, the distobuccal root is often narrower, and the lingual root shows little if any projection beyond the crown.

Occlusal Aspect (Fig. 5.27)

There are five noteworthy characteristics that differentiate the maxillary second molar from the first molar. The crown outline is rhomboidal but the MB and DL angles are more acute and the ML and DB angles are more obtuse (type trait). The DB cusp is not as prominent as in the first molar, and the talon and

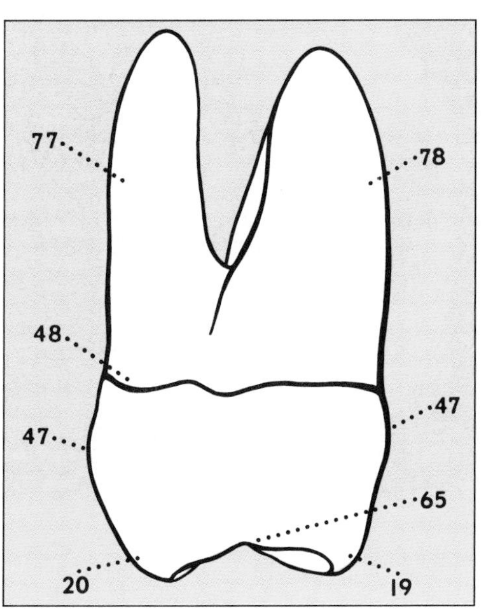

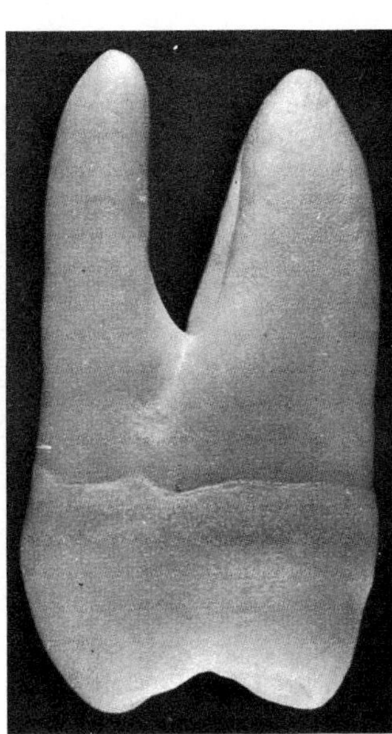

Figure 5.25
Maxillary left second molar (mesial aspect).

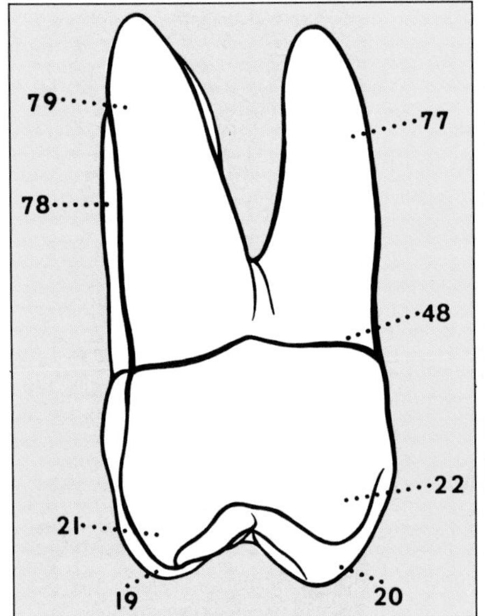

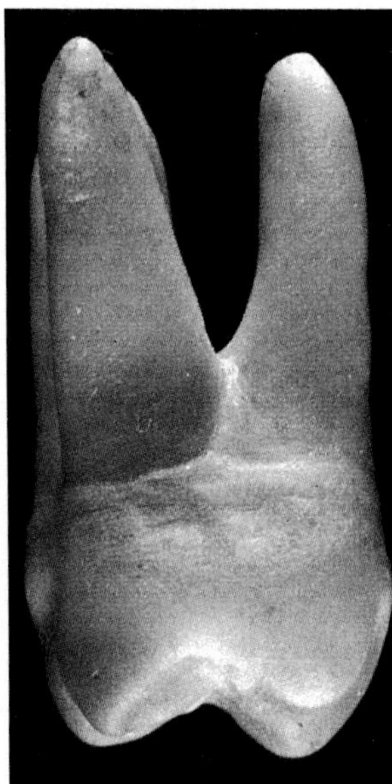

Figure 5.26
Maxillary left second molar (distal aspect).

oblique ridge are considerably reduced in size. There is a more variable pit-groove pattern, and the supplemental grooves are more numerous. The crown is generally more constricted mesiodistally.

Pulp (Fig. 5.28)

There is no significant difference between the first and second molar pulp cavities in mesiobuccal section. The same is true of the buccolingual section, although the canals are not as divergent in the second molar. In transverse section at the cervical line none of the three pulp canals can be detected.

Variations

The DL cusp is probably the most variable feature of the maxillary second molar. It may vary from complete absence, which is not rare, throuh various gradations of size or expression. Figure 5.29 shows occlusal views of three maxillary second molars: *a*, with complete absence of the DL cusp, *b*, with minimal expression of the DL cusp, and *c*, with major expression of the DL cusp. As can be seen, the crown outline of this molar varies from triangular (*a*) to rhomboidal (*c*) depending on the expression of the DL cusp.

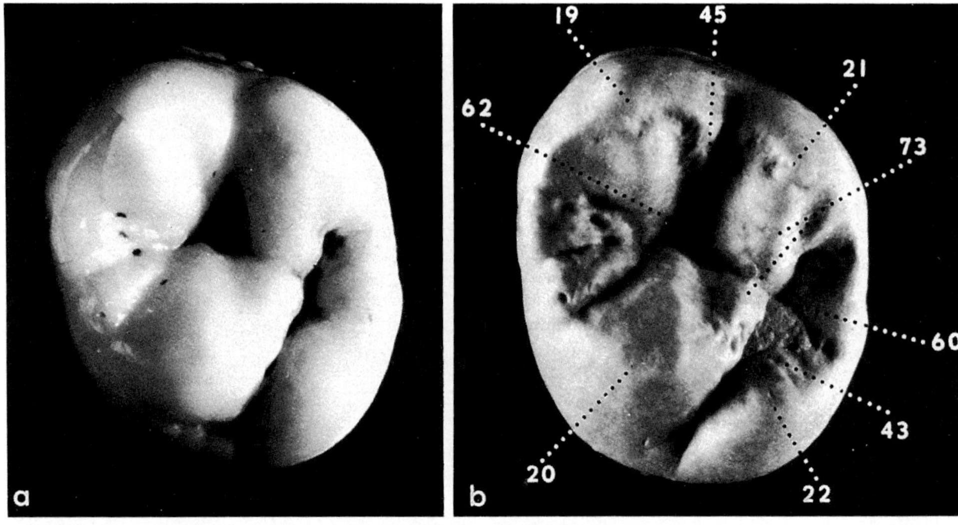

Figure 5.27
Maxillary left second molar (occlusal aspect): *a*, actual crown; *b*, cast.

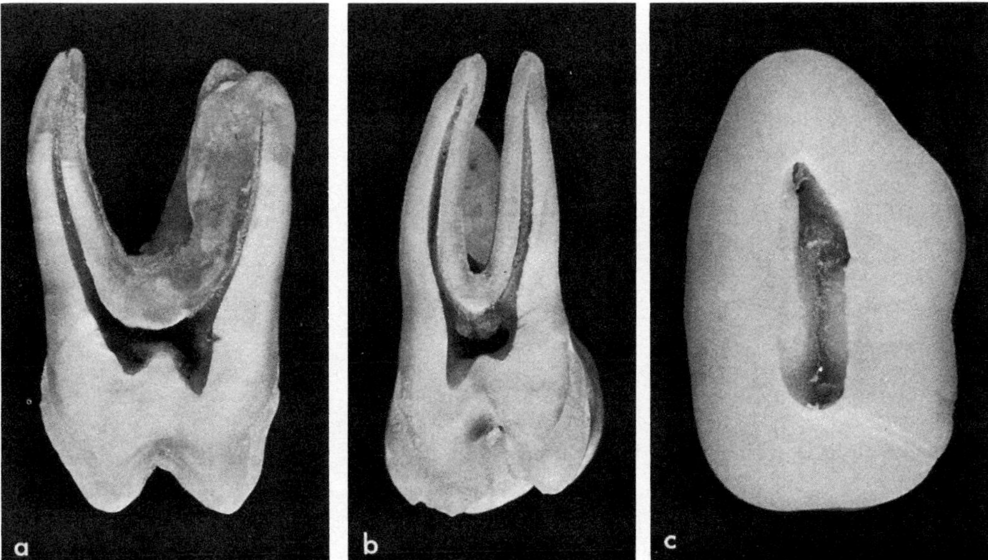

Figure 5.28

Pulp cavity of the maxillary left second molar: *a*, buccolingual section; *b*, mesiodistal section; *c*, transverse section at the cervix.

The occlusal surface shows a highly variable pit-groove pattern. It may resemble that of the first molar (Fig. 5.30*a*), be modified by the complete absence of the mesial and distal triangular fossae (Fig. 5.30*b*), show only a slight groove rather than a distal fossa (Fig. 5.30*c*), or show numerous well-defined supplemental grooves (Fig. 5.30*d*).

The roots of the maxillary second molar may be highly variable with regard to number, inclinations, and degree of fusion. Figure 5.31*a* shows a rare variation in the form of two mesiobuccal roots. The mesiobuccal and lingual roots may be fused (Fig. 5.31*b*) or all three roots may show a tendency to a partial fusion.

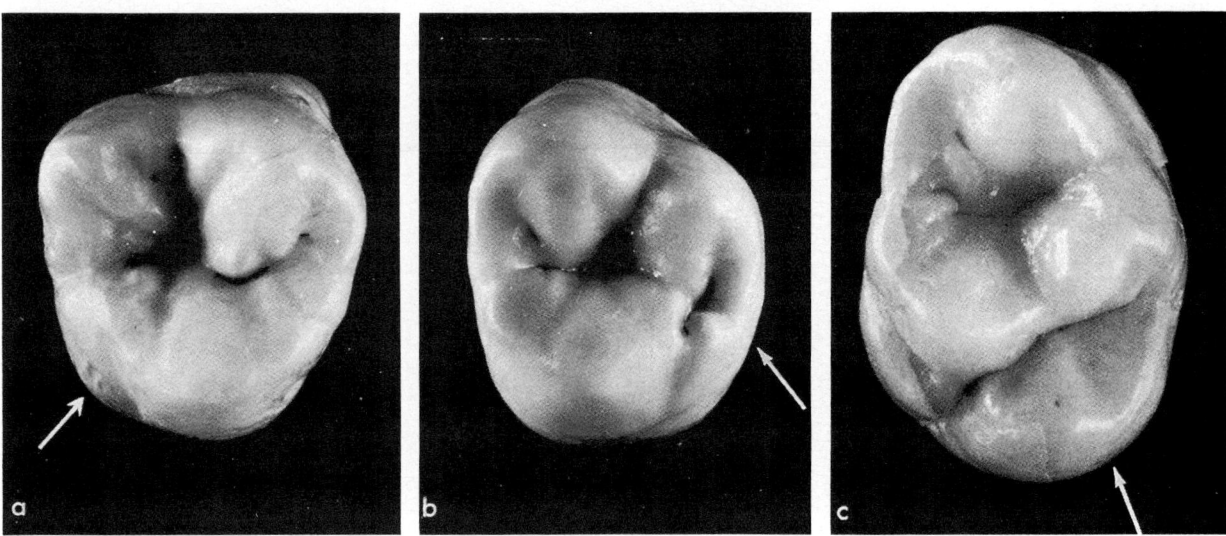

Figure 5.29

Variations in expression of the distolingual cusp (*arrows*), maxillary left second molars (occlusal aspect): *a*, complete absence of the cusp, triangular crown outline; *b*, minimal expression of the cusp; *c*, prominent expression of the cusp, rhomboidal crown outline.

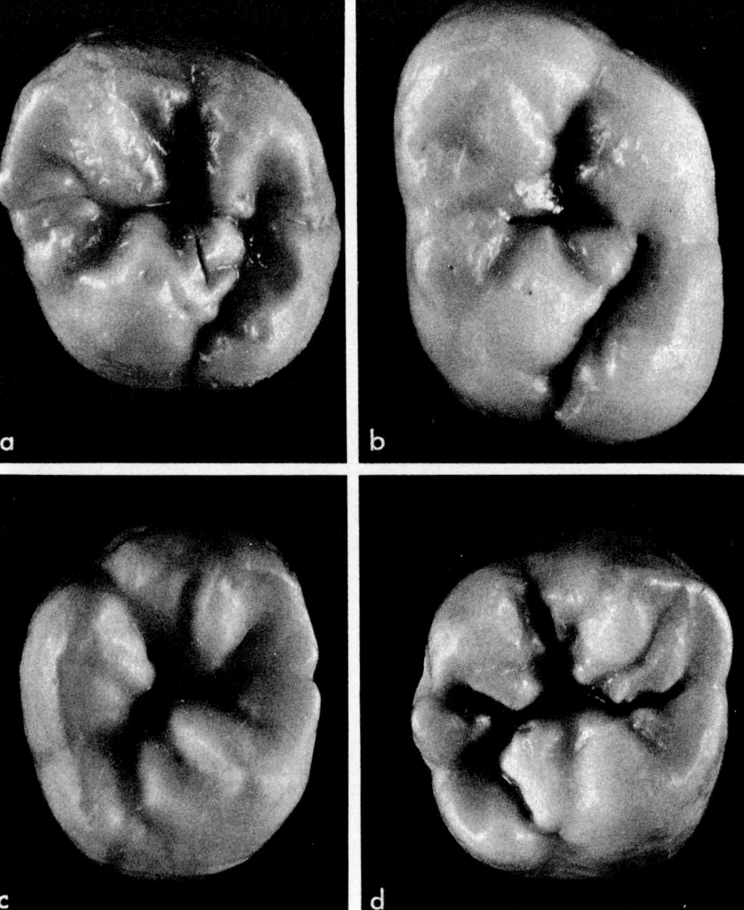

Figure 5.30

Variations in pit-groove pattern, maxillary second molars (occlusal aspect): *a*, patterns similar to that of first molar (left second molar); *b*, complete absence of mesial and distal triangular fossae; *c*, slight groove in place of a distal fossa; *d*, numerous supplemental grooves.

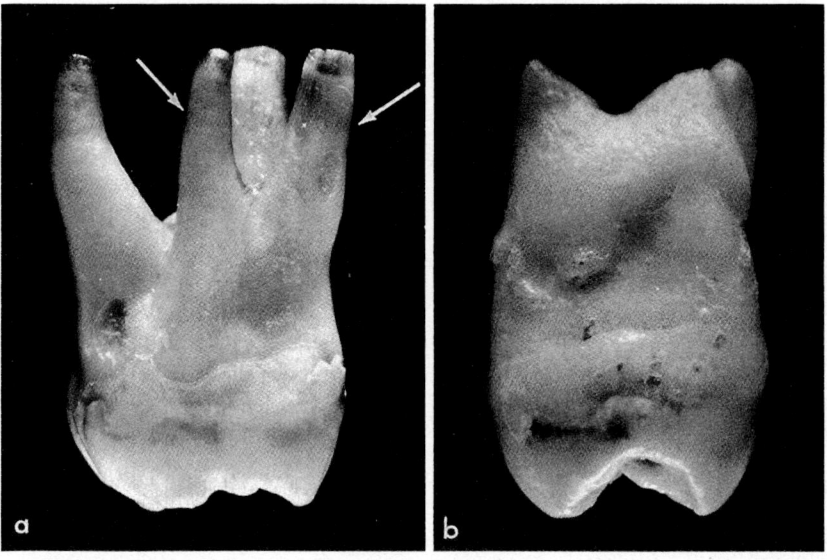

Figure 5.31

Variations in root form, maxillary second molar: *a*, presence of two mesiobuccal roots, left second molar (mesial aspect); *b*, fused mesiobuccal and lingual roots (*arrows*), left second molar (mesial aspect).

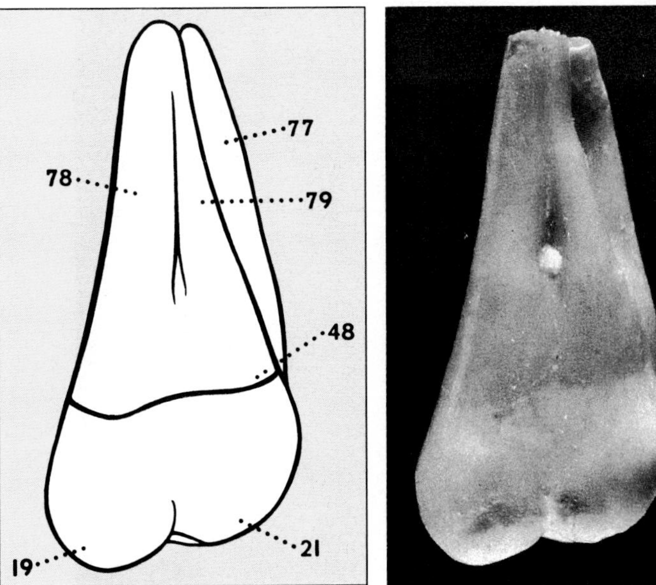

Figure 5.32
Maxillary left third molar (buccal aspect).

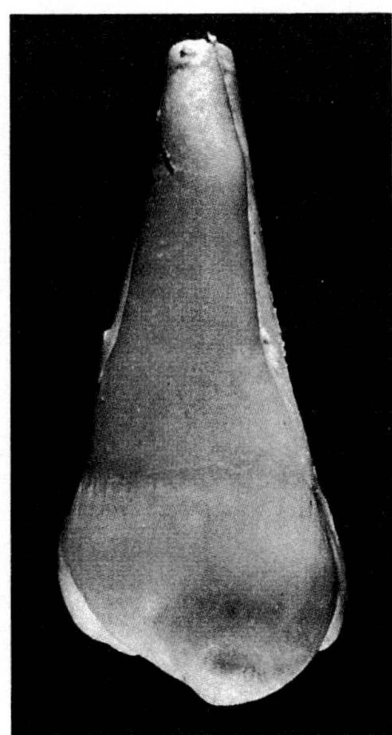

Figure 5.33
Maxillary left third molar (lingual aspect).

Third Molar

Buccal Aspect (Fig. 5.32)

The crown of the maxillary third molar is the smallest (both mesiodistally and cervico-occlusally) of the three maxillary molars (type trait). In addition, the roots are (1) much shorter in length (type trait), (2) commonly fused (type trait), and (3) generally show the most pronounced distal inclination of any of the three molars (type trait).

Lingual Aspect (Fig. 5.33)

The DL cusp is usually missing in the third molar (type trait) and the occlusal profile is made up of a single broad-based lingual cusp. In addition, the lingual root is usually fused with the buccal roots (type trait) and generally exhibits a more pronounced distal inclination than either of the other two molars.

Mesial Aspect (Fig. 5.34)

Fusion of the mesiobuccal and lingual roots is usually characteristic of the third molar in the maxillary dentition (type trait).

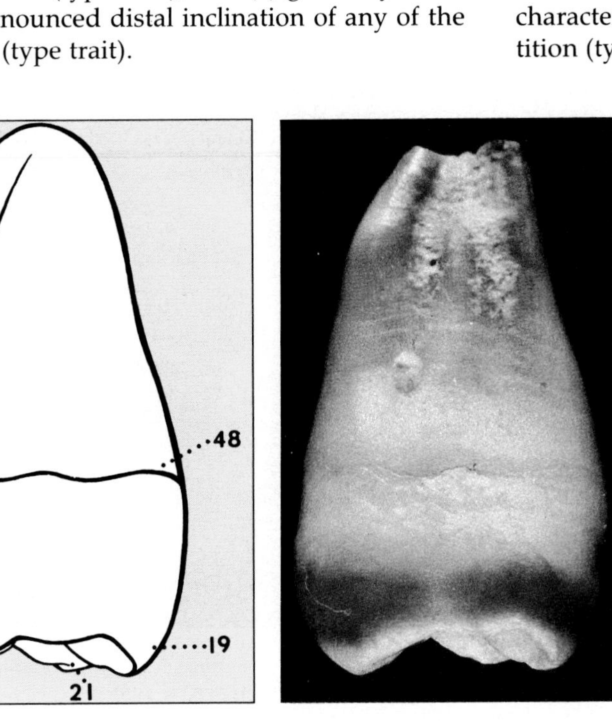

Figure 5.34
Maxillary left third molar (mesial aspect).

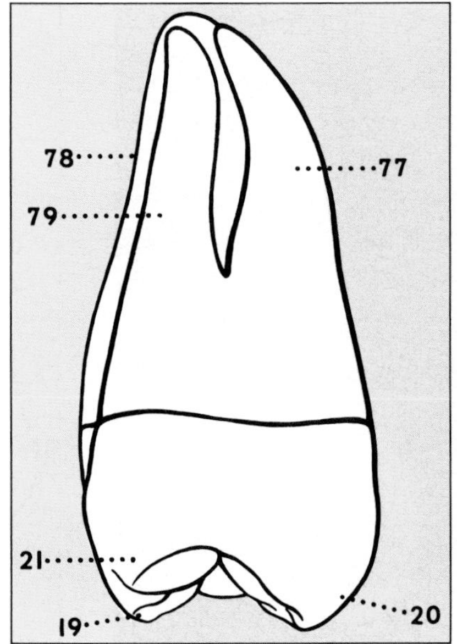

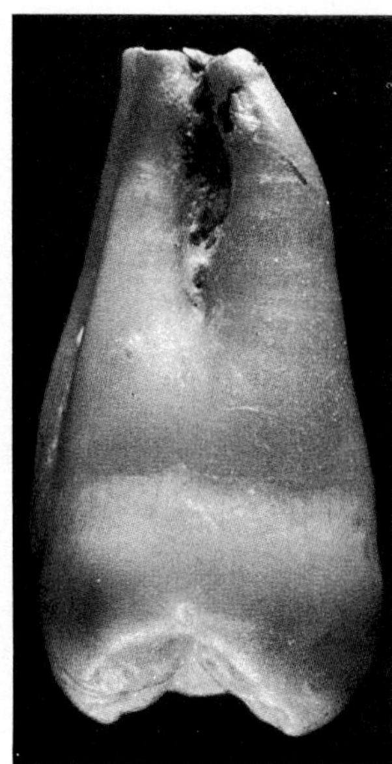

Figure 5.35
Maxillary left third molar (distal aspect).

The roots are invariably short (type trait) and the crown profiles may be quite irregular.

Distal Aspect (Fig. 5.35)

In the maxillary third molar the DL cusp is absent (type trait), the DB cusp is reduced in size (type trait), and more of the occlusal surface is visible than in the other molars (type trait).

Occlusal Aspect (Fig. 5.36)

Since the DL cusp is generally absent in the maxillary third molar, the crown profile assumes a triangular or heart-shaped outline (type trait). The DB cusp is now of minimal size (type trait). The occlusal surface is the smallest in area of the three maxillary molars (type trait). The oblique ridge, if not entirely absent, is barely visible at best (type trait). The pit-groove pattern is extremely variable and consists of numerous supplemental grooves.

Pulp (Fig. 5.37)

A mesiodistal section of the maxillary third molar shows a pulp chamber with a large mesiobuccal horn and a very diminutive distobuccal horn that appears to bulge off the side of the other horn. In buccolingual section the pulp cavity resembles an inverted carpet

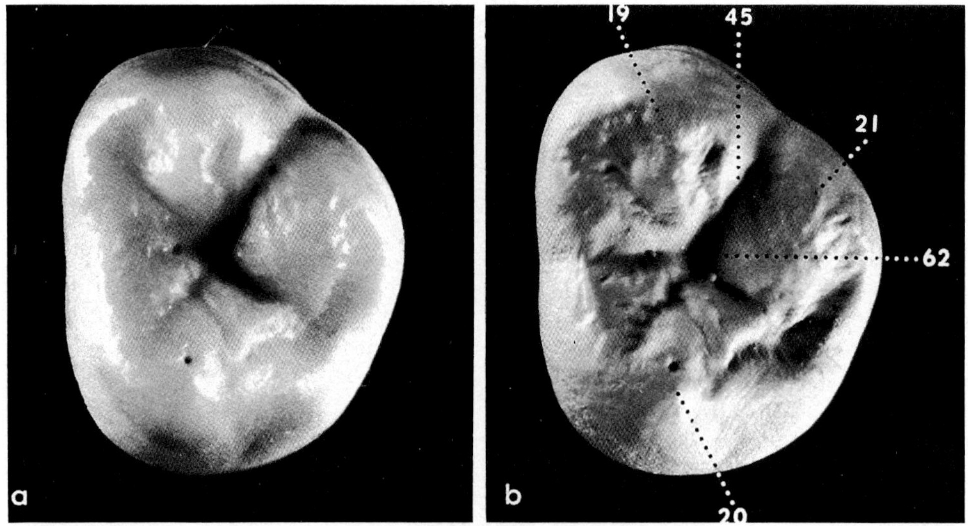

Figure 5.36
Maxillary left third molar (occlusal aspect): *a*, actual crown; *b*, cast.

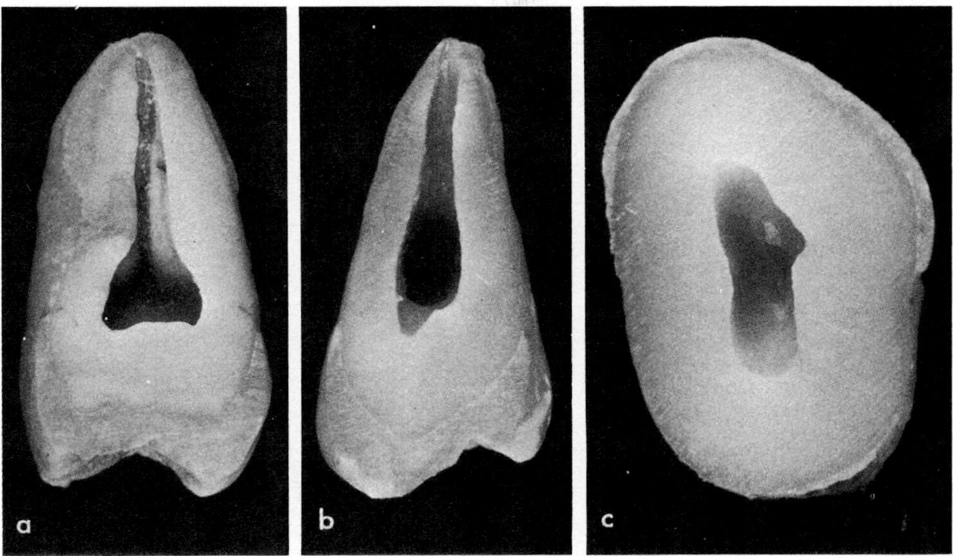

Figure 5.37
Pulp cavity of the left third molar: *a*, buccolingual section; *b*, mesiodistal section; *c*, transverse section at the cervix.

tack. The mesiobuccal and lingual pulp horns are widely separated and of equal prominence. In transverse section the pulp chamber is generally ovoid in shape, being narrow in the mesiodistal axis.

Variations

The third molars, mandibular and maxillary, are the most unpredictable teeth in the human dentition. They may fail to form at all (congenital absence) or, having completed their crown development, fail to erupt (impaction). Their time of eruption is highly irregular, some erupting as early as 16 years, others at 30 years or even later. Morphologically they run almost the whole gamut of possible molar types, including root and crown. They may have one, two, or three roots, or all three may be fused (Fig. 5.38*a*, *b*, and *c*). They may exhibit a single cusp or as many as eight cusps. This extreme range of variability applies mainly to Caucasians. Among the primitive peoples of the world the third molars are more regular in their development, time of eruption (about 18 years), and structure. Examples of oddly shaped third molars are presented in Figure 5.39.

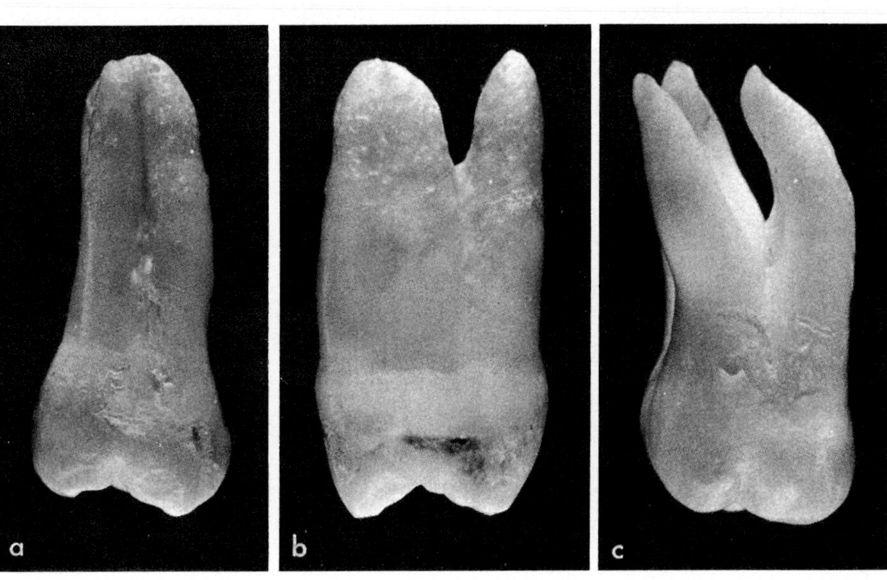

Figure 5.38
Root variations, maxillary third molars: *a*, single root (buccal aspect); *b*, two roots (mesial aspect); *c*, three roots (buccal aspect).

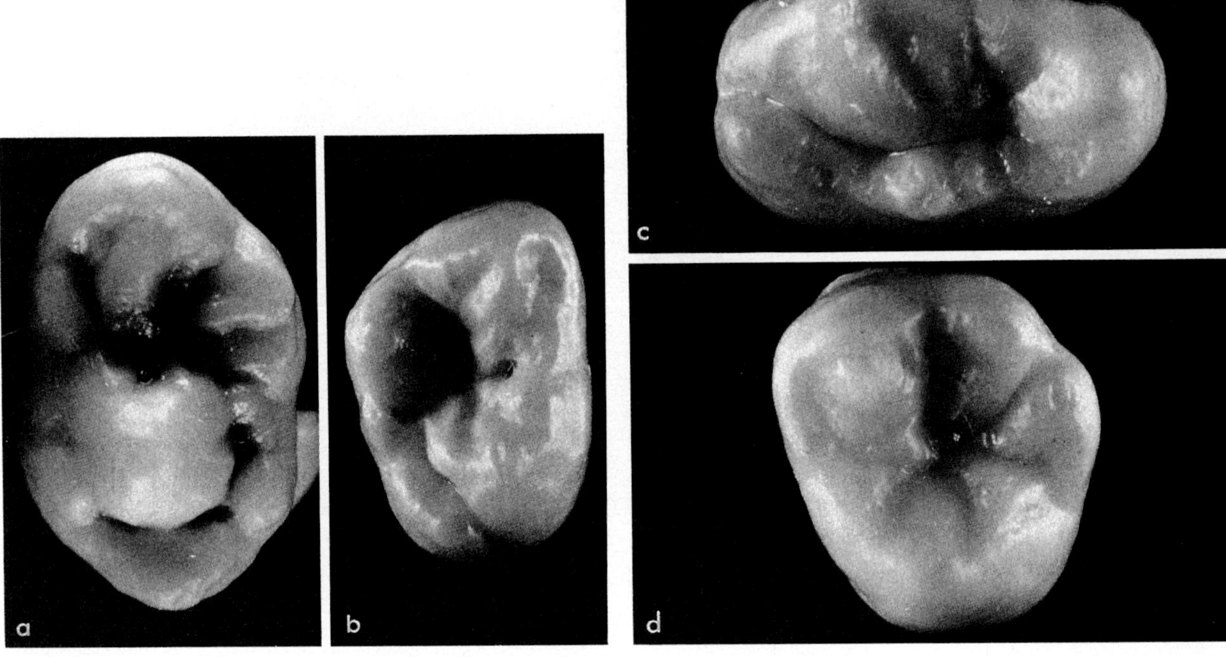

Figure 5.39
Variations in crown form, maxillary third molars (occlusal aspect).

Summary

Maxillary Molars—Arch Traits

1. There are generally three roots, two buccal and one lingual.
2. Generally there are three major cusps and a fourth of lesser size.
3. The crowns are always broader buccolingually than mesiodistally.
4. The distobuccal and mesiolingual cusps are, with few exceptions, connected by a ridge (the oblique ridge).
5. The mesiobuccal, distobuccal, and mesiolingual cusps are arranged in a tricuspate-triangular pattern.
6. The two buccal cusps are of unequal size, the MB being larger than the DB cusp.
7. The DL cusp is, at best, a minor elevation, and indeed may be greatly reduced or missing entirely.

Maxillary Molars—Type Traits

First Molar	Second Molar	Third Molar
Buccal Aspect		
Widest of the three Buccal cusps equal in height Apex of MB root directly in line with tip of MB cusp	Intermediate in width DB slightly shorter than MB MB root apex in line with center of crown	Smallest DB much shorter than MB Roots show pronounced distal inclination

First Molar	Second Molar	Third Molar
Lingual Aspect		
DL cusp largest of the three molars	DL cusp smaller in width and height	DL cusp usually missing
Lingual root wide mesiodistally	Lingual root narrower	Lingual root narrowest
Mesial Aspect		
Mesial marginal ridge tubercles numerous and pronounced	Mesial marginal ridge tubercles less numerous and less pronounced	Mesial marginal ridge tubercles absent
MB and lingual roots project beyond adjacent crown profiles	MB and lingual roots much less divergent	MB and lingual roots fused
Occlusal Aspect		
Crown outline square to rhomboidal	Rhomboidal form more pronounced in crown outline	Triangular or heart-shaped crown outline
Oblique ridge prominent	Oblique ridge smaller	Oblique ridge barely visible or absent
Large talon	Medium talon	Talon vestigial

The Mandibular Molars

Size and Eruption

Mandibular Molars	Crown Height (mm)	Mesiodistal Crown Diameter (mm)	Labiolingual Crown Diameter (mm)	Tooth Length (mm)	Age at Eruption (yr)
First	7.5	11.0	10.5	21.5	6
Second	7.0	10.5	10.5	20.0	12
Third	7.0	10.0	9.5	18.0	18+

Three molars occupy the posterior segment of each mandibular quadrant. Like their maxillary antagonists, the mandibular molars show a progressive diminution in size posteriorly. This is a characteristically human trait, since the molars of nonhuman primates increase in size posteriorly.

There are certain arch traits that differentiate mandibular from maxillary molars: (1) mandibular molars generally have two roots, one mesial and one distal. The only other units of the dentition that have two roots (i.e., the premolars) have one buccal and one lingual; (2) generally there are four major cusps and often a fifth of lesser size; (3) the crowns are always broader mesiodistally than buccolingually; (4) mandibular molars are the only units in the dentition in which the two major lingual cusps are of approximately equal size; (5) the mesio- and distobuccal cusps are approximately equal in size.

The mandibular first molar along with its maxillary counterpart is usually the first *permanent* tooth to appear in the oral cavity. It erupts at approximately 6 years of age just distal to the second primary molar. The appearance of the first permanent molars in the dental arches of the 6-year-old child marks the beginning of the "mixed dentition" period in which both primary and permanent teeth are present in the dental arch at the same time.

The first molar may be considered the "anchor tooth" of the mandibular dentition and exhibits, from a morphological standpoint the basic features that characterize molars. It is usually a five-cusped tooth.

First Molar

Buccal Aspect (Fig. 5.40)

The crown of the first mandibular molar has the widest mesiodistal diameter of all the molars (type trait). The occlusal profile is made up of three cusps, MB, DB, and distal (type trait). The MB is the widest of

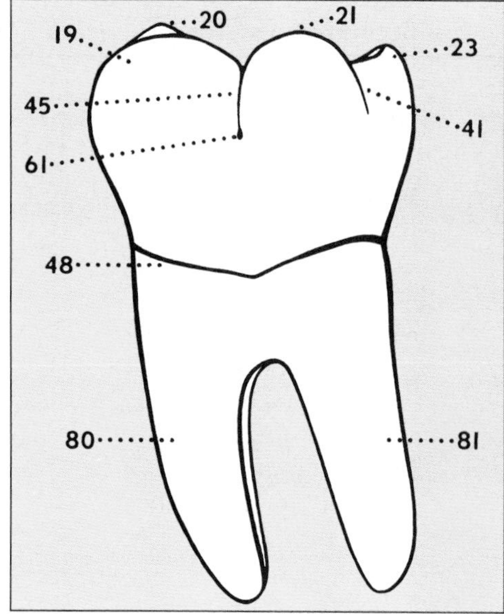

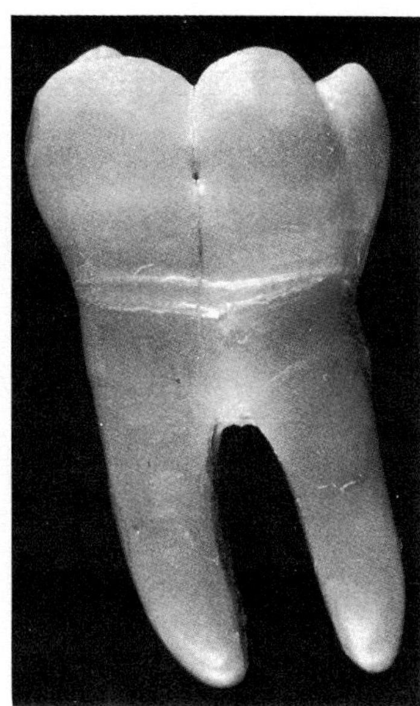

Figure 5.40

Mandibular left first molar (buccal aspect).

the three cusps and is followed in order of decreasing size by the DB and distal. The MB and DB cusps are approximately equal in height and are separated by the mesiobuccal groove. The distal cusp is much more conical in outline than the buccal cusps and occupies the extreme distobuccal corner of the crown. It is clearly demarcated from the DB cusp by the *distobuccal groove* (type trait).

The occlusal and middle thirds of the mesial profile are convex and the cervical third is concave. The entire distal crown profile is convex. Both mesial and distal crown profiles converge cervically. The cervical line is convex and extends, at its approximate midpoint, toward the root bifurcation in the form of a V-shaped point.

The cervical third of the crown consists of a bulbous prominence, the *buccal cervical ridge.* The rest of the buccal surface is relatively flat in the vertical plane. More or less prominent ridges extend cervically from the apices of the three buccal cusps. Two grooves run vertically down the buccal surface and demarcate the three buccal cusps (type trait). The *mesiobuccal groove* proceeds from the occlusal rim and ends approximately one-half of the way down the buccal surface in the *buccal pit.* The *distobuccal groove* separates the distobuccal and distal cusps and extends most of the length of the buccal surface.

Two roots, mesial and distal, are visible from the buccal aspect. They are widely separated (type trait) but share a common root base. A shallow depression, extending vertically down the midline of the root base, marks the beginning of the two roots. The mesial root runs almost straight vertically from the root base for almost half of its length, then curves toward the distal. Its apex lies almost directly in line with the tip of the MB cusp (type trait). The distal root shows little if any curvature and projects distally from the root base.

Lingual Aspect (Fig. 5.41)

Two cusps of equal size, ML and DL, constitute the occlusal profile of the first molar. They are clearly separated by a V-shaped notch, the *lingual groove.* The lingual cusps are noticeably higher and more conical than the buccal cusps. The apices of the two buccal cusps are visible in the background.

The greatest mesiodistal crown diameter is on the buccal aspect; accordingly, the buccal crown profiles and portions of the proximal surfaces are visible from the lingual aspect (type trait). The mesial and distal profiles of the lingual portion of the crown are both convex except for a slightly flattened or concave area just above the cervical line. Both profiles show a marked convergence cervically, and the mesiodistal crown width at the cervix is far less than its maximum diameter at the level of the contact areas (type trait).

The occlusal and middle thirds of the lingual surface are convex in both the vertical and horizontal planes, with the exception of that part of the surface in the region of the lingual groove, which is quite flat. The lingual groove is a shallow depression that extends down the lingual surface for a short distance and divides it into two moieties. The cervical third of the lingual surface, in contrast to the corresponding area of the buccal surface, is flat or concave.

A shallow depression reaches vertically down the root from the midpoint of the cervical line and marks the origin of the two roots. The lingual widths of the mesial and distal roots are less than their buccal widths. Accordingly, their proximal surfaces are vis-

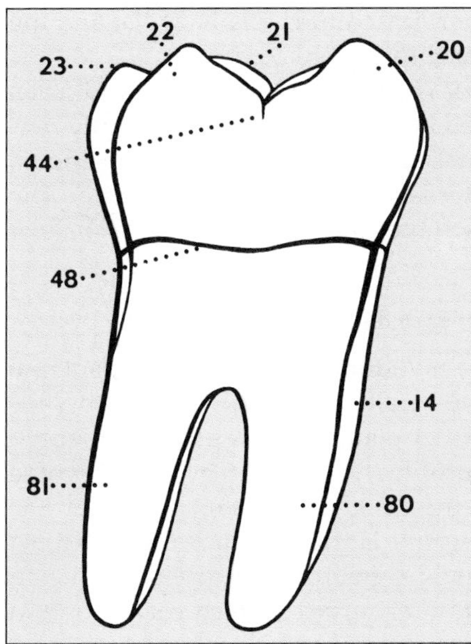

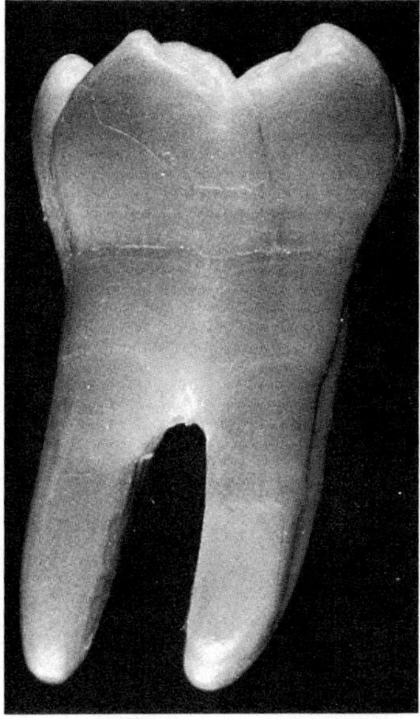

Figure 5.41
Mandibular left first molar (lingual aspect).

ible from the lingual aspect. The mesial root is marked by a deep concavity that extends vertically down the entire length of the mesial surface. A slight depression marks the corresponding surface of the distal root.

Mesial Aspect (Fig. 5.42)

Two cusps of unequal height, MB and ML, make up the occlusal profile of the mesial aspect of the mandibular first molar. The ML cusp is slightly higher than the MB, and both display prominent triangular ridges, extending toward the center of the occlusal surface. Just below the triangular ridges of the mesial cusps the mesial marginal ridge can be seen. It is a prominent crest and is marked, just lingual to its approximate midpoint, by a slight V-shaped notch, the *mesial marginal groove.*

The buccal profile is marked by a slight bulge in the cervical third that represents the *buccal cervical ridge,* which encircles the entire buccal surface. Above the ridge the buccal profile slopes sharply lingually to the MB cusp apex. This trait is common to all mandibular posterior teeth and distinguishes them from their maxillary antagonists.

The lingual profile is flat in its cervical third and uniformly convex to the apex of the ML cusp. The height of contour is located higher on the crown than on the buccal aspect, namely at the junction of the

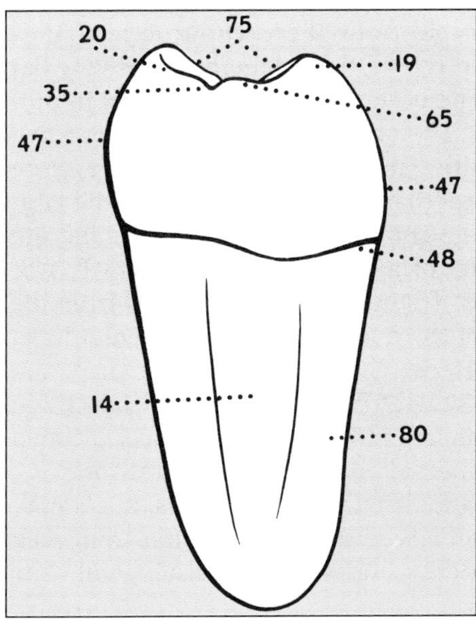

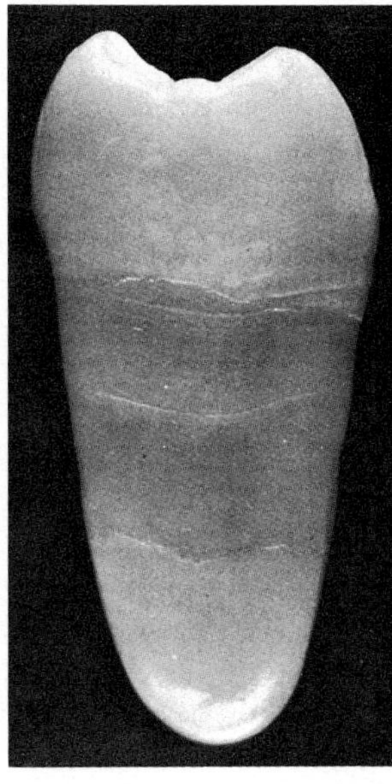

Figure 5.42
Mandibular left first molar (mesial aspect).

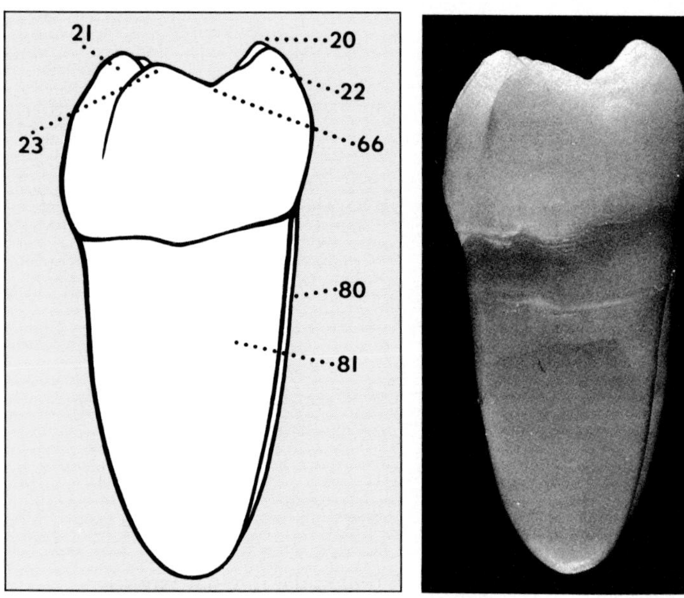

Figure 5.43
Mandibular left first molar (distal aspect).

middle and occlusal thirds. The cervical line is only slightly convex.

The mesial surface may be flat or concave in its cervical third and highly convex in its middle and occlusal thirds.

The mesial root is the broadest (buccolingually) of all the molars (type trait) and has a blunt apex. It is marked by a broad shallow concavity, the *proximal root concavity*, running longitudinally down the root surface for most of its length.

Distal Aspect (Fig. 5.43)

Three cusps are seen in occlusal profile of the mandibular first molar: the DB, distal, and DL. The DL cusp is the largest of the three and is followed in order of decreasing size by the DB and distal. The small distal cusp is situated lingual to the DB cusp and is separated from the latter by the *distobuccal groove* which extends approximately halfway down the buccal surface. A flattened or concave area lies just below the end of the groove. The distal marginal ridge is shorter than the mesial marginal ridge and has a V-shaped notch at its midpoint, the *distal marginal groove*. At least half of the buccal surface is visible from the distal aspect. The lingual profile, relatively flat in its cervical third, is highly convex in the middle and occlusal thirds. The cervical line is almost straight buccolingually.

The distal surface of the crown is far narrower buccolingually than the mesial surface. Almost half of the distal surface is made up of the distal cusp (type trait). The cervical third is relatively flat and the middle and occlusal thirds are convex.

The distal root is broad buccolingually and has a somewhat blunted apex (type trait). It is slightly narrower than the mesial root, however, and the lingual profile of the latter is visible in the background. The surface of the distal root may be marked by a shallow depression.

Occlusal Aspect (Fig. 5.44)

The crown of the mandibular first molar is pentagonal in outline (type trait). The total buccal profile is made of two distinct planes and is greater in length than the lingual profile (type trait). The mesial profile is far wider than the distal (Fig. 5.45).

The buccal profile is divided into three distinct and separate convex segments by two V-shaped constrictions of the buccal surface, which correspond in position to the mesiobuccal and distobuccal grooves. The buccal profile is most prominent in the region of the DB cusp, and the maximum buccolingual diameter of the crown is located just distal to the mesiobuccal groove (type trait). The buccal and mesial profiles meet in the form of a sharply defined angle (the *mesiobuccal angle*). The junction between buccal and distal profiles, on the other hand, is rounded and ill-defined. The mesial and distal profiles are relatively straight lines (type trait) and show a marked lingual convergence (type trait). The lingual profile forms a straight line which is interrupted at its midpoint by the *lingual groove*.

At least two-thirds of the buccal surface is visible from the occlusal aspect, a trait that is characteristic of all mandibular posterior teeth and serves to differentiate them from their maxillary counterparts. Prominent buccal ridges extend cervically from the apices of the three buccal cusps.

The occlusal third is the only portion of the lingual surface visible from the occlusal aspect. It is highly convex in the vertical plane but relatively flat mesiodistally. The occlusal table is hexagonal in outline (type trait). The occlusal surface consists of five cusps (type trait). The two lingual cusps are more pointed or conical than the others. They are the largest in terms of height and width (type trait) and are followed in order of decreasing size by the MB, DB, and distal cusps. Triangular ridges descend from the apices of each of the five cusps toward the middle of the occlusal surface. Those of the mesial cusps are directed almost straight buccolingually, whereas those of the other three are more or less obliquely inclined toward the geometric center of the occlusal surface.

The mesial and distal marginal ridges, in general, converge lingually (type trait). They differ from each other in prominence and width (buccolingual). The

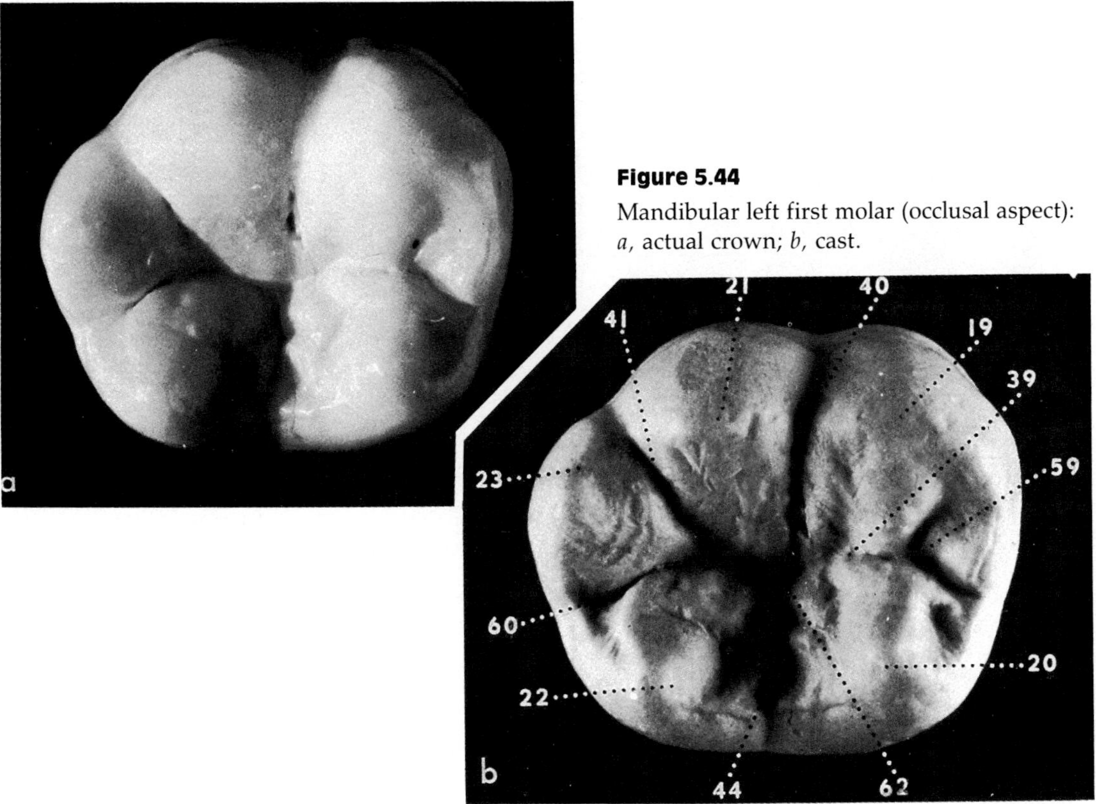

Figure 5.44
Mandibular left first molar (occlusal aspect): *a*, actual crown; *b*, cast.

mesial marginal ridge is a relatively wide, prominent elevation. The distal marginal ridge, on the other hand, is noticeably shorter and less prominent in height. Both ridges are interrupted at their midpoints by grooves that radiate from the occlusal surface.in the form of spillways.

The occlusal surface is marked by three distinct fossae: (1) a broad, relatively deep valley in the central area of the occlusal surface; (the *central fossa*); (2) a shallow triangle-shaped depression just within the confines of the mesial marginal ridge (the *mesial triangular fossa*); and (3) a slight depression just mesial to the central portion of the distal marginal ridge (the *distal triangular fossa*).

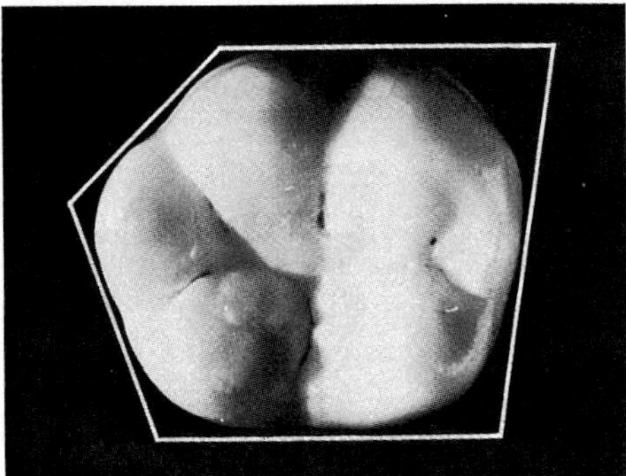

Figure 5.45
Pentagonal outline of crown, mandibular left first molar (occlusal aspect).

The five cusps of the occlusal surface are well set off by a distinctive pit-groove pattern. The *central groove* extends across the center of the occlusal surface and terminates in the *mesial* and *distal pits*. At the approximate midpoint of the occlusal surface the central groove is intersected by the *lingual* and *mesiobuccal grooves*. The lingual groove separates the triangular ridges of the two lingual cusps and continues on to the lingual surface. The mesiobuccal groove separates the MB and DB cusps and extends onto the buccal surface. The point of intersection of the central, mesiobuccal, and lingual grooves is marked by the *central pit*. Just distal to the central pit, the *distobuccal groove* (which divides the distal and DB cusps) intersects the central groove. The two buccal grooves and the lingual groove appear to form a Y in the central portion of the occlusal surface (type trait).

In addition to the main grooves described above, several supplemental grooves radiate from the mesial and distal pits. For example, two grooves are usually found in the region of the mesial pit, one extending toward the mesiobuccal corner of the crown, the other crossing the mesial marginal ridge.

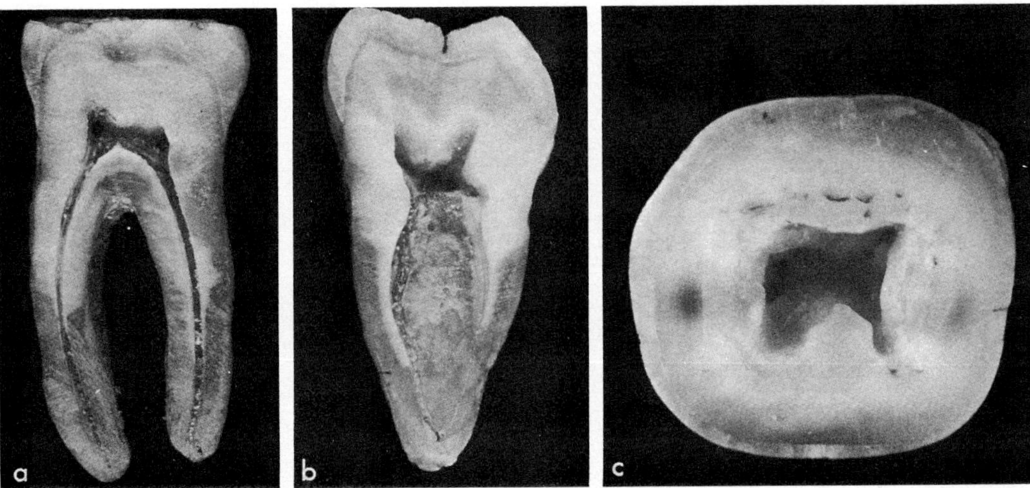

Figure 5.46
Pulp cavity of the mandibular left first molar: *a*, mesiodistal section; *b*, buccolingual section; *c*, transverse section.

Pulp (Fig. 5.46)

In the mandibular first molar two horns are seen in mesiodistal section: a mesiobuccal and a distobuccal. The former is invariably the larger. The two root canals are very narrow and follow the pincer-like shape of the mesial and distal roots. The buccolingual section likewise shows two horns, a mesiolingual and a mesiobuccal, the former being the larger. Although only one root can be seen in this view, there are usually two root canals (in the mesial root only). The pulp chamber itself is relatively small in comparison with the height of the two horns. In transverse section the pulp chamber is almost rectangular, the mesial and the distal boundaries being of equal length.

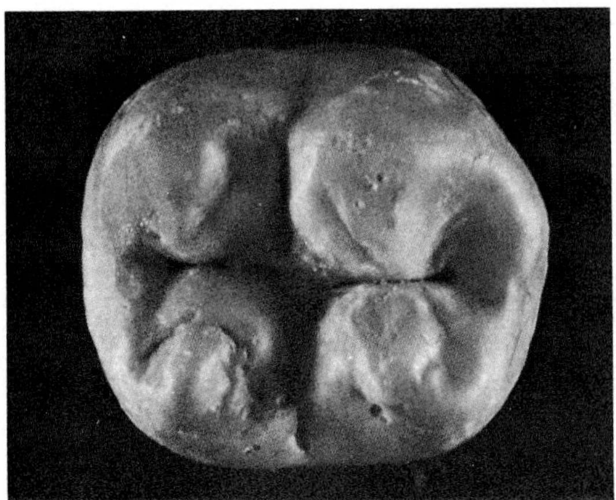

Figure 5.47
Absence of distal cusp, mandibular left first molar (occlusal aspect).

Variations

Mandibular first molars usually exhibit five cusps. However, sometimes the distal cusp may be missing entirely (Fig. 5.47). The structure is then markedly similar to that of the second molar. However, the four-cusped first molar may be distinguished from the second in that the widths (buccolingual) of trigonid (mesial portion) and talonid (distal portion) are approximately equal.

The *buccal pit* usually marks the cervical termination of the mesiobuccal groove. It may be a slight, almost undiscernible depression (Fig. 5.48*a*), a moderately conspicuous concavity (Fig. 5.48*b*), or a large deep pit in the middle of the buccal surface (Fig. 5.48*c*).

Two accessory cusps, the tuberculum sextum (C_6) and the tuberculum intermedium (C_7), may be present on the occlusal surface of mandibular molars. The *tuberculum sextum* (C_6) is located on the distal marginal ridge midway between the distal and DL cusps. It is believed to be of higher frequency in Mongoloid populations, and when present may vary greatly in size (Fig. 5.49).

Tuberculum intermedium (C_7) occurs characteristically as a small elevation on the distal ridge of the mesiolingual cusp (Fig. 5.50) or as a relatively prominent eminence on the lingual rim of the crown between the ML and DL cusps. Tuberculum interme-

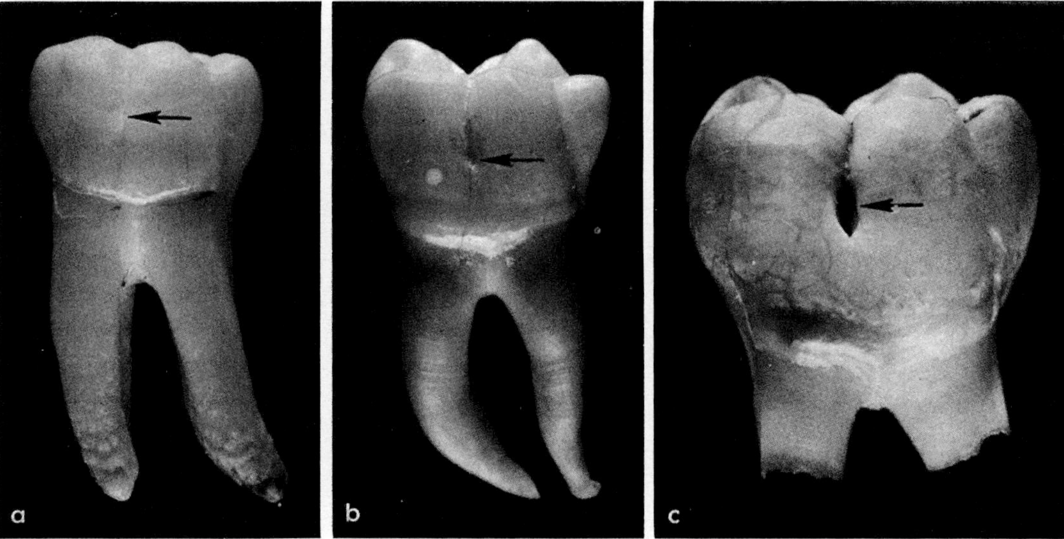

Figure 5.48

Variations in the buccal pit (*arrows*), mandibular left first molar (buccal aspect): *a,* slight depression; *b,* moderate fissure; *c,* wide pit.

dium is found in relatively high frequency among Negroid populations.

As with all other teeth the mandibular first molar may show a wide range of variation in size, inclination, number, and curvature of roots. Extreme curvature of the mesial root is particularly common (Fig. 5.51*a*), as are variations in the inclination and size of the distal root (Fig. 5.51*b*). The mesial root is frequently of unusual buccolingual width (Fig. 5.51*c*) and not uncommonly exhibits a "bifurcation" in its apical third (Fig. 5.51*d*). A comparatively rare root variation is the supernumerary distal root (Fig. 5.51*e*), which may be highly variable with regard to size and/or inclination.

Second Molar

Buccal Aspect (Fig. 5.52)

Four features of the buccal aspect differ in the mandibular second molar as compared with the first: (1) the second molar is smaller than the first but larger

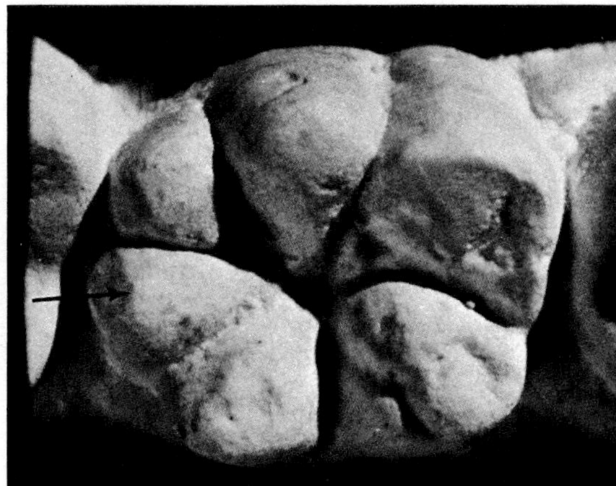

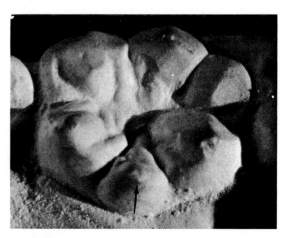

Figure 5.49

The tuberculum sextum (C_6) (*arrow*), mandibular left first molar (occlusal aspect).

Figure 5.50

Tuberculum intermedium (C_7) (*arrow*), mandibular left first molar (occlusal aspect).

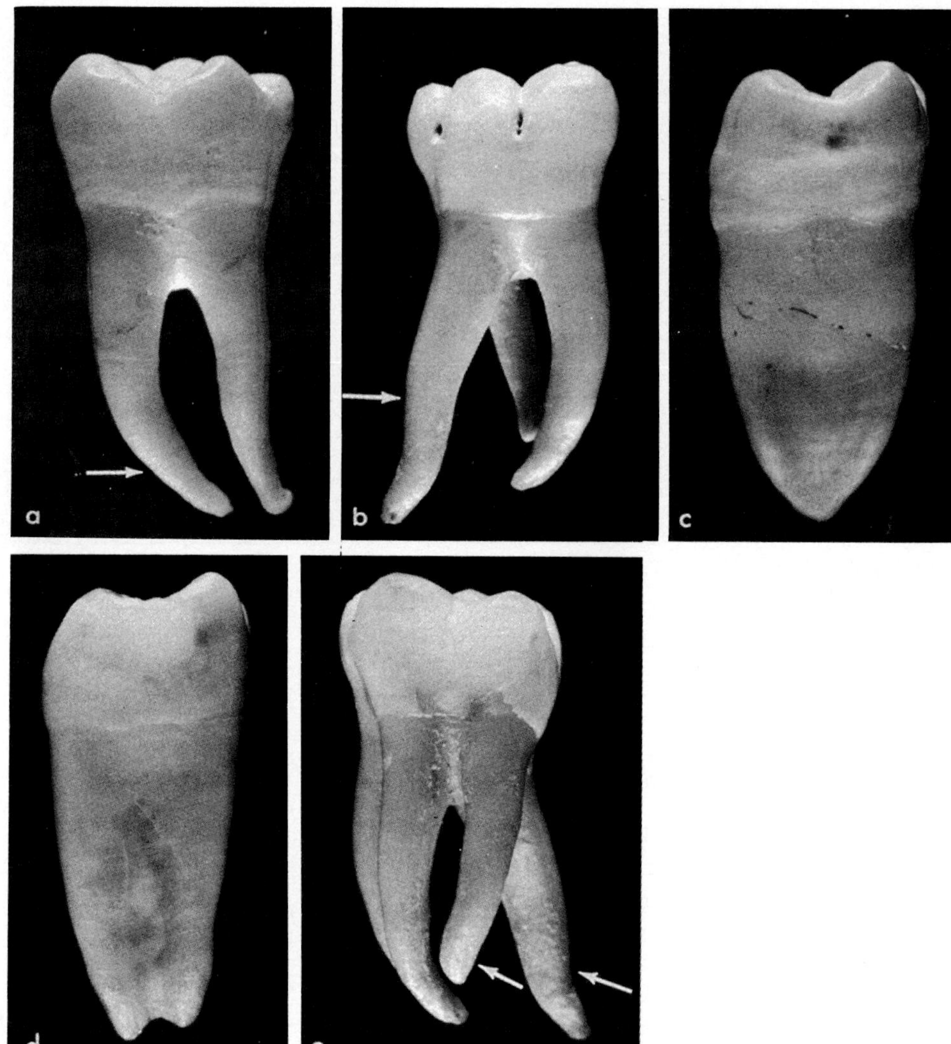

Figure 5.51

Variations in root morphology (*arrows*), mandibular first molar: *a*, extreme curvature of mesial root, right first molar (lingual aspect); *b*, long curved distal root, right first molar (buccal aspect); *c*, extreme buccolingual width of mesial root, right first molar (mesial aspect); *d*, bifurcation of mesial root in apical thirds, right first molar (mesial aspect); *e*, supernumerary distal root, right first molar (lingual aspect).

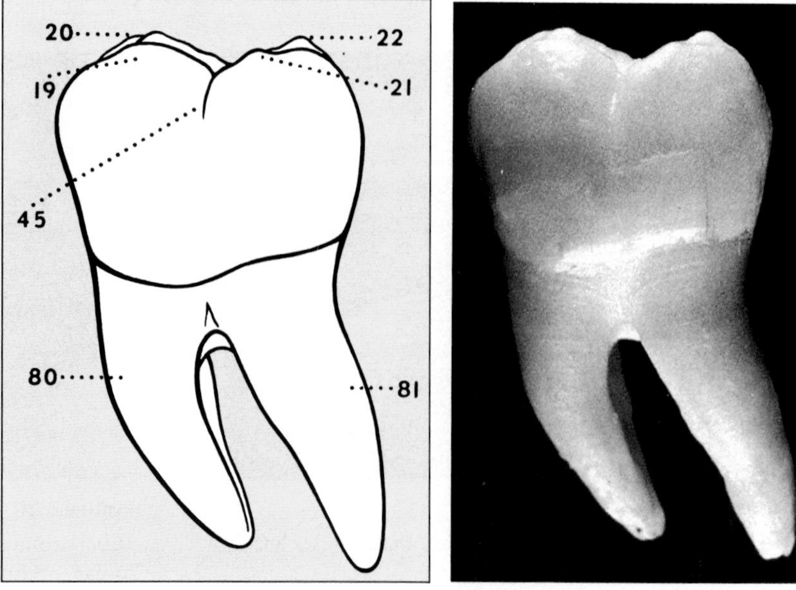

Figure 5.52

Mandibular left second molar (buccal aspect).

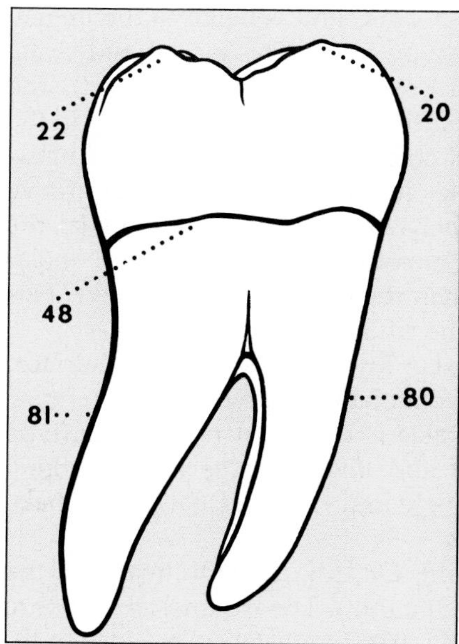

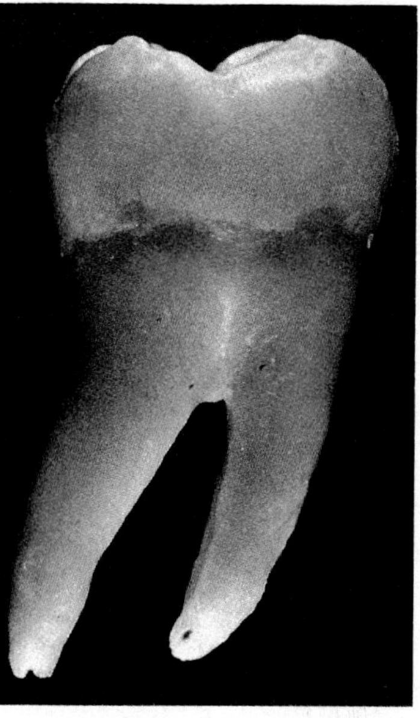

Figure 5.53
Mandibular left second molar (lingual aspect).

than the third in all dimensions (type trait); (2) in occlusal profile two cusps are prominent, MB and DB (type trait); (3) a *single* groove marks the buccal surface and separates the two cusps (type trait); (4) the roots are usually much closer together and show a greater distal inclination (type trait).

Lingual Aspect (Fig. 5.53)

This molar is differentiated from the first by four features: (1) the crown is noticeably shorter occlusocervically (type trait); (2) little if any of the mesial and distal surfaces are visible from the lingual aspect (type trait); (3) the mesial and distal crown profiles show far less cervical convergence (type trait); (4) the roots have a more pronounced distal inclination (type trait).

Mesial Aspect (Fig. 5.54)

The mesial aspect of the second molar crown closely resembles that of the first molar; in fact the crown profiles of the two are nearly identical. The root, however, is narrower than that of the first and forms a relatively sharp apex (type trait).

Distal Aspect (Fig. 5.55)

The following characteristics are peculiar to the second mandibular molar: (1) the distal cusp is missing (type trait); (2) far less of the buccal surface is visible

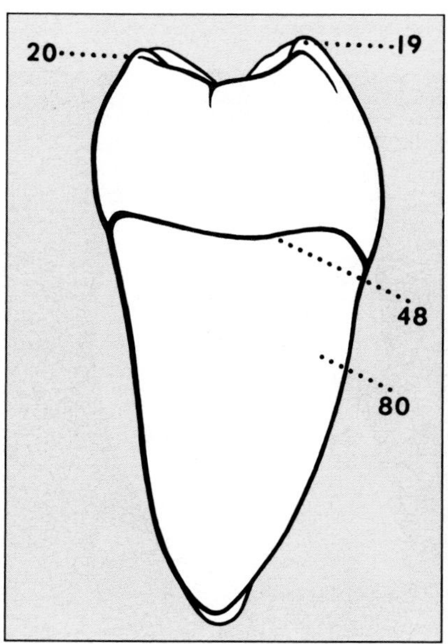

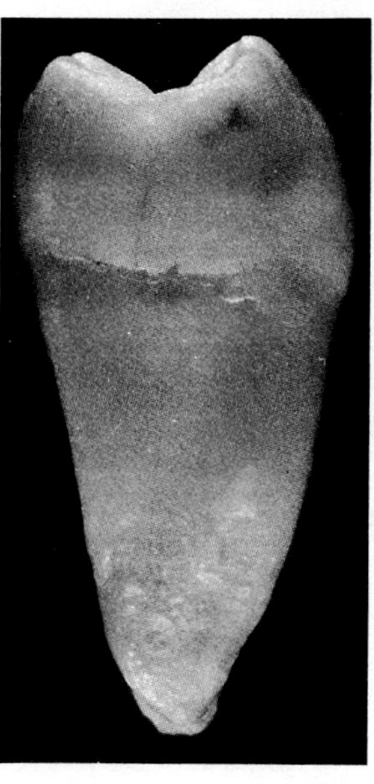

Figure 5.54
Mandibular left second molar (mesial aspect).

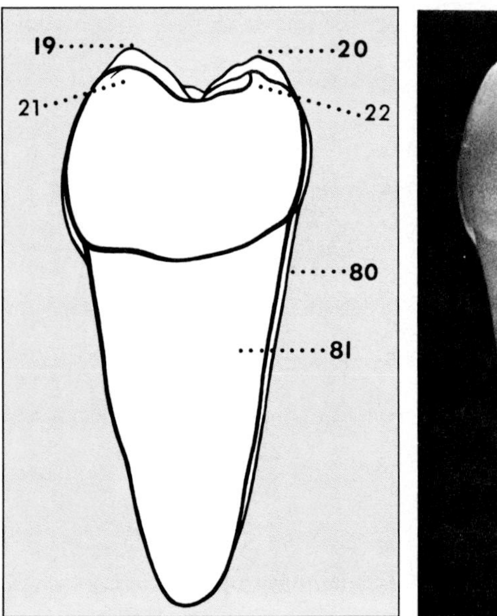

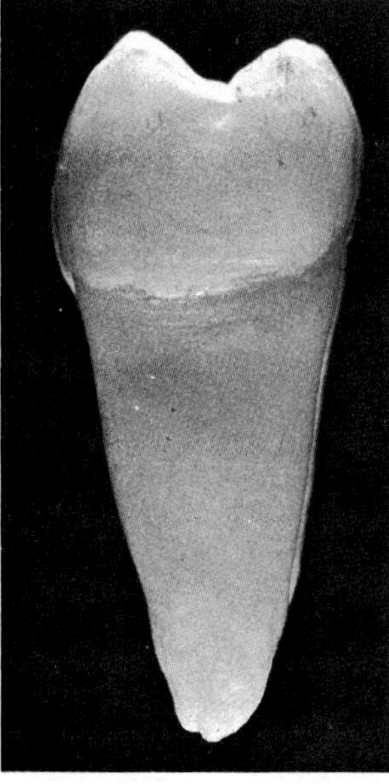

Figure 5.55
Mandibular left second molar (distal aspect).

from the distal aspect; (3) the distal surface is almost as large in area as the mesial surface (type trait); (4) the distal root is much narrower buccolingually than the first molar and has a pointed tip (type trait).

Occlusal Aspect (Fig. 5.56)

The crown of the mandibular second molar is rectangular in outline (type trait). The buccal profile lies in a single plane (type trait) and is equal to the lingual profile in width (type trait). The mesial and distal profiles are likewise similar in width (type trait). The most prominent portion of the buccal profile is in the region of the MB cusp; the maximum buccolingual crown diameter lies just mesial to the buccal groove (type trait). In other words, in the second molar the trigonid (mesial moiety of the mandibular molar crown) is wider than the talonid (distal moiety). This is the reverse of the situation in the first molar.

A single buccal groove crosses the buccal surface, dividing it into two moieties (type trait).

The occlusal table is rectangular in outline (type trait). The buccal and lingual cusps form the long sides of the rectangle and the marginal ridges make up the short sides.

Four cusps, MB, DB, ML, and DL, make up the occlusal surface (type trait). The two mesial cusps are wider mesiodistally than the distal cusps (type trait).

In contrast to the first molar, the mesial and distal marginal ridges of the second extend in a straight buccolingual direction with little if any convergence lingually (type trait). The mesial marginal ridge is slightly wider buccolingually. Neither ridge is crossed by a marginal groove.

The occlusal surface of the second molar is marked by the same kind of depressions seen in the first molar: the central, mesial triangular, and distal triangular fossae. The pit-groove pattern differs, however, in that a single *buccal groove* separates the

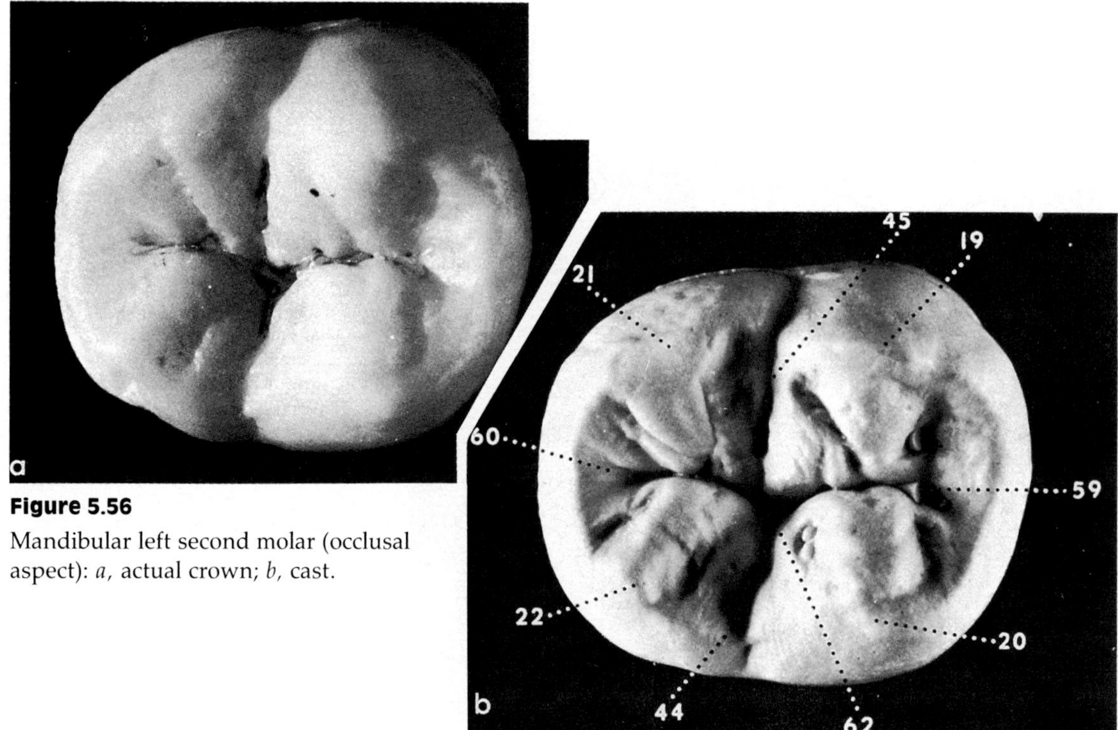

Figure 5.56
Mandibular left second molar (occlusal aspect): *a*, actual crown; *b*, cast.

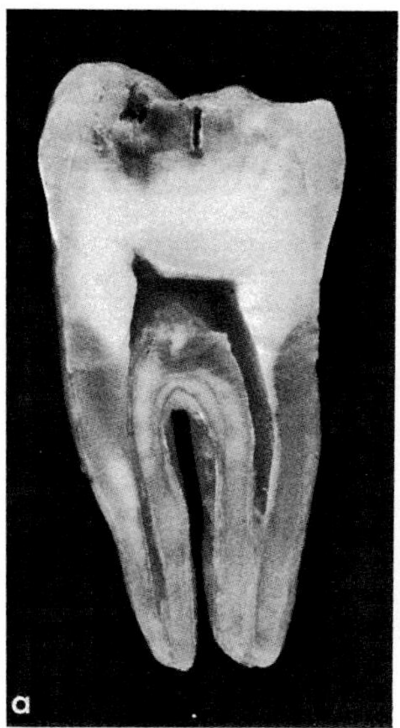

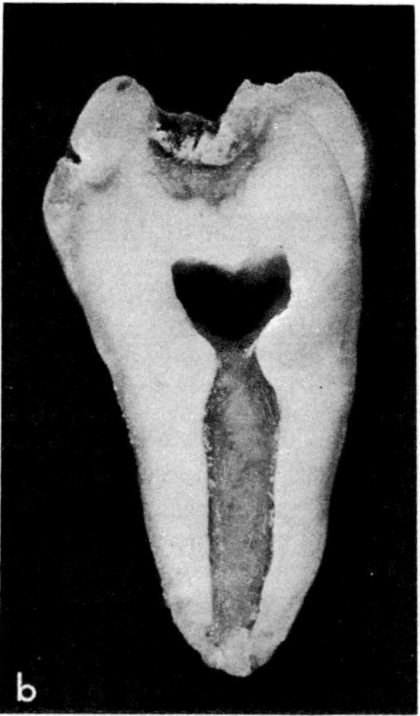

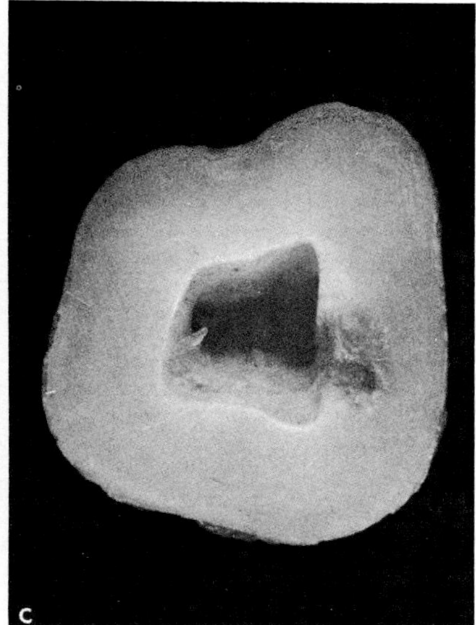

Figure 5.57

Pulp cavity of the mandibular left second molar: *a,* mesiodistal section; *b,* buccolingual section; *c,* transverse section.

two buccal cusps (type trait) and the buccal, lingual, and central grooves intersect in the middle of the occlusal surface to form the so-called "+4" pattern (type trait).* The groove pattern is complicated by the presence of numerous supplemental grooves radiating irregularly from the main ones.

Pulp (Fig. 5.57)

In mesiodistal section the outline of the pulp cavity of the second molar is similar to that of the first molar (Fig. 5.57*a*). In buccolingual section the paramount difference is in the single root canal seen in the mesial root (Fig. 5.57*b*), as compared with the double canal in the first molar. Another difference lies in the outline of the pulp chamber as seen in transverse section. The mesial dimension is considerably greater than the distal (Fig. 5.57*c*).

Variations

The five-cusp mandibular second molar is by no means uncommon (Fig. 5.58). Basically it is far more characteristic of Mongoloid and Negroid populations than Caucasoid. Its racial incidence is discussed at greater length in Section IV. The simplest expression of the distal cusp consists of slight bulge on the distobuccal corner of the crown (Fig. 5.59).

*The "+" refers to the groove pattern; the "4" refers to the number of cusps.

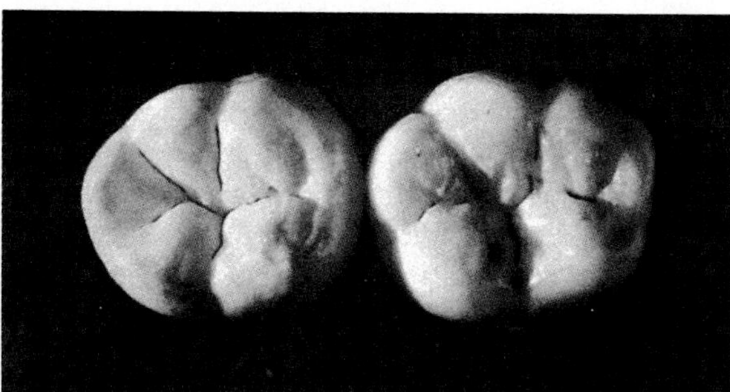

Figure 5.58

Mandibular left first and second molars (occlusal aspect), each showing five cusps.

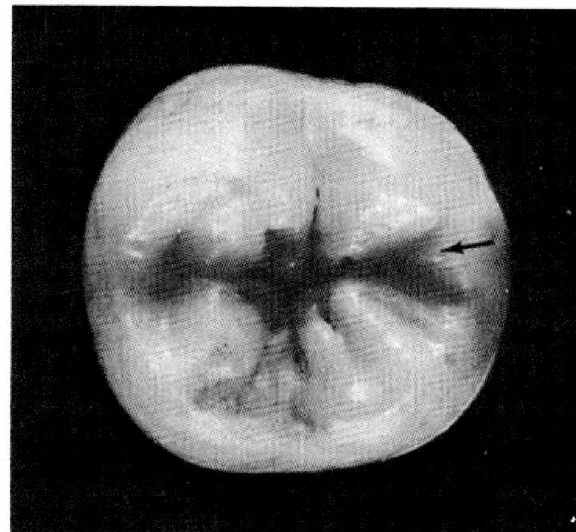

Figure 5.59

Minimal expression of distal cusp, mandibular right second molar (occlusal aspect).

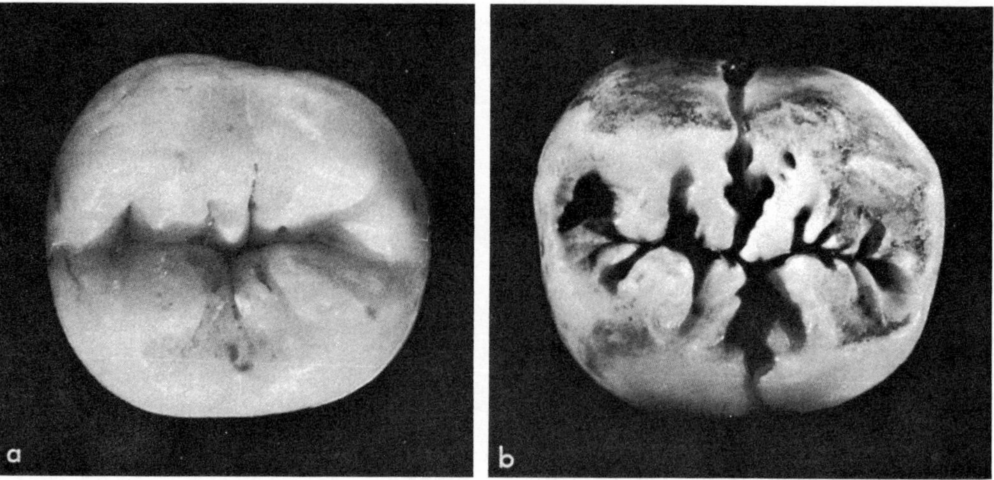

Figure 5.60

Variations in pit-groove pattern, mandibular right second molar (occlusal aspect): *a*, supplemental grooves parallel to triangular cusp ridges; *b*, crenulated appearance of occlusal surface.

There are occasionally supplementary grooves radiating from the main grooves and parallel to the triangular cusp ridges (Fig. 5.60*a*). These supplementary depressions may be both numerous and deep, imparting to the occlusal surface a crenulated appearance (Fig. 5.60*b*).

As in the first molar, a buccal pit of variable size and depth is frequently found.

The second molar may show a wide range of root variability. Usually the roots are narrower than those of the first molar and more distally inclined (Fig. 5.52), or they may be widely divergent with no distal

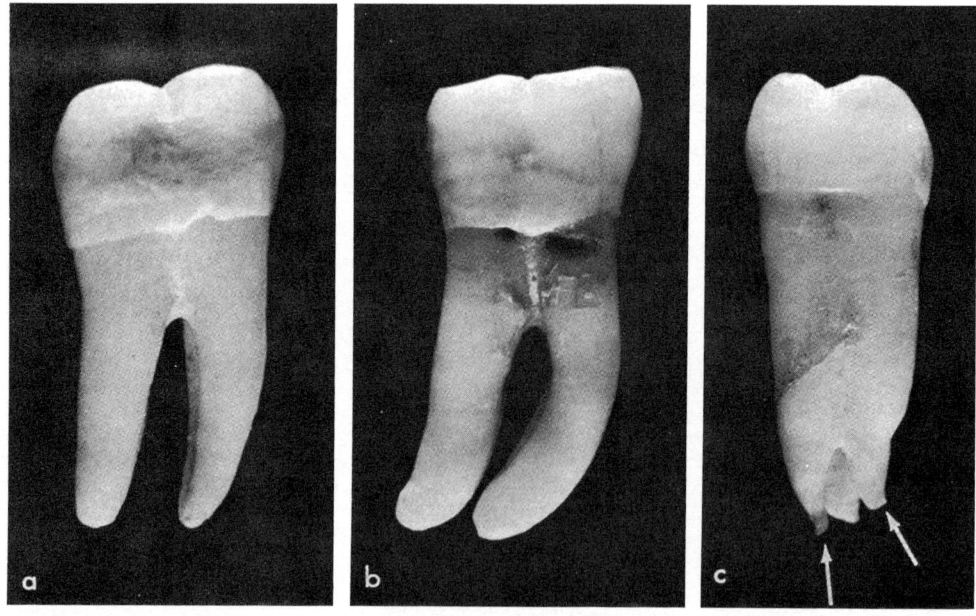

Figure 5.61

Variations in roots, mandibular second molar: *a*, widely divergent roots with no distal inclination, right second molar (buccal aspect); *b*, long roots with extreme distal inclination, right second molar (buccal aspect); *c*, bifid mesial root (*arrows*), right second molar (mesial aspect).

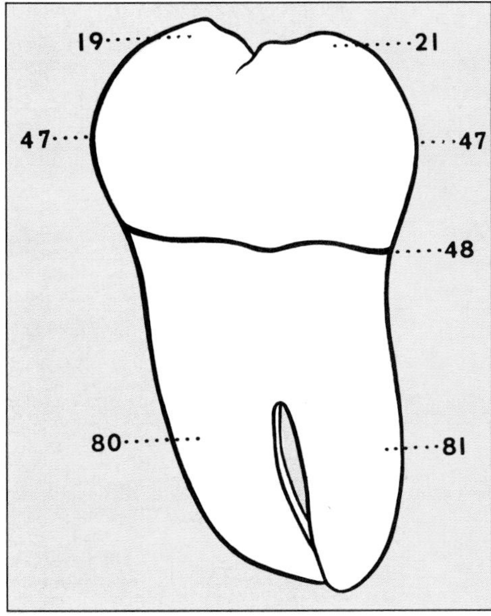

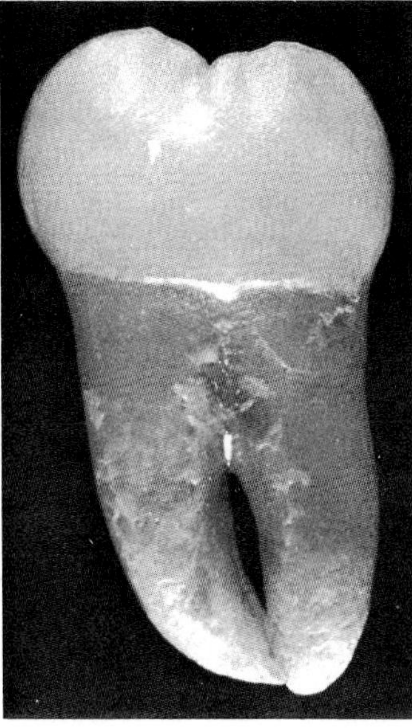

Figure 5.62
Mandibular left third molar (buccal aspect).

inclination (Fig. 5.61*a*). Frequently the roots are of unusual length with extreme distal inclination (Fig. 5.61*b*).

A common variation is the bifid or double apex of the mesial root (Fig. 5.61*c*). Extreme variations in length are also common.

Third Molar

Buccal Aspect (Fig. 5.62)

The crown of the third mandibular molar is so highly variable that it is impossible to identify constant characteristics. It may exhibit a high degree of morphological resemblance to the first or second molars. On the other hand, the crown may be readily identified by its short length and highly bulbous outline.

Possibly the most reliable distinguishing features are associated with the form and inclination of the roots. They are almost invariably short, fused, or compressed, and exhibit a marked distal inclination (type trait).

Lingual Aspect (Fig. 5.63)

The lingual aspect of the third molar may be hardly distinguishable from that of the first or second molars. On the other hand, it may be easily identified by irregularities, such as: (1) a short crown with a highly

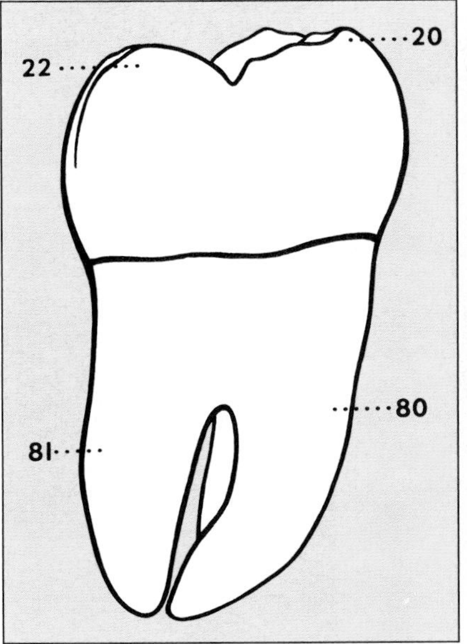

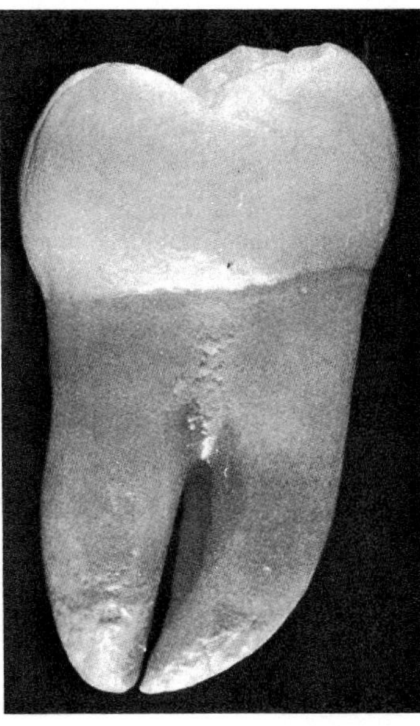

Figure 5.63
Mandibular left third molar (lingual aspect).

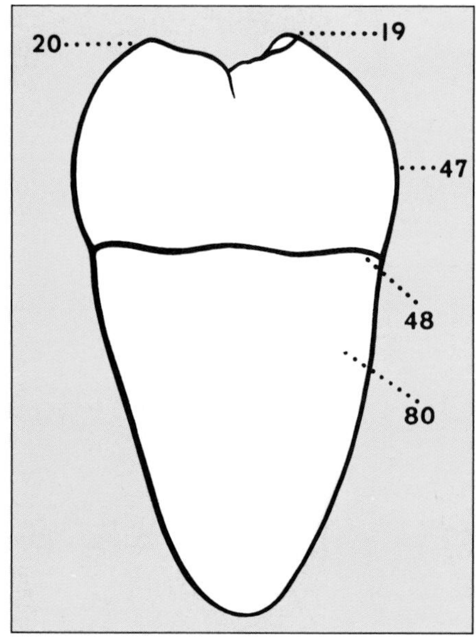

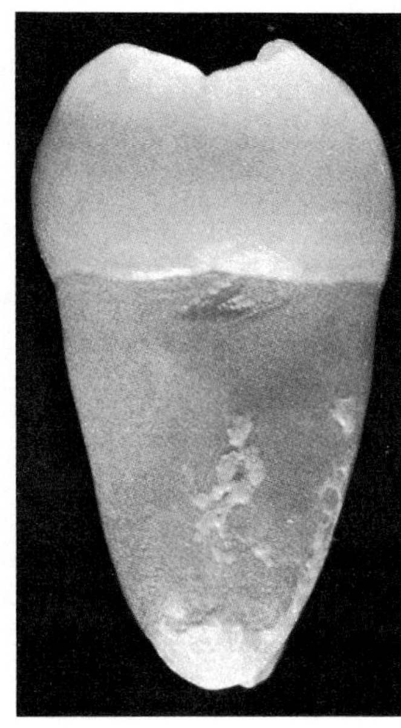

Figure 5.64
Mandibular left third molar (mesial aspect).

bulbous outline, (2) rounded cusps, and (3) short roots, close together or fused with a pronounced distal inclination.

Mesial Aspect (Fig. 5.64)

The crowns of mandibular third molars are often highly bulbous in outline. Both buccal and lingual crown profiles may be highly convex, with their respective heights of contour located in the middle third of the crown. In addition, the distance between the apices of buccal and lingual cusps is less than that of the first and second molars (type trait).

The mesial root is relatively broad buccolingually, but appears short compared with that of the first and second mandibular molars (type trait).

Distal Aspect (Fig. 5.65)

The distal outline of the mandibular third molar crown may be bulbous. The occlusal table is extremely constricted in area. Almost the entire buccal surface of the crown may be visible.

The distal root is usually the narrowest buccolingually and the shortest of all mandibular molar roots.

Occlusal Aspect (Fig. 5.66)

The mandibular third molar crown is often ovoid in outline.

The mesial moiety (trigonid) of the crown is much wider buccolingually than the distal portion

Figure 5.65
Mandibular left third molar (distal aspect).

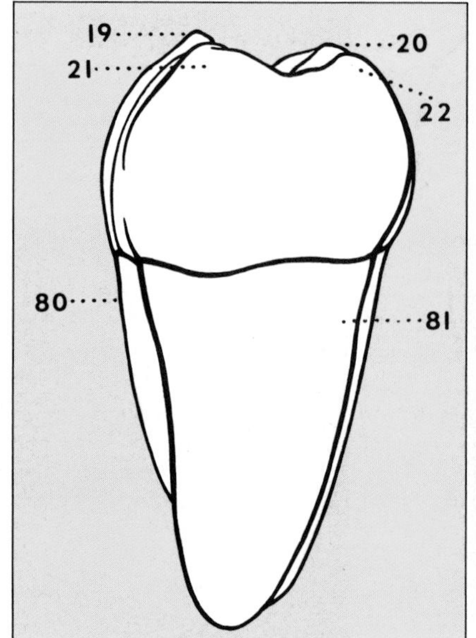

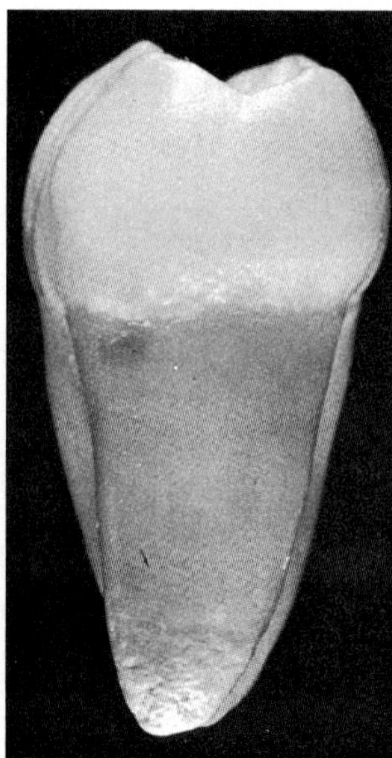

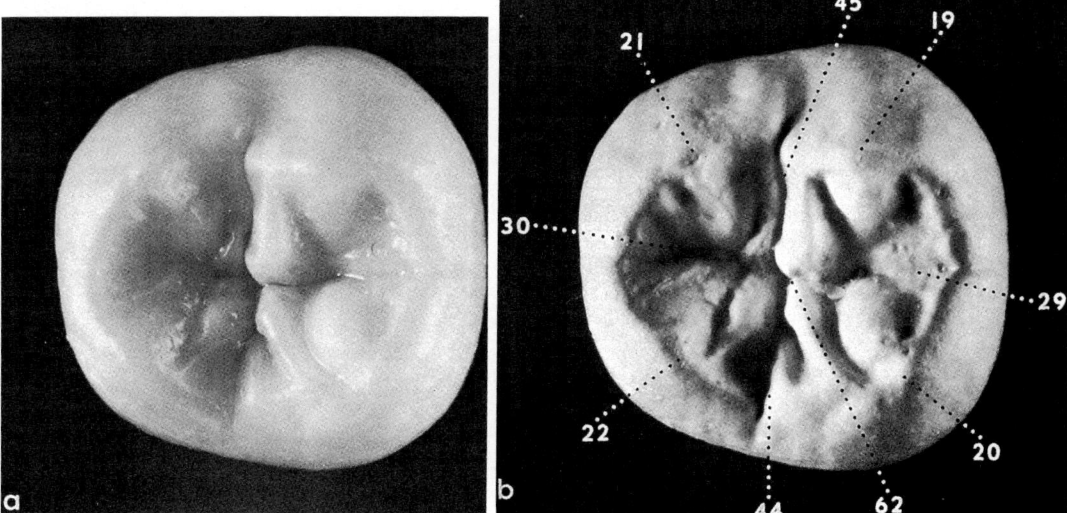

Figure 5.66
Mandibular left third molar (occlusal aspect): *a*, actual crown; *b*, cast.

(talonid). The more or less straight buccal and lingual profiles converge markedly toward the distal. Thus the trigonid is wider than the talonid, often to a greater degree than in the second molar.

The occlusal table is distinctly ovoid in outline (type trait). In addition it is highly constricted in area both buccolingually and mesiodistally relative to the total area of the crown as seen from the occlusal aspect (type trait).

There are generally four cusps, which are commonly narrow, irregular in form, and far less conical in shape when compared with the other molars.

The mesial and distal marginal ridges are not straight buccolingually but form highly convex arcs (type trait), which link the ridges of the buccal and lingual cusps.

The most distinctive feature of the occlusal surface is the irregularity of the pit-groove pattern (type trait). The main grooves are usually short in length and very irregular in direction. In addition, the entire occlusal surface is marked by numerous supplemental grooves, which are not unlike the *crenulations* seen on the occlusal surfaces of the molars of gorillas, chimpanzees, and orangutans.

Pulp (Fig. 5.67)

There is little difference between the second and third mandibular molars in all three types of sections.

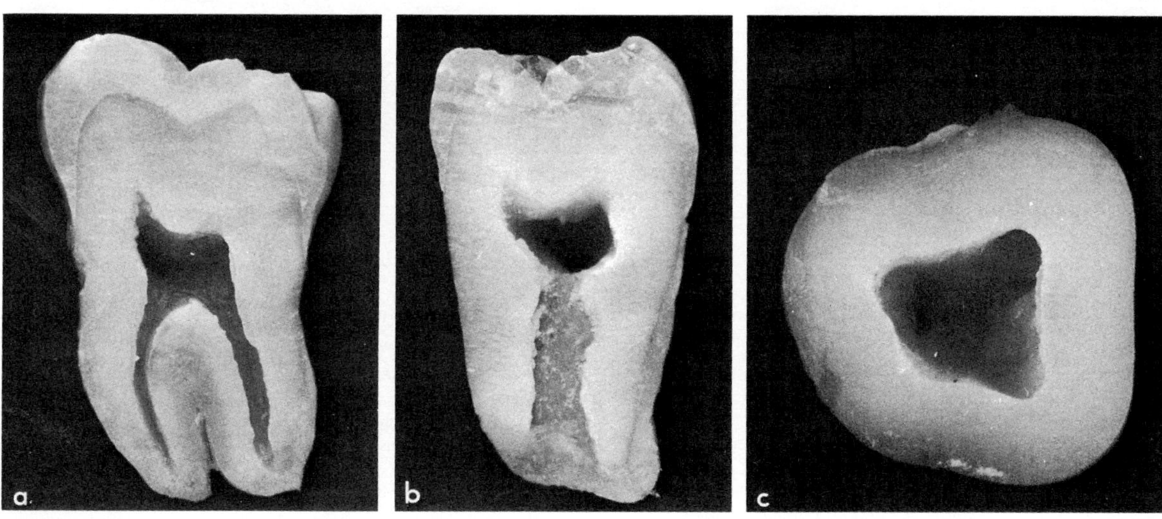

Figure 5.67
Pulp cavity of the mandibular left third molar: *a*, mesiodistal section; *b*, buccolingual section; *c*, transverse section.

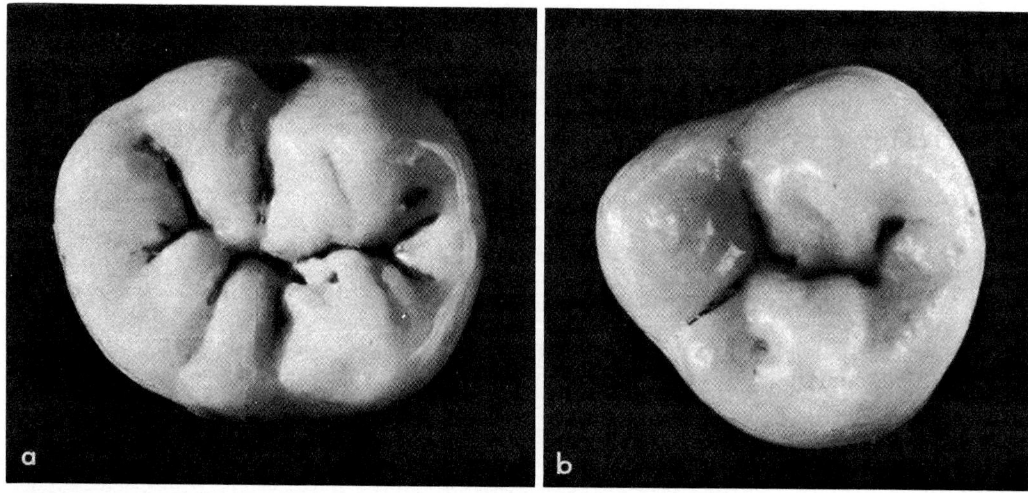

Figure 5.68
Variations in cusp pattern, mandibular left third molar (occlusal aspect): *a*, unusually large distal cusp; *b*, absence of distolingual cusp.

Variations

The mandibular third molar, like its maxillary antagonist, presents such a wide range of variation that an attempt at description would be endless. However, some of the frequently occurring variations may be seen in Figure 5.68. Four or five cusps may be present. When the distal cusp is present it may be larger in size than the adjoining distobuccal cusp (Fig. 5.68*a*). Not infrequently the distolingual cusp may be missing entirely or greatly reduced in size (Fig. 5.68*b*).

An accessory cusp, the protostylid, may be found on the buccal surface of the mesiobuccal cusp (Fig. 5.69). In addition, tuberculum sextum (C_6) and tuberculum intermedium (C_7) are commonly found on the third molar.

Roots of third molars are even more variable in number and form than is the crown. Extremes in length and inclination are common (Fig. 5.70*a* and *b*). Often they are fused (Fig. 5.71*a*); however, there may be as many as four large, distinct roots, as shown in apical view in Figure 5.71*b*. Small accessory roots, which appear to "branch off" a main root, are not uncommon (Fig. 5.71*c*).

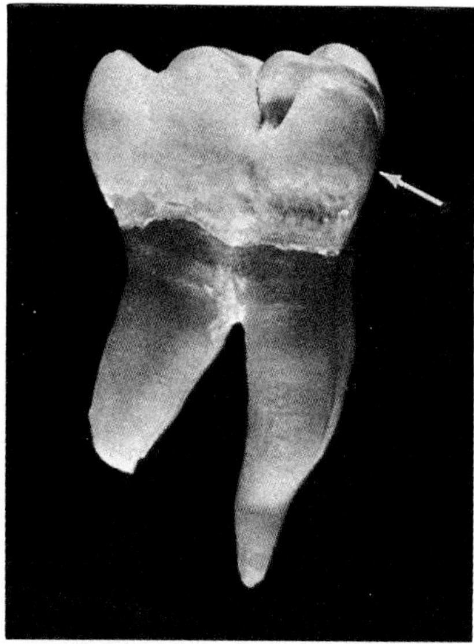

Figure 5.69
Unusually large protostylid (*arrow*), mandibular right third molar (buccal aspect).

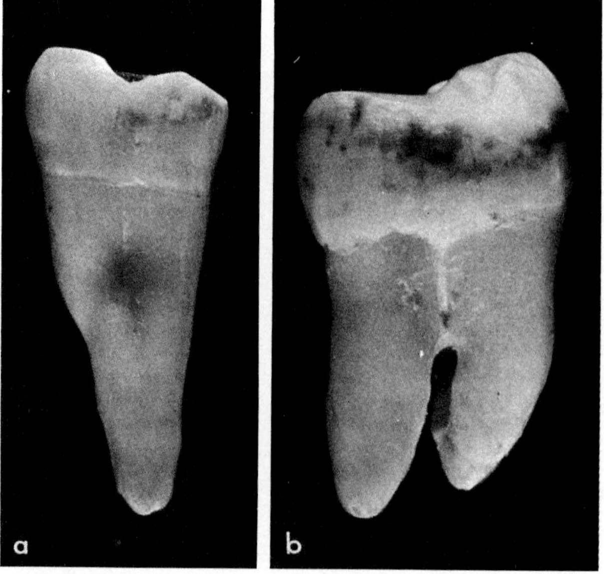

Figure 5.70
Extremes in root length, mandibular right third molar (buccal aspect).

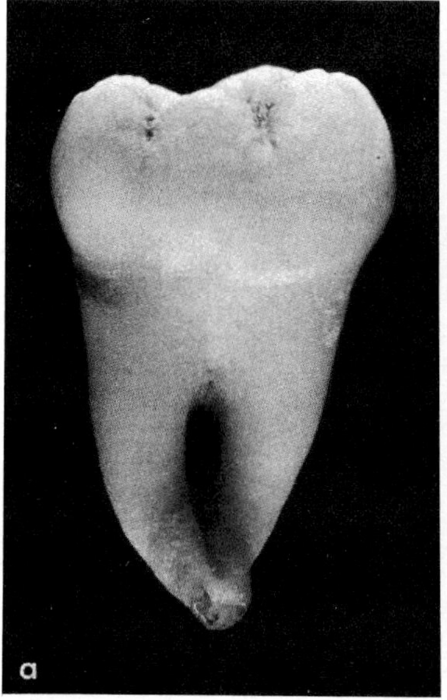

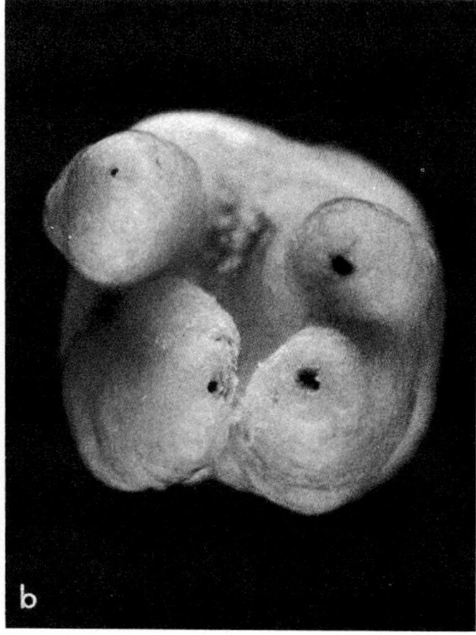

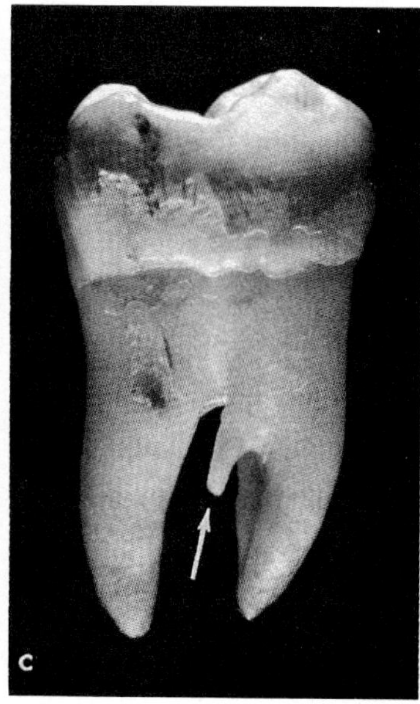

Figure 5.71

Variations in root number, mandibular third molar: *a*, fused roots, right third molar (buccal aspect); *b*, four large roots, right third molar (apical aspect); *c*, supernumerary root, right third molar (lingual aspect).

Summary

Mandibular Molar—Arch Traits

1. Generally there are two roots, one mesial and one distal.

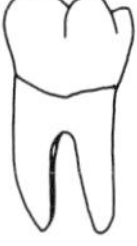

2. There are usually four major cusps, and often a fifth of lesser size.
3. The crowns are always broader mesiodistally than buccolingually.
4. Mandibular molars are the only units in the dentition in which the two major lingual cusps are of approximately equal size.
5. The mesio- and distobuccal cusps are approximately equal in size.

Mandibular Molars—Type Traits

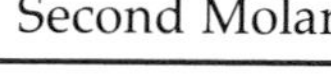

First Molar	Second Molar	Third Molar
Buccal Aspect		
Crown has widest mesiodistal diameter	Smaller crown than first 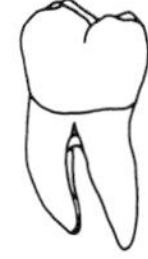	Smallest crown 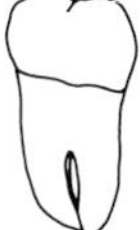
Three buccal cusps, MB, DB, and distal	Two buccal cusps, MB and DB	Two buccal cusps, same as second molar
Two buccal grooves	One buccal groove	One buccal groove
Roots widely separated and relatively vertical	Roots closer together and inclined distally	Roots short, fused, with marked distal inclination

continued

First Molar	Second Molar	Third Molar
Lingual Aspect		
Buccal profiles and proximal surfaces visible Crown narrower at cervix	Buccal profiles and proximal surfaces not visible Crown not as narrow at cervix	Buccal profiles and proximal surfaces not visible Same as second molar
Mesial Aspect		
Mesial root broad	Mesial root not as broad	Same as second molar
Occlusal Aspect		
Pentagonal outline Talonid and trigonid of equal breadth Mesial and distal profiles are straight and converge lingually	Rectangular outline Trigonid wider than talonid Mesial and distal profiles are curved; no lingual convergence	Ovoid outline Trigonid much wider than talonid Mesial and distal profiles highly curved; no lingual convergence
Main grooves form Y pattern Occlusal table is great relative to total crown area seen from occlusal	Main grooves form +4 pattern Occlusal table same as in first molar	Grooves show no set pattern Occlusal table least in relative area

The Molars—Clinical Applications

Thanks to the effectiveness of current preventive and patient education programs relative to oral hygiene, the molar dentition may survive intact for a considerable period of time (Figs. 5.72 and 5.73). However, the omnipresent clinical afflictions in the form of dental caries (Fig. 5.74), congenital malformation (Figs. 5.75 and 5.76), and wear and premature loss necessitate the placement of a wide variety of restorations in dental practice, all of which require an intimate knowledge of anatomic tooth form relative to proximal contours, occlusal surface anatomy, cusp form, marginal ridges, triangular ridges, groove pattern, and fossae location in order to result in long term successful restorative dentistry. Figures 5.77 to 5.88 illustrate typical clinical examples. All restorations illustrated were fabricated by undergraduate dental students.

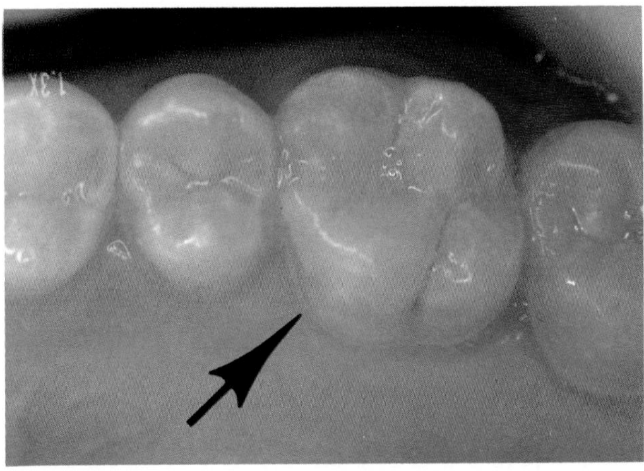

Figure 5.72
Intact maxillary first molar in a young adult patient.

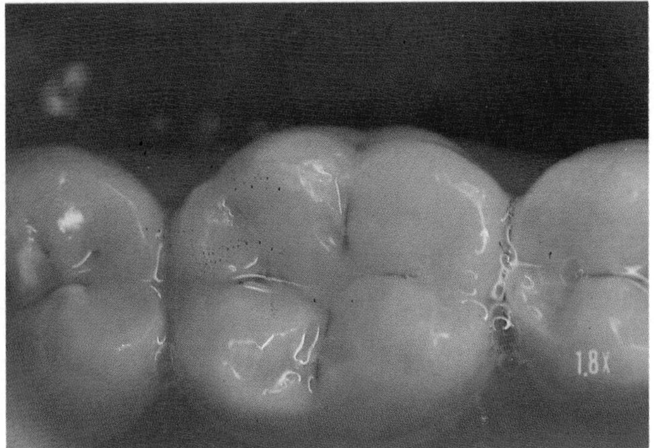

Figure 5.73
Intact mandibular first molar in an adolescent patient.

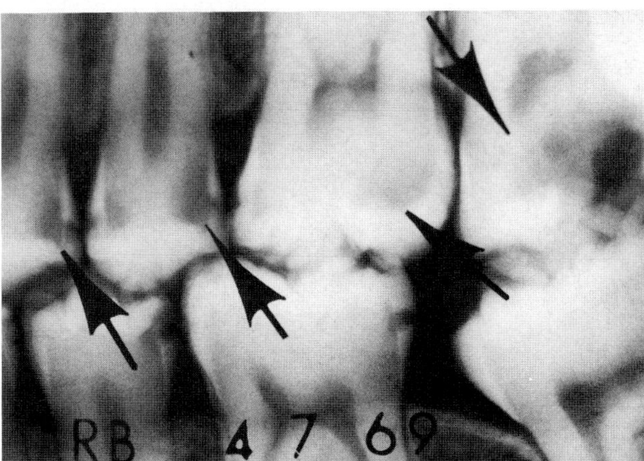

Figure 5.74
Bite wing radiograph showing extensive interproximal and occlusal caries in premolars and molars.

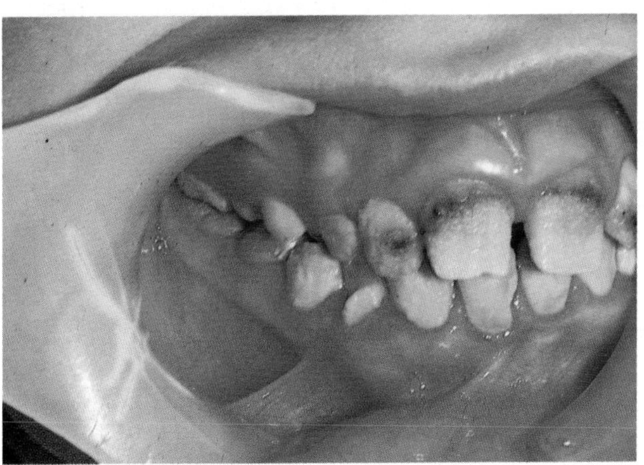

Figure 5.75
Fronto-lateral view of a patient afflicted with amelogenesis imperfecta.

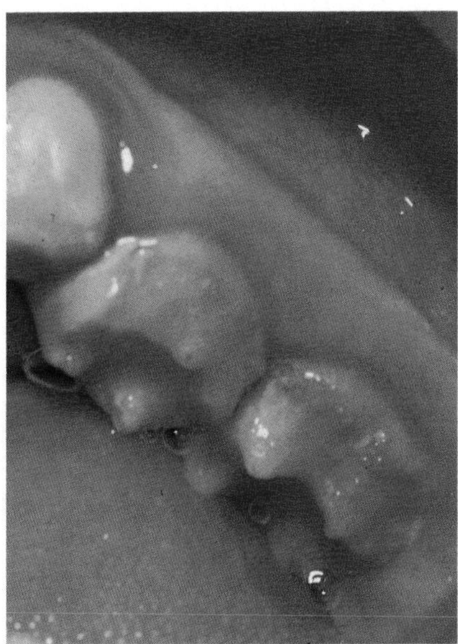

Figure 5.76
Mandibular molars of the same patient shown in Figure 5.75.

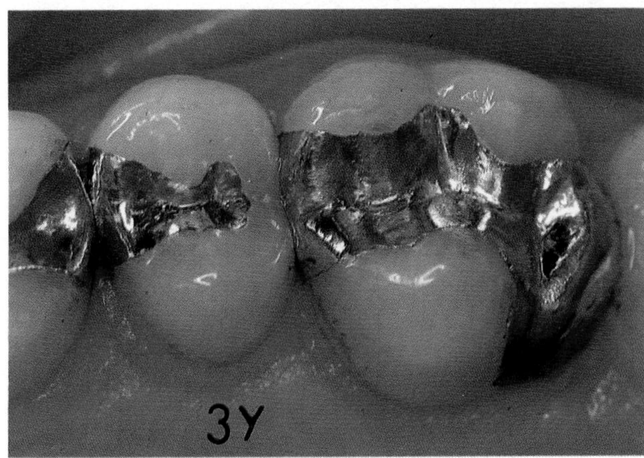

Figure 5.77
Class II proximo-occlusal amalgam restorations in the maxillary premolars and first molar.

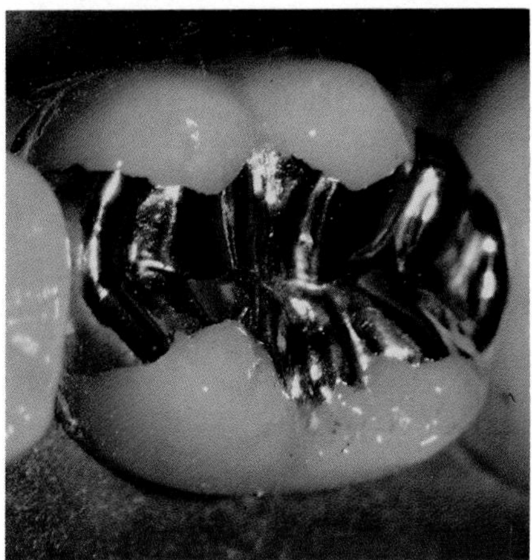

Figure 5.78
Mesio-occluso-distal silver amalgam restoration, mandibular first molar.

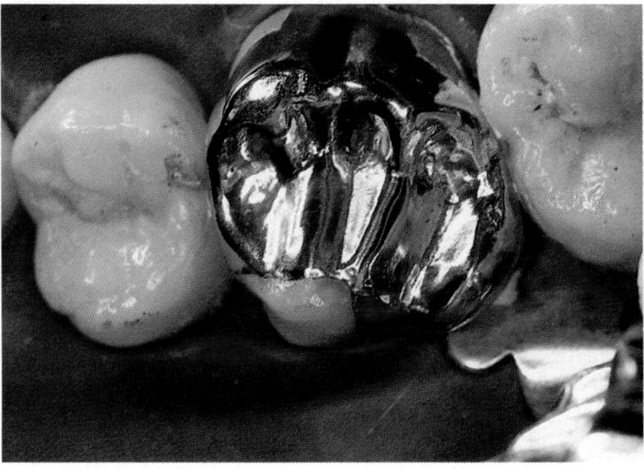

Figure 5.79

Extensive silver amalgam restoration in a maxillary first molar.

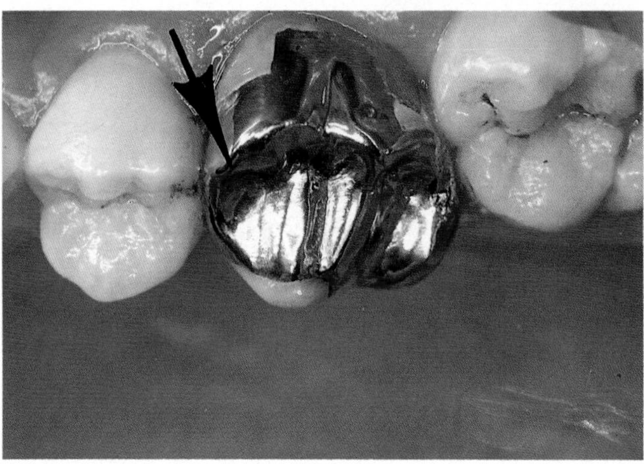

Figure 5.80

The same restoration as shown in Figure 5.79 from a buccal view. Note proper restoration of anatomic cusp form and contour.

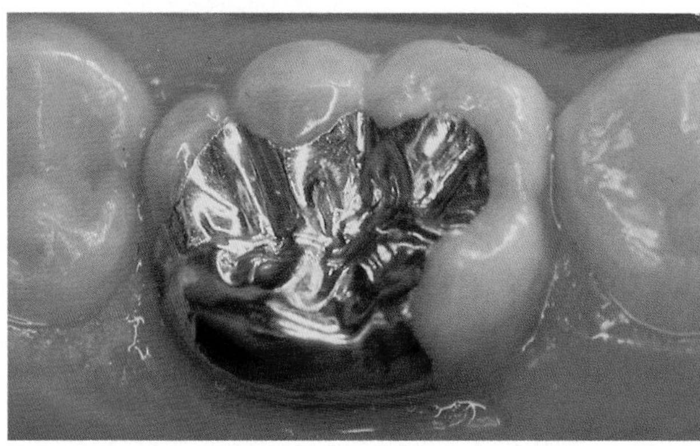

Figure 5.81

Occlusolingual amalgam restoration, mandibular first molar.

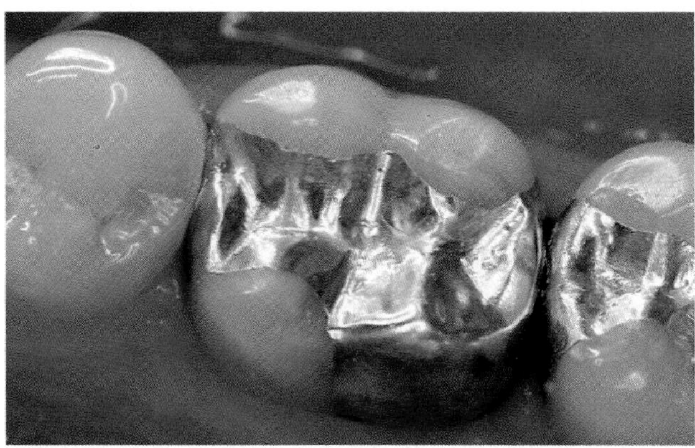

Figure 5.82

Mesio-occluso-distal amalgam restoration restoring the distolingual cusp of a mandibular first molar.

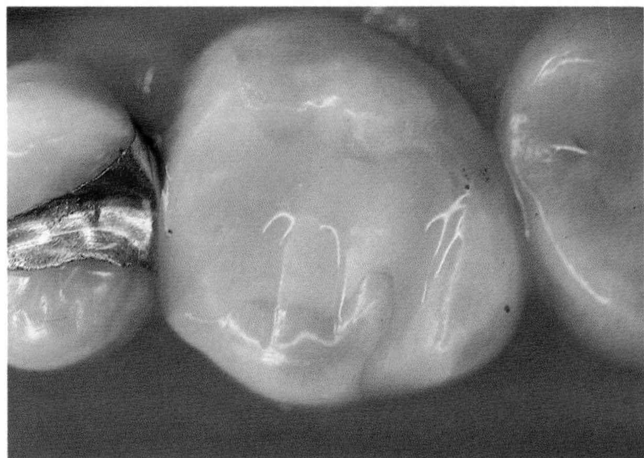

Figure 5.83

Extensive composite restoration resin (heat cured composite inlay) in a maxillary molar.

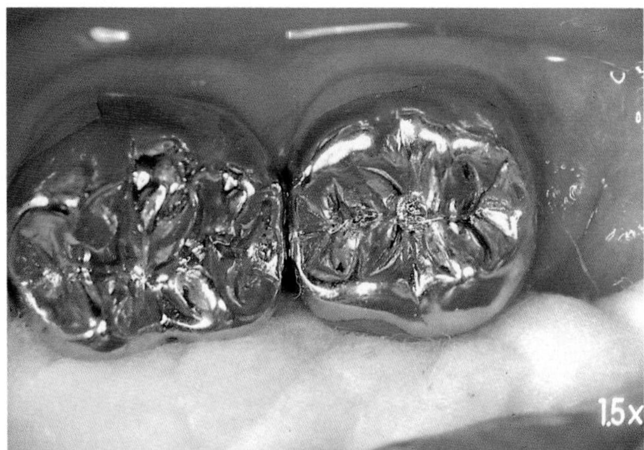

Figure 5.84

Cast gold occlusal onlays in the mandibular first and second molars.

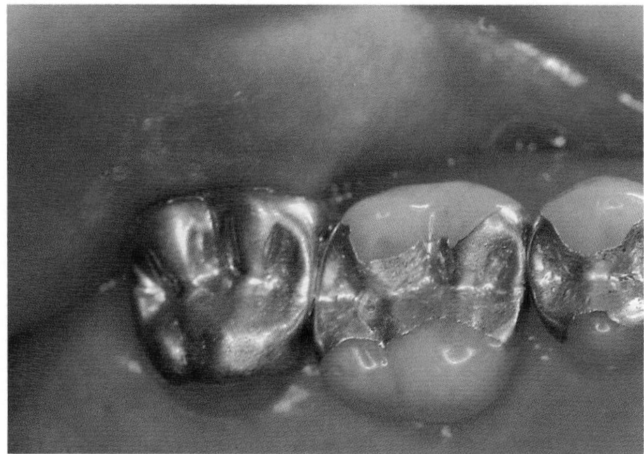

Figure 5.85

Cast gold inlay, maxillary first molar, and cast gold onlay, second molar at 18-year recall.

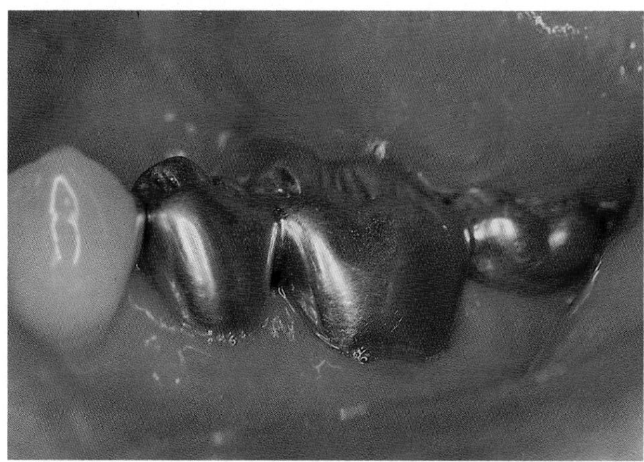

Figure 5.86

A three-unit cantilever fixed bridge replacing the mandibular second molar at 18-year recall (buccal view).

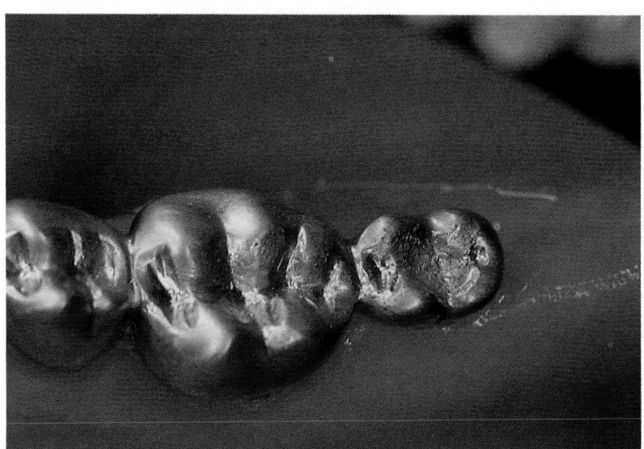

Figure 5.87

Occlusal view of the same fixed prosthesis as shown in Figure 5.86 at 18-year recall.

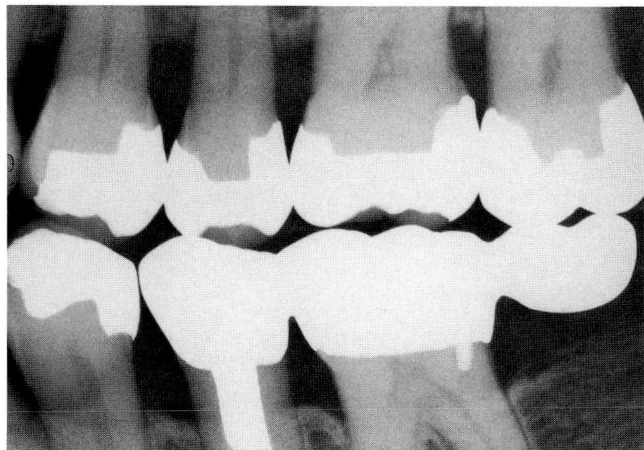

Figure 5.88

Bite wing radiograph of the same restoration shown in Figures 5.86 and 5.87 at 18-year recall. Note proper proximal contours.

The Primary Dentition

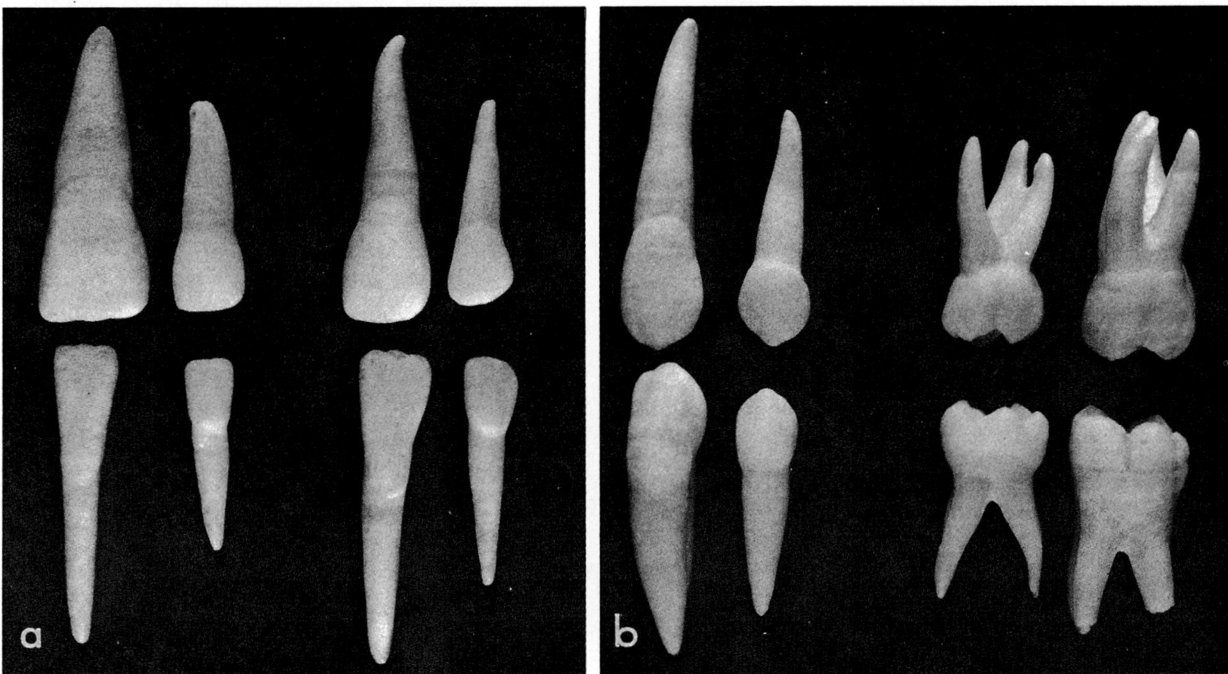

Figure 6.1

Comparison of primary and permanent teeth: *a,* the central and lateral incisors (labial aspect); *b,* the canines (labial aspect), second primary and first permanent molars (buccal aspect).

There are 20 primary teeth, five in each quadrant (see Fig. 1.3). As in the permanent dentition there are two incisors and one canine in each quadrant, but there are no premolars and only two molars. In the same person the primary teeth are much smaller than the permanent. Even if the teeth are mixed together, in a pile, as is the case in certain archaeological finds, it is relatively easy to sort out the primary teeth on the basis of what we may call *set traits*—traits that differentiate the primary set of teeth from the permanent. These set traits are described as follows.

1. In general, most primary teeth are smaller than the analogous permanent teeth. In Figures 6.1*a* and *b* the maxillary and mandibular primary and permanent teeth are shown side by side, grouped according to class. The differences in size of crown and root for each type of tooth are immediately apparent.

2. The crowns of primary teeth seem short compared with the permanent teeth; that is, relative to total length (crown and root) of the tooth, the crown height of each primary tooth appears to be significantly less than its succedaneous counterpart. This is substantiated in Table 6.1 in which the crown-length index (crown height—tooth length) is presented for the type of teeth in each set. The index should be interpreted as follows: an index of 0.446, for example, means that the crown height is 44.6 percent of the total length of the tooth (from root apex to tip of the crown).

3. The primary crowns also appear squat in relation to the permanent crowns. This can be expressed metrically in another index: the maximum mesiodistal crown diameter-crown height. Table 6.2 presents these indices for the primary and permanent

Table 6.1
Crown-Length Index of Permanent and Primary Teeth

Tooth Type	Permanent Tooth	Primary Tooth
Maxillary		
Central incisor	0.446	0.375
Lateral incisor	0.409	0.354
Canine	0.370	0.342
Molar*	0.375	0.326
Mandibular		
Central incisor	0.419	0.357
Lateral incisor	0.404	0.347
Canine	0.407	0.353
Molar*	0.349	0.293

*Indices are presented for the first permanent molar and the second primary molar.

Table 6.2
Crown Diameter–Crown Height of Permanent and Primary Teeth

Tooth Type	Permanent Tooth	Primary Tooth
Maxillary		
Central incisor	0.809	1.083
Lateral incisor	0.722	0.911
Canine	0.750	1.077
Molar*	1.333	1.438
Mandibular		
Central incisor	0.555	0.840
Lateral incisor	0.579	0.788
Canine	0.636	0.833
Molar*	1.467	1.800

*Indices are presented for the first permanent molar and the secondary primary molar.

teeth. For each type of tooth, the primary dentition consistently shows a greater mesiodistal diameter relative to height of the crown than its permanent successor. This difference in proportion accounts for the relatively "squat" appearance of the primary crowns.

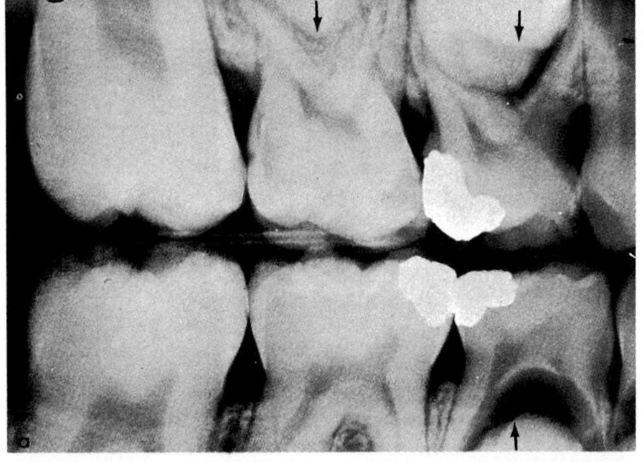

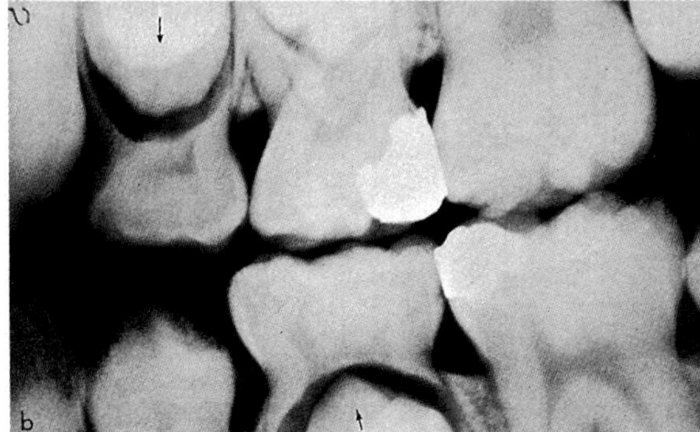

Figure 6.2
Position of the uninterrupted permanent crown relative to the roots of the primary molars.

4. In the anterior primary teeth the labial and lingual surfaces bulge conspicuously in the cervical third. These are termed the *cervical ridges.* This results in a marked constriction at the cervical line that is characteristic of these primary teeth.

5. In the primary molars only the buccal surfaces have a pronounced bulge (the so-called *buccal cervical ridges*). This gives a distinctive constricted appearance to the occlusal table when it is viewed from the occlusal aspect.

6. Primary molar roots are long and slender when compared with those of the permanent molars (Fig. 6.1*b*). In addition, they have a marked bowing or flaring outward. This unusually broad space provided between the primary molar roots is occupied by the crowns of the premolars during their formative phase. X-ray photographs (Fig. 6.2*a* and *b*) reveal the "tonglike" embrace of the permanent crown by

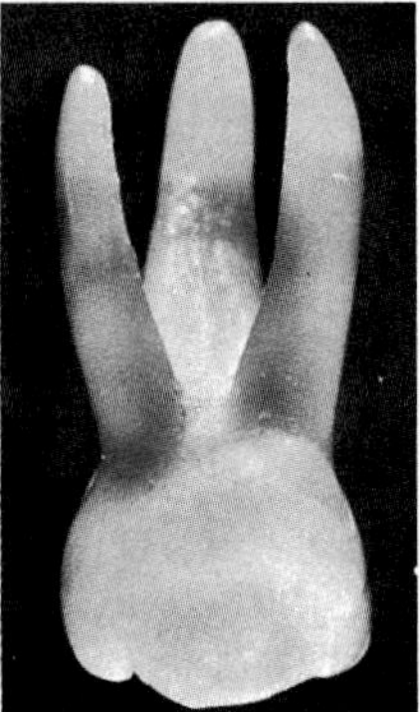

Figure 6.3
Absence of common root trunk, maxillary right first molar (buccal aspect).

the primary roots, which in an extreme case can become an "entrapment."

7. A striking difference between the two sets lies in the absence of a root base in the primary molars. The roots erupt directly from the crown and there is no *root trunk* (Fig. 6.3).

8. Primary crowns are milk-white in color.

9. The enamel is thinner in primary teeth and the pulp chamber is relatively large (more taurodont).

These are the basic traits that differentiate the primary from the permanent teeth (set traits). In the following section the various arch, class, and type traits are not emphasized as they were with the permanent dentition, since much the same arch, class, and type traits characterize the primary teeth. New type traits are confined, for the most part, to the primary molars and these are discussed in some detail.

The Incisors

The primary incisors are the first teeth to appear in the oral cavity, erupting between the ages of 6 and 8 months in the same sequence as do the permanent incisors (first, mandibular central; second, mandibular lateral; third, maxillary central; fourth, maxillary lateral). They are morphologically very similar to the permanent incisors and subserve the same cutting function, but they differ in one important trait. The newly erupted primary incisor does not show mammelons on the incisal margin.

Size and Eruption

Primary Incisors	Crown Height (mm)	Mesio-distal Crown Diameter (mm)	Bucco-lingual Crown Diameter (mm)	Tooth Length (mm)	Age at Eruption (mo)
Maxillary					
Central	6.0	6.5	5.0	16.0	7½
Lateral	5.6	5.1	4.0	15.8	8
Mandibular					
Central	5.0	4.2	4.0	14.0	6½
Lateral	5.2	4.1	4.0	15.0	7

Maxillary Incisors

The most characteristic feature of the *primary maxillary central incisor* (Fig. 6.4*a* to *e*) is the mesiodistal breadth of the crown. It is the only primary or permanent incisor with a mesiodistal diameter greater than its crown height. The mesial and distal margins of the crown profile appear to overhang the root profiles, particularly the distal. The labial surface is unmarked by grooves, depressions, or lobes, and is slightly convex both mesiodistally and incisocervically. The cingulum is a very prominent bulge, which extends much further incisally than in the permanent central incisor. Sometimes it may extend to the very incisal edge of the crown, in the form of a lingual ridge. The cingulum is not often marked by grooves or pits as in the permanent central incisor. The cervix, as a result of the bulging crown, appears constricted from all views. The cervical line from the labial and lingual views is only slightly convex apically, but from the proximal aspects it is more convex incisally. The root is conical and tapers to a rounded apex. The marginal ridges are clearly evident and blend into the lingual surface near the incisal edge.

The *primary maxillary lateral incisor* (Fig. 6.5*a* to *e*) is much smaller than the central incisor. The mesial and distal margin profiles are more in line with the profiles of the root. The distal incisal angle is more rounded. The labial surface, viewed from the incisal aspect, is more convex mesiodistally. The lingual fossa is deeper, since the marginal ridges are more pronounced. The cervical line is similar, from all four aspects, to that of the central incisor. The outline of the crown is viewed from the incisal aspect is almost circular in contrast to that of the central incisor, which is more diamond shaped.

Mandibular Incisors

The *mandibular central incisor* (Fig. 6.6*a* to *e*), viewed from the labial or lingual aspect, is bilaterally symmetrical. The mesio- and distoincisal angles are both sharp, forming almost 90-degree angles. The labial surface is unmarked and the incisal margin of the newly erupted tooth is perfectly straight in the horizontal plane. There are no mammelons or grooves visible. The root is almost three times the height of the crown and is narrow but conical, tapering to a relatively pointed apex. The lingual surface reveals a prominent overhanging cingulum with a lingual margin extending almost halfway up the crown and thence sending a ridgelike projection toward the in-

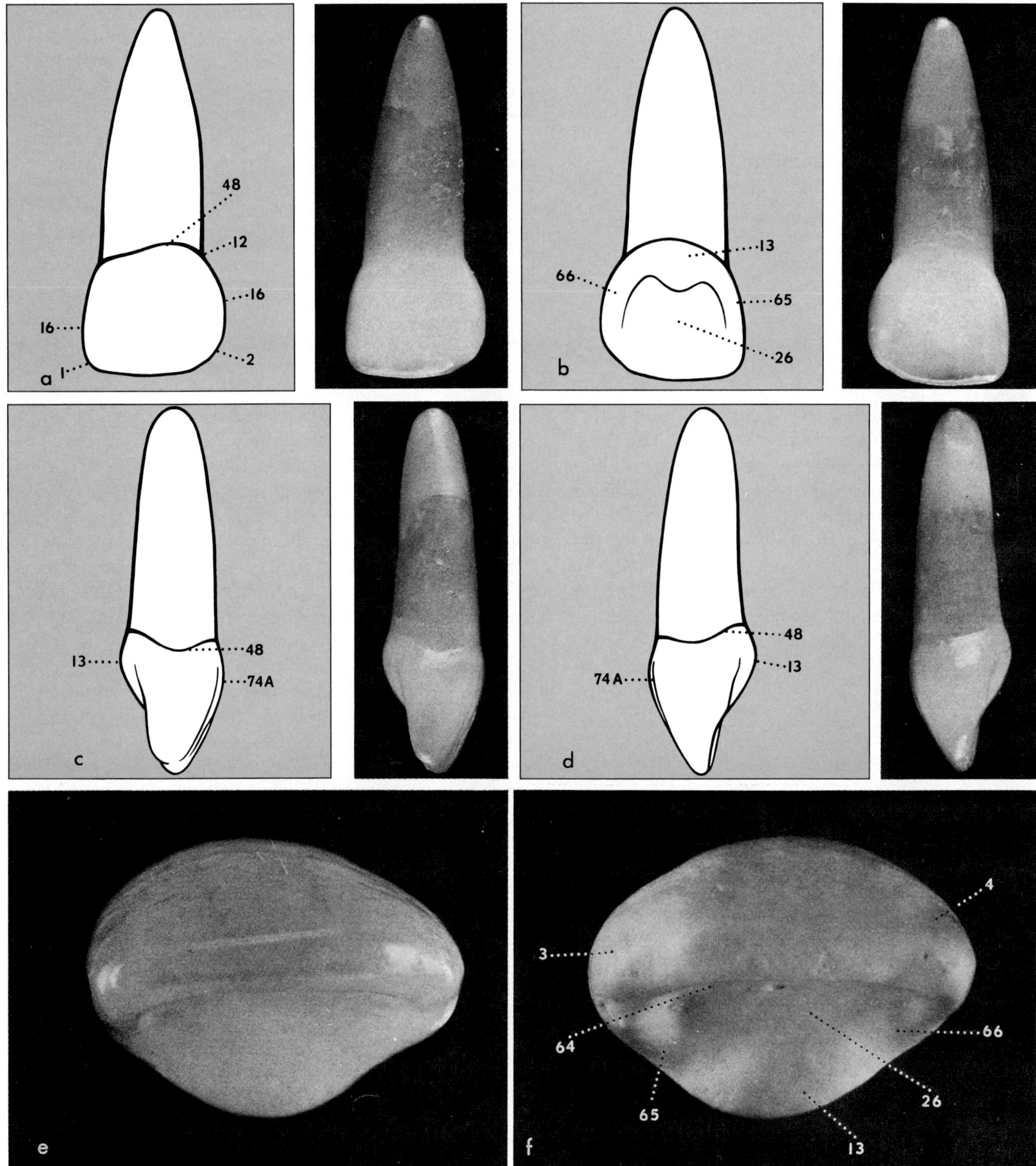

Figure 6.4

Primary maxillary left central incisor: *a,* labial aspect; *b,* lingual aspect; *c,* mesial aspect; *d,* distal aspect; *e,* incisal aspect (actual crown); *f,* incisal aspect (cast).

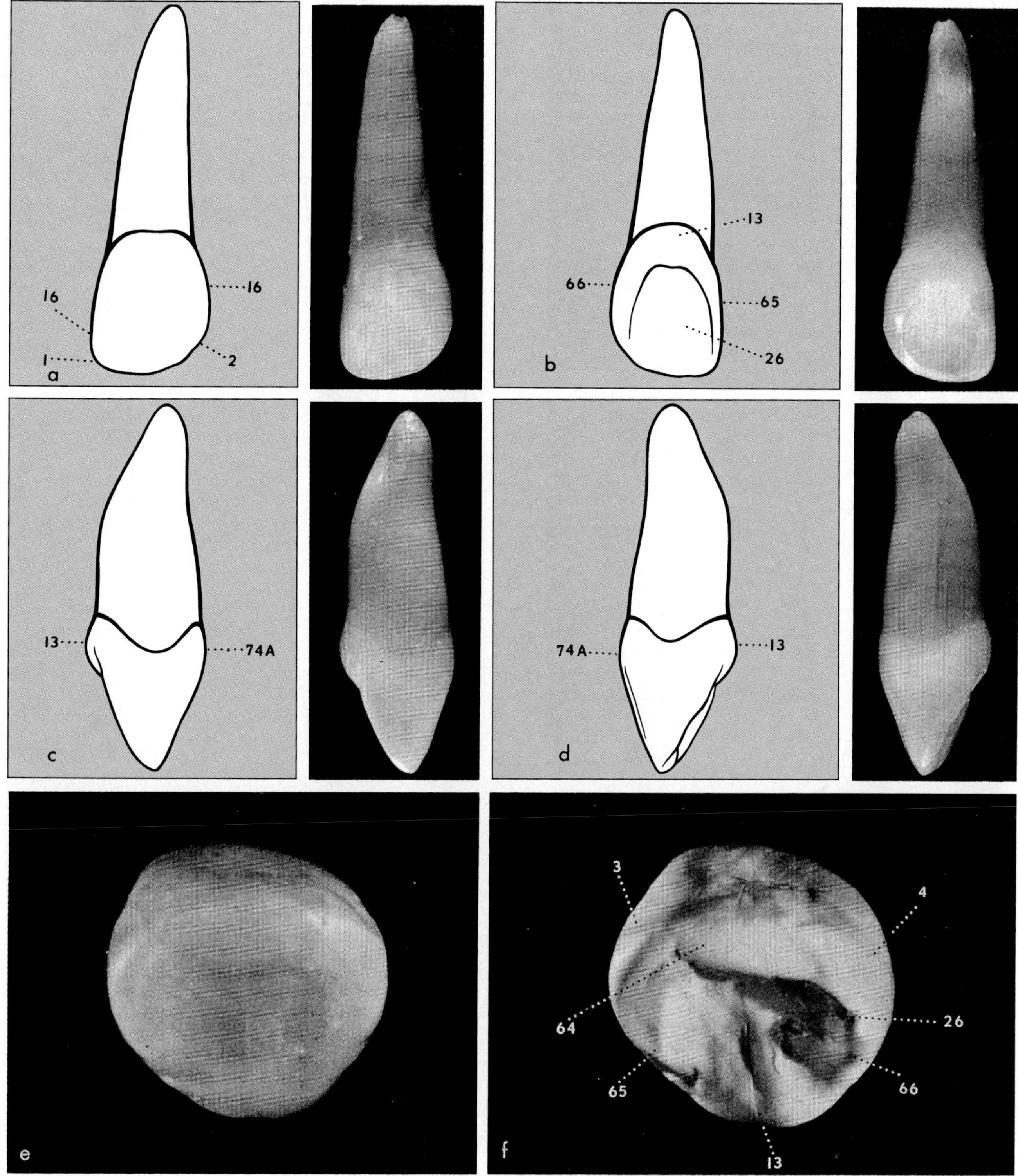

Figure 6.5

Primary maxillary left lateral incisor: *a*, labial aspect; *b*, lingual aspect; *c*, mesial aspect; *d*, distal aspect; *e*, incisal aspect (actual crown); *f*, incisal aspect (cast).

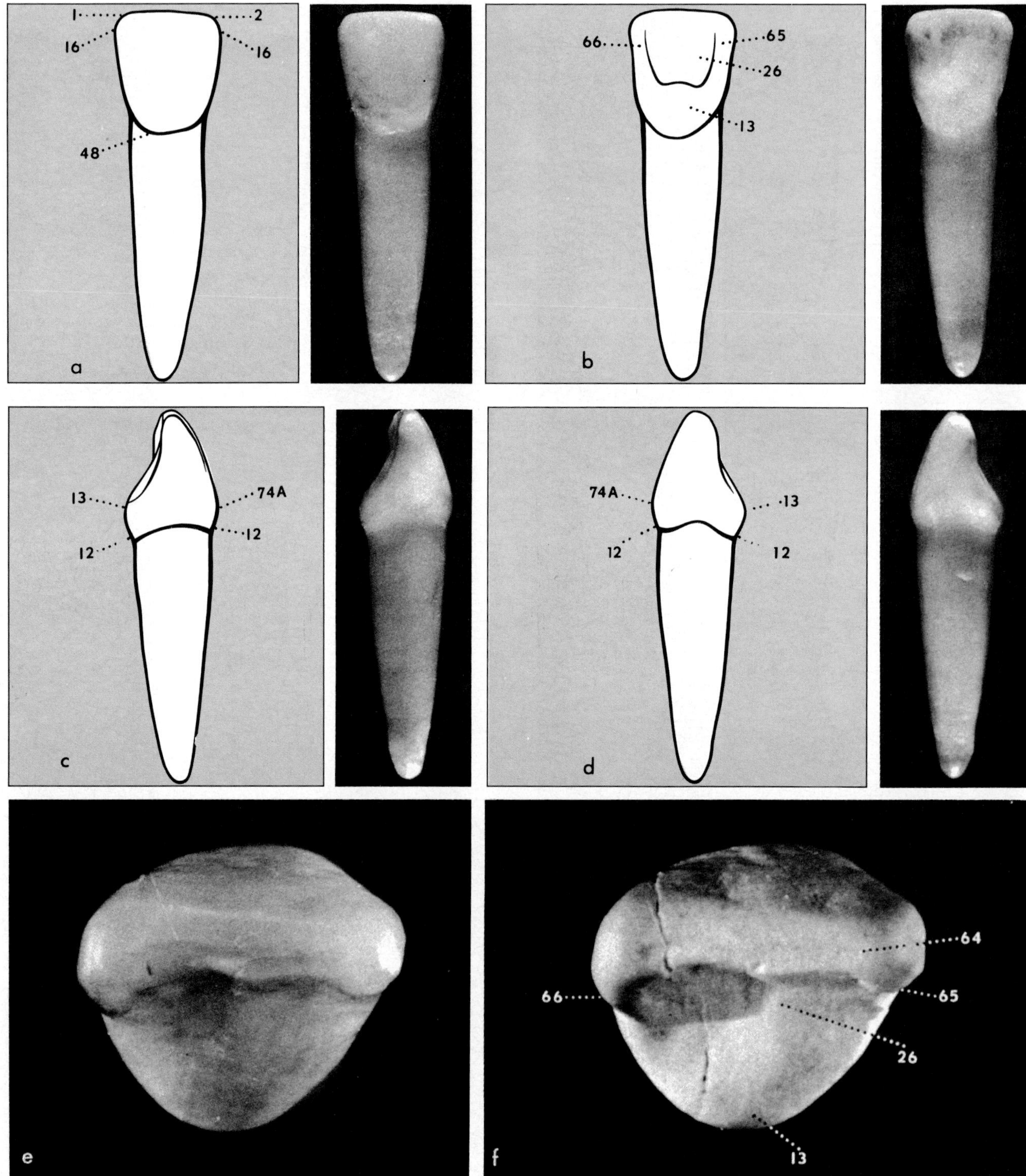

Figure 6.6

Mandibular left central incisor: *a,* labial aspect; *b,* lingual aspect; *c,* mesial aspect; *d,* distal aspect; *e,* incisal aspect (actual crown); *f,* incisal aspect (cast).

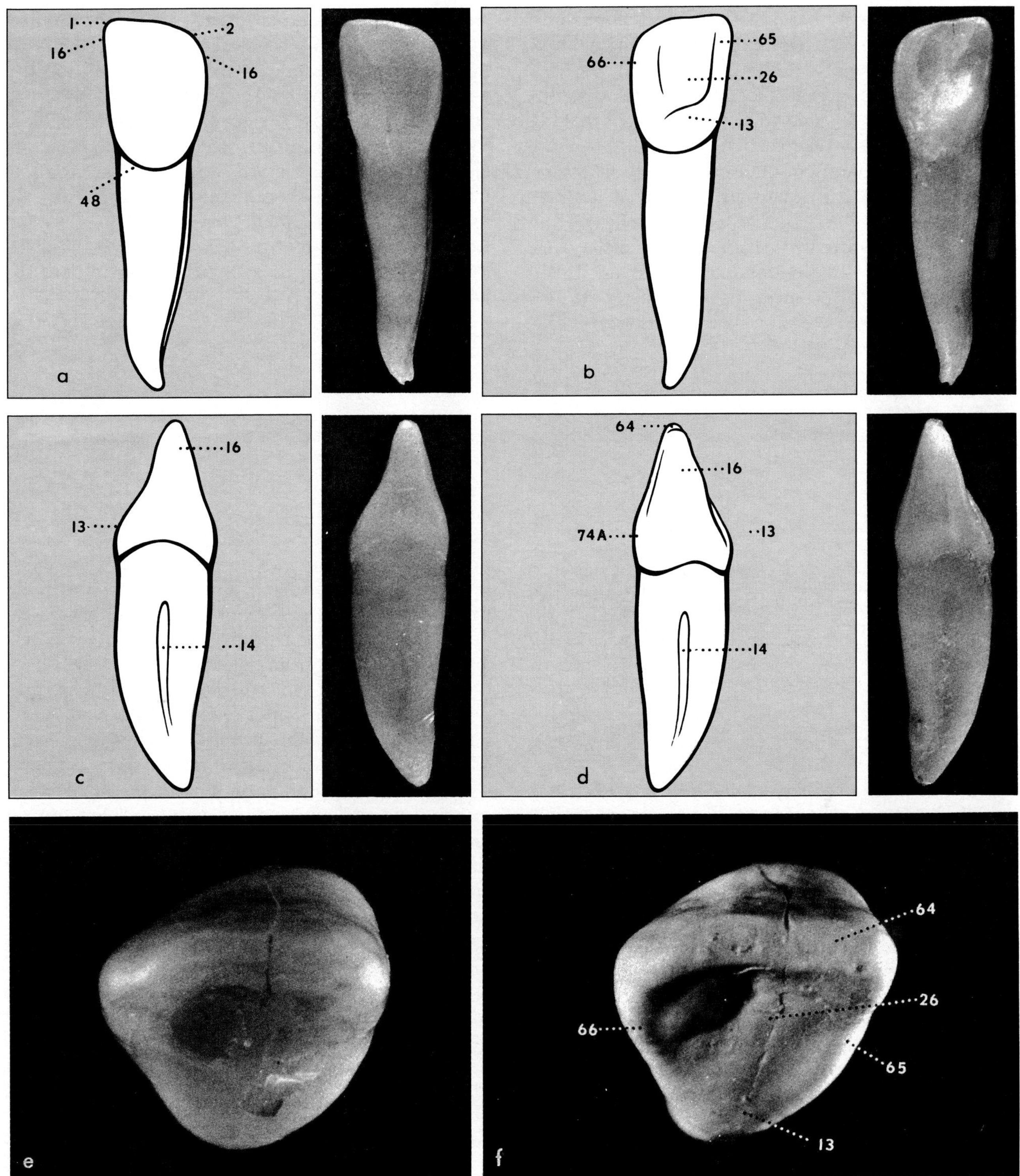

Figure 6.7

Mandibular left lateral incisor: *a*, labial aspect; *b*, lingual aspect; *c*, mesial aspect; *d*, distal aspect; *e*, incisal aspect (actual crown); *f*, incisal aspect (cast).

cisal edge. The marginal ridges are not as marked as they are in the maxillary incisors, and the lingual fossa is therefore more shallow. The labial surface, viewed from the incisal aspect, is flat mesiodistally. The cervical line is in no way different from that already described for the maxillary incisors.

The incisal margin of the *mandibular lateral incisor* (Fig. 6.7*a* to *e*) slopes downward distally, in contrast to the mandibular central incisor. Its distoincisal angle is rounded rather than sharp, and the distal margin of the crown is more rounded. The slightly greater height and lesser mesiodistal diameter of the crown as compared with the central incisor gives the crown a more rectangular, more narrow appearance. The root is narrow and conical but has a distinct distal inclination near its apex. From the distal aspect, a long, narrow depression separates the root into labial and lingual moieties. The cingulum is quite similar to that of the central incisor. The marginal ridges are also much like those in the central incisor. From the incisal view the crown outline shows its greatest dimension in the labiolingual axis and is not symmetrical as it is in the central. This is because the distal moiety of the crown bulges out more than does the mesial moiety.

The Canines

Size and Eruption

Primary Canines	Crown Height (mm)	Mesiodistal Crown Diameter (mm)	Labiolingual Crown Diameter (mm)	Tooth Length (mm)	Age at Eruption (mo)
Maxillary canine	6.5	7.0	7.0	19.0	16–20
Mandibular canine	6.0	5.0	4.8	17.0	16–20

The primary maxillary canine (Fig. 6.8*a* to *e*), unlike the maxillary central incisor, is greater in mesiodistal diameter than crown height. Also, like the central incisor, its crown margins bulge proximally so that they overhang the root profiles. This, in effect, gives the crown a diamond-shaped appearance when viewed labially or lingually. The bulging of the crown applies equally to the proximal views, wherein the cervical thirds of labial and lingual surfaces are markedly convex. The latter are the result of a prominent cingulum that occupies at least half of the height of the crown. Frequently a small tubercle occupies the incisal portion of the cingulum, on either side of which there is a crescent-shaped groove. The prominence of the marginal ridges is, like that in the permanent anterior teeth, related to race. In Caucasians the margins are minimal; in Mongoloids they reach their maximum expression. An unusual feature in the primary canines is the lack of styles on either mesial or distal cusp ridges. This gives the primary canine a "fang-like" appearance.

The *mandibular canine* (Fig. 6.9*a* to *e*) crown is proportioned quite the opposite from the maxillary. Its height is greater than its mesiodistal diameter. In addition it is arrow shaped rather than diamond shaped, since the cervical third of the proximal crown margins do not converge cervically. There are no grooves on the labial surface and no styles on the incisal margin. The mesial and distal heights of contour are much nearer the cervix than they are in the permanent mandibular canine. The labiolingual diameter of the crown is much smaller than that of the maxillary canine. This is because the cingulum is much reduced in size and prominence in the mandibular canine, and occupies less than the cervical third of the height of the crown. The marginal ridges are less pronounced. From the incisal aspect the crown outlines of both maxillary and mandibular canines are almost identical.

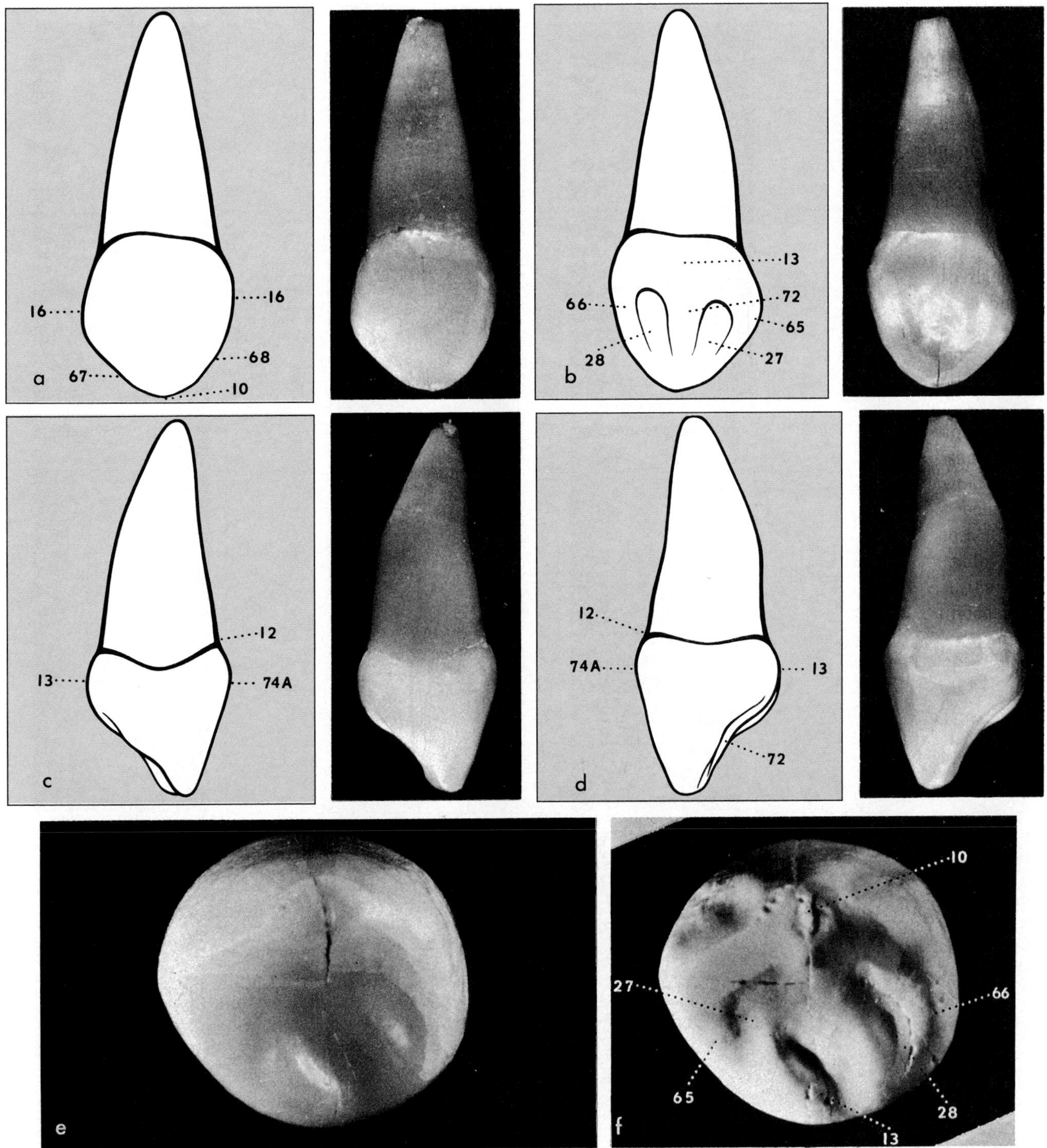

Figure 6.8

Maxillary left canine: *a,* labial aspect; *b,* lingual aspect; *c,* mesial aspect; *d,* distal aspect; *e,* incisal aspect (actual crown); *f,* incisal aspect (cast).

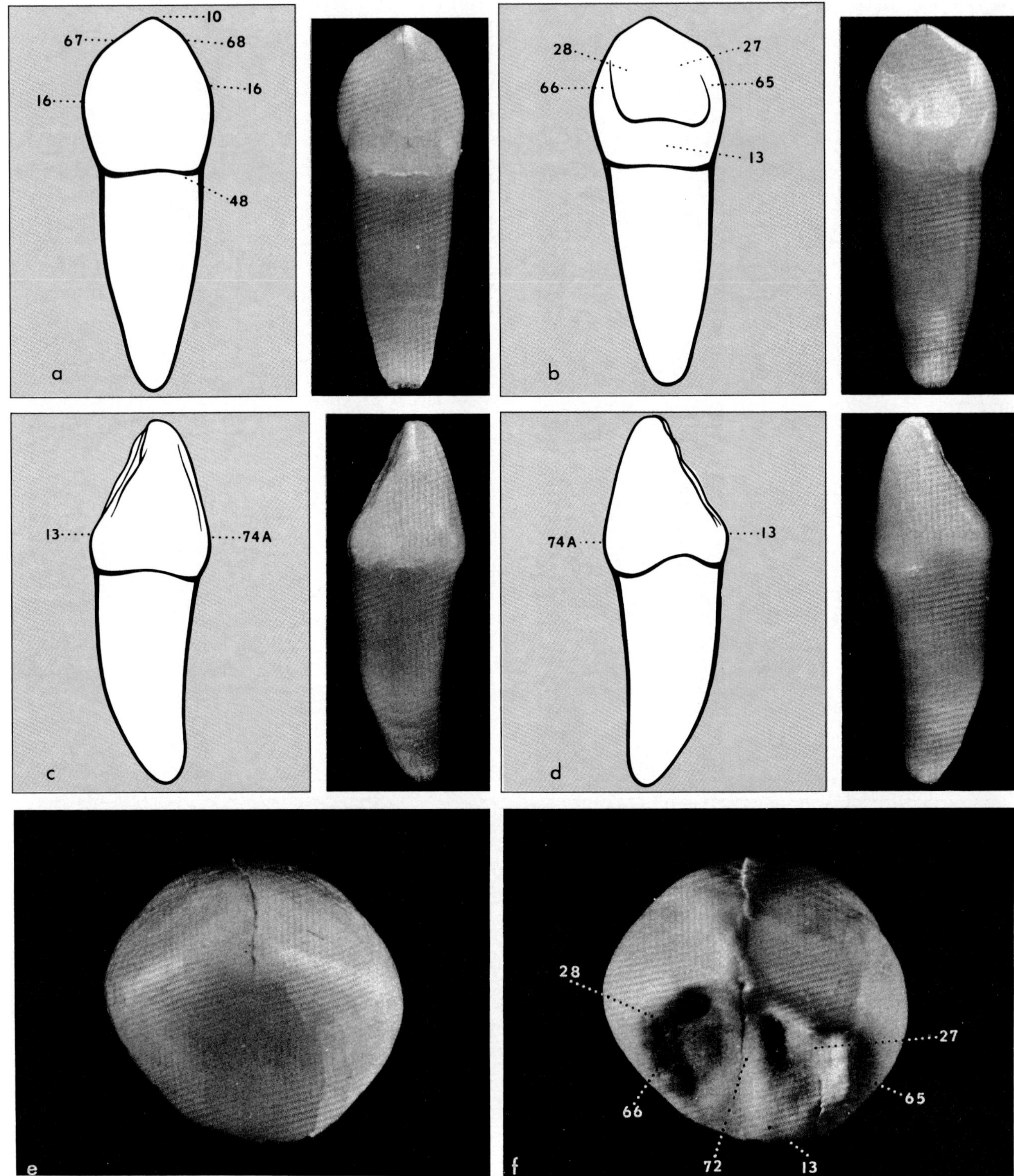

Figure 6.9

Mandibular right canine: *a*, labial aspect; *b*, lingual aspect; *c*, mesial aspect; *d*, distal aspect; *e*, incisal aspect (actual crown); *f*, incisal aspect (cast).

The Molars

Size and Eruption

Primary Molars	Crown Height (mm)	Mesio-distal Crown Diameter (mm)	Bucco-lingual Crown Diameter (mm)	Tooth Length (mm)	Age at Eruption (mo)
Maxillary					
First	5.1	7.3	8.5	15.2	12–16
Second	5.7	8.2	10.0	17.5	20–30
Mandibular					
First	6.0	7.7	7.0	15.8	12–16
Second	5.5	9.9	8.7	18.8	20–30

Maxillary Molars

The *maxillary first primary molar* (Fig. 6.10) is the most atypical of all the molars, primary or permanent. It appears to be intermediate in form and development between a premolar and a molar. In all dimensions except labiolingual diameter it is the smallest molar. Basically the final crown of this tooth is bicuspid (two cusped). From embryological studies it can be determined that the two cusps present are the mesiobuccal (MB) and the mesiolingual (ML). A third cusp, the distobuccal (DB), is frequently present as a style on the distal ridge of the mesiobuccal cusp. Never does it approach the latter in size. A smaller style is frequently found on the mesial ridge of the same cusp. This is given the name *parastyle.*

A distolingual (DL) cusp rarely occurs as such on the first molar. In some cases, however, the lingual portion of the distal marginal ridge bears a nodular tubercle that seems to resemble a distolingual cusp.

From the buccal aspect the crown appears squat since the mesiodistal diameter is considerably greater than the crown height. The mesial moiety of the crown has a greater height in consequence of its more cervical projection onto the root area. This results in a cervical line that is higher mesially than distally. As in all primary molars there is a marked cervical constriction of the crown.

There is very little root trunk and the three roots are strongly divergent. From the buccal aspect the lingual root is positioned exactly midway between the two buccal roots.

In mesial view the mesial marginal ridge groove is sharp and deep in profile and continues in the form of a shallow, narrow depression up the crown surface toward the cervical line. From this view the crown appears even more squat than from the buccal. The lingual height of contour is immediately below the cervical line and the buccal is only slightly lower. The cervical third of the buccal margin bulges very prominently and is called the *buccal cervical ridge.* It is always more prominent in the maxillary and mandibular first molars. From the proximal views the buccal roots appear straight and are directed slightly toward the buccal. The lingual root, on the other hand, is banana shaped with a definite lingual projection but a strong buccal curvature in its apical third.

From the occlusal view the crown outline appears trapezoidal, the mesial and distal margins being straight with a slight lingual convergence. The buccal margin is longer than the lingual and relatively straight with a pronounced lingual inclination distally. The lingual margin is narrow and markedly convex toward the lingual. The occlusal surface is dominated by the buccal cusp, which has a prominent triangular ridge terminating in the center of the surface. The lingual cusp is smaller with a less conspicuous triangular ridge. The DB style (or cusp) is separated from the MB cusp by a deep *buccal groove,* which crosses the buccal margin, forms the distal boundary of the triangular ridge of the MB cusp, and meets the *central groove* to form the *central pit.*

Between the buccal groove and the distal marginal ridge a small transverse ridge is frequently found. This has been called the *oblique ridge.* Although it occupies a position similar to that of the oblique ridge in the maxillary permanent molars, developmentally it is not actually the same structure.

The occlusal pit-groove pattern is most frequently H shaped, with the central groove forming the cross bar. A *mesial pit* is located just distal to the midpoint of the mesial marginal ridge. Another pit, the *distal pit,* occupies a similar position in relation to the distal marginal ridge. From each pit, extending bucally and lingually there may be found supplemental grooves. In addition, a groove crossing each marginal ridge at its midpoint may be found.

The *maxillary second primary molar* (Fig. 6.11*a* to *e*) is morphologically almost a model for the maxillary first permanent molar. This interesting fact has long been noted by dental morphologists. If one has the second primary molar one can easily predict in detail what the first permanent from the same quadrant will look like. Even unusual variations in minor features are faithfully reproduced in the permanent first molar. This morphological concordance between both

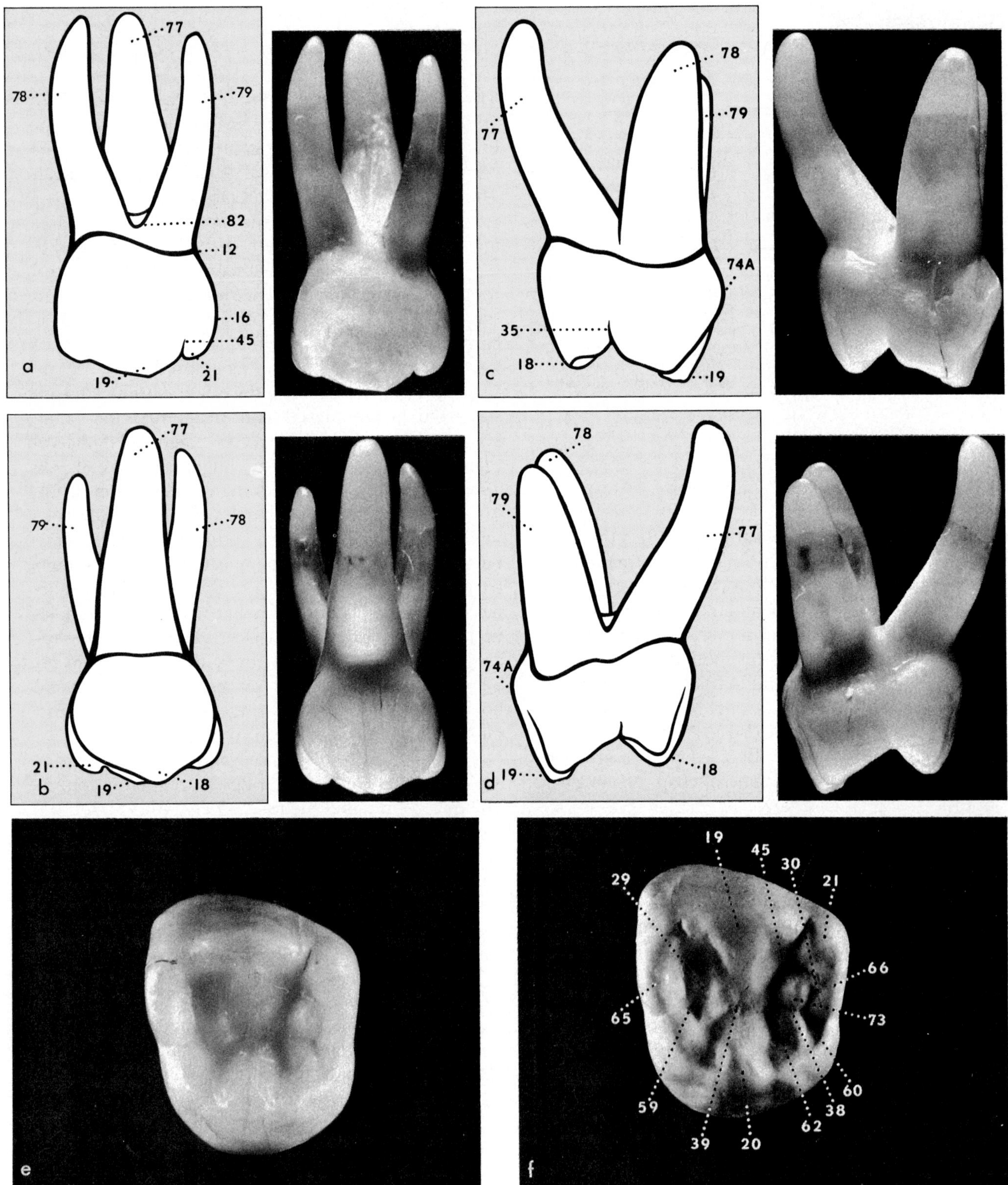

Figure 6.10

Maxillary left first molar: *a*, buccal aspect; *b*, lingual aspect; *c*, mesial aspect; *d*, distal aspect; *e*, occlusal aspect (actual crown); *f*, occlusal aspect (cast).

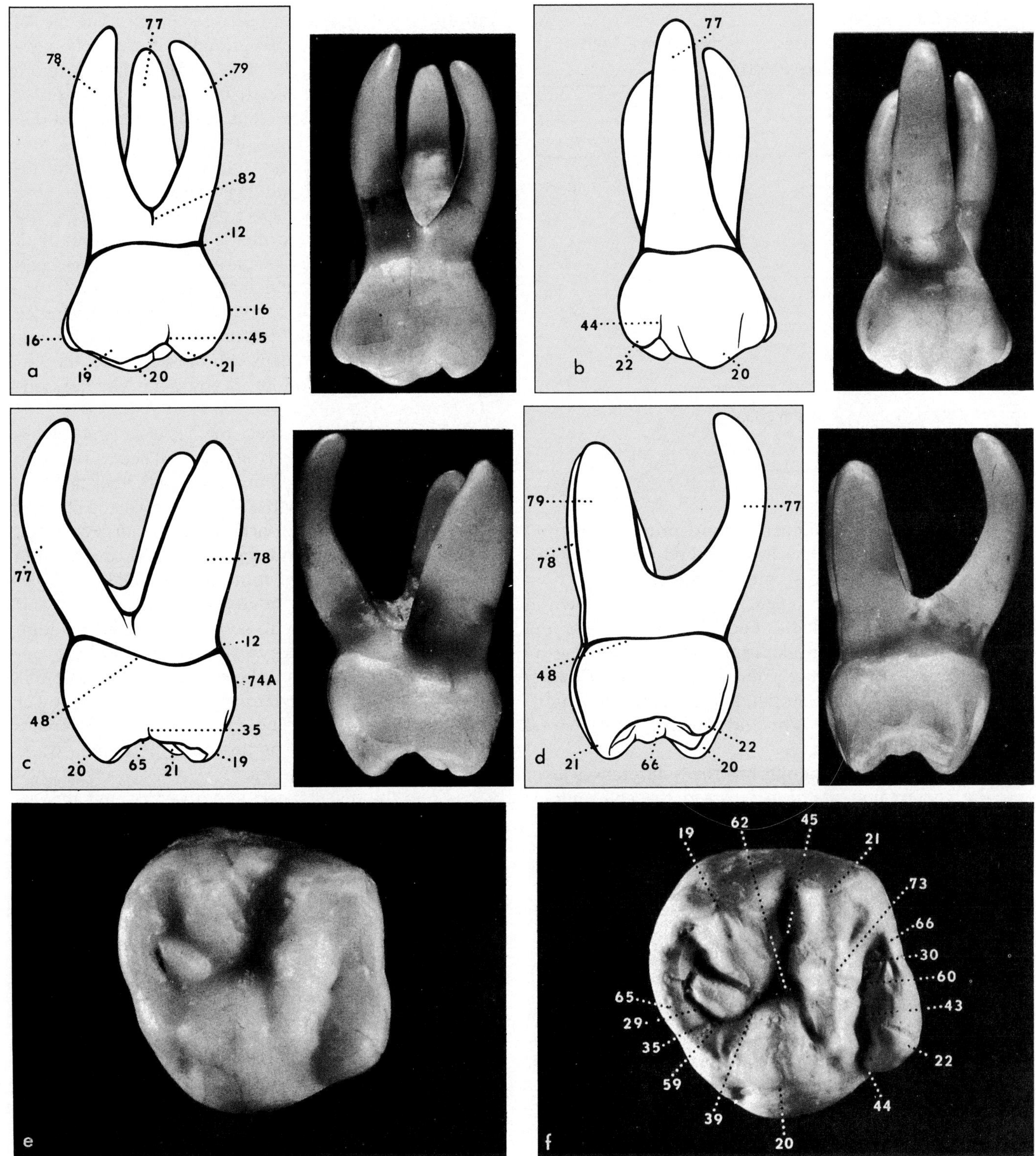

Figure 6.11

Maxillary left second molar: *a*, buccal aspect; *b*, lingual aspect; *c*, mesial aspect; *d*, distal aspect; *e*, occlusal aspect (actual crown); *f*, occlusal aspect (cast).

Table 6.3
Comparison of the Indices for Second Primary and First Permanent Maxillary Molars

	Maxillary Molars	
Indices	*Second primary*	*First permanent*
BL crown diameter / MD crown diameter	1.22	1.10
MD crown diameter / Crown height	1.44	1.33
Crown height / Total tooth length	0.33	0.38
BL crown diameter / Crown height	1.75	1.47

BL, buccolingual; MD, mesiodistal

maxillary and mandibular second primary and first permanent molars has been termed *isomorphy.* Primarily the differences between the second primary and first permanent molars are small, as is shown in Table 6.3. If we call the buccolingual diameter the "breadth" and the mesiodistal diameter the "length" of the crown, then the primary second molar crown is broader relative to length, longer relative to height, broader relative to height, and shorter relative to total length of the tooth.

The only other significant crown differences lie in the constriction of the cervix and the concomitant bulging of the buccal surface. In addition, there is relatively little common root trunk as compared with the permanent first molar, and the roots are thinner and more divergent.

Mandibular Molars

The *mandibular first primary molar* (Fig. 6.12*a* to *e*) is indeed molariform, unlike the maxillary first, but has a number of unique features when compared with either the mandibular permanent molars or the first primary molar. It is usually a four-cusped tooth, with two buccal and two lingual cusps.

From the buccal aspect a great discrepancy in size between the mesial and distal moieties of the crown can be seen. The former projects higher occlusally and occupies at least two-thirds of the crown area. The MB cusp has a short mesial ridge and a longer, more steeply inclined distal ridge. The same applies to the smaller DB cusp, so that the occlusal crown profile presents a sort of serrated shape. The mesial profile is almost vertically straight and scarcely overhangs the root profile. The distal profile is more curved and projects slightly beyond the root profile.

There are two divergent roots, a mesial and distal. The former is almost invariably the longer and thicker. The cervical line is relatively straight and inclines downward slightly from distal to mesial.

From the lingual aspect one sees two cusps, the ML and the DL. The former is the most conical of all molar cusps, primary or permanent. This has been regarded by some dental anatomists as a very "primitive" feature. The DL cusp is a bulging protuberance on the distal margin of the occlusal surface. The outlines of both buccal cusps can be seen from the lingual view. The cervical line is straight in the horizontal plane.

From the mesial aspect the *buccal cervical ridge* is a striking feature of the crown since it seems to droop over the root profile, almost in "potbelly" fashion. From the apex of the MB cusp there is a steep straight incline to the buccal cervical ridge. A *transverse ridge,* connecting the MB and the ML cusps, can be seen from the mesial aspect forming the occlusal profile. The mesial marginal ridge is very prominent and uplifted to a great extent, so that it resembles a high rampart. The *mesial marginal groove* separates the mesial marginal ridge from the ML cusp ridge. The cervical line is convex toward the occlusal and is lower on the buccal end. The mesial root is extremely broad, in fact, almost as broad as the crown. Most frequently it has a bifid apex.

From the distal aspect all four cusps and the entire profile of the mesial root as well are visible. The buccal profile of the DB cusp does not have the bulbous protuberance that distinguishes the buccal profile of the MB cusp. The distal marginal ridge is not as elevated or as prominent as the mesial marginal ridge. The cervical line is straight and horizontal.

From the occlusal, the profile of the crown would be rectangular if it were not for the buccal cervical ridge which makes the profile of the mesial moiety (trigonid) of the crown broader than the distal (talonid). This is an interesting fact since just the opposite proportions characterize this tooth in its early stages of crown development. The MB cusp is the largest of the four cusps and is followed by the ML, DB, and DL cusps in order of decreasing size. The triangular ridges of the MB and ML cusps together form a more or less continuous crest (the *transverse ridge*). This ridge is interrupted at its midpoint by the *central groove,* which extends mesiodistally across the center of the occlusal surface and terminates mesially in the *mesial* pit. Two supplemental grooves radiate

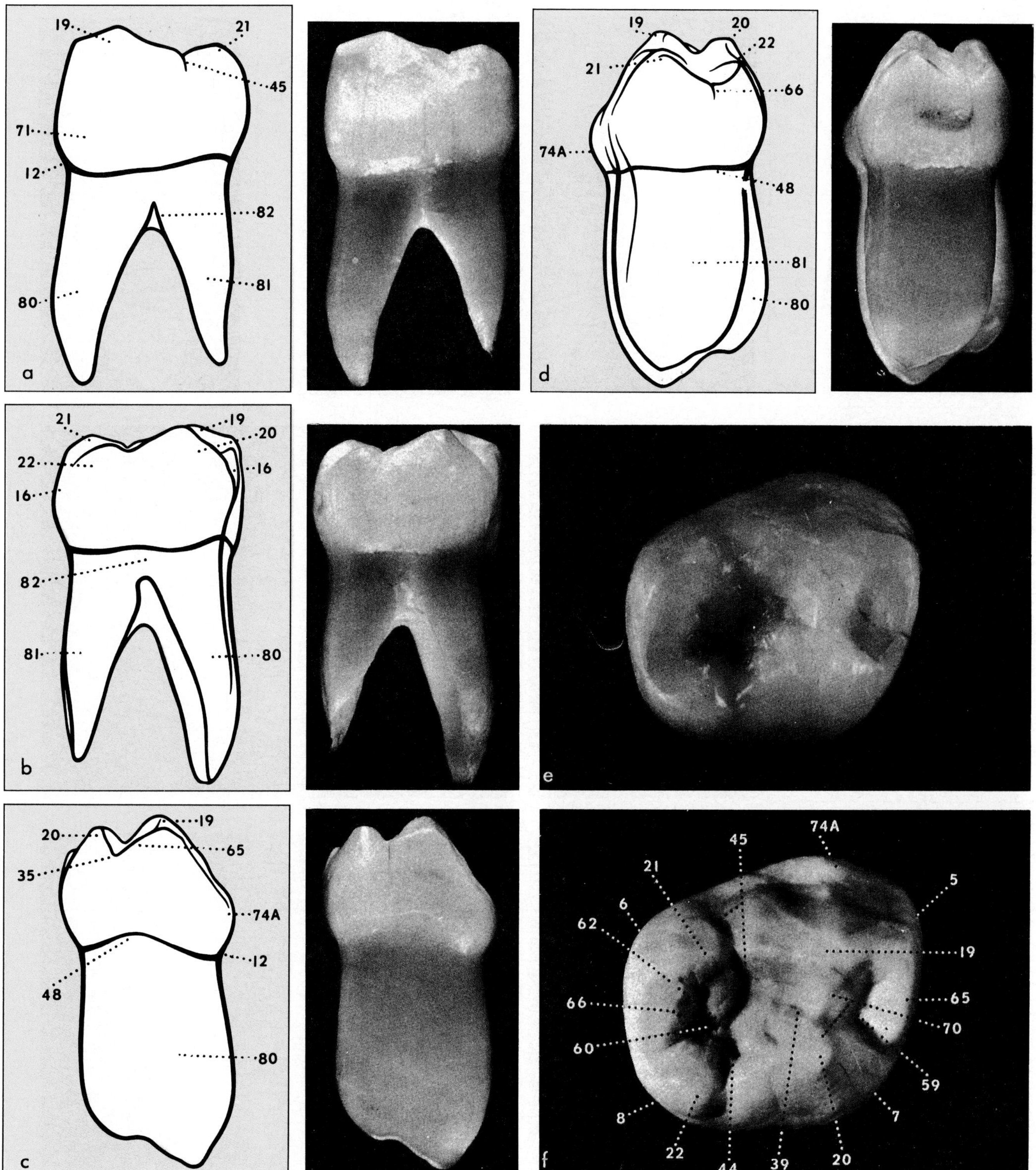

Figure 6.12

Mandibular left first molar: *a,* buccal aspect; *b,* lingual aspect; *c,* mesial aspect; *d,* distal aspect; *e,* occlusal aspect (actual crown); *f,* occlusal aspect (cast).

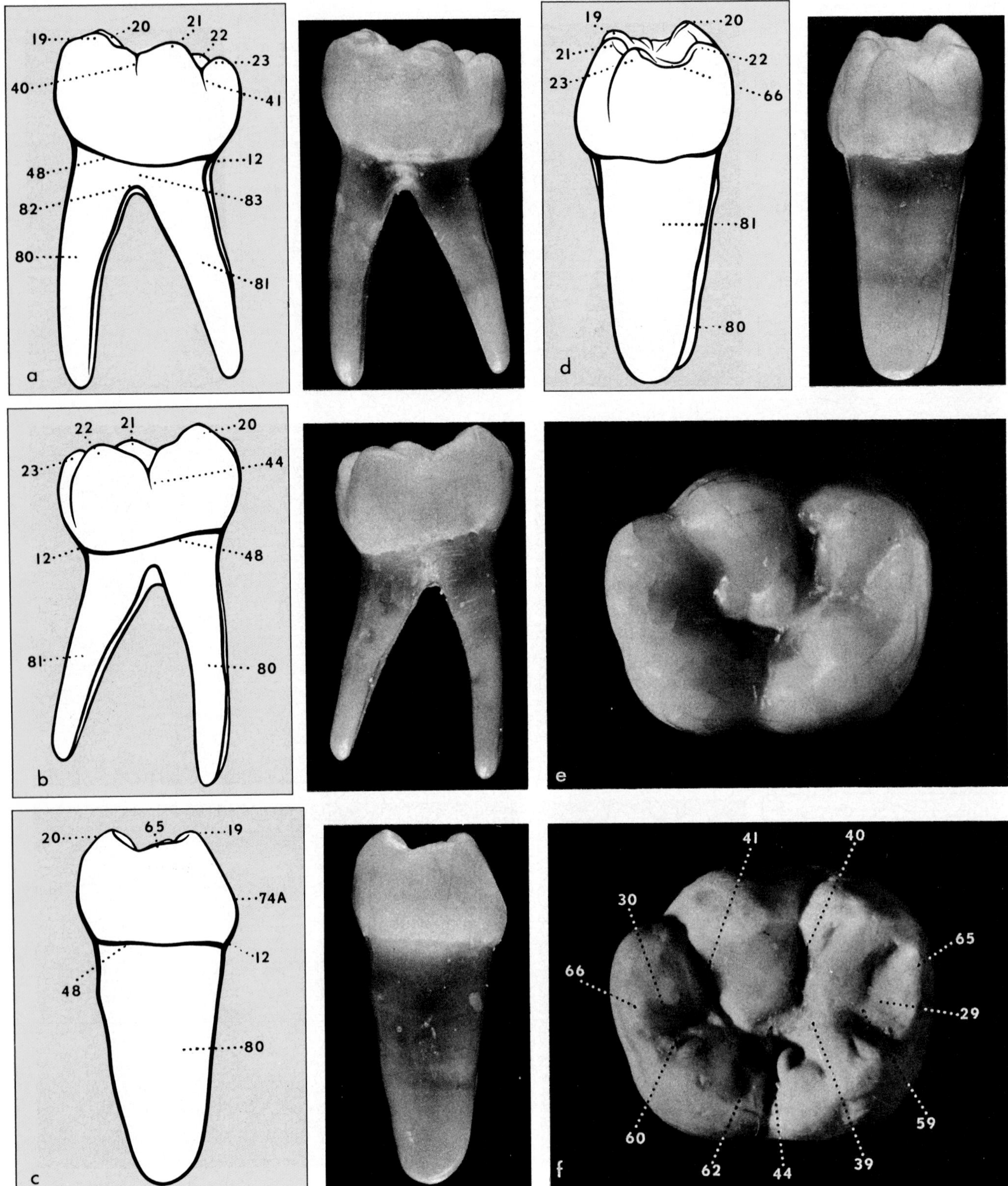

Figure 6.13

Mandibular left second molar: *a*, buccal aspect; *b*, lingual aspect; *c*, mesial aspect; *d*, distal aspect; *e*, occlusal aspect (actual crown); *f*, occlusal aspect (cast).

Table 6.4
Comparison of the Indices for Second Primary and First Permanent Mandibular Molars

	Mandibular Molars	
Indices	*Second primary*	*First permanent*
BL crown diameter / MD crown diameter	0.88	0.95
MD crown diameter / Crown height	1.80	1.47
Crown height / Total tooth length	0.30	0.35
BL crown diameter / Crown height	1.58	1.40

BL, buccolingual; MD, mesiodistal

from the mesial pit, one toward the mesiobuccal corner of the occlusal surface, the other extending over the marginal ridge onto the mesial surface. The distal termination of the central groove is marked by the *central pit,* which forms a deep valley in the distal portion (talonid) of the crown. Two grooves run from the central pit, one buccally (the *buccal groove*) and one lingually (the *lingual groove*). Often a distal pit may be found just mesial to the distal marginal ridge.

The *mandibular second primary molar* (Fig. 6.13*a* to *e*) as is the case with its antagonist is almost a duplicate of the adjoining permanent molar. The number and disposition of cusps, grooves, ridges, pits, and other crown characteristics conform remarkably. Only in crown and root proportions are the two dissimilar, as is demonstrated by Table 6.4.

The nature of the proportional dissimilarities is basically like that which distinguishes the two maxillary molars, with one exception. The mandibular permanent molar is broader relative to crown length than the mandibular primary. In the other three proportionate indices the relationship between the two is the same as between the maxillary two molars. It might be pointed out, however, that the mesiodistal length of the maxillary second molar crown is almost twice the height of the crown, giving the crown, from the buccal aspect, an extremely elongated appearance.

Like the other primary molar crowns, the mandibular second shows the usual cervical constriction and the concomitant bulging surfaces. The two roots are extremely narrow mesiodistally and very broad buccolingually. They are quite divergent and are less curved than those of the mandibular first molar. The occlusal pit-groove pattern, as noted above, is in no way different from that of the mandibular permanent first molar.

The chronology of morphogenetic stages in the development of the four primary molars before birth is presented in Tables 6.5 to 6.8.

Table 6.5
Chronology of Maxillary First Primary Molar Crown Development

Stage	Calcification	C-R Range (mm.)	Mean C-R	No.	Approximate Age (wk)
I	—	73–95	85	5	12½
II	—	77–95	85	17	12½
III	—	75–115	94	10	13
IV	—	90–125	110	6	14½
V	—	114–135	120	8	15
VI	1 cusp	118–136	127	14	15½
VII	1 cusp	113–150	131	27	16
VIII	1 cusp	124–185	158	10	17½
IX	2 cusps	150–207	174	43	19
X	3 cusps	200–230	216	13	22
XI	Buccal and lingual ridges	200–300	264	26	27
XII	Buccal and lingual ridges joined	265–320	288	10	30
XIII	Mesial and distal marginal ridges	287–350	326	4	28–32
XIV	Two pits uncalcified	205–340	295	12	28–32
XV	Occlusal surface calcified	268–370	328	21	32+
				Total 226	

Reprinted by permission from Kraus BS, Jordan RE. Human dentition before birth. Philadelphia: Lea & Febiger, 1965.

Table 6.6
Chronology of Maxillary Second Primary Molar Crown Development

Stage	Calcification	C-R Range (mm.)	Mean C-R	No.	Approximate Age (wk)
I	—	73–95	83	15	12½
II	—	84–115	100	3	13½
III	—	88–125	106	6	14
IV	—	91–122	106	2	14
V	—	103–136	118	21	15
VI	—	110–144	130	14	16
VII	—	124–150	138	10	16½
VIII	—	124–164	140	8	17
IX	1 cusp	135–224	173	40	19
X	2 cusps	200–270	226	5	23
XI	3 cusps	200–328	266	46	28
XII	4 cusps	251–300	275	15	28½
XIII	1st coalescence	275–350	294	7	30½
XIV	2nd coalescence	268–340	309	6	32
XV	Trigon cups joined	280–350	312	20	32
XVI	Lingual cusps joined	285–364	320	11	33
XVII	2 pits uncalcified (mesial and distal)	300–390	353	10	36
XVIII	Distal pit uncalcified	340–360	350	2	36
XIX	Occlusal surface calcified	370	370	1	38
				Total 242	

Reprinted by permission from Kraus BS, Jordan RE. Human dentition before birth. Philadelphia: Lea & Febiger, 1965.

Table 6.7
Chronology of Mandibular First Primary Molar Crown Development

Stage	Calcification	C-R Range (mm.)	Mean C-R	No.	Approximate Age (wk)
I	—	70–88	79	8	12
II	—	73–95	83	9	12½
III	—	76–125	107	6	14
IV	—	90–132	112	29	14½
V	1 cusp	113–146	126	15	15½
VI	1 cusp	124–150	136	16	16
VII	1 cusp	110–164	136	12	17
VIII	1 cusp	130–168	151	5	17½
IX	1 cusp	136–210	171	8	19
X	2 cusps	195–270	225	32	23
XI	3 cusps	200–285	237	25	24
XII	4 cusps	200–258	229	11	24
XIII	5 cusps	245–260	253	6	26
XIV	1st coalescence	251–301	275	4	28
XV	2nd coalescence	252–328	285	10	29½
XVI	3rd coalescence	251–381	296	43	30½
XVII	4th coalescence	287–340	314	9	32
XVIII	5th coalescence	268–362	307	37	32
XIX	Occlusal surface calcified	295–390	343	32	36+
				Total 314	

Reprinted by permission from Kraus BS, Jordan RE. Human dentition before birth. Philadelphia: Lea & Febiger, 1965.

Table 6.8
Chronology of Mandibular Second Primary Molar Crown Development

Stage	Calcification	C-R Range (mm.)	Mean C-R	No.	Approximate Age (wk)
I	—	76–95	82	14	12½
II	—	75–100	89	10	13
III	—	88–122	107	11	14
IV	—	91–132	118	5	15
V	—	103–136	118	14	15
VI	—	130–146	137	10	16
VII	—	109–143	127	10	16
VIII	—	124–176	146	13	17
IX	1 cusp	145–178	160	12	18
X	1 cusp	178–270	207	26	22
XI	2 cusps	200–246	221	7	23
XII	3 cusps	200–328	252	12	26
XIII	4 cusps	256–300	274	10	28
XIV	5 cusps	251–285	270	16	28
XV	1st coalescence	268–310	290	9	30
XVI	2nd coalescence	265–350	308	17	±32
XVII	3rd coalescence	270–307	291	12	±32
XVIII	4th coalescence	290–362	324	8	32–36
XIX	5th coalescence	320–370	347	10	36
XX	Occlusal surface calcified	300–390	350	4	36+
				Total 230	

Reprinted by permission from Kraus BS, Jordan RE. Human dentition before birth. Philadelphia: Lea & Febiger, 1965.

Part Two

Histology of the Teeth and Their Investing Structures

7

The Enamel

Enamel is the hard, vitreous-like substance that covers the outer regions on the tooth crown. In an oversimplified sense it can be pictured as the cap that covers and protects the underlying tissues (Fig. 7.1). In its mature state, enamel is highly mineralized, containing 96 percent inorganic substance by weight. Its most abundant mineral component (90 percent) is hydroxyapatite, which is crystalline in nature. Other minerals are present in much lower quantities in conjunction with a wide variety of trace metals. Water and organic substances, both of which are functionally important components, comprise the remaining 4 percent.

Structurally, enamel is composed of millions of calcified rods or prisms that traverse uninterruptedly the entire width of the enamel. These repetitive units constitute the bulk of the enamel. The submicroscopic component of the prism is the apatite crystallite, and it is the extremely tight packing and distinct pattern of orientation of these crystals that give the rods their structural identity and strength. An organically rich rod periphery and other important structural components comprise this very hard substance.

Hardness is an important property, since enamel must provide a protective covering for the softer underlying dentin, as well as serve as a unique masticatory surface on which crushing, grinding, and chewing of nutrient particles can be accomplished. To understand how tooth enamel can withstand the masticatory forces that it must continually bear, it is first necessary to consider its physiochemical, structural, and ultrastructural features.

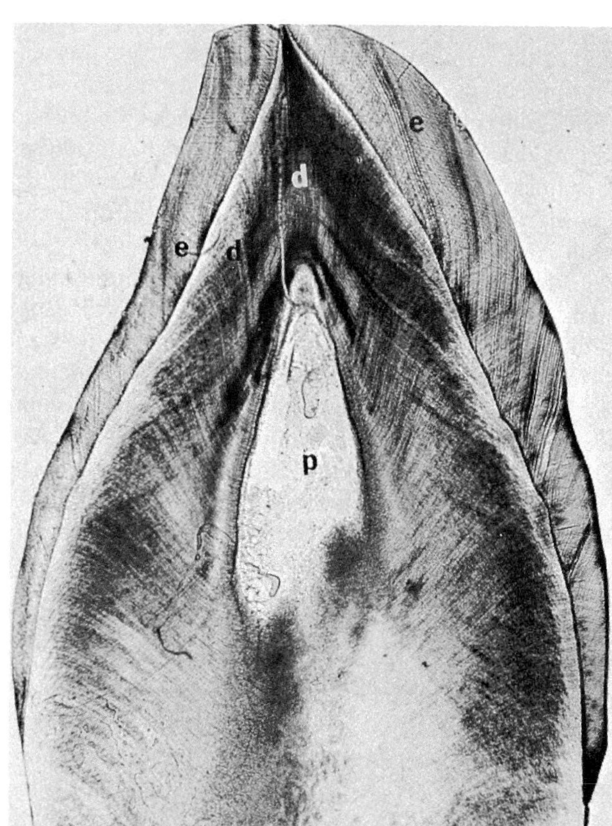

Figure 7.1

Longitudinal section of an incisor. *e*, enamel; *d*, dentin; *p*, pulp.

Physical Properties

Hardness

Since the *hardness* of tooth enamel can be expressed in terms of its ability to withstand deformation by indentation or scratching, several such measuring systems have been used to measure the hardness of enamel. As measured by the Moh's 10-point hardness scale, which is based on the hardness of diamond (Moh's no. 10), enamel demonstrates a range of 5 to 8 Moh. Several comparable, but more precise measurements of hardness have been reported with the Knoop hardness number (KHN, ratio of a given load to area of indentation expressed in kg/mm^2) microindentation tests. These studies indicate that there is considerable variability in enamel hardness (200 to 500 KHN). The wide variability is attributed to the

Table 7.1
Effect of Plane of Section and Location on Enamel Hardness (± Standard Deviation)*

	Labial Surface		Near Surface		Near Dentinoenamel Junction	
Tooth No.	*Intact*	*Polished*	*Transverse section*	*Longitudinally sectioned buccolingually*	*Transverse section*	*Longitudinally sectioned buccolingually*
10	363 ± 42	326 ± 13	324 ± 19	283 ± 13	284 ± 8	268 ± 15
12	392 ± 29	289 ± 26	328 ± 15	268 ± 14	272 ± 22	252 ± 20
G1		338 ± 9	314 ± 11		287 ± 11	
G2		342 ± 9	317 ± 23	285 ± 16	270 ± 11	280 ± 22

*Enamel hardness expressed in Knoop hardness number (KHN). Hardness varies according to the plane of section. Surface hardness is greater than subsurface area. KHN is lowest near the dentinoenamel junction.

Reproduced from Newbrun E. Variations in the hardness of enamel. Dent Progr 1962;2:21–27; by permission of *Dental Progress*.

fact that hardness of enamel can vary according to the plane in which it is tested (Table 7.1). Nevertheless, it seems evident that there are regional differences in hardness within a single tooth, the peripheral regions of the tooth being harder than the deeper regions (Table 7.1). Such regional differences have been suggested by radiopaque tracings and can be explained in part on the basis of regional differences in calcification. However, structural differences in these regions involving degree of calcification, prism and crystallite orientation, and distribution of metallic ions greatly influence the final hardness of enamel. Knowledge of tooth enamel hardness has value not only in assessing its plastic properties in relation to masticatory forces, but also as a consideration in the selection and use of restorative materials as well.

Density

The *density* of teeth has been measured directly using a technique capable of yielding absolute instead of relative values. It has been demonstrated that density values decreased from the surface of the enamel to the dentinoenamel junction. Similar distribution of values was obtained with an indirect microradiographic procedure, thus confirming the results of previous investigators. However, this increase in density, according to the more recent study, lies consistently within the narrow range of 3.00 to 2.84 g/ml (Fig. 7.2). Moreover, in permanent teeth it was shown that the density of upper incisors was greater than that of premolars and lower incisors; molars appeared to lie somewhere in between. The lowest density measurements of all human teeth studied were those of the deciduous teeth. It has also been shown that the density of enamel increases progressively during development, reaching its normal value after eruption into the oral cavity.

Enamel reaches its final thickness before eruption of the tooth. In general, the thickness of enamel varies throughout different regions of the tooth and from one type of tooth to another; over the cusps of molars it attains an average thickness of 2.6 mm, over the cusps of premolars it is 2.3 mm, and over the incisal edge of incisors it is approximately 2.0 mm thick. The

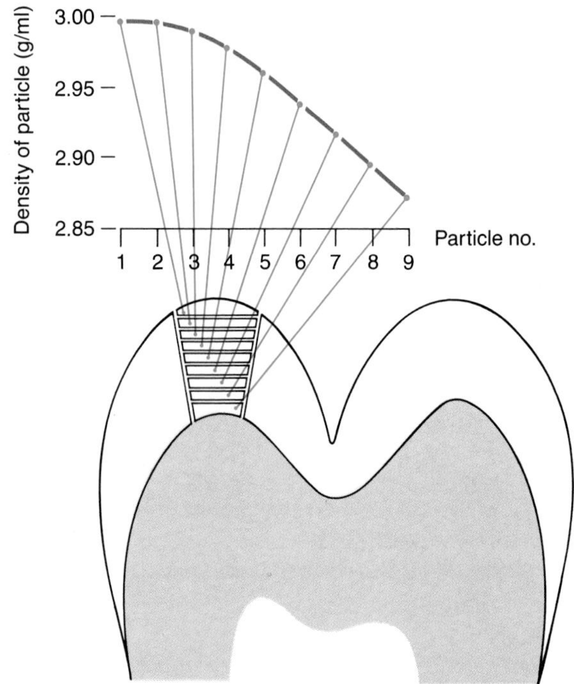

Figure 7.2
Density of enamel from the surface to dentinoenamel junction. Density of enamel decreases from the surface to the dentinoenamel junction. (Modified from Weidemann SM, et al., Variations of enamel density in sections of human teeth. Arch Oral Biol 1967; 12:85–97; by permission of Pergamon Press.)

enamel becomes progressively thinner toward the cervical regions and decreases even further as it approaches the cementoenamel junction where it terminates.

Color

Since it is semitranslucent in nature, the *color* of enamel is partly dependent upon the thickness of the enamel. For this reason, enamel frequently assumes the various hues of the underlying structures. That is, where enamel is thicker and more opaque, it will appear grayish or bluish white, thus reflecting its inherent coloration. Where enamel is relatively thin, it will be yellow-white in appearance, reflecting the underlying yellow dentin. This variation in the appearance of the enamel should not be confused with the yellowish layer or coating that accumulates on the tooth for lack of cleansing. Such colorations are due to the formation of dental plaque, which is an organic layer of film containing bacteria, leukocytes, and epithelial cells mixed with organic substances. Frequently brown or white spots mottle the enamel surfaces. This condition appears to be related to local changes in enamel such as subsurface decalcification, a loss in carbonate content, or an increase in nitrogenous compounds. Other variations in enamel coloring have also been reported. It can be seen from this cursory account that enamel coloration can be of considerable importance in revealing underlying physiochemical changes of normal and abnormal conditions of dental health.

Tensile Strength and Compressivity

Enamel must be hard to function properly as a masticatory tissue. Yet, hardness alone is not sufficient for it to withstand the hundreds of pounds of pressure brought to bear on each tooth during mastication. Quite the contrary, its hardness, as reflected in its brittleness, represents a structural weakness, since it is prone to splitting and chipping. Enamel does, however, have sufficient strength to withstand masticatory pressures and this is in great part due to the cushioning effect of the underlying dentin. *Tensile strength* and *compressivity* measurements on enamel reveal this physical relationship. Enamel has been shown to possess a high *elastic molulus* (19×10^6 PSI), which indicates that it is extremely brittle, and a relatively low tensile strength (11,000 PSI), which means it is a rigid structure. Dentin, on the other hand, is a highly compressive tissue (40,000 PSI), and can therefore act as a cushion for the overlying enamel. Thus, in addition to the conditions mentioned earlier, the ability of the tooth to withstand great masticatory force appears to be related to the structural and physical interrelationship between enamel and dentin.

Solubility

Enamel *solubility* is an important clinical consideration. When enamel is exposed to an acid medium it is subject to dissolution. Dissolution is not uniform throughout the enamel. Certain ions and molecules influence the solubility rate of enamel under acidic conditions. It is well known, for instance, that fluorides, when applied to the enamel surface, will reduce the solubility of the surface enamel. Other ions (silver nitrate, zinc chloride, indium nitrate, and stannous sulfate) similarly applied will do the same; however, in the latter instances, the anticariogenic effect that is characteristic of fluoride is absent. It remains to be elucidated exactly what role the various ions play in retarding solubility of enamel and preventing caries. It is clear, however, that protection is offered mainly to the surface regions, since subsurface regions of the tooth are much less affected by the fluoride treatment and are readily attacked by the acids.

It was mentioned earlier that carbonates decrease the solubility of enamel. Studies have shown that this ion is distributed more generously in the deeper regions of the enamel than in the surface areas. Accordingly, it would be expected that the enamel in the deeper region is more subject to dissolution than that of the surface. This has in fact been demonstrated. Enamel taken from the surface regions of the tooth was shown to be less soluble in acids than that taken from the deeper regions. The difference in solubility was not gradual, since the surface enamel was several times less soluble than the subsurface regions. However, from the subsurface region to the deepest regions near the dentinoenamel junction a gradual increase in solubility has been observed.

The organic matrix is also believed to play some role in enamel solubility. Earlier studies showed that areas of higher organic content were more resistant to the action of acids than those of the highly mineralized areas, as mentioned previously. These observations have led to the notion that the organic matrix may play some protective role, since removal of the organic matrix followed by acid treatment results in accelerated demineralization. Because of this it has been suggested that the organic matrix may also play some role in the defense against the acidogenic bacterial action which accompanies dental caries. Evidence bearing on this point is not, however, conclusive.

Permeability

Fluids of the oral cavity constitute the natural environment for tooth enamel. It might be expected, therefore, that some of the elements comprising this environment will *permeate* the enamel to varying degrees. Suggestive of this possibility is the fact that fluorides, which are present in human saliva, are found in greatest concentration at the surface of the enamel. This selective deposition along the enamel surface has been amply demonstrated in topical application procedures as well as under normal conditions. Fluorides are limited in their penetrability into the surface enamel, although reports indicate that with repeated application of the ion to the tooth surface its subsurface deposition is further enhanced. Despite this increased penetration, it seems evident that fluoride penetrability is limited. This is attributable to the fact that fluorides can be incorporated into the crystalline lattice of the apatite crystals. Such an exchange may also involve increased crystal growth and result in a decreased intercrystalline space, thus further restricting the transport of ions and molecules at the surface regions. This condition at the surface areas would then, presumably, act as a barrier to the influx of other ions and molecules, thus restricting permeability.

Early experiments used organic dyes to demonstrate enamel permeability. After the application of various organic dyes to the surface of the enamel, microscopic observations revealed that the enamel was, to varying degrees, permeable, and that the route of passage occurred mainly via the zone immediately surrounding the prism (rod sheath). The dye was also observed in enamel defects such as cracks or lamellae, as well as in the enamel tufts. All of the above-named structures are relatively rich in organic content. Although the mechanism by which diffusion occurs is not known, it is clear from this and other experiments that such organic dyes can indeed penetrate the enamel, particularly through structural units which are hypomineralized, or rich in organic content.

Subsequent studies have shown that the lamellae and other gross structural units are not the only passageways of ion or molecular transport. This can be demonstrated by connecting the root of an extracted tooth to a rubber tube that is in turn attached to a glass barometer containing saline. When the tooth is placed in water, the saline level in the capillary tube rises. The results indicate that the water passes through the enamel as though it were selectively permeable. Similar results are obtained when the tooth is placed in saline instead of water, although the rate of flow is considerably reduced.

Evidence for ion transport in enamel is also supported by early studies with radioactive tracers. These studies clearly indicated that certain pathways must be open to diffusing ions and molecules since tagged or radioactive substances penetrated the tooth to varying degrees. For example, NaI^{131}, I^{131}, nicotinamide, urea, thiourea, and acetamide were found in histological sections of human enamel 30 minutes after topical application. However, enamel is not freely permeable to all the ions and molecules tested; for example, radioactive calcium, zinc, and silver could not be detected in the enamel except in regions revealing cracks or other defects.

The importance of these findings lies not only in the necessary assumption that submicroscopic avenues or passageways of molecular transport must exist in tooth enamel but also in the possibility that the fluids (water) can possibly act as the transporting medium or agent for ions and molecules contained within the structural complex of enamel. The organically rich interstices of enamel contain a loosely bound fraction of water, which could facilitate ion and molecular transport through the restrictively small intercrystalline spaces. Under experimental conditions, it has, in fact, been demonstrated that water travels through the enamel at a fairly rapid rate (4 $mm^3/cm^2/$24 hours). Since enamel is not endowed with a "nutrient" supply system such as found in cellular tissues, the presence of an analogous "circulatory" system delivering ions and molecules to various regions of the enamel would be of some importance in influencing the structural integrity of the crystallite as well as that of the organic matrix.

There exists evidence which indicates that the organic matrix must play an important role in maintaining the permeability properties of young, healthy enamel. In deciduous teeth undergoing exfoliation, it has been demonstrated that permeability properties are progressively lost during the advanced stages. A loss of permeability has also been noted in aging permanent teeth, although in the latter case it is not complete and basic permeability is maintained. The exact reason for decreased permeability has not been ascertained but there is evidence that changes in the enamel matrix may be a contributing factor. This is suggested by experiments in which diffusion of sodium through enamel was measured before and after heat treatment. As is shown in Figure 7.3, the diffusion of sodium is sharply curtailed after heating or boiling of enamel. This has been explained on the ba-

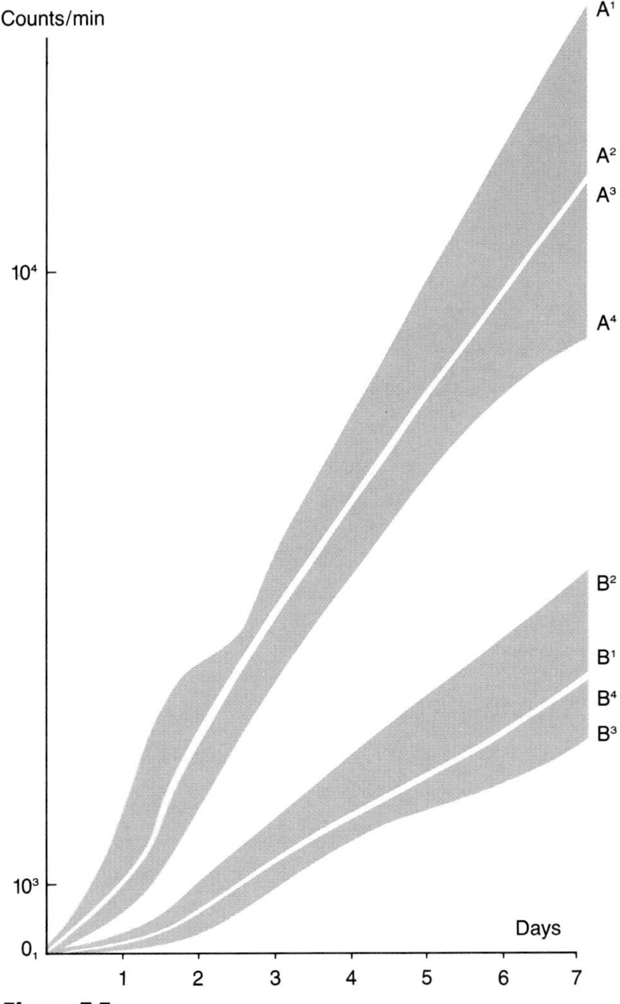

Figure 7.3

Na^{22} diffusion rate of freshly extracted tooth (*A*'s) and boiled (*B*'s) contralateral premolar crowns. (From Arwill ETG. Formal contributions: Discussion of fourth session. In: Stack MV, Fearnhead RW, eds. Tooth Enamel: Its Composition, Properties, and Fundamental Structure. Guilford, England: Butterworth-Heinemann, 1965.)

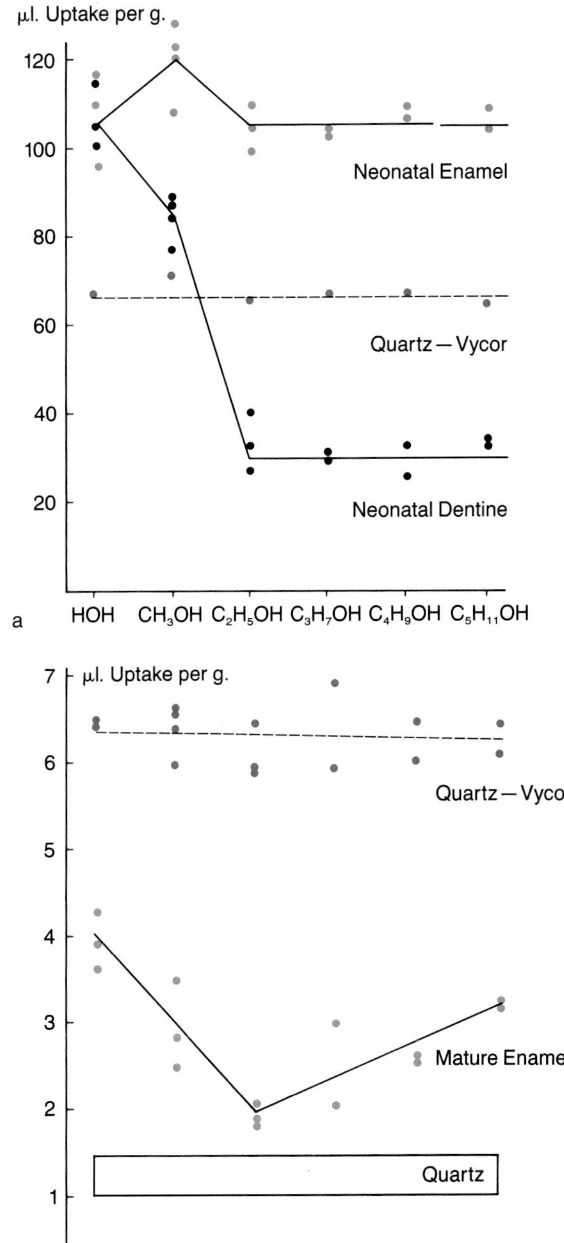

Figure 7.4

a, volume uptake of *n*-alcohols by developing enamel and dentin. *b*, volume uptake of *n*-alcohols by mature enamel. (Reproduced from Poole DFG, Stack MV. In: Stack MV, Fearnhead RW, eds. Tooth Enamel: Its Composition, Properties, and Fundamental Structure. Guilford, England: Butterworth-Heinemann, 1965.)

sis that the organic content of enamel undergoes denaturation, which involves a loss of permeability.

From previously cited permeability studies, particularly those dealing with molecular transport and diffusion of water and permeable ions, it is believed that water and ions pass, via osmosis, through the enamel substance proper as though it were a selectively permeable membrane; from this it has been deduced that enamel possesses a submicroscopic pore system. Attempts have been made to localize and determine the diameter of such pores using liquids with molecular dimensions graduated in size, such as methyl, ethyl, and propyl alcohols (Fig. 7.4*a* and *b*). The results indicated that enamel is capable of taking up molecules and ions comparable in size to that of the pores since the larger molecules failed to be imbibed. It was therefore suggested that enamel possesses a pore system similar to that of a molecular sieve. It is not presently known how such a pore system is distributed in enamel; x-ray diffraction, electron microscopy, and phase-contrast studies have been suggestive in this regard, pointing to the interprismatic and intercrystalline spaces as possible pore sites. Unfortunately, the organic substance occupying such spaces complicates the understanding of the pore system hypothesis and makes it difficult to evaluate without further intensive study. Despite these difficulties, it seems safe to say that enamel is, to varying degrees, porous, but that the organic matrix and the type of penetrant, its molecular size, and ionic character must all be considered as factors influencing enamel permeability.

Chemical Composition

Inorganic Content

Major Constituents

Calcium and phosphate are by far the two largest inorganic elements in tooth enamel. X-ray diffraction studies indicate that both of these constituents along with hydroxyl ions are present in the form of a crystalline lattice that is apatite ($Ca_{10}(OH)_2(PO_4)_6$) in character (Fig. 7.5). The apatites in enamel are somewhat variable in nature because they can bind and incorporate a variety of ions into their crystalline structure. The incorporation of such ions usually involves the displacement and substitution of an existing ion. Experiments indicate that strontium, radium, vanadium, and carbonate can exchange with the phosphates in the lattice. Such exchanges can frequently alter the properties and the crystalline structure. Most notable in this respect is the *effect of fluoride on tooth enamel.* This exchange reaction leaves the enamel apatites more resistant to acid dissolution and has been shown to be clearly anticariogenic in nature.

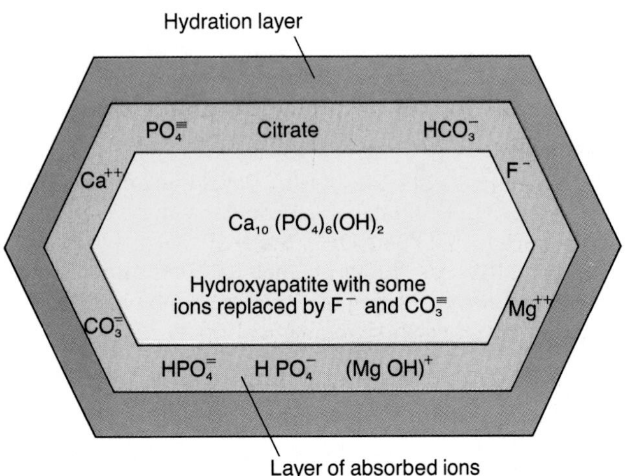

Figure 7.5

Diagrammatic structure of apatite crystals.

Opposite effects are seen, however, when carbonates associate with or incorporate into the apatite crystalline lattice. In this instance, the tooth enamel becomes much more soluble in acids and less resistant to cariogenic processes. Knowledge of these facts has led to widespread use of fluorides in drinking water to combat dental caries.

Minor Constituents

A considerable number of minor inorganic constituents have been detected in human enamel. Fluoride,

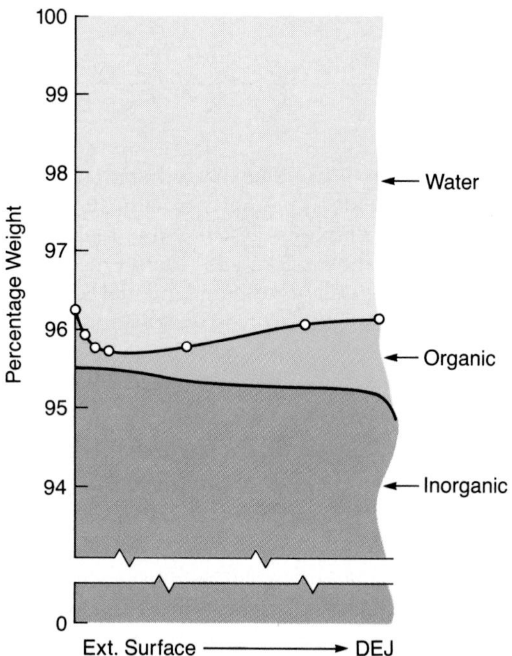

Figure 7.6

Distribution of water and organic and inorganic substances from the surface to the dentinoenamel junction (*DEJ*). (From Brudevold F, et al. Inorganic and organic components of tooth structure. Ann NY Acad Sci 1960; 85:110–132; by permission of *Annals of the New York Academy of Science.*)

silver, aluminum, barium, copper, magnesium, nickel, lead selenium, strontium, titanium, vanadium, and lead are among those elements which are present. Of course, fluoride and zinc appear to be present in greatest quantities (about 2000 parts per million), whereas the remainder are present in sufficiently low amounts to be considered trace elements. These minor inorganic components are not all uniformly distributed throughout the enamel, but rather appear to show some degree of stratification. For instance, F, Pb, Zn, Fe, and Sr appear in higher concentration near the surface of the enamel. On the other hand, Na, Mg, and CO_2 are found in increasingly higher concentrations near the dentinoenamel junction or the innermost region of the enamel.

It is not clear why many of these inorganic components stratify in the manner described. However, there are sufficient differences (contact with oral fluids versus tissue fluids; an uneven distribution of water, organic content, and minerals) (see Fig. 7.6) existing between surface and deep enamel which conceivably could influence the deposition of these minor constituents in a preferential manner.

Organic Content

Amino Acid Content of Mature Enamel Matrix

Less than 1 percent of deciduous and permanent tooth enamel is composed of organic matter, and of this 1 percent, only 0.4 percent contains proteins. The remaining 0.6 percent consists of carbohydrates, lipids, and other organic substances. It is generally agreed that most of this organic matter is derived from the organic matrix that is laid down by the ameloblasts during their secretory period. The exact nature of these proteins is as yet an unsettled question. This is partly because the analysis of the enamel matrix presents a constellation of special technical obstacles difficult to overcome. First of all, enamel proteins are available in such limited quantities (0.4 percent) that enormous amounts of enamel are required for study. Secondly, it has until recently been difficult to isolate pure enamel from the remainder of the tooth, making contamination difficult to avoid. Thirdly, a large fraction of the enamel matrix is not readily soluble; upon its hydrolysis a soluble component is removed by the very agents that are capable of breaking down the relatively insoluble matrix into amino acid fragments. Notwithstanding these and other technical difficulties, a general picture of the enamel matrix proteins has been obtained.

The amino acid profile of the enamel matrix is not identical to any of the known proteins (Table 7.2). Yet its relatively high glycine content and the presence of lysine, histidine, and arginine in small but significant amounts have led a number of investigators to believe that the enamel proteins may belong to the family of keratin-type proteins. The latter suggestion is based on the fact that the keratins, though a heterogeneous group, are generally endowed with large amounts of glycine and may contain lysine, arginine, and histidine in a ratio not dissimilar to that seen in enamel proteins. Also, both the enamel matrix and keratins are epidermal in origin, show similar histochemical staining patterns, and are relatively insoluble in acids and with certain enzymes. Despite these and other similarities, there appear to be significant differences between keratins and proteins of the enamel matrix. Glycine, for instance, is not present in amounts quantitatively comparable to those seen in most keratins. Usually keratins contain much higher amounts of glycine. Perhaps the most disconcerting data regarding the classification of enamel matrix proteins is the presence of hydroxyproline. The amino acid is generally regarded as indicating the presence of collagen, an extracellular fibrous protein. Yet electron microscope studies reveal no collagen fibers in the enamel matrix. In addition, neither infrared analysis nor histochemical stains, both of which can detect collagen, yield data or results that can be interpreted as indicating the presence of this protein.

On the basis of the foregoing evidence, some investigators have proposed that the enamel matrix may contain a keratin-like protein, although the quantitative aspects of its amino acid profile are distinct from other known keratins. It has been suggested in addition that the protein may be able to incorporate hydroxyproline as an integral part of its structure since this amino acid is invariably found to be present in the absence of collagen. Alternatively, there is the suggestion that hydroxyproline is a persistent and unavoidable contaminant derived from the dentin and cementum (two major sources of collagen). Countering the view that the enamel matrix is a keratin, it has been claimed that the criterion for identifying keratins rests on too broad and ill-defined a basis and is prejudiced by an earlier histologic notion that epithelial derivatives are *carte blanche* keratin producers.

Efforts to establish the identity of the enamel matrix proteins have been attempted with x-ray diffraction procedures. Such a technique can give valuable information regarding the tridimensional configuration of the enamel proteins. The x-ray pattern obtained indicates that the peptide chain arrangement resembles the structure of several other keratogenous proteins. There is, however, lack of agreement on whether the enamel proteins have an alpha (stretched) or beta (folded) configuration. This uncertainty stems

Table 7.2
Comparison of Amino Acid Composition of Mature Enamel Matrix (Numbers of Amino Acid Residues per 1,000 Total Residues)

	Insoluble Mature Enamel				Water Soluble	EDTA Soluble	Insoluble	Enamel, Human Fetal
	Hess et al. *(1953)*	*Battistone and Burnett (1956)*	*Stack (1954)*	*Rodriguez (1963)*	*Lofthouse (1961)*			*Eastoe (1961)*
Hydroxyproline	47.3	42.5	32.4	70.6	12.0	14.1	54.1	0
Aspartic acid	45.8	44.0	24.2	55.6	60.2	59.4	58.9	30.3
Threonine	44.8	41.5	79.3	26.0	31.8	54.8	37.8	38.1
Serine	75.5	71.6	81.0	39.2	55.0	55.1	50.1	62.5
Glutamic acid	78.0	76.9	25.3	91.6	113.0	119.0	88.9	142.0
Proline	47.0	39.6	74.9	92.6	82.9	124.0	106.0	251.0
Glycine	304.0	336.0	71.9	282.4	146.0	105.0	173.0	65.0
Alanine	111.0	131.0	80.5	101.7	60.0	42.3	80.6	20.3
Cystine		2.6		3.8		4.6	2.4	2.3
Valine	33.8	33.5	35.4	42.0	22.8	35.7	42.2	39.6
Methionine	8.3	7.3	10.4	11.8		14.4	4.0	42.3
Isoleucine	16.3		20.6	22.0	13.7	20.2	16.5	32.7
Leucine	41.9	99.5	61.8	47.6	35.9	64.0	50.5	91.3
Phenylalanine	45.8		52.4	22.0		15.7	12.8	23.4
Tyrosine	6.9	6.5	16.1	5.3	32.3	28.8	18.6	53.4
Hydroxylysine				4.2	10.7	7.2	3.9	
Lysine	31.2	19.0	25.5	28.8	36.9	29.2	32.5	17.7
Histidine	9.0	4.0	6.0	6.6	9.2	15.0	9.7	64.5
Arginine	47.0	43.7	76.1	45.0	104.0	22.3	47.9	23.3
NH_3			226.0		173.0	171.0	110.0	146.0

Adapted from Weidmann SM, Hamm SM. In: Stack MV, Fearnhead RW, eds. Tooth Enamel: Its Composition, Properties, and Fundamental Structure. Guilford, England: Butterworth-Heinemann, 1965.

from the fact that the alpha form is readily converted into the beta form through a wide variety of conditions that induce denaturation of the protein. It is therefore uncertain whether the commonly observed folded configuration truly exists in its native state or whether it represents an artificially induced interconversion.

It must be clear from the foregoing discussion that enamel proteins have not as yet been clearly characterized. On the one hand they have features in common with other keratogenous and fibrous proteins, while on the other hand they are not identical to any protein thus far known. On this basis, they have been considered as being keratin-like in nature. Perhaps this is a temporary designation which awaits modification. With improved methods of solubilization, purifying, and separating the components of enamel proteins, a more definitive classification will doubtlessly emerge.

Amino Acid Content of Developing Enamel Matrix

In contrast to the rather low percentage of organic content of mature enamel, fetal or developing enamel matrix contains a relative abundance of organic substances. Deciduous human enamel contains 15 to 20 percent protein by weight, a figure similar to that found in pig enamel (Fig. 7.7). It appears to contain a number of proteins that are as yet unidentified. From an analysis similar to that described for the adult enamel matrix, it can be seen that developing enamel bears no strict resemblance to any of the known keratins. It is toward the latter phase of enamel matrix development that the points of comparison become obvious. This resemblance is acquired through a change in relative proportions of the amino acid content. That is, the proline and histidine content decreases whereas glycine, hydroxyproline, serine, and aspartic acid increase in amounts. There are data to indicate that an inversion of the lysine:histidine: arginine (L:H:A) ratio occurs (Fig. 7.8). Histidine, which is initially present in increased amounts, drops precipitously during maturation, whereas arginine, which is initially low, is substantially increased. Lysine almost doubles in value during the developmental period. At present, it is not clear why there is a selective loss in certain amino acids and an increase

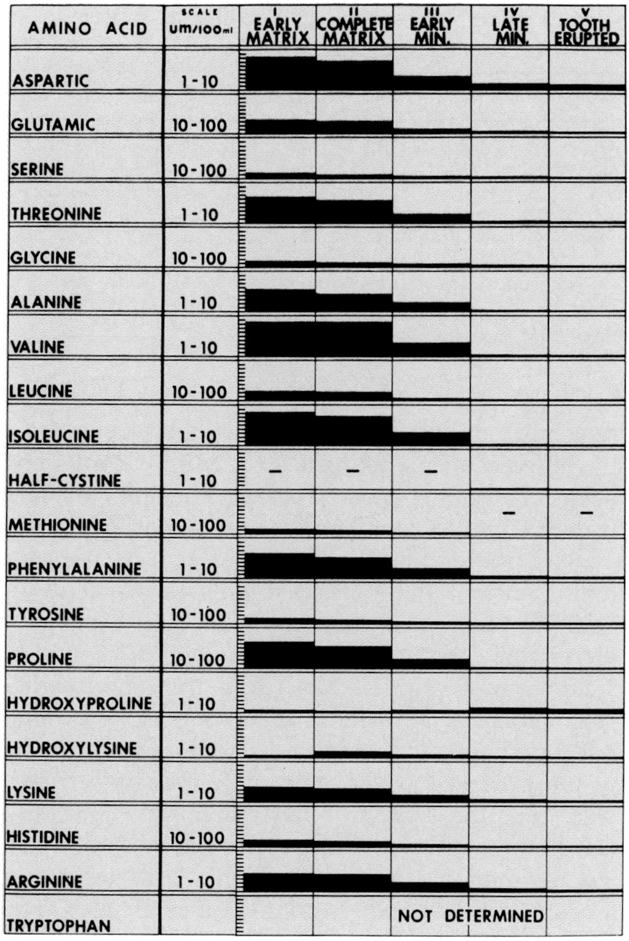

STAGE OF ENAMEL FORMATION
AMINO ACID
SCALE um/100ml
I EARLY MATRIX
II COMPLETE MATRIX
III EARLY MIN.
IV LATE MIN.
V TOOTH ERUPTED
ASPARTIC 1-10
GLUTAMIC 10-100
SERINE 10-100
THREONINE 1-10
GLYCINE 10-100
ALANINE 1-10
VALINE 1-10
LEUCINE 10-100
ISOLEUCINE 1-10
HALF-CYSTINE 1-10
METHIONINE 10-100
PHENYLALANINE 1-10
TYROSINE 10-100
PROLINE 10-100
HYDROXYPROLINE 1-10
HYDROXYLYSINE 1-10
LYSINE 1-10
HISTIDINE 10-100
ARGININE 1-10
TRYPTOPHAN
NOT DETERMINED

Figure 7.7

Change in relative proportions of amino acid during development. (Drawn with modification from Burgess RC, Maclaren C. Proteins in developing bovine enamel. In: Stack MV, Fearnhead RW, eds. Tooth Enamel: Its Composition, Properties, and Fundamental Structure. Guilford, England: Butterworth-Heinemann, 1965.)

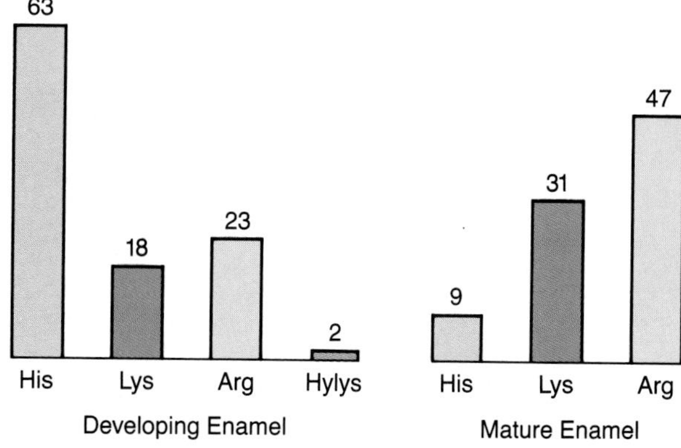

Figure 7.8

Developing enamel. Alteration in lysine:histidine:arginine (L:H:A) ratio during development. (From Eastoe JE. The amino-acid composition of proteins from the oral tissues. Arch Oral Biol 1963; 8:633–652; by permission of Pergamon Press.)

in others. There is general agreement that overall losses in protein content are not due to technical procedures, although some loss probably occurs. It has been postulated that the total decrease in organic content together with the change in relative proportions of amino acids may be associated with the concomitant mineralization or maturation process.

Some cytologic studies suggest that the ameloblasts are instrumental in bringing about such losses. Throughout most of the phases of mineralization, the ameloblast functions as a secretory cell, laying down the enamel matrix. This is evidenced by the fact that new matrix is always seen in association with the receding cell surface of the ameloblast. Yet when mineralization increases considerably, the ameloblast undergoes morphologic changes in the cell surface not unlike those seen in other cells of the body known to be absorptive in function. The ameloblast begins to develop a pseudopod type of cell surface which is seen to acquire small granules similar in density to organic substances in the extracellular mineralizing zone. These cytologic events have been interpreted as indicating the withdrawal of organic substances from the enamelized regions of the tooth (Fig. 7.9).

Water Content of Enamel

Relative to the amount of organic material present in enamel, water is present in considerable abundance. It is not, however, uniformly distributed. The deeper region of enamel contains more water than the peripheral region. Recent studies indicate that the enamel of permanent teeth contains a minimum of 4 percent water by weight. This is a significantly high figure; if calculated by volume, water would occupy as much as 11 percent of the tooth enamel.

It is estimated that about 25 percent of the water is present in a form loosely associated with that of the crystallite, since it is readily freed when subjected to thermal radiation. Because of this, it is believed to be associated with the organic component of the enamel. It is conceivable that the fraction of the water component may act as the media by which ions and molecules can be transported through enamel. The significance of this possibility will be discussed further in conjunction with studies on enamel permeability.

The greater portion of the water present in enamel appears to be associated with the mineral component and is believed to be present as a hydrated shell surrounding the apatite crystallite. The

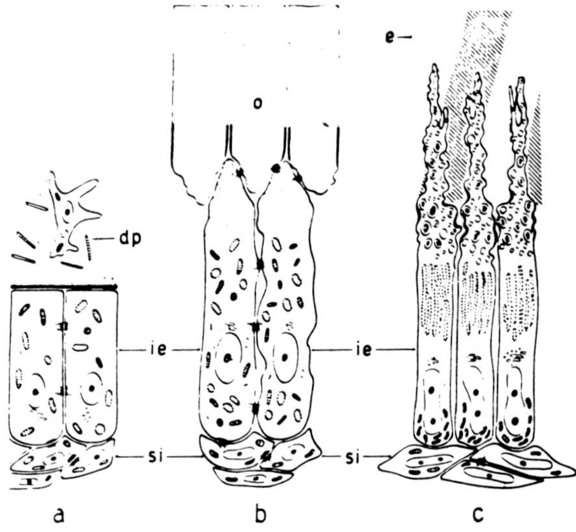

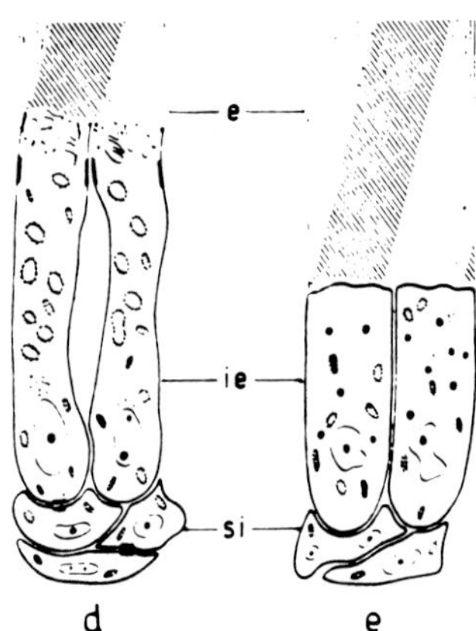

Figure 7.9
Schematic diagram of inner enamel epithelium illustrating the initial differentiation and final involution of the ameloblasts. *ie,* inner enamel epithelium; *si,* stratum intermedium; *e,* enamel. (From Pannese E. Ultrastructure of the enamel organ. Int Rev Exp Pathol 1964; 3:198; by permission of Pergamon Press.)

mechanism of this attachment is as yet unknown, but it is clear from the more recent studies that the water is tightly bound. The presence of a hydrated layer around the hydroxyapatite crystals may be of importance in facilitating both ion exchange reactions and ion and molecular transport.

Carbohydrates

It has been demonstrated that the enamel matrix contains several hexoses with traces of two pentose sugars. Galactose was found in greatest abundance, glucose next, and mannose least. The trace sugars were identified as fucose and xylose. A fraction containing hexuronic acid was also isolated. The latter fraction was believed to contain glucosamine and galactosamine. Earlier studies by Stack (1955) on hexose content of enamel matrix indicate the presence of glycogen. However, histochemical techniques capable of identifying glycogen and glycoproteins are found to yield faintly positive results, except during the earlier stage of matrix deposition. A subsequent histochemical investigation yielded similar results with respect to the presence of acid mucopolysaccharide stains. Here too, the reaction appeared positive during a stage in mineralization and became fainter upon matrix maturation. These histochemical studies are in accord with the radioisotope studies that demonstrated the incorporation of radioactive sulfate in maturing enamel matrix. The results of these studies therefore indicate the presence of carbohydrates during the earlier phases of mineralization, whereas its presence during the latter or mature phase of enamel matrix development is not readily evident. This can be accounted for either by a generalized loss of organic substances during maturation as pointed out previously, or possibly by a linking up of the carbohydrate moiety with proteins or even minerals which make their histochemical detection more difficult. Whatever the reason, it is clear that the decreasing stainability of carbohydrates parallels the loss in organic content. It has therefore been associated with the mineralization process which inversely increases with the loss of organic substance.

Table 7.3
Percentage of Mineral, Organic Matter, and Water in Human Enamel by Weight and Volume

Phase	Weight	Volume
	%	%
Mineral	95.0	87
Organic	1.0	2
Water	4.0	12

Reproduced from Brudevold and Söremark. In: Miles AEW, ed. Structural and Chemical Organization of Teeth II. New York: Academic Press, 1967.

Lipids

There are several areas of investigation which indicate that the organic matrix contains *lipoidal substances.* By chemical analysis, as much as 0.6 percent total lipids in enamel matrix with traces of cholesterol and noncholesterol lipids were detected. Also, x-ray diffraction patterns of enamel have been interpreted as revealing the presence of lipoidal materials. At present, there have been no definitive studies to identify the basic type of lipids that may be glycerides or masked or protein-bound forms. It has been suggested that such lipids may play some role in the calcification process as well, since lipoidal substances stainable by organic dyes are found to be present in greater amounts in the latter stages of matrix mineralization development than in the earlier stages. It should be noted that the presence of lipoidal substance in organic matrix is not inconsistent with the view that enamel matrix contains a keratin type of protein since this protein is frequently found in conjunction with lipoidal substances.

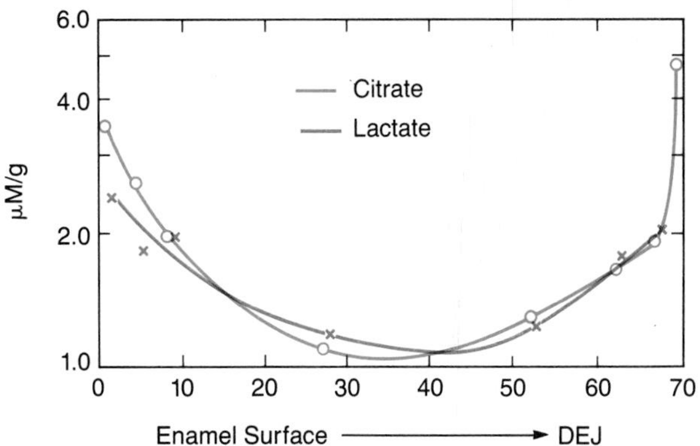

Figure 7.10

Citrate and lactate distribution in enamel of persons under 20 years of age. Concentration of both constituents are higher at the surface and the dentinoenamel junction (*DEJ*) than at the middle. (Modified from Burdevold F, et al. Inorganic and organic components of tooth structure. Ann NY Acad Sci 1960; 85:110–132; by permission of *Annals of the New York Academy of Science*.)

Citrate

Citrate has its importance in relation to the tricarboxylic acid cycle in that it can provide electrons and energy to be used for biological energy transactions. However, it is likely that it serves in some other capacity in relation to enamel. Since citrate is well known to possess the ability to bind with calcium, and is found in association with other calcifying tissues, it is believed to play some role in mineralization.

Citrate is present in enamel matrix and represents about 0.1 percent of the nonprotein organic content. It has been postulated that the anion is in some way associated with an inorganic lattice, possibly serving to influence crystal formation and growth. As is shown in Figure 7.10, citrate is present in greater amounts at the surface of the enamel than its interior although there is a notable increase at the dentinoenamel junction. Citrate is present in human saliva, particularly after the intake of carbohydrate material. Similar observations have been made with regard to the presence of lactate; the latter is present in smaller amounts in enamel than citrate.

Structural Components of Enamel

Enamel Prisms

The fundamental morphologic unit of enamel is the calcified rod or prism. When observed in longitudinal section with the light microscope, prisms are seen to arise from the dentinoenamel junction, which borders the underlying dentin and proceeds uneruptedly to the external surface of the tooth (Fig. 7.11*a*). However, they initially follow an undulating or sigmoidal path through one-third of the enamel; for the remaining two-thirds, the enamel follows a more direct path to the surface. In histologic section, however, this continuity is often difficult to follow, since the rods curve out of the place of section. In general, however, enamel rods are aligned perpendicularly to the dentinoenamel junction (Fig. 7.11*b* and *c*) except in the cervical regions of permanent teeth (Fig. 7.11*a*).

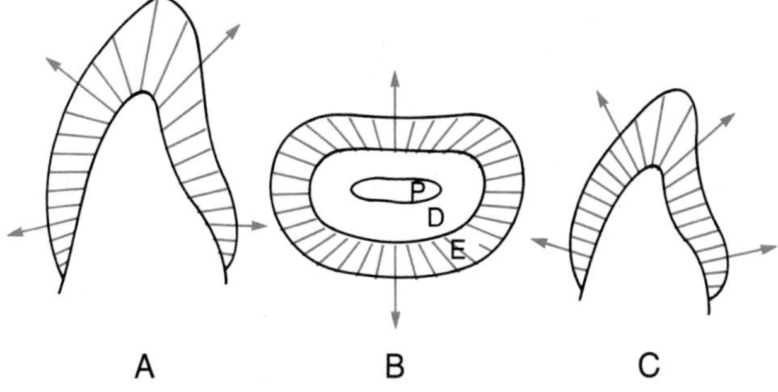

Figure 7.11

a, direction of enamel rods in permanent teeth, long section. Rods in cervical areas are directed apically. *b*, cross-section of enamel showing the direction of rods. *c*, direction of enamel rods in deciduous teeth. Rods are oriented more or less perpendicular to dentinoenamel junction. *P*, pulp; *D*, dentin; *E*, enamel.

In the latter case, the rods are oriented somewhat apically (Fig. 7.11*a*). Groups of enamel rods that follow a highly serpentine and tortuous path in their ascent to the surface are called parazones and diazones. In the cuspal region these zones contribute to enamel. In the cervical region rod arrangement is highly irregular.

Measurements of rod width indicate that rods near the dentinal borders have a smaller diameter (approximately 4 μm) than those nearer the surface (8 μm). A number of studies report that the actual dimensions may vary although the ratio of the polar ends is approximately 2:1. The explanation for this difference is attributed to the secreting ameloblast surface, which widens as it recedes to the surface during the development of the crown. Hence, the width of the matrix and mineralization path follows the change in the secreting surface of the ameloblast.

Along the length of most rods, *cross-striations* can be observed. These striations are spaced at variable intervals (3 to 10 μm), thus giving the rod a segmented appearance (Fig. 7.12). This feature can best be observed using the higher-power microscope objectives, though it is also visible at lower magnification. Cross-striations are believed to represent transverse zones or areas of increased organic content and will stain selectively with organic dyes after partial decalcification of the section. Some investigators suggest that crystallite orientation or localized width difference creates the optical effect of striated markings. It has been suggested that striations may also mark the site of a complex pore system that will selectively permit the flow or penetration of certain-sized molecules. The suggestion that cross-striations represent a micropore system is based upon imbibition (uptake of various fluids) studies with the light, phase contrast, and polarizing microscopes. As yet, however, no direct morphologic evidence confirming the existence of a pore system (associated with cross-striations) has been obtained with the electron microscope.

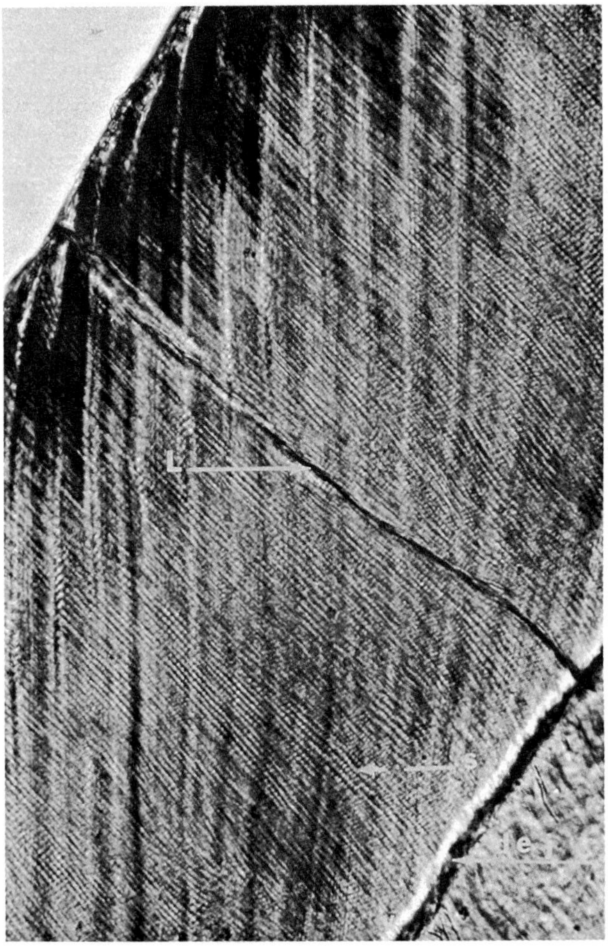

Figure 7.12

A portion of enamel showing the dentinoenamel junction (*dej*), direction of rods, striations (*s*), lamellae (*L*).

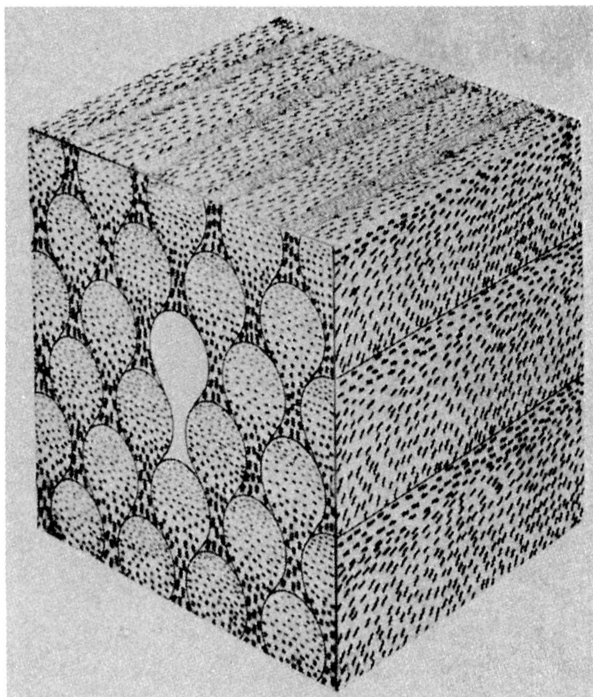

Figure 7.13

Cardboard model illustrating keyhole shape of enamel prisms in cross-section. Orientation of crystallites in "head" region is more or less longitudinal with long axis of prism. Crystallites in "tail" region perpendicular to long axis (based on electron micrographs of enamel prisms). (From Meckel AH, et al. Ultrastructure of fully calcified human dental enamel. In: Stack MV, Fearnhead RW, eds. Tooth Enamel: Its Composition, Properties, and Fundamental Structure. Guilford, England: Butterworth-Heinemann, 1965.)

Classically, enamel rods or prisms in cross-section have been described as being either round or hexagonal, but more frequently horseshoe shaped. More recent studies with the electron microscope reveal that the prisms, in cross-section, are not simply scalariform or horseshoe shaped but rather possess a configuration that is roughly similar in shape to that of a keyhole (Figs. 7.13 to 7.16). It is doubtful that this is a constant pattern, since variations in the schematic keyhole shape have also been observed. Nevertheless, these prisms are frequently assembled in such a manner as to suggest some functional arrangement since they form a repetitive series of interlocking structures. The rounded portion of each prism (5 μm) lies between the "tail" (5 μm long) of two adjacent prisms. Such an interlocking arrangement can conceivably provide the enamel with added strength and durability. The prism is oriented so that the rounded portion is oriented in the occlusal direction and the tail is oriented toward the cervical regions of the crown. If some functional significance were to be attributed to this orientation it might indicate that the head region bears the brunt of the masticatory impact, whereas the tail, which is distributed over a wider surface, may act to distribute and dissipate the impact. Despite this possibility, it is perhaps premature to attribute any functional significance to rod shape, since the extent of rod shape variability is itself not presently known.

The enamel prism is composed of innumerable crystallites that vary in size as well as shape. Some electron microscope studies indicate that the mature crystals are either ribbon-like, needle-shaped, or hexagonal rods (Figs. 7.17 and 7.18). In all instances noted, they appear elongated. So far as can be determined at present there is no constant size, ranging from 2,000 to 10,000 Å in length or perhaps longer. X-ray diffraction studies on crystal length indicate an average length of about 1,600 Å, and a width of 200 to 400 Å.

The crystallites within the prism are closely aggregated and show a definitive orientation. Schematically they can be visualized as tiny rodlets that are oriented in accordance with the area in the prism in which they are located. Crystallites in the round part

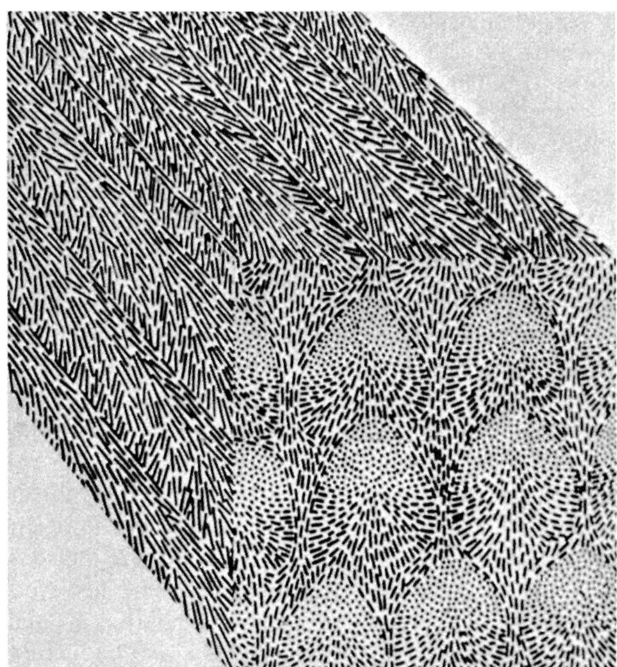

Figure 7.14

Conceptual model of prism shape and crystallite orientation. Modified keyhole shape based upon x-ray diffraction and polarization microscopy. (From Carlstrom D. Polarization microscopy of dental enamel. Adv Oral Biol 1964; 1:255–296; by permission of Academic Press.)

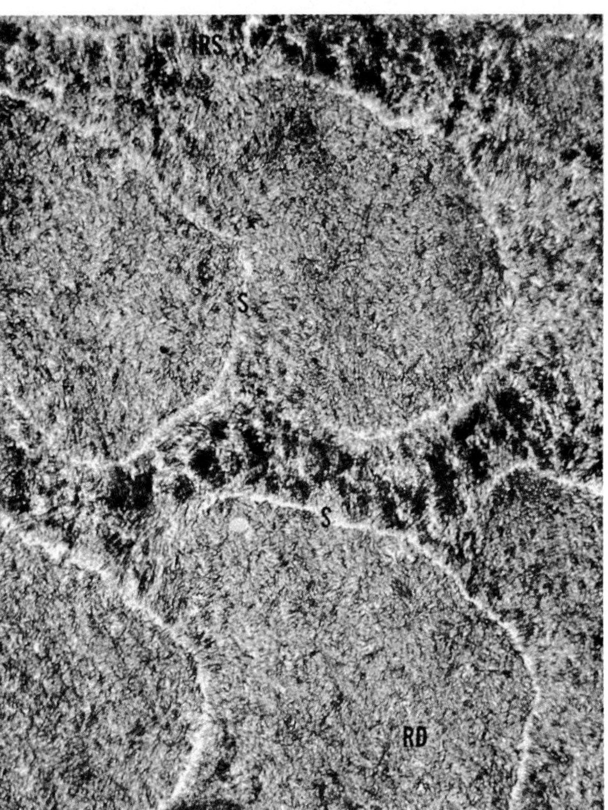

Figure 7.15

Electron micrograph of enamel prisms in cross-section. *RD*, rod; *S*, sheath; *IRS*, interprismatic zone. (Reproduced from Nalbandian J, Frank RM. Microscopic electronique des gaines, des structures prismatiques et interprismatiques de l'email foetal humain. Bull Group Int Rech Sci Stomatol Odontol 1962; 5:523–542; by permission of the *Bulletin du Groupement International pour la Recherche Scientifique en Stomatologie et Ondontologie*.)

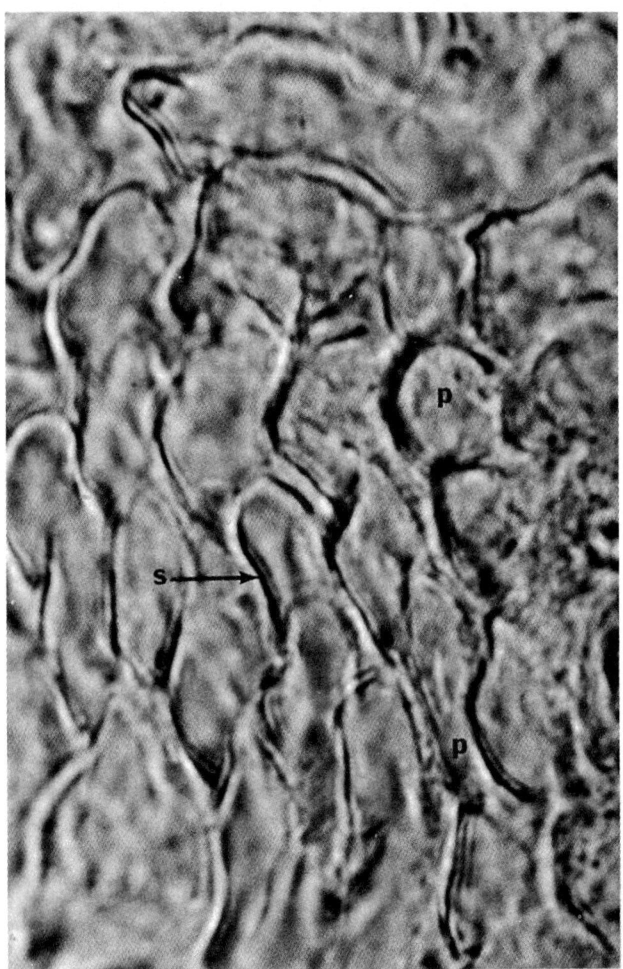

Figure 7.16

Light micrograph of enamel prism in cross-section and tangential. Note similarities in shape with Figure 7.15. *s*, sheath; *p*, prism.

of the prism are oriented in the direction of the long axis of the prism. Crystallites in the tail region deviate in varying degrees from the long axis and frequently lie almost perpendicular to the long axis of the rod (Figs. 7.13 and 7.14).

Prism Sheath

The *prism sheath*, according to light-microscopic observations, has been described as a distinct structure or sheath enveloping an enamel prism or rod. Its existence as a distinct structure has been surmised from its ability to stain with dyes, its paucity in mineral content, its refractive index, and its ability to withstand or resist acid attack. More recent electron microscopic studies reveal, however, that the rod sheath is not a discrete structural entity but rather an organically rich interspace between prisms that is essentially devoid of apatite crystals (Fig. 7.19). Some investigators believe, however, that it may also contain "subfibers," although this has not been unequivically demonstrated. It has been determined by light microscopy that the sheath may or may not be present. Its variable presence or absence can be explained on the basis of an increase in crystal size at the very boundaries between adjacent rods; as a result of this crystal growth the interspace between adjacent rods narrows until it ceases to exist (Fig. 7.19).

Interprismatic Substance

The interrod or interprismatic substance has hitherto been considered as the cementing substance for rods. With the revised concept of the structure of the enamel prism, that is, its resemblance to a keyhole-shaped structure, it has been shown that interrod substance is in fact an extension or tail of the adjacent rod. As mentioned previously, the crystallite orientation in the tail region differs from that seen in the head region; hence, this explains in part the earlier presumption that interrod material is a separate cementing substance (see Fig. 7.15).

The Incremental Lines of Retzius

When a tooth is viewed in longitudinal (ground) section under the light microscope, one observes a concentric series of brown lines, which transverse the cuspal or incisal areas of the tooth in an arclike pattern resembling a pontiff's hat (Fig. 7.20). Each of the brown lines forming the arc descends symmetrically to the cervical region and terminates at various levels along the dentinoenamel junction. Near the cervical region, these parallel brown striae fan out at a somewhat more acute angle toward the enamel surface and do not complete the arc.

Lines of Retzius which terminate at the enamel surface and fail to complete the arc, form a series of alternating grooves that are referred to as the *imbrication lines of Pickerill* (Figs. 7.21 and 7.22). The elevations between the grooves are known as *perikymata*. The surface enamel, under normal masticatory pressure, undergoes attrition particularly in the incisal or cuspal region. Therefore, such areas will rapidly lose their original surface characteristics. Toward the less affected cervical regions, however, the imbrication lines of Pickerill and perikymata are readily seen.

The lines of Retzius are formed first in the incisal or cuspal regions during the early periods of enamel formation. The concentric layers arise first, just above

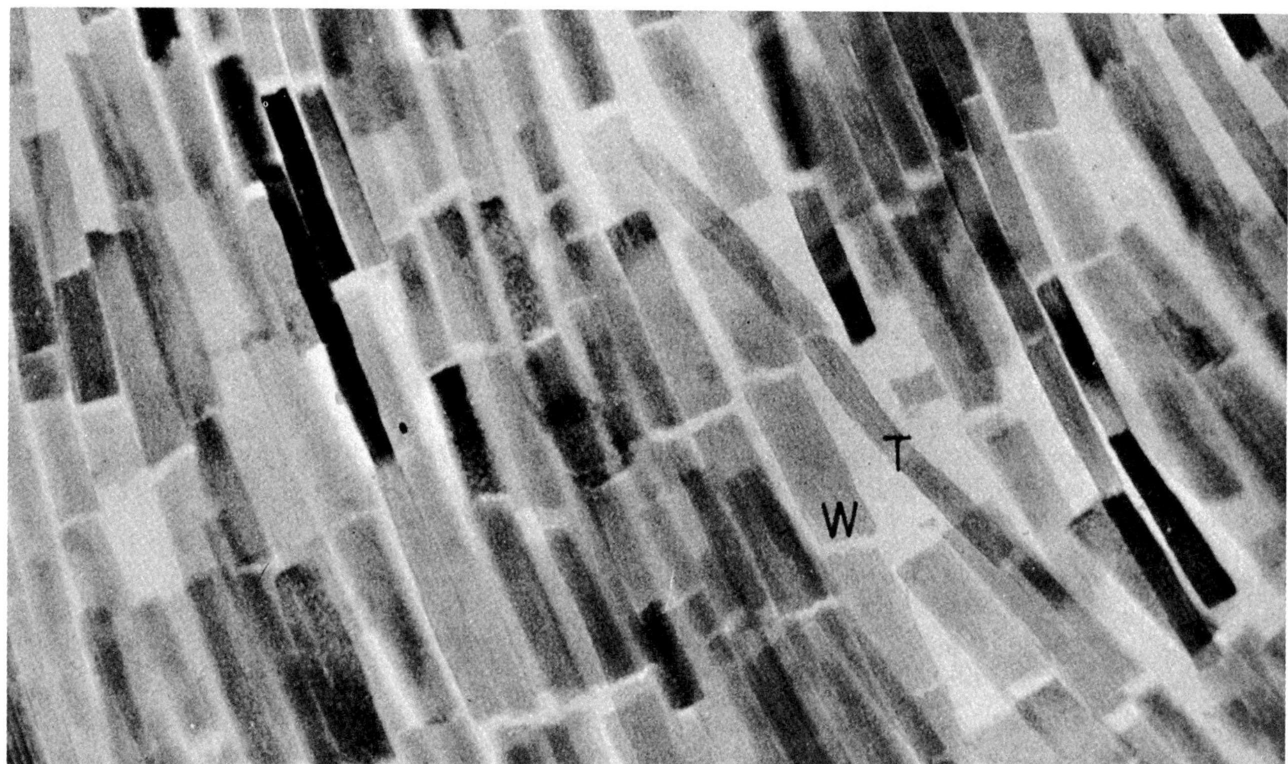

Figure 7.17

Electron micrograph of crystallites showing segmented ribbon-like shape. (Reproduced from Nylen MV, et al. Crystal growth in rat enamel. J Cell Biol 1963; 18:109–123; by copyright permission of the Rockefeller University Press.)

the dentinal cusp or incisal areas, with each successive layer encircling a larger and larger area (see Fig. 7.20). Each of these layers marks the receding path of the ameloblast as it approaches the enamel surface.

In deciduous teeth and first molars, the striae of Retzius are not uniform throughout the entire thickness of the enamel. The inner regions of the enamel are marked off from the outer regions by a dense line that divides the enamel crown into two clearly different zones. This dense line of demarcation, though it may be considered as an accentuated line of Retzius, is referred to as the neonatal line (Fig. 7.23). It divides the prenatal enamel from that produced after birth. Microscopic observations on decalcified and stained sections reveal the inner zone of enamel to be richer in organic material than that of the outer regions; also, it is more homogeneous than the outer regions. The fact that caries infiltration is slowed down or retarded as it approaches and invades this zone has led some investigators to believe that the high organic content of prenatally formed enamel serves as a protective shield (protecting the underlying dentin) against the progressive incursion of the caries lesion.

Hunter-Schreger Bands

Hunter-Schreger bands are a series of alternating dark and light bands seen in enamel (long section) when viewed by reflected light. They emanate from the dentinoenamel junction and run more or less perpendicularly or obliquely to the striae of Retzius (Figs. 7.24 and 7.25). The bands appear most prominent toward the dentinoenamel junction and diminish in contrast farther toward the enamel surface. The dark bands are referred to as the diazones, whereas the light bands are referred to as parazones. Diazones represent the cross-sectional cut of the prisms, and the parazones represent the rods in longitudinal section (Fig. 7.26). Optically, the density would be greater in rods that were transversely sectioned where light is absorbed; on the other hand, rods running in a longitudinal direction reflect rather than absorb light rays. It has been suggested that this alternating arrangement of rods serves to reinforce the strength of the enamel, thus allowing it to serve as a more durable masticatory apparatus.

Explanations of the Hunter-Schreger bands on the basis of alternation of rod paths have, in general,

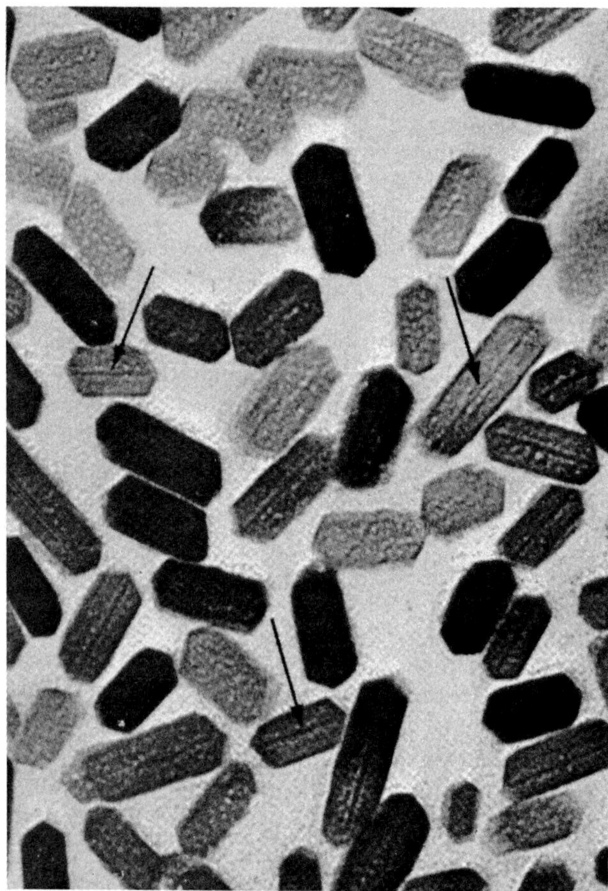

Figure 7.18

Electron micrograph of hexagonally shaped crystallites (*arrows*). (Reproduced from Nylen MV, et al. Crystal growth in rat enamel. J Cell Biol 1963; 18:109–123; by copyright permission of the Rockefeller University Press.)

been accepted by most investigators. Some authors suggest, however, that there are differences in the degree of mineralization between the light and dark bands. Thus far, the evidence for this thesis has not been entirely conclusive.

Enamel Tufts

Projecting into the enamel from the dentinoenamel junction are the enamel tufts (Figs. 7.27 and 7.28). These tasseled or unbraided projections possess basal stems that appear to be inserted into the dentinoenamel junction but actually extend down into the dentin. This can best be seen in transverse (ground) sections of the teeth. They are referred to as enamel tufts because their tufted terminals project into the enamel proper. The tufted portions of these projections follow the curvilinear path of the enamel rods (see Fig. 7.27). There is some disagreement about what structural units make up these tufted structures, that is, whether they are composed of rods, sheaths, and interrod substance combined, or only the sheaths and interrod substance. Whatever the case may be, it is agreed that enamel tufts are hypomineralized structures and therefore rich in organic material. Their role in the caries process has been imputed by some investigators although some others maintain that they are tubular structures with a function circulatory in nature. Thus far, however, there is no strong evidence for their precise function.

Enamel Spindles

The slender projections that traverse the dentinoenamel junction from the underlying odontoblast are called enamel spindles (Fig. 7.29). These hair-like processes are believed to be the elongated odontoblastic processes that have insinuated between ameloblasts during the formative period of enamel production. Such processes project at right angles to the dentinoenamel junction and thereby form an oblique angle with respect to the direction of the enamel rods. A number of studies have suggested that the penetration of the odontoblastic processes may in some way make these serve as pain receptors of the enamel proper. The receptivity of these processes to pain and irritants would explain the sensitivity experienced by the patient as excavation of the enamel nears the dentinoenamel junction (see Pulp, Innervations).

Cementoenamel Junction

It will be recalled that the cervical regions of the tooth demonstrate the thinnest deposits of enamel. If the enamel covering this region is followed microscopically in the apical direction, it will be noted that the enamel terminates, and that a different type of external covering forms a junction with the enamel. This latter covering encloses the apical or root region of the tooth and is called the cementum. Quite naturally, the junction between these two surface coatings is referred to as the cementoenamel junction.

Enamel Lamellae

Lamellae are defects in the enamel resembling cracks or cleavages that traverse the entire length of the crown from the surface to the dentinoenamel junction (see Fig. 7.12). Occasionally they are observed to penetrate into the underlying dentin. Hitherto, they

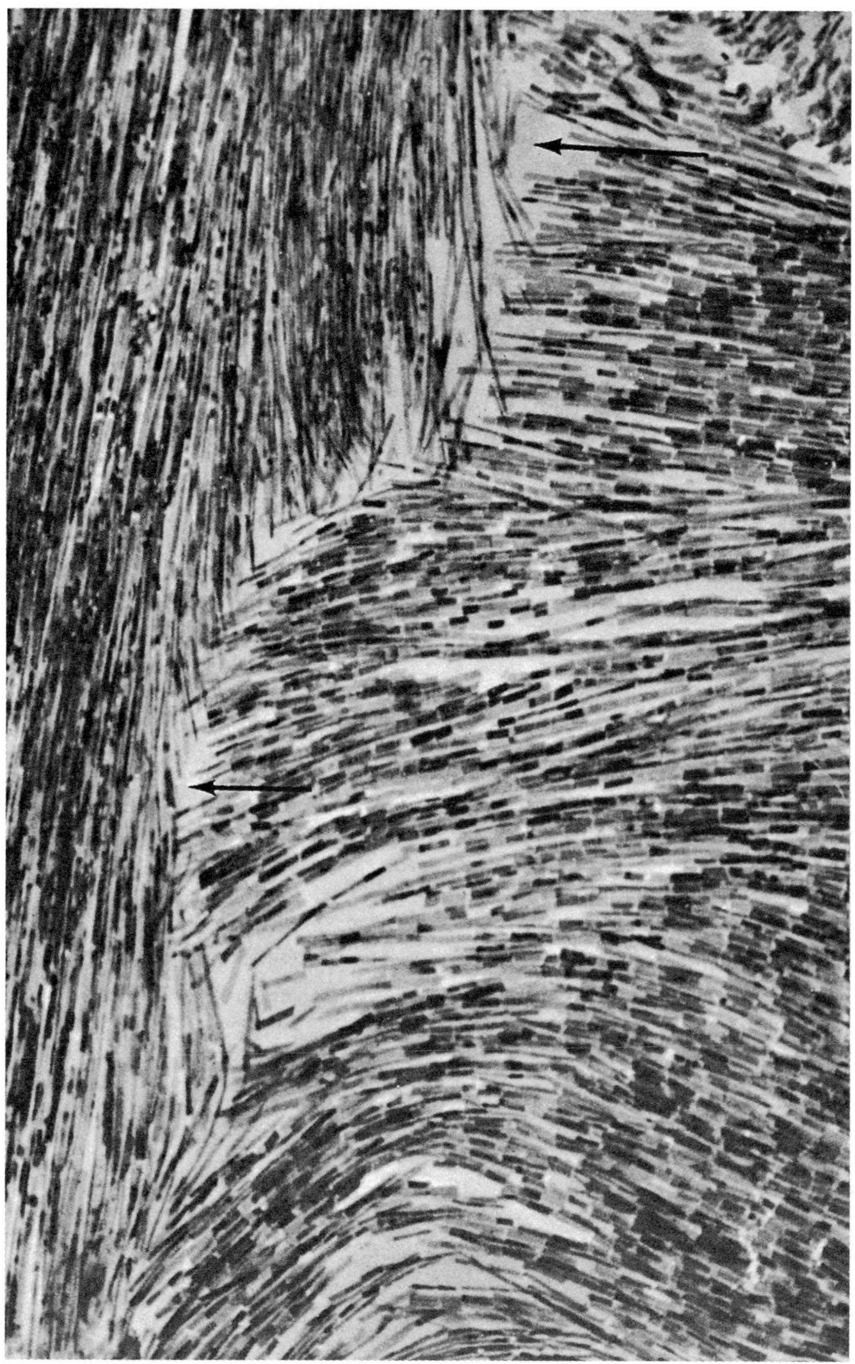

Figure 7.19

Electron micrograph of adjacent prisms. Note differing orientation of crystallites between adjacent prisms. Clear interspace presumably filled with organic material separates prisms (*arrow*). (Reproduced from Nylen MV, et al. Crystal growth in rat enamel. J Cell Biol 1963; 18:109–123; by copyright permission of the Rockefeller University Press.)

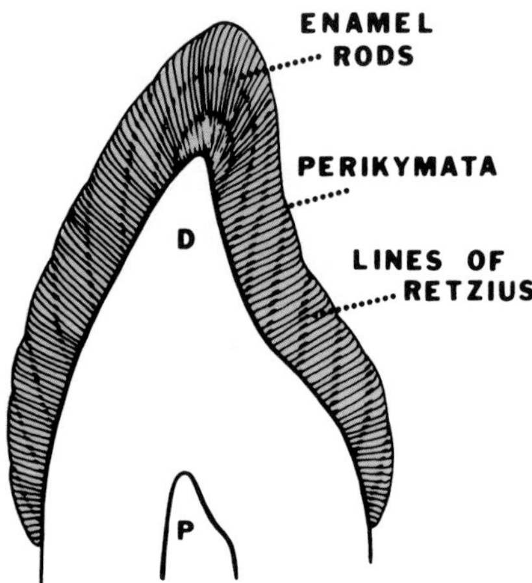

Figure 7.20

Diagrammatic representation of enamel indicating direction of rods, lines of Retzius, and perikymata. *D,* dentine; *P,* pulp.

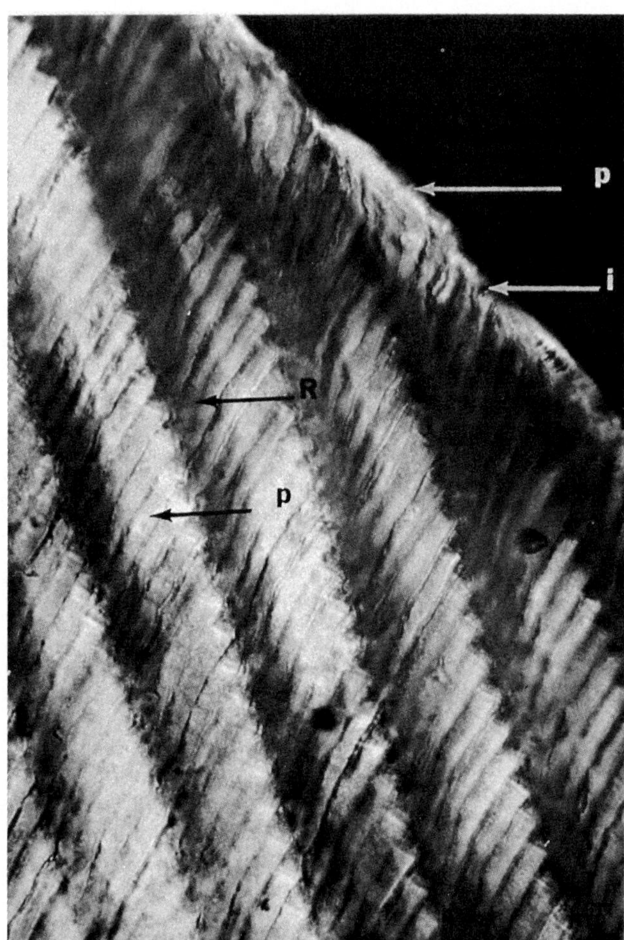

Figure 7.21

Light micrograph demonstrating lines of Retzius (*R*), perikymata (*p*), and imbrication lines of Pickerill (*d*).

were believed to be artifactitious in nature, but it is now commonly accepted that they are indeed real structures occurring either preeruptively or posteruptively. These lamellae can be distinguished from artifactitious cracks by decalcification techniques, since such procedures leave intact an organic matrix residue that marks the site of this structure. Inasmuch as the lamellae are defects that penetrate the surface of the enamel, they readily collect organic matter from the oral cavity. Some investigators believe that such defects are to an extent corrected, since the oral desquamations and organic matter seal the defect: some degree of secondary mineralization of this organic matrix material is believed possible. Another view holds that the lamellae are preferential foci for caries; that is, since enamel lamellae represent a defect in the enamel surface, they may be a possible site of entry for proteolytic bacteria and hence caries attack. The defect is a hypomineralized area containing cellular debris and other particles derived from the oral cavity. This is verified by the fact that it stains readily with organic dyes.

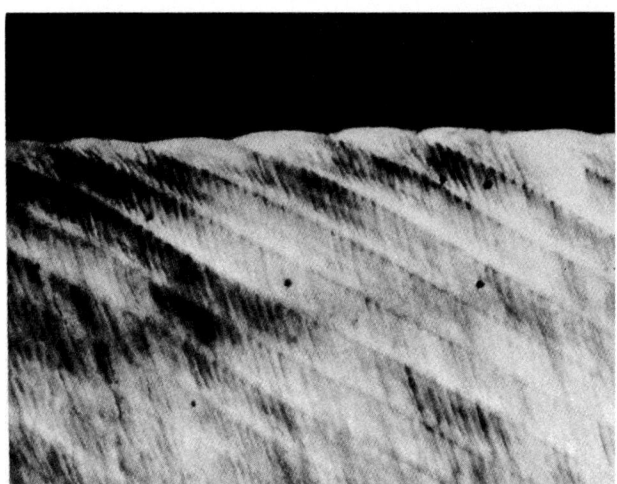

Figure 7.22

Stria of Retzius terminating at surface forming the imbrication lines of Pickerill and perikymata.

The Dentinoenamel Junction

The interface separating enamel crown or cap from the underlying dentin is called the dentinoenamel junction. In mesiolongitudinal section, the dentinoenamel junction is contoured like a pointed feather (see Fig. 7.1). In cross-section, it runs more or less

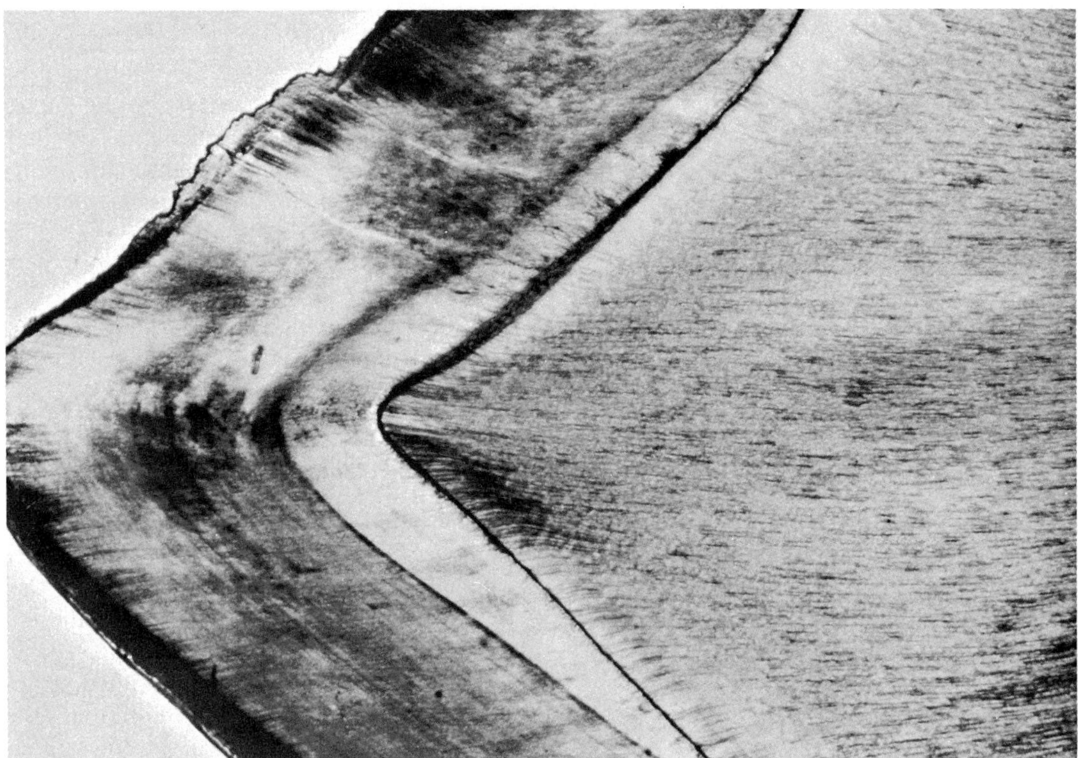

Figure 7.23
Neonatal line. A homogeneous zone running parallel to dentinoenamel junction.

concentrically with the external surface of the enamel; however, although the interface is circular, it is seen to be wavy in outline with the crests of the waves penetrating the apposed enamel surface. This interdigitation is believed by some investigators to contribute to the firm attachment between the dentin and enamel. On the same basis, it might be ventured that the enamel tufts which are partially mineralized serve a similar function, although there is no concrete evidence to support either of these hypothetical notions. With the same degree of speculation it may also be pertinent to mention that the dentinoenamel junction is a hypermineralized zone, but whether this in fact contributes to firm attachment between these two structures is not known at present.

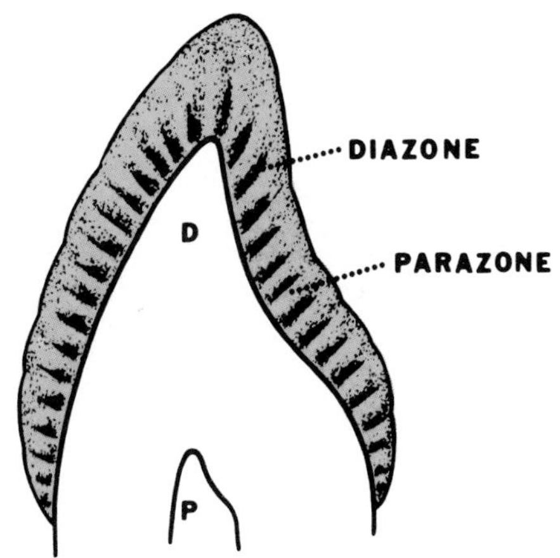

Figure 7.24
Diagrammatic representation of enamel demonstrating diazones and parazones. Dentin (*D*); pulp (*P*).

Nasmyth's Membrane

Just before eruption and soon after the enamel crown is formed, the ameloblasts undergo degenerative changes consisting of a loss of Tomes' processes, vacuolization, formation of irregular cell contours, and

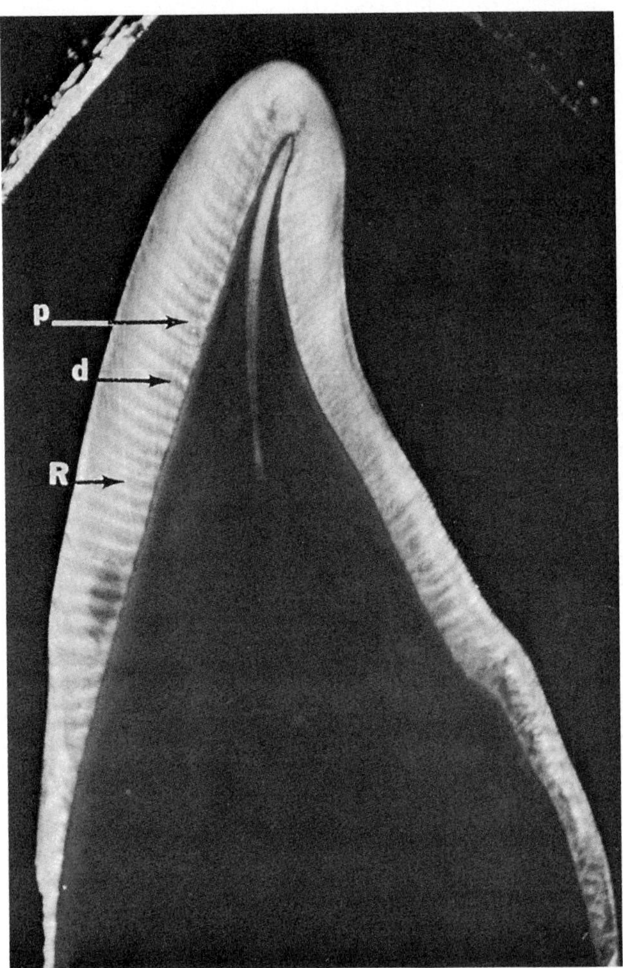

Figure 7.25
Light micrograph of enamel (reflected light). Diazones (*d*); parazones (*p*) of the Hunter-Schreger bands; lines of Retzuis (*R*).

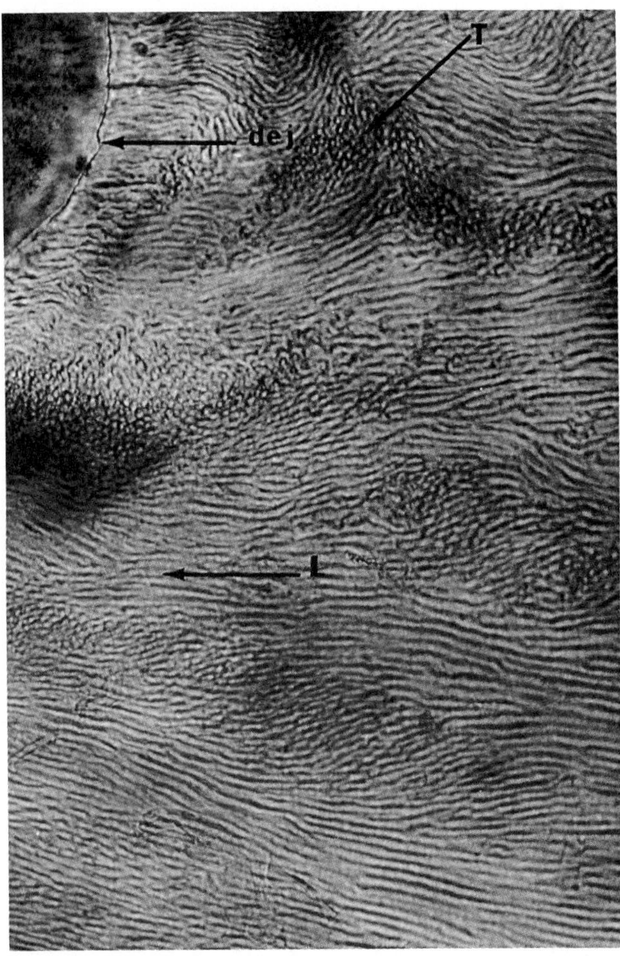

Figure 7.26
Light micrograph of enamel demonstrating longitudinal (*L*) and transverse (*T*) orientation of rods which yield the Hunter-Schreger band images (transmitted light). Dentinoenamel junction (*dej*) at upper left.

shortening into cuboidal shape. It is during this period that one observes the formation of an eosinophilic-staining membrane that appears to border the surface of the enamel. This membrane is frequently observed to develop in conjunction with the final deposition of a basophilic-staining organic matrix. However, this basophilic interface in unerupted teeth appears to be developmental in nature and soon disappears after full mineralization, leaving only the thin eosinophilic, structureless membrane that is referred to as the acellular portion of Nasmyth's membrane. Above this membrane lies the remaining cellular portion of the membrane; the latter consists of cells of the reduced enamel epithelium. The acellular layer serves to unite the overlying cells of the reduced enamel epithelium to the underlying enamel surface.

Primary Cuticle

The acellular portion of Nasmyth's membrane appears to develop in association with the ameloblasts during the final stages of amelogenesis; this is believed to represent their final secretion product. Some investigators have referred to the acellular component of the membrane as the primary cuticle (Fig. 7.30). However, full agreement on what constitutes the "primary cuticle" is at present lacking.

A recent comparison of serial sections of the "primary cuticle" by phase contrast and electron microscopy has revealed contradictory information regarding its nature and dimensions. Under phase-contrast microscopy, a dense, 1-μm structure is seen separating the reduced enamel epithelium from the underlying enamel surface. This observation is in accord

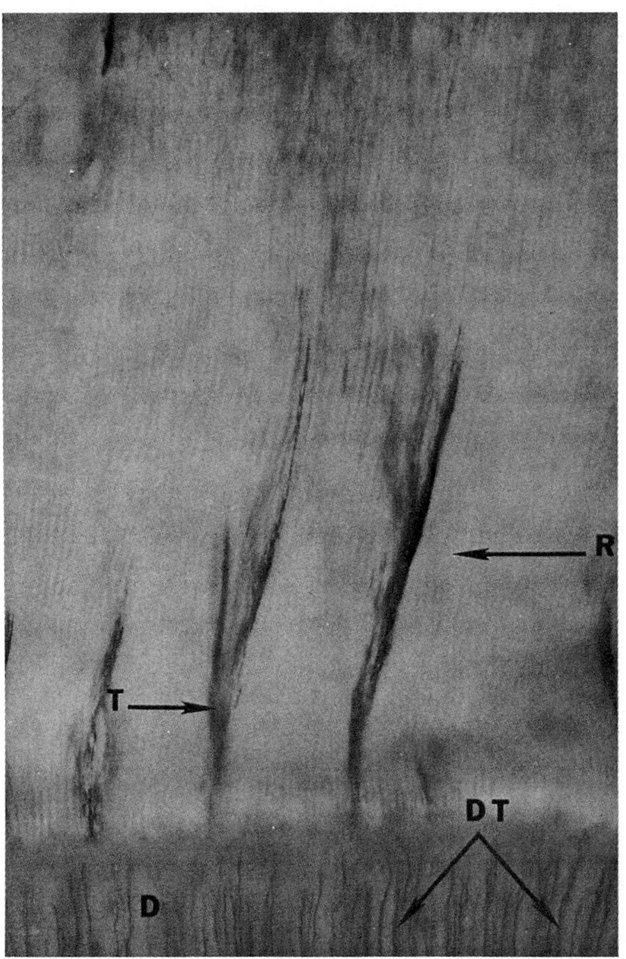

Figure 7.27
Enamel tufts (*T*) oriented in the direction of the enamel rods (*R*). Dentinotubules (*DT*); dentin (*D*).

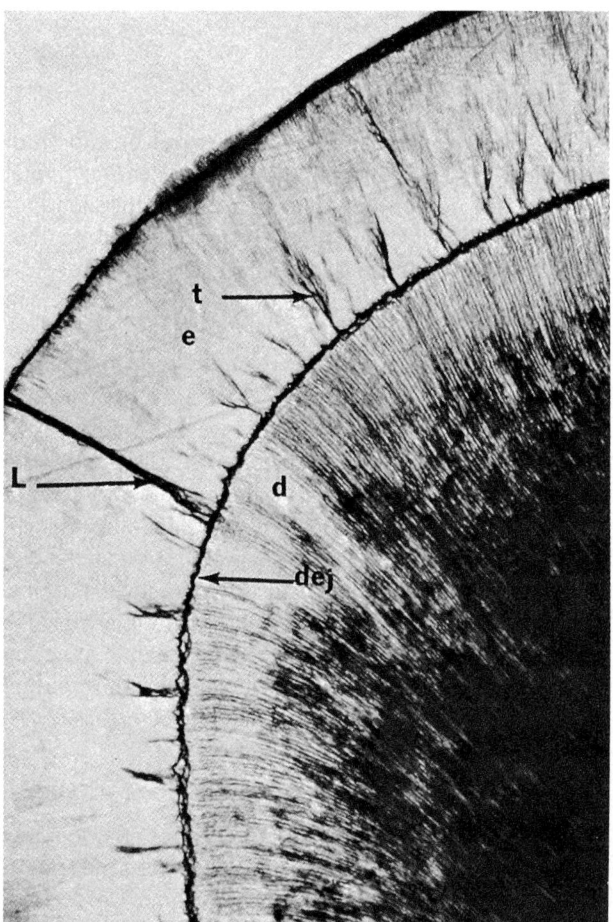

Figure 7.28
Transverse section of enamel (*e*). Tufts (*t*) project from dentinoenamel junction (*dej*); lamellae (*L*); dentin (*d*).

with the classic description of the structure. However, when alternate thin sections of the same material were observed under the electron microscope, it was not possible to identify the 1-μm cuticle observed previously. Instead, a 200-Å amorphous layer covered the enamel interface and was observed to be essentially no different from the basement lamina commonly seen in other epithelial cells. The disparity between observations obtained with the phase-contrast microscope and those obtained with the electron microscope can be explained as the result of an optical effect; structures below the limit of resolution of the light or phase-contrast microscope can be seen because of unusual optical properties. It can be further explained on the basis that the relatively thick sections used for conventional microscopy appear to increase the inherent dimensions of the structure, particularly if the structure is tangentially sectioned. Moreover, staining such a structure with various dyes may result in dye deposition not only upon the structure itself but extending along its surface, thus exaggerating its real dimensions. It is not clear precisely which factors are involved in making the 200-Å basement lamina visible under the light microscope (which has a theoretical limit of resolution of 0.2 μm), but it seems clear nevertheless that the classic concept which holds that a 1-μm cuticle covers the enamel surface must be modified in view of the results obtained with the electron microscope.

The basement lamina, it will be recalled, frequently separates epithelial, endothelial, and muscle fibers from underlying or surrounding fibrous or connective tissue elements. Under the light microscope, the lamina is seen as a thin acellular layer; it is known to be rich in mucopolysaccharides as shown by its strong affinity for periodic acid-Schiff stain. It has been suggested that such structures have the capacity to bind and exchange ions, and thus it may be that

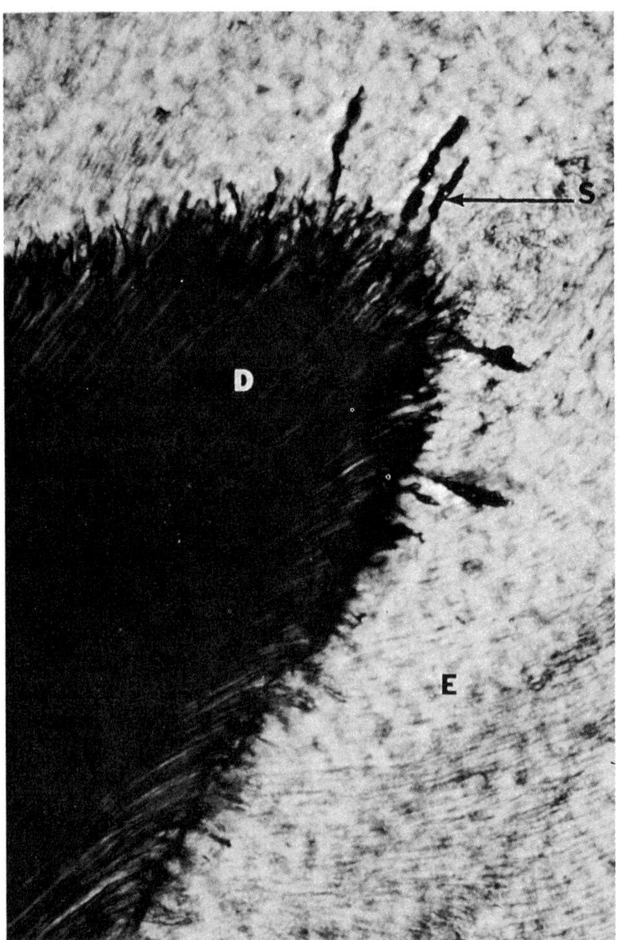

Figure 7.29
Enamel spindles (*S*); enamel (*E*); dentin (*D*).

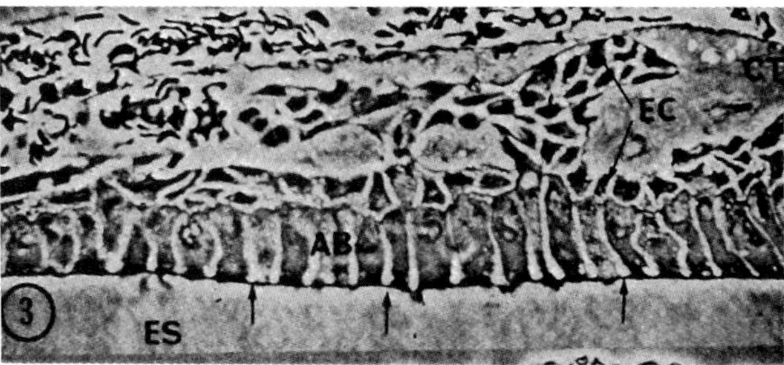

Figure 7.30
Primary (*arrows*) and secondary cuticle. *AB*, ameloblasts; *CT*, connective tissue; *ES*, enamel space; *EC*, epithelial cells. (Reproduced from Listgarten MA. Phase contrast and electron microscopic study of the junction between reduced enamel epithelium and enamel in unerupted human teeth. Arch Oral Biol 1966; 11:999–1016; by permission of Pergamon Press.)

the so-called primary cuticle can in some way control or modify the ionic character of the subjacent enamel rods by controlling the selection and rate of ionic or molecular exchange. The basement lamina does not appear to be a permanent structure of the tooth surface, since it is partially shorn off by occlusal forces (except in the more protected cervical areas) soon after eruption. Hence, its mediating effect would therefore appear to be optimally functional during the preeruptive stages, when the last layer of matrix is being deposited.

The cellular portion of Nasmyth's membrane consists of the reduced enamel epithelium, and overlies the acellular or basement lamina. It has been suggested by earlier studies that this stratified squamous layer represented by the outer enamel epithelium, stratum intermedium, and ameloblastic layer becomes cornified and acts as a protective covering for the enamel after eruption. It has frequently been described as being keratogenous in nature. Recent histochemical studies, however, indicate that the reduced enamel epithelium is probably not keratin, but rather possesses a protein-associated, carbohydrate moiety. It is believed that the reduced enamel epithelium plays some role in passive eruption of the tooth, as well as protecting the tooth from bacterial invasion and caries attack after eruption. The latter view, although it has currency in some scientific circles, remains as yet disputed.

Reduced Enamel Epithelium

As is described above, the ameloblasts, during the final stage of amelogenesis, progressively lose their elongated form and become virtually indistinguishable from the overlying cells of the stratum intermedium. With the intervening stellate reticulum completely resorbed at this stage of development, the stratum intermedium makes intimate contact with the outer enamel epithelium. These layers, which eventually merge with the overlying oral epithelium, together constitute the *reduced enamel epithelium* (Fig. 7.31). According to one classic view, the organic union of these three celullar layers eventually becomes hornified or keratinized in preparation for the eruption of the tooth.

Secondary Cuticle

This "horned" layer of cells has been regarded by some as the *secondary enamel cuticle* and was considered to be the most important part of the enamel cuticle since it appeared to play a role in the emergence of the tooth into the oral cavity; the horned cuticle

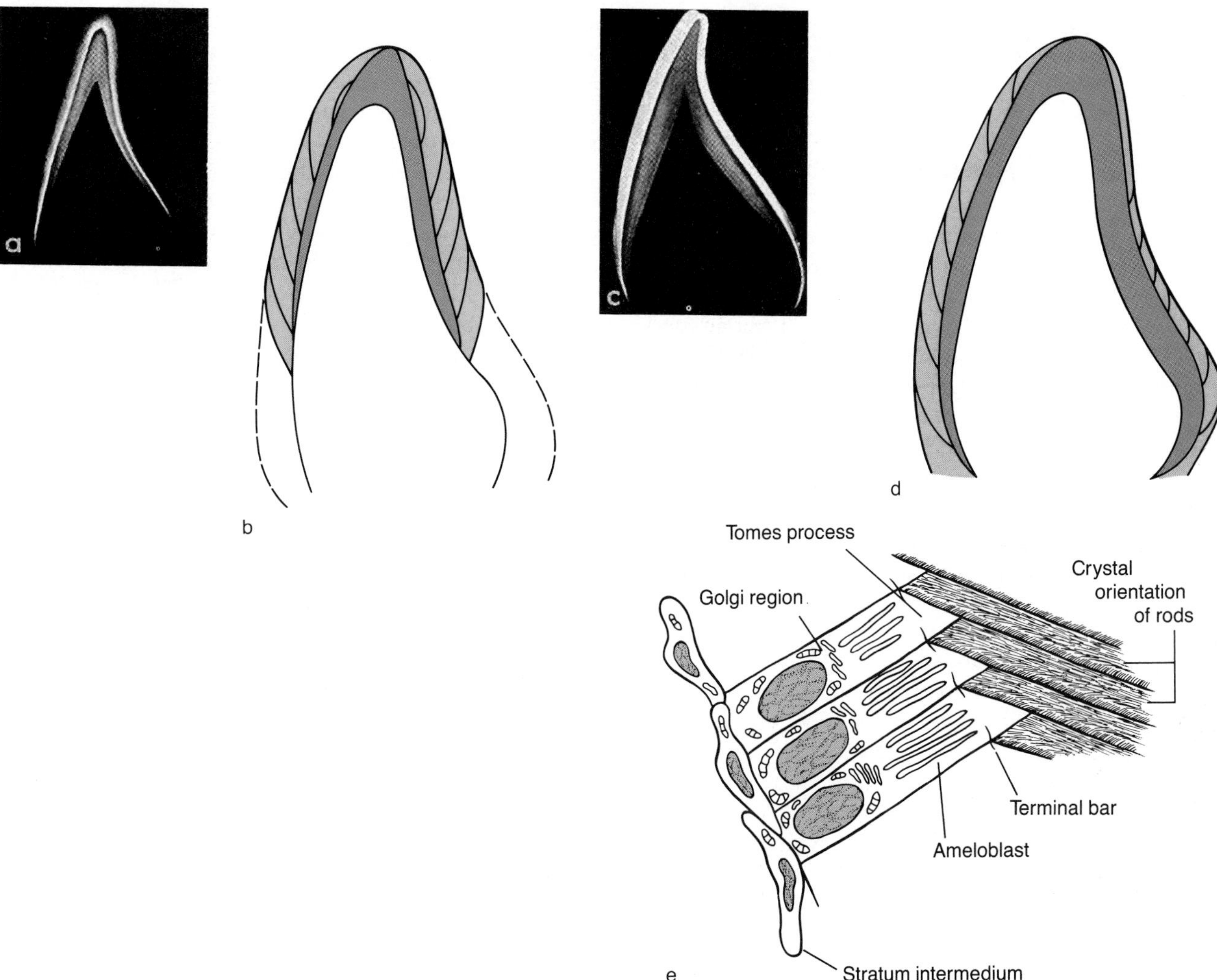

Figure 7.31

a, microradiograph of deciduous upper central incisor in 28-week-old fetus. Zone of mineralization heaviest at incisal region. (Reproduced from Allan. In: Miles AEW, ed. Structural and Chemical Organization of Teeth, 1967, by permission of Academic Press, Inc., New York.) *b,* calcified region (*black*) in relation to incremental matrix deposits (*lined areas*). (Modified from Crabb HSM. The pattern of mineralization of human dental enamel. J R Soc Med 1959; 52:118; with permission.) *c,* microradiograph of deciduous upper central incisor 9 weeks after birth. Zone of heavy mineralization extends to cervical region but is greatest at incisal area. (Reproduced from Allan. In: Miles AEW, ed. Structural and Chemical Organization of Teeth, 1967, by permission of Academic Press, Inc., New York.) *d,* calcified regions (*black* in relation to incremental matrix deposits (*lined area*)). Note enamelized region is thicker, particularly at the incisal region. (Modified from Crabb, HSM. The pattern of mineralization of human dental enamel. J R Soc Med 1959; 52:118; with permission.) *e,* a conceptual version showing crystallite orientation with cell surface of ameloblasts (Tomes process). (Drawn with modification from Ronnholm E. An electron microscopic study of the amelogenesis in human teeth. J Ultrastruc Res 1962; 6:229–248; by permission of Academic Press.)

purportedly protects the surface of the erupted tooth from bacterial invasion, particularly in the area of the gingival crevice (Fig. 7.31).

Amelogenesis and Matrix Production

The tooth germ develops as an inpocketing of the oral epithelium into the underlying mesenchymal region during the sixth week of embryonic life. With further development, the basal portion of the flask-shaped layer of cells begins to indent to form a cap-like structure; hence, the name "cap stage" has been applied to designate this phase of development. This stage of development is succeeded by the "bell stage" and involves the breakdown of the dental lamina and the further indentation of the basal zone. By this stage four distinct cell layers can be distinguished: (1) the outer enamel epithelium, which is cuboidal in shape, (2) the fusiform and stellate cells of the stellate reticulum, (3) the cuboidal cells of the stratum intermedium, and (4) the cuboidal cells of the inner enamel epithelium. The orientation of these cellular layers is such that the inner enamel epithelium is most deeply embedded into the mesenchyme and is therefore most distant from the oral epithelium. The outer enamel epithelium, on the other hand, is superficially embedded in the mesenchyme and is therefore closest to the oral epithelium. It is the cell layer most deeply embedded in the mesenchyme that is intimately associated with the formation of enamel. The cells constituting this layer, upon further differentiation, are referred to as ameloblasts.

The contours of the ameloblastic cell layer are of vital importance to the formation of the crown since they establish the fundamental pattern of the tooth structure. Thus, the deepening ridges formed by this layer of cells presages the final morphologic contours peculiar to the tooth formed. It can be said that the diversity in crown structure is attributable to varied patterns assumed by the ameloblastic layer during development.

A variety of organellar changes are associated with ameloblast differentiation and their ability to secrete matrix. Initially cells of the inner enamel epithelium are low columnar or cuboidal in shape and possess an ovoid nucleus. Dispersed within the cytoplasm are mitochondria and innumerable ribonucleoprotein particles that account for the intensely basophilic character of the cytoplasm. Another important cytoplasmic organelle is the Golgi apparatus, which is characteristically located in the juxtanuclear region on the basal or nonformative side of the cell. With further development, the cells of the inner enamel epithelium develop into high columnar cells, and the nuclei elongate and migrate toward the basal end of the cell. Accompanying the nucleus to the basal region are aggregates of mitochondria. The Golgi apparatus, previously in the juxtanuclear region on the basal side of the cell, migrates over to the juxtanuclear region on the distal side of the cell. Along with these morphologic changes, the ameloblast acquires a system of tubules or canaliculi which are studded with ribonucleoprotein particles on its external surface. These tubules line up parallel to the long axis of the cell, and with these cytologic changes the cell begins to assume its secretory function, that is, the laying-down of the organic ground substance or matrix. This is evidenced by the fact that new ground substance is always seen in association with newly acquired distal protoplasmic extensions called Tomes' processes.

Electron-microscopic evidence suggested that this organic matter is elaborated in the cytoplasm by the ribonucleoprotein particles; the proteinaceous material is then transported via the endoplasmic reticulum and Golgi apparatus into the regions of the Tomes' processes and is released into the adjacent extracellular spaces. The actual mode of secretion as indicated by electron microscope studies involves the migration of the dense organic materials in the form of particles to the cell membrane of the distal regions of the cell or Tomes' process. Fusing with the cell membrane, the particle is temporarily enclosed and finally released into the extracellular spaces. After expulsion of the dense organic substance, the cell membrane resumes its previous condition.

Ameloblasts do not all become secretory at the same time; this is because there exists a gradient of cell differentiation. Cells in the presumptive incisal or cuspal regions are more differentiated than those cells more laterally and cervically placed. Correspondingly, it is the incisal and cuspal region that contains the advanced organic front in which mineralization will subsequently occur. As matrix material is secreted, the mature ameloblasts recede in a stepwise manner toward the outer enamel epithelium, thus forming the lines of Retzius in the cells of the stellate reticulum, until finally this cellular zone is almost entirely occupied by matrix material, ameloblasts, and cells of the stratum intermedium. Just before the deposition of the final layer of organic matrix, the ameloblasts undergo a series of morphologic changes. The Tomes' processes become shorter and more irregular, vacuoules are formed, and most notably, there is a shortening and widening of the cell. These are degenerative signs indicating the cessation of matrix production. It is during this period, when the crown pattern is complete, that the ameloblasts secrete their final product, the primary cuticle (see Fig. 7.30). The primary cuticle is also referred to as the acellular portion of Nasmyth's membrane. As mentioned previously, the primary cuticle appears to be identical to the basement membrane seen in other tissues. Its function is believed to be related to ion exchange and transport.

It can be seen from the foregoing account and elsewhere in this chapter that the ameloblasts execute several important functions: they fulfill the determinant growth pattern of the enamel crown, induce development of the odontoblasts, lay down the organic matrix and the primary cuticle, conceivably resorb the organic matter and water during mineralization, and lastly may participate in the functional role of the reduced enamel epithelium.

Mineralization

Earlier studies on enamel have established that mineralization proceeds from the dentinoenamel junction to the surface of the tooth. Mineralization is most decidedly advanced, however, at the incisal and cuspal regions, with a decreasing gradient of mineralization towards the cervical areas. The pattern of mineral deposition and growth appears to follow rather closely the incremental layers of the lines of Retzius, laid down by the matrix-secreting ameloblasts. It will be recalled that the incremental lines of Retzius traverse the cuspal and incisal zones in an arc-like fashion and end bisymmetrically at the cervical regions of the dentinoenamel junction. Following these lines, the mineralized zone advances peripherally and to a lesser extent cervically until complete mineralization has been attained (see Fig. 7.31*a* and *b*).

The microradiographic pattern of the above sequence could be somewhat misleading to the student since it might suggest that the matrix radiotranslucent (black) areas contain no mineral content. However, electron-microscopic studies indicate that as soon as the matrix is deposited by the ameloblast, tiny crystallites are indeed present. These crystallites grow in size subsequent to the peripheral retreat of the secreting ameloblasts cell layer. Hence, newly deposited matrix contains smaller and more dispersed crystallites than that of matrix which was deposited previously. Accordingly, it would be expected that the more peripheral regions, which include the ameloblasts and newly secreted matrix, would be more radiotranslucent than the more centrifugally located zones of deposition. The microradiographic pattern shown in Figure 7.31*a*, *b*, and *c* illustrates this gradient mineralization. During the earlier period a zone of hypermineralization is seen along the dentinoenamel junction (see Fig. 7.31*a* and *b*). In subsequent stages, this radiodense zone extends peripherally, starting at the incisal and cuspal regions (see Fig. 7.31*c* and *d*).

It might be asked how, or from whence come the crystallites? Although they appear to be formed in conjunction with the secreting ameloblasts cell surface, they are not, in the usual sense, a secretion product. There is at present no answer available. Once formed, however, they grow in size. It is clear that if such growth is to be sustained, there must be a source of minerals available in the matrix. Earlier studies indicated that the primary source of minerals to the organic zones is via the blood vessels of the pulp, through the dentin, to the dentinoenamel junction, and finally to the organic front where mineralization is occurring. However, it has since been demonstrated that even when the pulp is occluded so that capillary circulation to the enamel organ is restricted, mineralization of the organic zones can nevertheless occur. It was suggested that the pulp is not the primary pathway by which calcium enters the organic zone. Rather, it is believed that this route is peripheral via the enamel organ.

Whether the route taken by minerals is pulpal or via the enamel organ, or both, it seems evident that the flow of calcium is from the area of the dentinoenamel junction to the peripheral regions of the tooth. It would seem therefore that the crystallite formed earliest would have, at least initially, greater access to the minerals than that of crystallite more distant from the dentinoenamel junction. This and other factors during development may conceivably account for the preferential crystal growth in zones distant from the newly deposited organic front. However, other factors must come into play after the completion of the enamel crown, because crystallites are larger in the surface regions of the enamel. Calcium and phosphate ions in the tissue fluids surrounding the crown during the preeruptive period may account for this increased crystal growth. This is undoubtedly augmented by fluids of the oral cavity after eruption.

The determining factors involved in crystallite formation, orientation, and growth have been subject to considerable speculation. In view of earlier studies on dentin and bone, it was thought that a fibrous ground substance determined the crystallite orientation. In bone and dentin, the matrix contains collagenous fibers which provide the seeding surfaces upon which crystallites readily deposit. Deposition of the crystallites occurs in such a way that they are deposited along the transverse periodic bands which are marked off perpendicular to the long axis of the fiber. In enamel matrix, however, collagen fibers are not present, so far as can be determined. Much to the contrary, the organic matrix appears to be highly amorphous in nature, yet it provides a surface upon which nucleation and seeding can occur. In view of the absence of collagenous fiber, some investigators maintain the existence of a macromolecular protein stroma that determines crystallite deposition and orientation. On the other hand, crystallite nucleation and orientation may depend upon the molecular configuration of the protein matrix itself. At present, the process by which nucleation occurs in the matrix remains unknown. There is, however, some suggestive evidence which indicates that the crystallite orientation is determined in part by the secreting cell surface of the ameloblasts since crystallites are frequently seen to be deposited perpendicular to the ameloblast cell surface (see Fig. 7.31*e*). But whatever the governing factors in crystallite nucleation and orientation may be, it seems evident from the various electron-microscopic studies that once crystallites are deposited they increase in size. As was mentioned previously, crystal growth is said to occur either by fusion of smaller crystallites or as a result of addition of individual atoms. The latter view appears to be more in accord with the known chemical behavior of crystallites and is thus more generally accepted.

A number of other important problems regarding the role of the organic matrix remains unsolved. It is not known, for instance, how an insignificantly small quantity of organic material weight (1 percent) can conceivably fill all the interstices between crystallites as well as provide the matrix in which crystallites are embedded. Even with the tight packing of crystallites, the available volume to be filled is indeed considerable. Fibrous proteins, because of their relatively contracted structure, may not have sufficient bulk to occupy the available interstitial enamel volume. On the other hand, a protein gel, although low in weight, could conceivably occupy a disproportionately large volume. This latter view has received considerable attention since it not only provides an explanation of how small amounts of matrix proteins can occupy a relatively inordinate volume but would also provide an explanation for the rapid loss of organic material which accompanies maturation. Gels are known to be thixotrophic (capable of gelation and solation) and could readily interconvert with proper stimulus to form either an expanded gel or reduced sol, the latter of which would hypothetically be subject to absorption by ameloblasts. The ramifications of the various other functional properties of this type of matrix would also have to be considered. These include matrix involvement with crystallite initiation, ion and molecular permeability, and crystallite growth and decay. At present virtually nothing is known about the mechanisms of these various functional activities of the protein matrix. To gain further insights into these interrelationships it is first necessary to ascertain the matrix amino acid composition, sequence, molecular configuration, and ionic characteristics. This information, considered in juxtaposition to the theoretical constructs of the crystallite structure, ionic character, and chemistry, may lead to experimentation which will shed further light on the above-mentioned problems.

Aprismatic Enamel

Commonly in the cervical region of permanent teeth and the buccal and proximal surfaces of the primary dentition, the outermost enamel appears histologically devoid of prisms (Fig. 7.32). Enamel prisms can be traced to within 25 μm of the surface, after which a structurally homogeneous zone of aprismatic enamel is seen. In contrast to the three-dimensional spread of crystallites in the prismatic enamel, those in the aprismatic layer run parallel to each other and perpendicular to the enamel surface. The denser packing of crystallites in the aprismatic layer confers an increase in radiodensity compared to the underlying enamel. Although the structure of aprismatic enamel can be explained on the basis of ameloblast relationships in the final stages of amelogenesis, the role of this enamel is not clearly understood.

Bonding Resins to Enamel

The bonding of polymeric resins to enamel, mediated by chemical conditioning of the tissue, has had a profound impact on the way dentistry is currently practiced. An understanding of the morphologic and micromorphologic structure and properties of enamel set forth in this chapter have helped formulate and develop resin systems, which under the consummate skill of the clinician have led to new approaches to treatment. Some of these have replaced or supplemented conventional procedures. Indeed some spe-

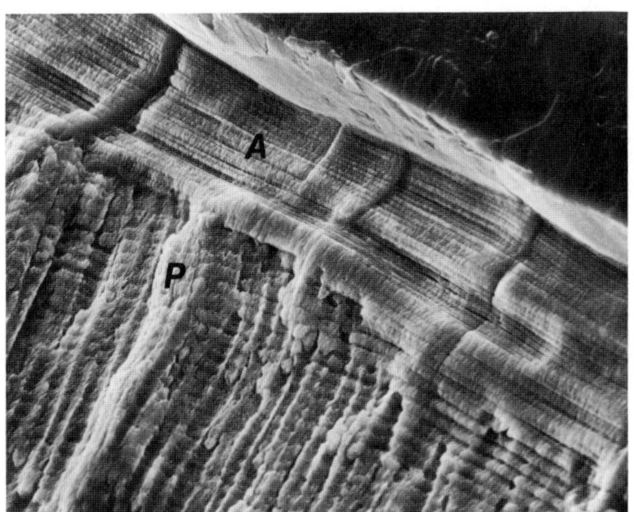

Figure 7.32

Parallel, incremental lines punctuate the aprismatic enamel (*A*); *P*, prismatic enamel.

cialties, for example orthodontics, have been radically altered by the development of bonded brackets, which have largely displaced the bulky, unphysiologic, and uncomfortable circumferential metal bands. Although bonding techniques demand skill and understanding, if properly understood, they are no more demanding than conventional procedures.

It is clear that the enamel is morphologically, chemically, and physiologically complex. Furthermore, the surface with which bonding is to take place is equally complex. Clinically, the enamel has a low surface energy; its surface is relatively inert, is fully reacted, and under normal conditions is homeostatic with its salivary environment.

The enamel surface, after tooth eruption, acquires a biofilm called pellicle. Microorganisms colonize this proteinaceous film to form plaque. In addition to its complexity, therefore, the enamel surface is also contaminated. Summarily, it is not conducive to bonding and requires modification. The objective is to remove the surface contaminants and raise the surface energy or reactivity of the enamel surface. More than 30 years ago, Buonocore pioneered a method called the acid-etch technique; its protocol involves a dental prophylaxis, site isolation, phosphoric acid conditioning, washing to remove reaction products, and placement of resin in an isolated dry field.

The dental prophylaxis is predicated upon the need to remove gross deposits such as materia alba, plaque, and calcific accretions from the enamel. Achieved with conventional methods and using a watery slurry of flour of pumice, a thorough cleaning of the surface, combined with acid conditioning can raise bond strengths to enamel as much as 50 percent.

After appropriate isolation of the treatment site, acid conditioning is usually conducted with phosphoric acid in either solution or gel form. Commercially available acids range in concentration from 30 to 50 percent. Although no clinically significant differences exist among these concentrations, there is a preponderance of products using concentrations in the 30 percent range. The conditioning is carried out for 60 seconds, although there is an increasing body of laboratory and clinical evidence to support shorter etching times, for example 15 seconds. The effect of acid conditioning is several-fold: it removes old and fully reacted enamel, it removes residual pellicle and cuticle to expose the inorganic crystallite components of enamel, it enhances enamel porosity, and it increases surface area and creates polar phosphate groups as potential binding sites. The partial dissolution of approximately 30 to 50 μm of enamel results in a variety of morphologic patterns. These patterns vary from site to site (Fig. 7.33) on the tooth as well as tooth to tooth. The most common pattern involves the preferential loss of prism cores with peripheral regions relatively intact (Fig. 7.34). The next most common is the preferential loss of peripheral material from the prisms with the cores relatively intact (Fig. 7.35). These differences clearly reflect variations in solubility of the prisms, which in turn probably relate to chemical compositional differences, the orientation and packing of the crystallites, and accompanying microporosity. Approximately 25 μm of the outermost enamel in the region of pits and fis-

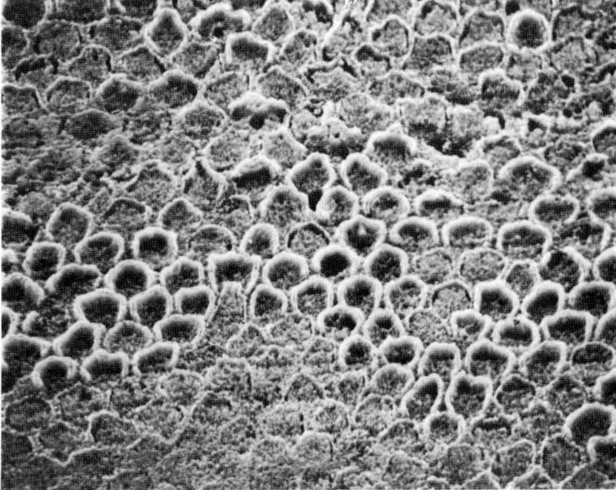

Figure 7.33

Variation in prism etching patterns from site to site on the same tooth. Original magnification 2,000 ×.

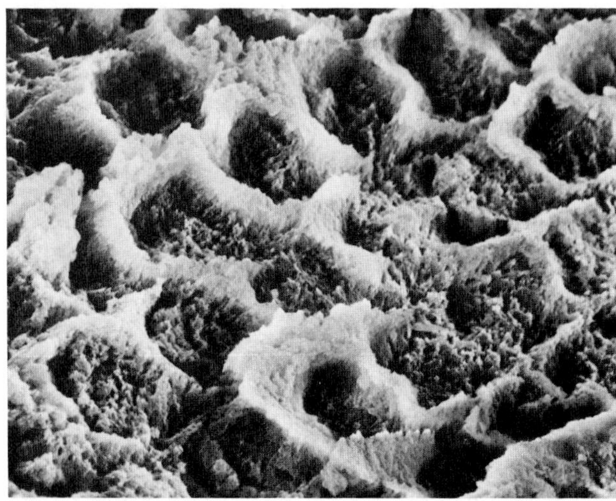

Figure 7.34
Preferential dissolution of prism cores. Original magnification, 5,000 ×.

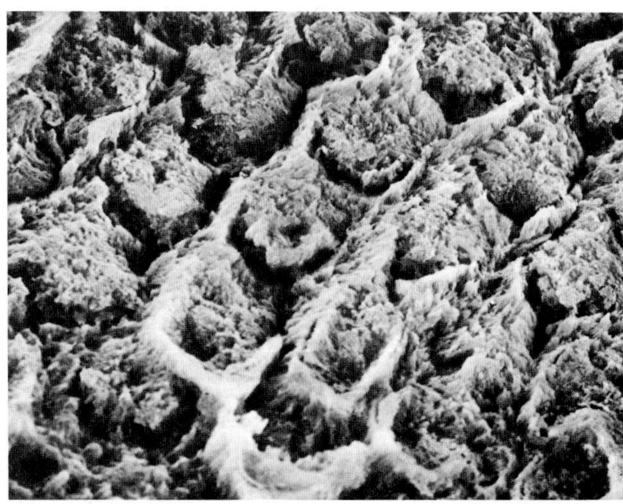

Figure 7.35
Preferential dissolution of prism peripheral regions. Original magnification, 5,000 ×.

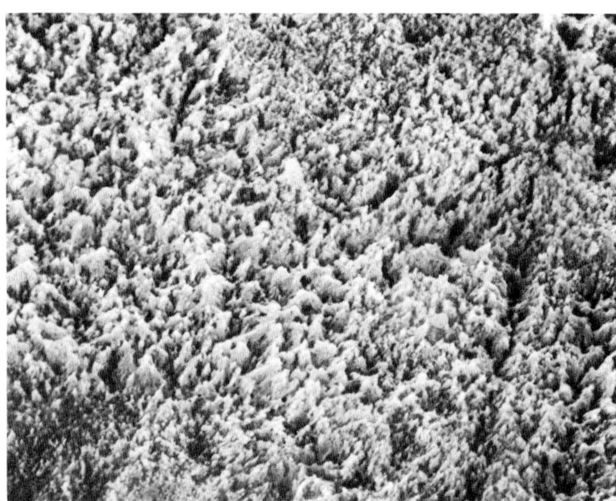

Figure 7.36
Characteristic porosity following dissolution of prismless enamel. Original magnification, 5,000 ×.

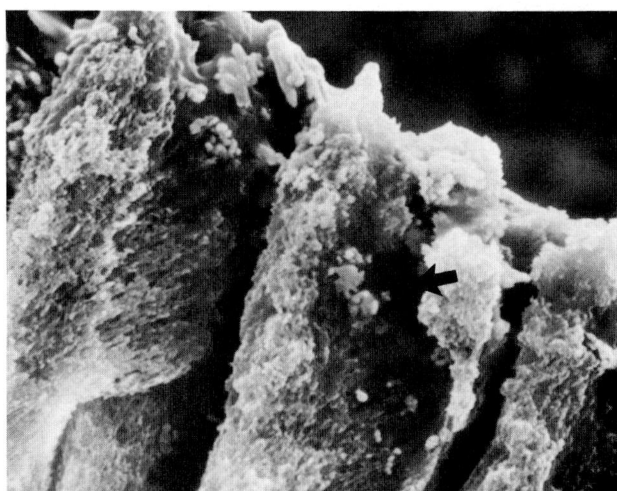

Figure 7.37
Resin (*arrow*) located within enhanced prism micropores. Original magnification, 10,000 ×.

sures, and the buccal and cervical regions may be devoid of typical, histologic prism structure. Such an occurrence is more common in the primary dentition. This aprismatic or prismless enamel is rendered porous after acid conditioning but contrasts with the preferential dissolution patterns seen for prismatic enamel (Fig. 7.36). There is no evidence to suggest that these patterns confer differences in bond strength or clinical performance.

Acid conditioning increases both the volume and the size of existing enamel micropores present in the outermost layer of enamel. Application of a low-viscosity resin to the conditioned enamel results in its rapid infiltration into the microspaces. After polymerization by either chemical or photoactivation, the resin forms a micromechanical link (Fig. 7.37) between the enamel and the subsequent placement of restorative or other resins. The resulting bond strength is sufficient to withstand normal masticating forces.

Suggested Reading

Angmar B, Carlstrom D, Glas JE. Studies on the ultrastructure of dental enamel. IV. The mineralization of normal human enamel. J Ultrastruct Res 1963; 8:12–23.

Apostolopolos AX, Buonocore MG. Comparative dissolution rates of enamel, dentin and bone. I. Effect of the organic matters. J Dent Res 1966; 45:1093–1100.

Atkinson HF, Saunsbury P. An investigation into the hardness of human enamel. Br Dent J 1953; 94:82–83.

Barkmeier WW, Shaffer SE, Gwinnett AJ. Retentive and morphological characteristics of enamel following 15 and 60 second acid conditioning. J Oper Dent 1986; 11:111–116.

Battistone GD, Burnett GW. The amino acid composition of human enamel protein. J Dent Res 1956; 35:260.

Belanger LF. Autoradiographic detection of radiosulfate incorporated by the growing enamel of rats and hamsters. J Dent Res 1955; 34:20–27.

Berggren H. Experimental studies on the permeability of enamel and dentine. Svensk. Tandlak T 1947; 40:5–110.

Bergman G. Microscopic demonstration of liquid flow through human dental enamel. Arch Oral Biol 1963; 8:223.

Bergman G. Techniques for microscopic study of the enamel fluid in vitro. Odont Rev Lund 1963; 14:1–7.

Bergman G, Siljestrand B. Short communication. Water evaporation in vitro from human dental enamel. Arch Oral Biol 1963;8:37.

Bhussey BR. Chemical and physical studies of enamel from human teeth. II. Specific gravity, nitrogen content and hardness rating of discolored enamel. J Dent Res 1958; 37:1045–1053.

Bhussey BR. Chemical and physical studies of enamel from human teeth. III. Specific gravity, nitrogen content, and histological characteristics of opaque white enamel. J Dent Res 1958; 37:1054–1059.

Bhussey BR, Bibby BG. Surface changes in enamel. J Dent Res 1957; 36:409.

Block RJ, Horwitt MK, Bolling D. Comparative protein chemistry: The composition of the protein of human teeth and fish scales. J Dent Res 1949; 28:518–524.

Bonar LC. In: Stack MV, Fearnhead RW, eds. Tooth enamel: its composition, properties, and fundamental structure. Baltimore: Williams & Wilkins, 1965: 147–153.

Brudevold F, Steadman LT. A study of copper in human enamel. J Dent Res 1955; 34:209–216.

Brudevold F, Steadman LT, Gardner DE, Rowley J, Little MF. Uptake of tin and fluoride by intact enamel. J Am Dent Assoc 1956; 53:159–164.

Brudevold F, Steadman LT, Smith FA. Inorganic and organic components of tooth structure. Ann NY Acad Sci, 1960; 85:110–132.

Brudevold F, Steadman LT, Spinelli MA, Amdur BH, Gron P. A study of zinc in human teeth. Arch Oral Biol 1963; 8:135–144.

Buonocore MG. A simple method of increasing the adhesion of acrylic filling materials to enamel surfaces. J Dent Res 1955; 34:849–855.

Buonocore MG, Bibby BG. The effect of various ions on enamel solubility. J Dent Res 1945; 24:103–108.

Burgess RC, Maclaren C. Proteins in developing bovine enamel. In: Stack MV, Fearnhead RW, eds. Tooth enamel: its composition, properties, and fundamental structure. Baltimore: Williams & Wilkins, 1965: 74–82, 109–110.

Burgess RC, Nikiforuk G, Maclaren C. Chromatographic studies of carbohydrate components in enamel. Arch Oral Biol 1960; 3:8.

Caldwell RC, Muntz ML, Gilmore RW, Pigman W. Microhardness studies of intact surface enamel. J Dent Res 1957; 36:732–738.

Carlstrom D, Glas JE, Angmar B. Studies on the ultrastructure of dental enamel. V. The stage of water in human enamel. J Ultrastruct Res 1963; 8:24–29.

Crabb HSM. The pattern of mineralization of human dental enamel. Proc Roy Soc Med 1959; 52:118–122.

Crabb HSM, Darling AI. The gradient of mineralization in developing enamel. Arch Oral Biol 1960; 2:308–318.

Crabb HSM, Darling AI. The pattern of progressive mineralization in human dental enamel. In: Ant Ser Monographs on Oral Biol, Vol 2. Oxford: Pergamon Press, 1962.

Darling AI, Mortimer KV, Poole DFG, Ollis WD. Molecular sieve behavior of normal and carious human dental enamel. Arch Oral Biol 1961; 5:251–273.

Deakins M. Changes in the ash water and organic content of pig enamel during calcification. J Dent Res 1942; 21:429–435.

Deakins M, Volker JF. Amount of organic matter in enamel from several types of human teeth. J Dent Res 1941; 20:117–121.

Decker JD. A light and electron microscope study of the rat molar enamel organ. Arch Oral Biol 1963; 8:301–310.

Eastoe JE. Organic matrix of tooth enamel. Nature (London) 1960; 187:411.

Eastoe JE. The amino-acid composition of proteins from the oral tissues. Arch Oral Biol 1963; 8:633–652.

Eastoe JE. Formal contributions: Discussion of second session. In: Stack MV, Fearnhead RW, eds. Tooth enamel: its composition, properties, and fundamental structure. Baltimore: Williams & Wilkins, 1965:91–98.

Engfeldt B, Bergman G, Hammarlund E. Studies on mineralized dental tissues. I. A microradiographic and autoradiographic investigation of teeth and tooth germs of normal dogs. Exp. Cell Res 1954; 7:381–392.

Fincham AG, Graham GN, Pautard FGE. The matrix of enamel and related calcified keratins. In: Stack MV,

Fearnhead RW, eds. Tooth enamel: its composition, properties, and fundamental structure. Baltimore: Williams & Wilkins, 1965:117–121.

Frank RM, Nalbandian J. Comparative aspects of development of dental hard structures. J Dent Res 1963; 42:422–437.

Frank RM, Sognnaes RF. Electron microscopy of matrix formation and calcification in rat enamel. Arch Oral Biol 1960; 1:339–348.

Fullmer HM. Histochemical protein reactions in human developing teeth. Lab Invest 1959; 7:48–51.

Fullmer HM, Alper N. Histochemical polysaccharide reactions in human developing teeth. Lab. Invest 1958; 7:163–170.

Geller JH. Metabolic significance of collagen in tooth structure. J Dent Res 1958; 37:276–279.

Glas JE, Omnell KA. Studies on the ultrastructure of dental enamel. I. Size and shape of the apatite crystallites as deduced from x-ray diffraction data. J Ultrastruct Res 1960; 3:334–344.

Gwinnett AJ, Buonocore MG. Adhesives and caries prevention. Br Dent J 1965; 119:77–82.

Gwinnett AJ. The ultrastructure of the prismless enamel of deciduous teeth. Arch Oral Biol 1966; 11:1109–1115.

Gwinnett AJ. The ultrastructure of the prismless enamel of permanent teeth. Arch Oral Biol 1967; 12:381–387.

Gwinnett AJ, Matsui A. A study of enamel adhesives: the physical relationship between enamel and adhesive. Arch Oral Biol 1967; 12:1615–1620.

Gwinnett AJ. Histologic changes in human enamel following treatment with acidic adhesive conditioning agents. Arch Oral Biol 1971; 16:731–738.

Gwinnett AJ. Human prismless enamel and its influence on sealant penetration. Arch Oral Biol 1973; 18:441–444.

Hartles RL. Role of citric acid in mineralized tissues. Br Dent J 1961; 111:322–331.

Hartles RL, Leaver AG. Citrate in mineralized tissues. Arch Oral Biol 1961; 5:38.

Hess WC, Lee CY. The amino acid composition of proteins, isolated from the healthy enamel and dentin of carious teeth. J Dent Res 1954; 33:62–64.

Hormati AA, Fuller JL, Denehy GE. Effects of contamination and mechanical disturbance on the quality of acid etched enamel. J Am Dent Assoc 1980; 100:34–39.

Irving JT. Sudanophil inclusions in ameloblasts, odontoblasts, and cells of the oral epithelium. Nature (London) 1958; 181:569.

Irving JT. Calcification of the organic matrix of enamel. Arch Oral Biol 1963; 8:773–774.

Isaac S, Brudevold F, Smith FA, Gardner DE. Solubility rate and natural fluoride content of surface and subsurface enamel. J Dent Res 1958; 37:254–263.

Jansen MT, Visser JB. Permeable structures in normal enamel. J Dent Res 1950; 29:622.

Johansen E, Parks HF. On the three-dimensional morphology of crystallites in developing deciduous human enamel. J Dent Res 1961; 40:702.

Kallenluch E, Sandborn E, Warshawsky H. The Golgi apparatus of the rat at the stage of the enamel matrix formation. J Cell Biol 1963;16:629–632.

Kanthak FF, Benedict HC. The effect of dilute acids on the enamel surface as disclosed by the reflecting microscope. Dent Cosmos 1932; 74:429–441.

Leblond CP, Belanger LF, Greulich RC. Formation of bones and teeth as visualized by radiography. Ann NY Acad Sci 1955; 60:629–659.

Listgarten MA. Phase contrast and electron microscopic study of the junction between reduced enamel epithelium and enamel in unerupted human teeth. Arch Oral Biol 1966; 11:999–1016.

Little MF, Cueto ES. Some chemical and physical properties of "altered" enamel. J Dent Res 1959; 38:674–675 (Abstract).

Little MF, Cueto ES, Rowley J. Chemical and physical properties of altered and sound enamel. I. Ash, Ca, P, Co_2, N, water, microradiolucency and density. Arch Oral Biol 1962; 7:73–184.

Lowater F, Murray MM. Chemical composition of teeth. V. Spectrographic analysis. Biochem J 1937; 31:837–841.

Manly RS, Bibby BG. Substances capable of decreasing the acid solubility of tooth enamel. J Dent Res 1949; 28:160–171.

Marsland EA. A histological investigation of amelogenesis in rats. I. Matrix formation, Br Dent J 1951; 91:251–261.

Marsland EA. A histological investigation of amelogenesis in rats. II. Maturation. Br Dent J 1952; 92:109–119.

Meckel AH, Griebstein WJ, Neal RJ. Structure of mature human dental enamel as observed by electron microscopy. Arch Oral Biol 1965; 10:775–783.

Meckel AH, et al.: Ultrastructure of fully calcified human dental enamel. In: Stack MV, Fearnhead RW, eds. Tooth enamel: its composition, properties, and fundamental structure. Baltimore: Williams & Wilkins, 1965: 160–162.

Miura F, Nakagawa K, Ishizaki A. Scanning electron microscope studies of the direct bonding system. Bull Tokyo Med Dent Univ 1973; 20:245–249.

Myrberg (cited by Arwill ETG). Formal contributions: Discussion of fourth session. In: Stack MV, Fearnhead RW, eds. Tooth enamel: its composition, properties, and fundamental structure. Baltimore: Williams & Wilkins, 1965:212.

Nalbandian J, Frank RM. Microscopie electronique des gaines, des structures, prismatiques et interprismatiques de l'email foetal humain. Bull Group Int Rech Sci Stomat 1962; 5:523–542.

Neuman WF, Newman NW. The chemical dynamics of bone mineral. Chicago: University of Chicago Press, 1958.

Newbrun E. Variations in the hardness of enamel. Dent Progr 1962; 2:21–27.

Nylen MV, Eanes ED, Omnell KA. Crystal growth in rat enamel. J Cell Biol 1963; 18:109–123.

Osborn JW. The nature of Hunter-Schreger bands in enamel. Arch Oral Biol 1965;10:929–933.

Pannese E. Observations on the ultra-structure of the

enamel organ. I. Stellate reticulum and stratum intermedium. J Ultrastruct Res 1960; 4:372–400.

Pannese E. Observations on the ultra-structure of the enamel organ. II. Involution of the stellate reticulum. J Ultrastruct Res 1961; 5:328–342.

Pautard FGE. Formal contribution: discussion of third session. In: Stack MV, Fearnhead RW, eds. Tooth enamel: its composition, properties, and fundamental structure. Baltimore: Williams & Wilkins, 1965:136, 137, 155.

Poole DFG, Stack MV. The structure and physical properties of enamel. In: Stack MV, Fearnhead RW, eds. Tooth enamel: its composition, properties, and fundamental structure. Baltimore: Williams & Wilkins, 1965:172–176.

Poole DFG, Tailby PW, Berry DC. The movement of water and other molecules through dental enamel. Arch Oral Biol 1963; 8:77.

Reith EJ. Ultrastructure of enamel organ of rat's incisor. Anat Rec 1959; 133:327–328.

Reith EJ. The ultrastructure of ameloblasts from the growing end of rat incisors. Arch Oral Biol 1960; 2:253–262.

Reith EJ. The ultrastructure of ameloblasts during matrix formation and the maturation of enamel. J Biophys Biochem Cytol 1961; 9:825–840.

Reith EJ. The ultrastructure of ameloblasts during early stages of maturation of enamel. J Biophys Biochem Cytol 1963; 9:825–840.

Reith EJ, Cotty VF. Autoradiographic studies on calcification of enamel. Arch Oral Biol 1962; 7:365–372.

Reith EJ. Ultrastructure of enamel organ of rat's incisor. In: Stack MV, Fearnhead RW, eds. Tooth enamel: its composition, properties, and fundamental structure. Baltimore: Williams & Wilkins, 1965:108.

Ronnholm E. An electron microscopic study of the amelogenesis in human teeth. I. The fine structure of the ameloblasts. J Ultrastruct Res 1962; 6:229–248.

Ronnholm E. The amelogenesis of human teeth as revealed by electron microscopy. II. The development of enamel crystallites. J Ultrastruct Res 1962; 6:249–303.

Ronnholm E. The structure of the organic stoma of human enamel during amelogenesis. J Ultrastruct Res 1962; 6:368–389.

Scott DB. The electron microscopy of enamel and dentin. Ann NY Acad Sci 1955; 60:575–585.

Scott DB, Nyles MU. Changing concepts in dental histology. Ann NY Acad Sci 1960; 85:133–144.

Scott DB, Ussing MJ, Sognnaes RF, Wyckoff RNG. Electron microscopy of mature human enamel. J Dent Res 1952; 31:74–84.

Silverstone LM, Saxton CA, Dogon IL. Variations in the pattern of acid etching of human dental enamel by SEM. Caries Res 1975; 9:373–379.

Stack MV. Soluble protein and peptide fractions from human dental enamel. Abstr 3rd Int Congr Biochem, Brussels, 1955, No. 2–14, Secr. Gen., Liege, Belgium, 1955.

Stack MV, Fearnhead RW, eds. Tooth enamel: its composition, properties, and fundamental structure. Baltimore: Williams & Wilkins, 1965.

Stein G, Boyle PE. Studies on enamel. I. The yellow color of the incisor teeth of the albino rat. J Dent Res 1941; 20:261–262.

Symons, NBB. Lipid distribution in the developing teeth of rat. Br Dent J 1958; 105: 27–30.

Ten Cate AR. The distribution of hydrolytic enzymes and lipids in the enamel epithelium of man and the macaque monkey. Arch Oral Biol 1963; 8:755–763.

Thewlis J. The structure of teeth as shown by x-ray examination. MRC Spec Rep Ser, 1940; 238.

Turner EP. The integument of the enamel surface of the human tooth. Dent Pract 1958; 8:341–348, 373–382.

Tyldesley WR. The mechanical properties of human enamel and dentine. Br Dent J 1959; 106.

Ussing M. The development of the epithelial attachment. Acta Odont Scand 1955; 13:123–154.

Vallotton CF. An acquired pigmented pellicle of the enamel surface. I. Review of the literature. J Dent Res 1945; 24:161–169.

Wainwright WW. Penetration of teeth by radioactive materials. J Dent Res 1954; 33:767, 34:28.

Wainwright WW, Lemoine FA. Rapid diffusion penetration of intact enamel and dentin by carbon^{14}-labeled urea. J Am Dent Assoc 1950; 41:135.

Walkaug J. Enamel cuticle. J Dent Res 1956; 35:313–322.

Watson ML. The extracellular nature of enamel in the rat. J Biophys Biochem Cytol 1960; 7:489–492.

Weidmann SM. Enamel density measurements using density gradients. J Dent Res 1965; 44:1170 (Abstract).

Weidmann SM, Hamm SM. Studies on the enamel matrix of mature teeth. In: Stack MV, Fearnhead RW, eds. Tooth enamel: its composition, properties, and fundamental structure. Baltimore: Williams & Wilkins, 1965:83–90, 111–113.

Weidmann SM, Weatherell JA, Hamm SM. Variations of enamel density in sections of human teeth. Arch Oral Biol 1967; 12:85–97.

Wertheimer FW, Fullmer HM. Morphologic and histochemical observations on the human dental cuticle. J Peridont 1962; 33:29–39.

Yardini J, Gedalia D, Kohn M. Fluoride concentration of dental calculus, surface enamel and cementum. Arch Oral Biol 1963; 8:697–701.

Young RW, Greulich RC. Distinctive autoradiographic patterns of glycine incorporation in rat enamel and dentine matrices. Arch Oral Biol 1963; 8:509–521.

Zipkin I, Piez KA. The citric acid content of human teeth. J Dent Res 1950; 29:498–505.

8

The Dentin

Dentin constitutes the main portion of the tooth structure, extending almost the entire length of the tooth. It is covered by enamel on the crown and by cementum on the root. The internal surface of the dentin forms the walls of the pulp cavity, which is primarily occupied by the pulpal tissue. This internal wall closely follows the outline of the external surface of the dentin (Fig. 8.1).

The odontoblast cells that are found in the pulp cavity are believed to play a significant role in the production of dentin. During dentinogenesis these cells form protoplasmic extensions, which become entrapped in the ground substance of the dentin. Their cell bodies remain outside this matrix with the cellular elements of the pulp (Fig. 8.2). The protoplasmic extensions are called the *odontoblast processes* and they extend up to the outer periphery of the dentin on a more or less perpendicular course from the pulp cavity. This arrangement differs from bone and cementum in that the tissue-forming cells and their processes are completely embedded in the matrix.

Because of the existence of the odontoblast processes in the dentinal matrix, the dentin is considered a living tissue, with the capacity to react to physiologic and pathologic stimuli. These stimuli may produce changes within the dentin, such as secondary dentin, sclerotic dentin, and dead tracts. A thorough explanation of these changes is given later in this chapter.

Chemically, dentin is composed of organic and inorganic matter. The inorganic components comprise chiefly calcium phosphate in the form of hydroxyapatite ($Ca_{10}(PO_4)_6(OH)_2$), whereas the organic matter, for the most part, is collagenous material.

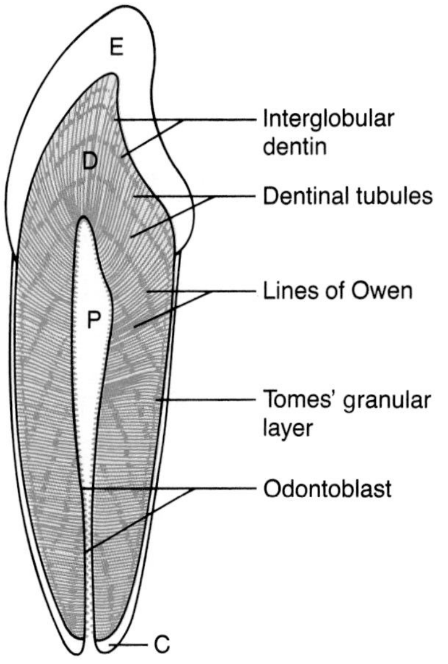

Figure 8.1

Diagrammatic illustration of a longitudinal sectional of the dentin (*D*) with the enamel (*E*) covering the crown portion and cementum (*C*) on the root. The internal wall of the dentin closely follows the outline of the external surface forming the pulp cavity (*P*).

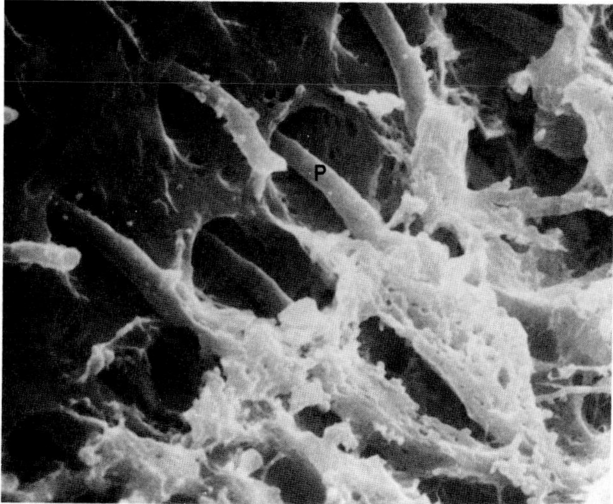

Figure 8.2

Protoplastic extensions (*P*) from the odontoblasts entering the dentinal tubules at the pulpo-dentinal interface.

Physical Properties

The *color* of dentin is yellowish white and may differ in primary and permanent dentitions. The former seem to have a lighter coloration.

The *hardness* of dentin is known to be less than that of enamel but greater than either bone or cementum. Measurements have shown different microhardness values in the different layers of dentin. The Knoop method is most frequently used for measuring microhardness of dentin. This procedure uses an indenting tool made from diamond which cuts into the material that is being tested. These indentations are then measured and a mathematical formula applied to the results, yielding the Knoop hardness number (KHN). The highest microhardness values of an intact dentin occur at the area approximately 450 μm from the dentinoenamel junction, with an average KHN of 70. The lowest value (approximately 20 KHN) is found at the innermost layer of dentin at a distance of 100 μm from the pulp. With advancing age the microhardness of dentin increases. Comparison of the microhardness value of dentin to other hard tissues and restorative dental materials is shown in Table 8.1.

Although the dentin is considered a hard structure, it also has elastic properties, which are important for the support of the brittle, nonresilient enamel of the tooth as described in the previous section. In dentin, the modulus of elasticity has been found to be 1.67×10^6 PSI. The tensile strength of dentin (6,000 PSI) is less than that of compact bone. The compressive strength may be as high as 40,000 PSI.

The presence of numerous dentinal tubules and odontoblast processes in the matrix makes the dentin highly permeable. This property can be studied by means of the diffusion of dyes and radioactive materials. Permeability of dentin decreases with advancing age.

Table 8.1
Comparison of Microhardness Value of Dentin to Other Materials

Materials	KHN
Dentin	65
Enamel	300
Silicate cement	70
Gold (pure)	32
Amalgam	90

Reproduced from Skinner EW, Phillips RW. The Science of Dental Materials. 6th ed. Philadelphia: WB Saunders, 1967; by permission.

Chemical Composition

According to the chemical balance sheet of Eastoe, human dentin is composed, by weight, of 75 percent inorganic and 20 percent organic materials. The remaining 5 percent represents the retained water, error, and other materials (Table 8.2).

Inorganic Composition

The principal inorganic constituents of dentin are calcium, phosphorus, and in lesser amounts carbonate, magnesium, sodium, and chloride. The trace inorganic elements of dentin are aluminum, barium, platinum, potassium, silver, silicone, tin, titanium, tungsten, rubidium, vanadium, and zinc.

The concentration and distribution of these elements have been studied by several workers, and they all agree that the principal elements (calcium, carbonate, phosphorus, and magnesium) are higher in concentration in the dentin than in either cementum or bone, but lower than in enamel. This also holds true with sodium and chloride. As to the distribution of these principal elements, there are no conclusive data available, but it is believed that they are more concentrated at the crown portion of the dentin.

Although dentin is considered a hard structure, it is less mineralized than enamel but more so than

Table 8.2
Chemical Balance Sheet for the Organic Constituents of Normal Human Dentin*

	Range	Average	Total
Inorganic matter (ash + CO_2)†			75
Ash	71.5–72.4	72.0	
CO_2		3.0	
Organic matter			20
Collagen	17.5–18.5	18.0	
Water soluble	0.5–0.9		
Citrate	0.86–0.89	0.89	
Lactate		0.15	
Resistant protein		0.2	
Lipid	0.044–0.36	0.2	
Chondroitin sulfate	0.2–0.6	0.4	
Other mucosubstances	?	?	
Unaccounted for (water retained at 100°C, error, etc.)			5

*Values are given as percentage by weight of dentin which has been dried at 100°C.

†Residue from KOH-glycol extraction (77.8).

Reproduced from Eastoe JE. Chemical organization of the organic matrix of dentine. In: Miles AEW, ed. Structural and Chemical Organization of Teeth. New York: Academic Press, 1967; by permission.

either cementum or bone. The calcium : phosphorus ratio in dentin is usually lower than that of enamel and is believed to be more variable.

Of the several trace inorganic materials detected in dentin, only fluoride, zinc, and lead are found in quantities sufficient to allow determination of their concentration and distribution. Fluoride is considered to be an important inorganic trace element of dentin and enamel since its presence reduces the solubility of the teeth. Because of this, it plays an important role in the reduction of dental caries. It has been shown that people living in a community with a high content of fluoride in the water supply will have teeth that are more resistant to dental caries than will those people living in an area with a lower concentration of fluoride. This was also demonstrated in vitro (see Chapter 6). The concentration of fluoride in dentin is between two and three times the amount found in enamel and is higher in the permanent than in the primary teeth. As to location, fluoride is more concentrated near the pulp, decreasing toward the dentinoenamel junction. This might be attributed to its proximity to the circulating body fluid. Although the incorporation of fluoride in the dentinal matrix occurs during the process of calcification, the concentration of this mineral is increased with advancing age through the ingestion of food and drinking water, as well as topical application of this element.

The trace elements, zinc and lead, have been found to increase in concentration with age. The amount, however, is dependent on the level of ingestion. The content of dentin, when compared with that in other tissues in the body, has a higher concentration. The distribution of zinc in dentin is similar to that of fluoride, whereas lead seems to be evenly distributed with a slight elevation at the area near the pulp. The role of these elements is not known.

In general it is agreed that the mineral content of dentin increases with age.

Organic Composition

The organic portion of dentin is made up mainly of dentinal protein. This protein is similar to collagen, which is characterized by four amino acids, glycine, alanine, proline, and hydroxyproline, which represent two-thirds of the amino acid content. When compared with other mammalian collagen, dentin has a similar composition except that there is a difference in hydroxylysine and lysine ratio. The dentinal collagen appears to be richer in hydroxylysine and poorer in lysine. The higher hydroxylysine content in dentin is believed to play some role in the mineralization process.

Table 8.3
Composition of Human Dentin Collagen

Amino Acids	Permanent Teeth	Deciduous Teeth (Developing)
Alanine	112	108*
Glycine	319	308
Valine	25	27
Leucine	26	27
Isoleucine	10	12
Proline	115	115
Phenylalanine	14	15
Tyrosine	2.3	4.9
Serine	38	41
Threonine	19	20
Methionine	5.2	6.8
Arginine	47	51
Histidine	5.3	6.5
Lysine	23	25
Aspartic Acid	55	51
Glutamic Acid	73	75
Hydroxyproline	101	98
Hydroxylysine	8.4	8.1
Amide	41	54

*Values are expressed as numbers of units of each amino acid per 1000 units of all types.

Reproduced from Eastoe JE. Chemical organization of the organic matrix of dentine. In: Miles AEW, ed. Structural and Chemical Organization of Teeth. New York: Academic Press, 1967; by permission.

Dentinal collagen as a whole is thought to be a seeding agent in the formation of apatite crystals (see Table 8.3).

Other Organic Constituents

Lipid materials have also been found in dentin. They are cholesterol, esterified cholesterol, and phospholipids. The presence of these lipids seems to be related to the calcification process, since these substances, through specific staining methods, have been found in areas where calcification is taking place.

Chondroitin sulfuric acid, similar to that found in cartilage, has also been isolated in dentin. Other carbohydrates are found, such as hexosamine in the odontoblast process and sulfated acid mucopolysaccharides in the peritubular areas. The histochemical changes that accompany mineralization, such as metachromasia (staining with many tints) and basophilia (staining readily with basic dyes), suggest that carbohydrates also play a role in calcification.

Because enzymatic processes are involved in calcification of bone, cartilage, and dentin, the enzyme alkaline phosphatase becomes bound with the organic matrix of mature dentin. This has been observed also in the predentinal and dentinal tubules.

Other organic substances of the dentin are citrate and lactate (see Table 8.2). Citrate appears to be distributed evenly in the crown and root portion of the dentin with the exception of a greater concentration in the area adjacent to the pulp. This is in contrast to the concentration of lactate, which is high near the periphery of the dentin and low in the area near the pulp. The function of these organic substances is not yet clear; however, they too may play an important part in the calcification process.

Structural Components

The basic structural components of dentin are of two kinds: (1) the odontoblasts and their processes and (2) the dentinal matrix (Fig. 8.3). Since the odontoblast cells are located in the pulp cavity, discussion of these cells is reserved for the next chapter.

Odontoblast Processes (Tomes' Fibers) and Innervation

The odontoblast processes are cytoplasmic extensions traversing the body of the dentin from the main protoplasmic mass of the odontoblast cells (Fig. 8.4). In several areas, they may extend into the enamel structure as enamel spindles (Fig. 8.5). The lengths of these processes range from 2 to 3 mm from the odontoblast nucleus to the surface, with a diameter of approximately 1.0 to 1.5 μm. These processes also give off lateral branches penetrating the dentinal matrix in a direction radiating diagonally toward the outer dentinal surface (Fig. 8.6). Anastomoses of these branches are often seen between the processes. Terminal branches are also present and extend to the dentinoenamel and dentinocemental junction (see Figs. 8.4 and 8.5).

Structurally, each odontoblast process is limited by a cell membrane (Fig. 8.7). The cytoplasm of each process contains organelles such as mitochondria, endoplasmic reticulum vesicles, ribosome-like gran-

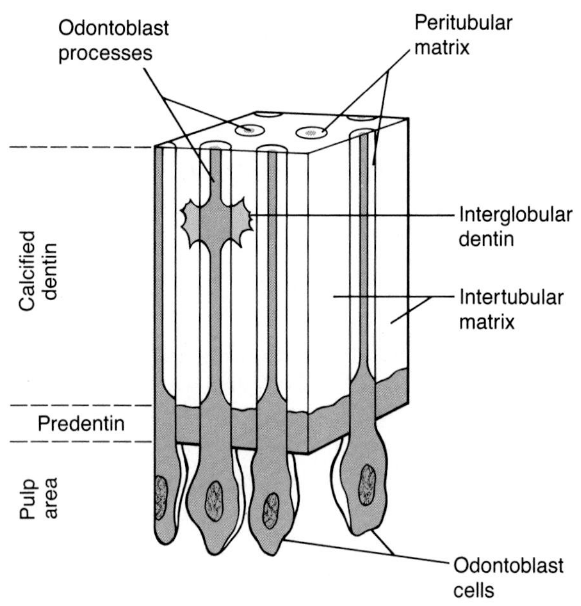

Figure 8.3

Schematic illustration of the odontoblast cells and their processes, and the dentinal matrix. Note that the odontoblast cell bodies are found in the pulp area, whereas the processes are included in the dentinal matrix. The peritubular areas are absent in the predentinal layer and interglobular dentin. (Drawn with modification from Blake GC. The peritubular translucent zones in human dentine. Br Dent J 1958; 104:57–67; by permission of the *British Dental Journal.*)

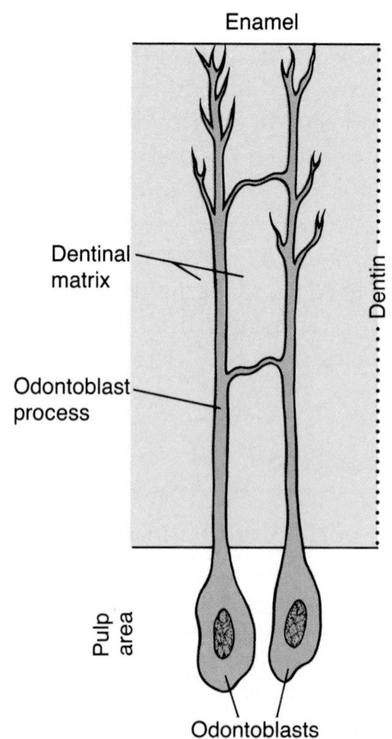

Figure 8.4

Schematic illustration of the odontoblast processes penetrating the dentinal matrix with lateral and terminal branches. Note the anastomosis of these processes.

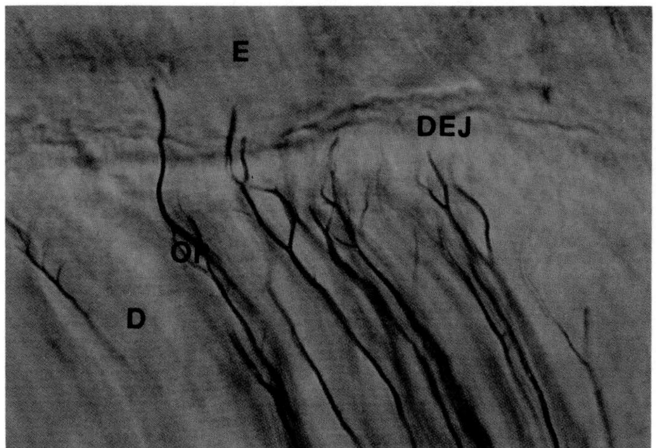

Figure 8.5

A longitudinal ground section of the dentin (*D*) with the odontoblast processes (*OP*) extending to the enamel proper (*E*) as enamel spindles cross the dentinoenamel junction (*DEJ*). The processes also show lateral and terminal branches. Original magnification, 700 ×.

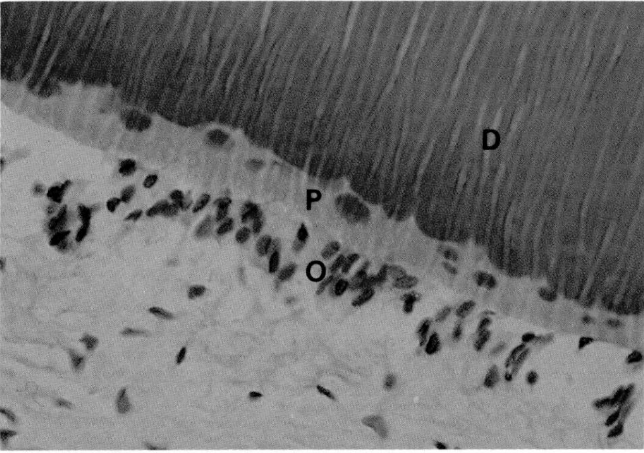

Figure 8.6

Longitudinal stained section of the pulpo-dentinal interface showing the odontoblasts (*O*), predentin (*P*) and the tubular structure of mature dentin (*D*).

ules, and vacuolar structures. The organelles are found at different levels within the process. A large vacuole is located centrally in cross-section, and is farther removed from the cell body than the organelles and the smaller vacuoles (Fig. 8.8). The presence of the above ultramicroscopic structures suggests that metabolic activity occurs in the cytoplasm of the odontoblast process. The vacuoles found in the process are believed to secrete materials related to calcification of the matrix immediately surrounding the process (*peritubular matrix*). This secretion is thought to be found in the periodontoblastic space located between the odontoblast process and the calcified wall of the dentinal tubule (Fig. 8.9). Fine collagenous fibrils may exist in this space. However, these fine fibril materials are without cross-striations, indicating that they may not be collagen. Up to the present time there has been no definite resolution of the nature of the material that exists within the periodontoblastic space.

As the odontoblast process approaches the periphery of the dentin, it seems to taper off to a smaller diameter and only the large vacuole, surrounded by a thin annular layer of cytoplasm, is seen (see Fig. 8.8). Other organelles have not been identified in this area.

Histochemically, the odontoblast process as a whole reacts positively to the periodic acid-Schiff procedure and stains with Sudan black B, indicating the presence of phospholipid material. The vacuoles of the odontoblast process may contain lipid material.

Nerve fibers originating from the pulp have been shown to accompany some of the odontoblast pro-

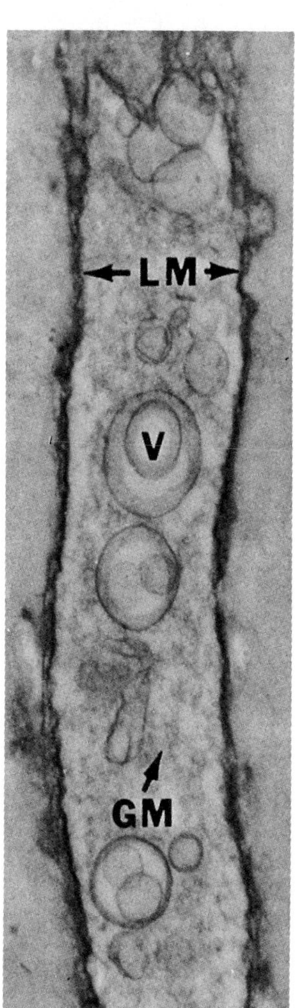

Figure 8.7

Odontoblast process showing limiting cell membrane (*LM*), flocculant or granular material (*GM*) and vesicular structure (*V*). Original magnification, 21,000 ×. (Courtesy of Kaye and Herold.)

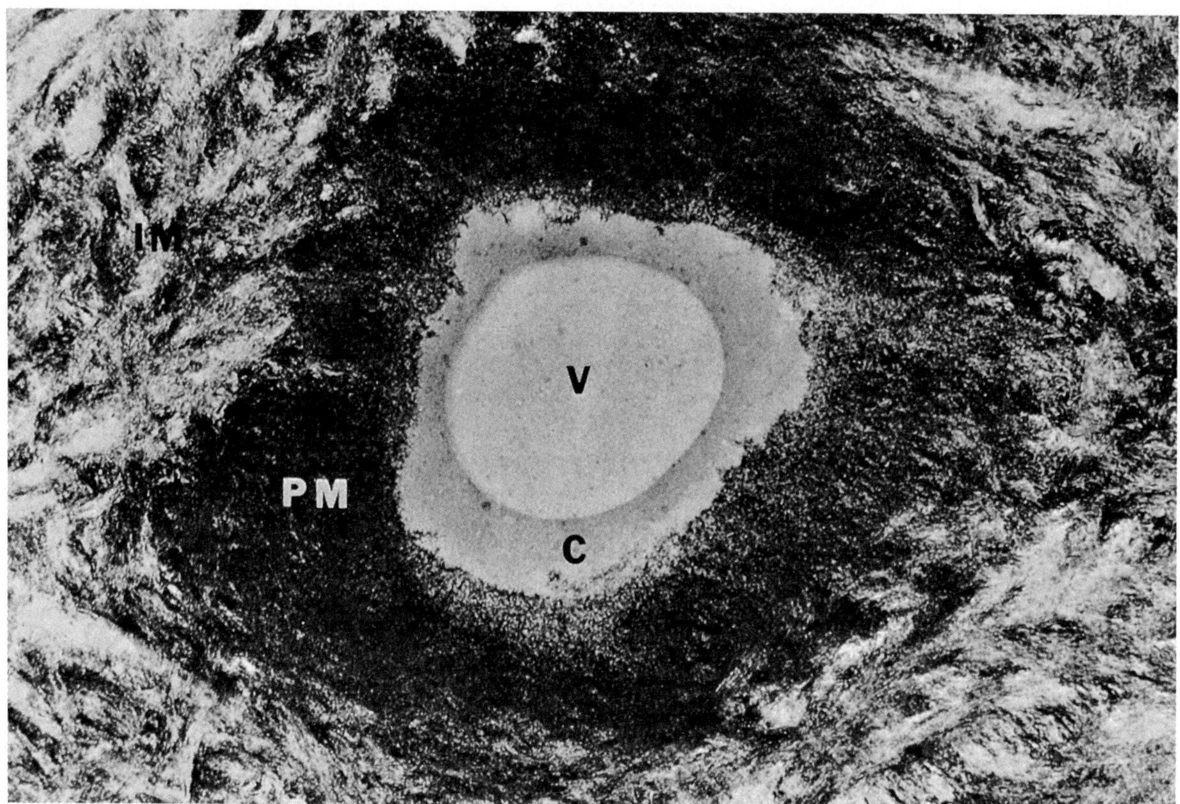

Figure 8.8

A transverse section of a dentinal tubule with the odontoblast process showing a centrally located vacuole (*V*) and a thin annular layer of cytoplasm (*C*). Note the electron-dense, dark peritubular area (*PM*) surrounding the process. The peritubular organic materials also appear to be in continuity with the intertubular matrix (*IM*). Original magnification, 35,000 ×. (Reproduced from Frank RM, in *The Proceedings of the Third European Symposium on Calcified Tissue*. New York: Springer-Verlag, 1966; by permission.)

cesses into the predentinal layer (Fig. 8.10). However, whether or not nerve fibers extend into the calcified dentin remains a controversial subject, and further investigation is needed. By means of the silver impregnation technique, some have maintained that nerve fibers do extend into the calcified portion of the dentin; others are of the opinion that nerve endings terminate at the predentinal layer and do not extend into the calcified dentin. It is believed that fibers in the predentinal layer undergo a degenerative process as calcification progresses in the dentin. If nerve fibers can be shown to be present in the calcified dentin the extreme sensitivity of newly exposed dentin could then be easily explained, since fibers could then function as direct sensory pathways from the dentin to the nerves in the pulp. But if nerve fibers are nonexistent in this area, other explanations must be given for dentin sensitivity. The main theories that attempt to explain the transmission of stimuli *without* neural connections fall into two general classes: physical and chemical. Of the physical theories the most widely known is the *hydrodynamic transmission theory*. This theory attempts to attribute the transmission stimulus effect through the dentinal tubules to a sudden flow of the fluid contained within them. This surge of fluid is caused by capillary forces induced by physical changes in the dentin such as drying and changes in temperature. The pressure change caused by this fluid movement exerts itself upon the pulp, which is rich in nerve endings, thereby creating a pain sensation. The chemical theory relies upon the fact that the specific neurotransmitting agent, cholinesterase, has been found in the odontoblast processes and at the dentinoenamel junction. It is thought, therefore, that the odontoblast process itself may be a pain receptor, with the cell body making a synaptic connection with the nerves in the pulp.

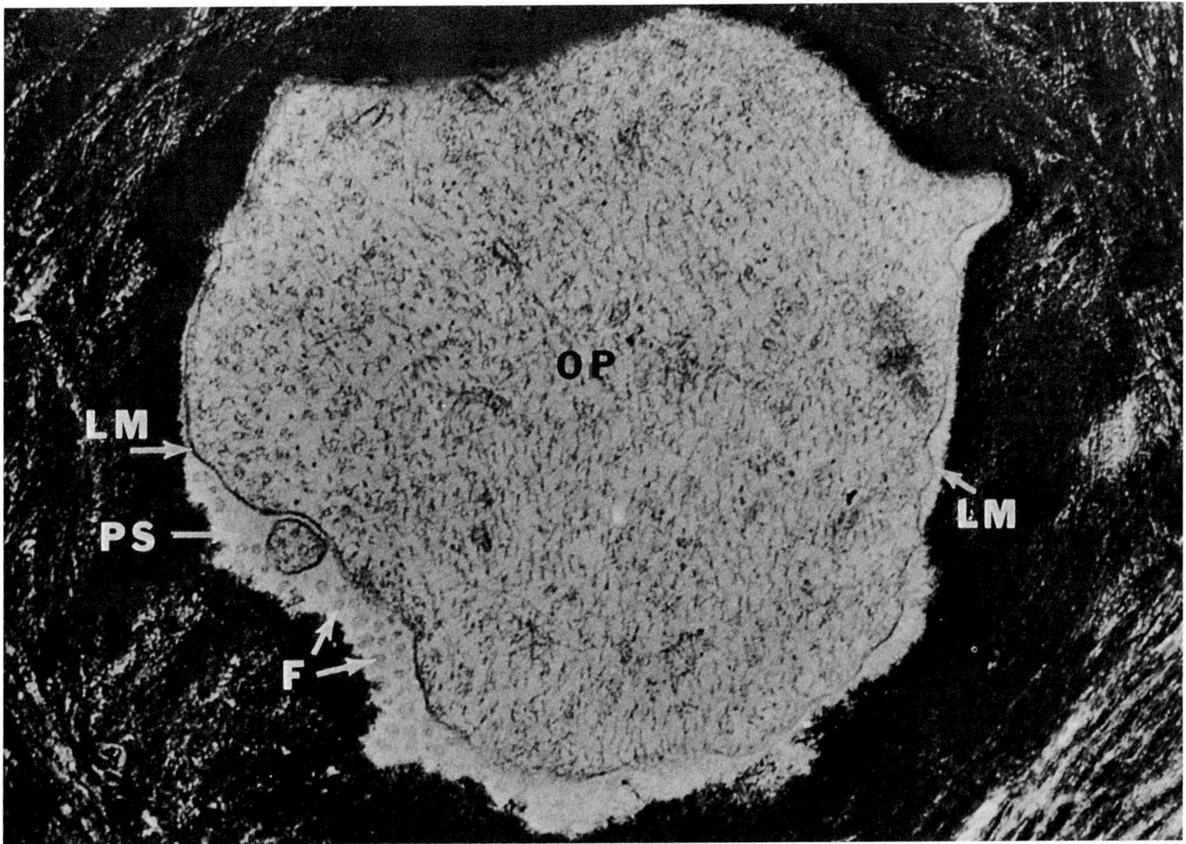

Figure 8.9

A transverse section of a dentinal tubule with the odontoblast process (*OP*) showing the periodontoblastic space (*PS*) containing a cross-section of fibril materials (*F*) and lateral branch of the process. The process is limited by a thin cell membrane (*LM*). Original magnification, 52,000 ×. (Reproduced from Frank RM, in *The Proceedings of the Third European Symposium on Calcified Tissue.* New York: Springer-Verlag, 1966; by permission.)

Dentinal Matrix

The dentinal matrix is a calcified network of collagenous fibrils that is penetrated by the odontoblast processes. The passageways occupied by the processes are called the dentinal tubules. The matrix immediately surrounding each odontoblast process has been shown to be more mineralized than the adjacent matrix and to have different histochemical properties. In accordance with these structural and chemical differences, the two areas of the dentinal matrix have been designated as peritubular and intertubular matrices (see Fig. 8.3).

Peritubular Matrix

The peritubular matrix is variously referred to as the *translucent area, calcified canalicular sheath, peritubular dentin, peritubular translucent zone,* and the *periprocess solid area.* This matrix is an annular, hypercalcified zone around the odontoblast process; however, these zones are absent in some areas so that the wall of the tubule is directly formed by the intertubular matrix. An example of this arrangement is at the area of interglobular dentin (Figs. 8.3 and 8.11). Under electron microscopy and through radiographic studies, it has been demonstrated that the peritubular matrix is not present at the predentinal layer. The thickness of this matrix varies from 0.4 to 1.5 μm with a diameter of approximately 3.0 μm.

It has been well documented that the peritubular matrix is more highly mineralized than the neighboring intertubular matrix. It is composed mainly of inorganic material in the form of apatite crystals with a small amount of organic substance. This has been indicated by the fact that the peritubular matrix is more electron opaque and easily lost under decalcifying solution (Figs. 8.8 and 8.12). The organic portion of this

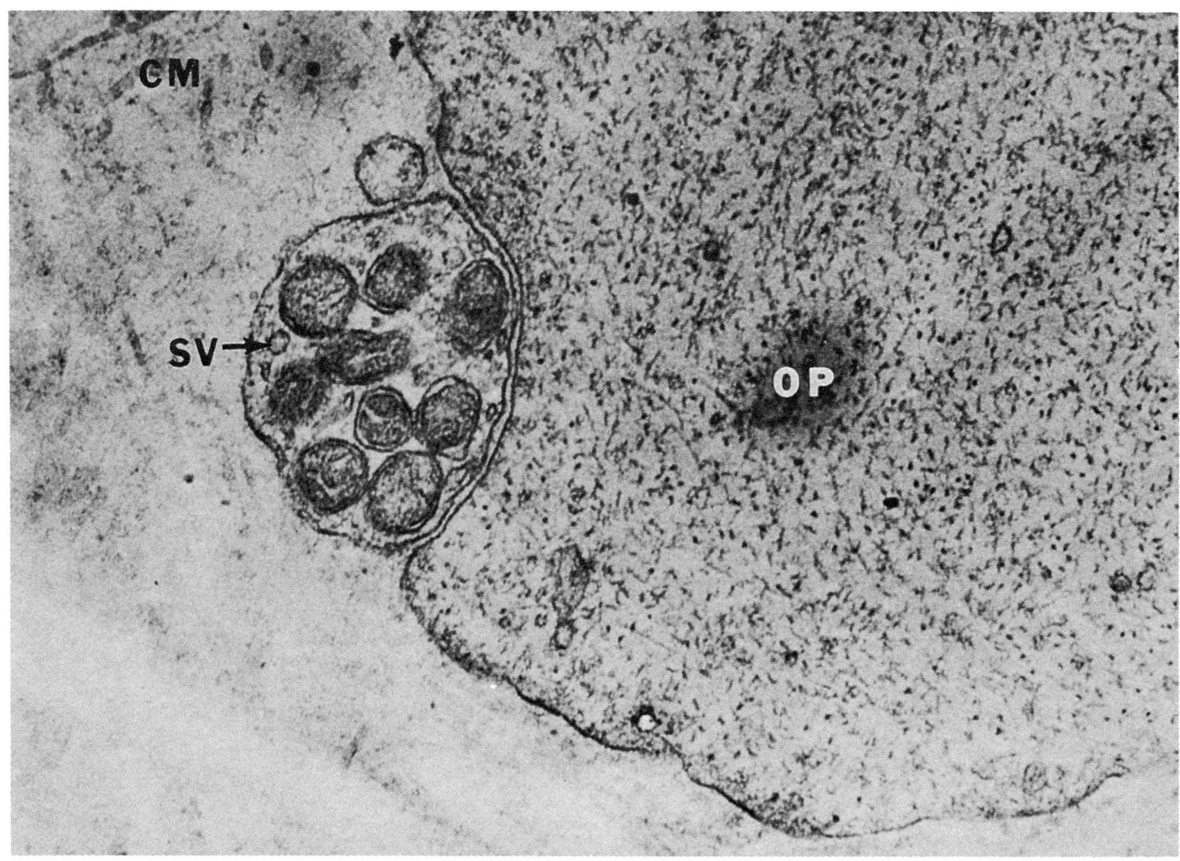

Figure 8.10

A transverse section of the odontoblast process (*OP*) in the predentin layer showing a cross-section of unmyelinated nerve fiber that runs in close association with the process containing synaptic vesicle-like structures (*SV*). Note the noncalcified collagenous matrix (*CM*). Original magnification, 67,000 ×. (Reproduced from Frank RM, in *The Proceedings of the Third European Symposium on Calcified Tissue.* New York: Springer-Verlag, 1966; by permission.)

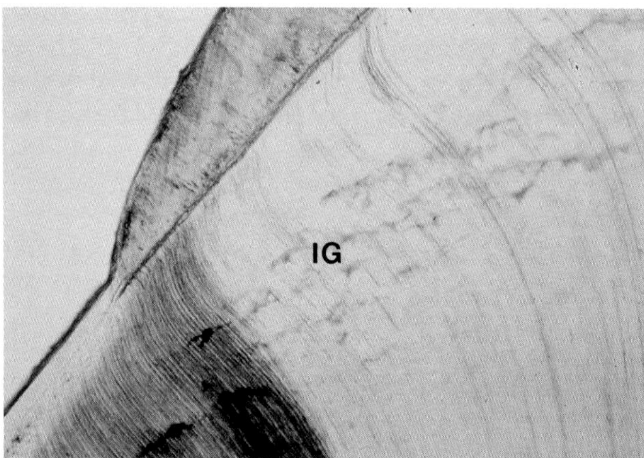

Figure 8.11

Longitudinal ground section through dentin viewed by polarization microscopy. A zone of interglobular dentin (*IG*) lies just below the mantle dentin (*M*).

matrix is very scarce and can be destroyed easily by a regular decalcifying method (Figs. 8.12 and 8.13).

The question of whether the organic substance in the peritubular matrix contains collagenous material is still unsettled. Some investigators have found collagenous material "sparsely distributed" in the peritubular matrix. Others found only some fine nonstriated fibers which appear to be of a "structureless filamentary substance." Regardless of the true nature of these fibers, they are in continuity with the collagenous fibers of the intertubular matrix (Fig. 8.8).

Histochemically, the peritubular matrix contains a large amount of acid mucopolysaccharides indicated by metachromatic and basophilic stain at low pH. The presence of mucopolysaccharides may be responsible for binding positively charged metals, such as calcium, and may trigger crystal formation in the calcification process of the peritubular matrix.

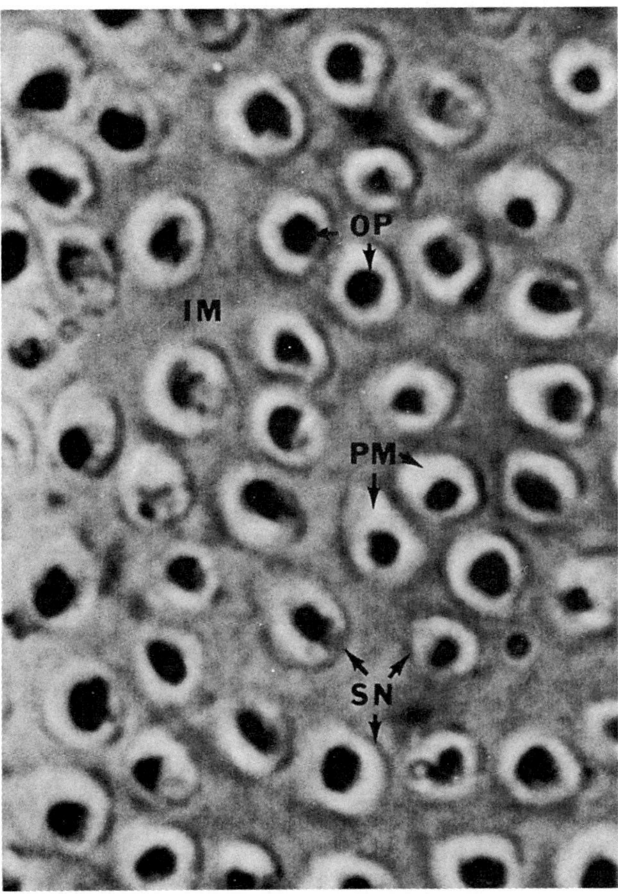

Figure 8.12

Decalcified transverse section of the dentin showing odontoblast processes (*OP*) encased in the tubules. The white areas surrounding the processes are the peritubular matrix (*PM*). Because of their high mineral content, they are easily destroyed under regular decalcifying methods. The intertubular matrix (*IM*) and the odontoblast processes (*OP*), being rich in organic substance, are retained after decalcification. Note the location of the sheath of Neumann (*SN*). Original magnification, 1575 ×.

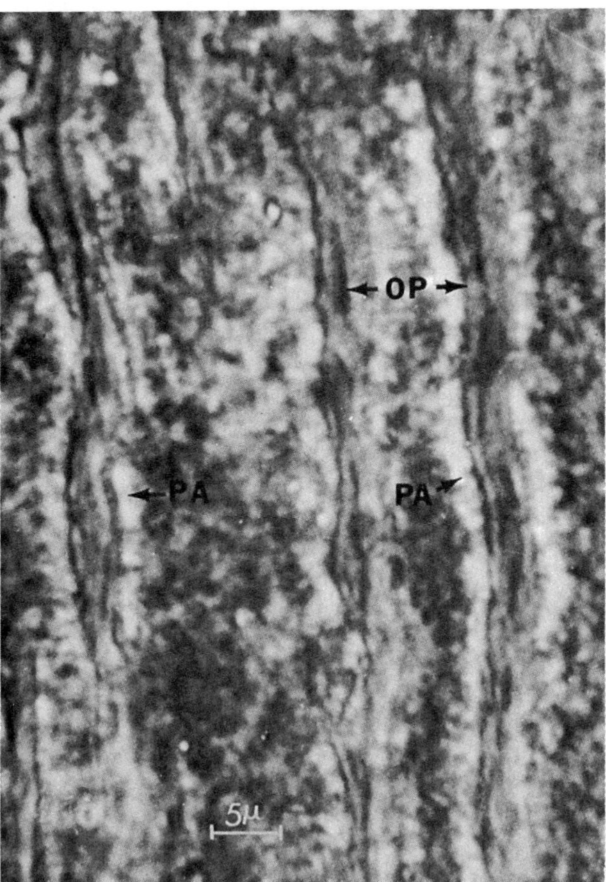

Figure 8.13

A longitudinal decalcified section of the dentin showing odontablast processes (*OP*) accompanied by translucent peritubular areas (*PA*). Original magnification, 3,000 ×. (Courtesy of Kaye and Herold.)

Intertubular Matrix

The intertubular matrix is also known as *intercanalicular dentin* or *intertubular dentin*. This matrix constitutes the main structural component of the dentin that surrounds the lumen of the dentinal tubule in areas where no peritubular dentin is present. It also fills the region between the outer parts of the peritubular zone (see Fig. 8.2). The intertubular dentin consists mainly of collagenous material with amorphous, organic ground substance and smaller amounts of apatite crystals (Fig. 8.14). These collagenous fibers resemble collagen found in tendons and other types of connective tissue, and are characterized by cross-striations at 640-Å intervals with a diameter of 600 to 700 Å. These fibers form interlacing bundles running in a crisscross manner or trellis-like arrangement between dentinal tubules (Fig. 8.14). The direction is generally parallel to the surface of the dentin, i.e., at right angles or oblique to the dentinal tubules. The arrangement near the dentinoenamel junction, however, is different, and the fibrils are generally oriented at right angles to the dentin surface. It was also shown that some fine fibrils may project into the prism sheath or interprismatic substance and it was suggested that these fibrils probably provide the mechanism for anchoring the enamel to the dentin. The fibrils beneath the cementum have the same arrangement except that these fibrillar bundles are coarser and they tend to join at the end, giving rise to a looped or lace-like appearance. Recent investigations have revealed that the orienta-

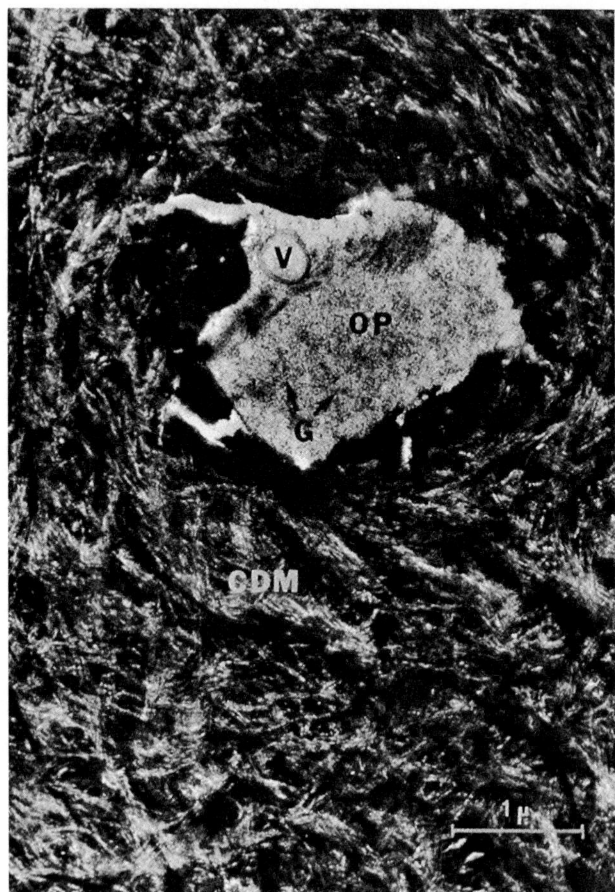

Figure 8.14

A transverse ground section of the odontoblast process (*OP*) and collagenous dentinal matrix (*CDM*) characterized by cross-striation. The collagenous fibers appear to form interlacing bundles running in a crisscross manner or "trellis-like" arrangement. Note that the process contains small vesicle (*V*) and fine granular material (*G*). Original magnification, 23,000 ×. (Courtesy of Kaye and Herold.)

tion of these collagenous fibers of the intertubular matrix may be influenced by and may follow the direction of the lateral branches of the odontoblast processes (see Fig. 8.6).

The apatite crystallites are believed to be arranged roughly parallel to the collagenous fibers. Morphologically, the crystallites are plate-like structures with a maximum length of 1,000 Å and a 20 to 35 Å thickness. The sizes vary according to the location. The crystallites located near the pulp or at the area close to the dentin-predentin junction are of smaller size and are less densely distributed.

Histochemically, the intertubular matrix stains with methylene blue and toluidine blue at pH 2.6 and 3.6. However, the density of the stain varies at different zones; it has been shown that the innermost layer stains intensely and decreases its affinity toward the periphery. The staining indicates an acid mucopolysaccharide content of the intertubular matrix. The degree of staining, however, is less in the intertubular than in the peritubular matrix, which is richer in acid mucopolysaccharide.

Sheath of Neumann

For many years the sheath of Neumann has been described as a structure or simply an optical artifact around the inner wall of the dentinal tubule and in close apposition to the contained odontoblast process. The annular space between the sheath and the odontoblast process was believed to be due to shrinkage of the process during decalcification. In reality, the annular space in decalcified sections was occupied in vivo by the highly mineralized peritubular matrix. The sheath of Neumann, if present at all, could therefore be located only between the peritubular and intertubular matrices (see Fig. 8.12).

On the basis of studies involving electron microscopy, and microradiography, there are indications that the sheath of Neumann does not exist as such. However, by replica study, collagenous fibrils have been found between the peritubular and intertubular matrices. These fibers are intimately connected to the two matrices by a series of interlacing fibrils and are not considered to constitute a solid and definite sheath. Some workers have described a "sharp border line" separating the two zones (peritubular and intertubular), but the sheath of Neumann was not observed. Other investigators consider this structure to be an optical artifact, and the sheath of Neumann as a structural entity to be nonexistent.

Incremental, Contour, and Neonatal Lines

Incremental lines mark the sites of transition between alternating periods of accelerated and decelerated growth. The annual rings in trees, with their varying widths, are an example of differential amounts of tree growth *each year.* In dentin, the incremental lines reflect periods of *varying durations* of fast and slow growth rates. They are seen as fine lines oriented perpendicular to the dentinal tubules, and are referred to as *imbrication lines* or *incremental lines of von Ebner* (Fig. 8.15). In humans, the average distance between these increments measures approximately 4 μm. This represents the rate of dentin deposition in 24 hours. Some of the increments also follow the contour lines of Owen, which are heavier and have a wider distance between them (Figs. 8.1 and 8.16). It should be clearly understood, however, that the contour lines

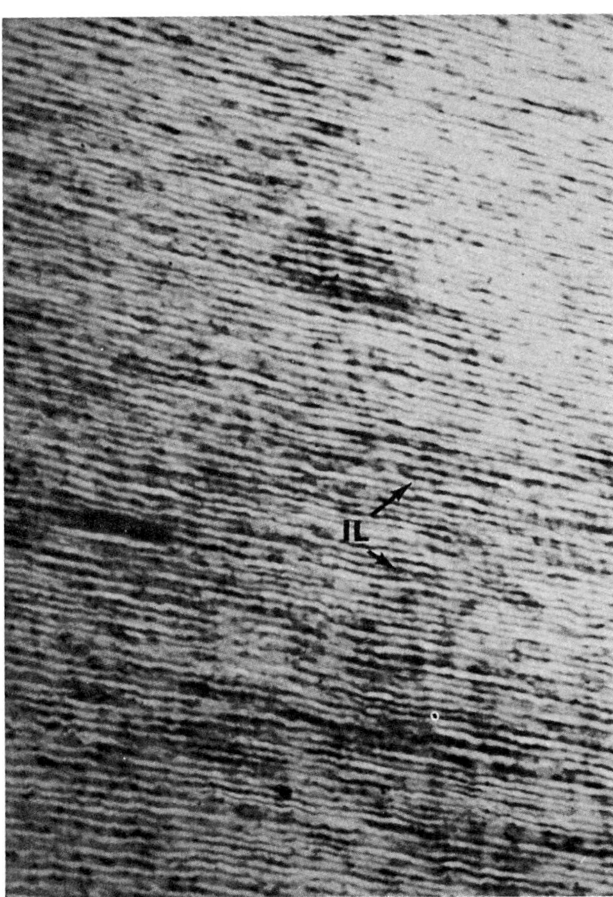

Figure 8.15

A longitudinal decalcified section of the dentin showing the incremental lines of von Ebner (*IL*). Original magnification, 187.50 ×.

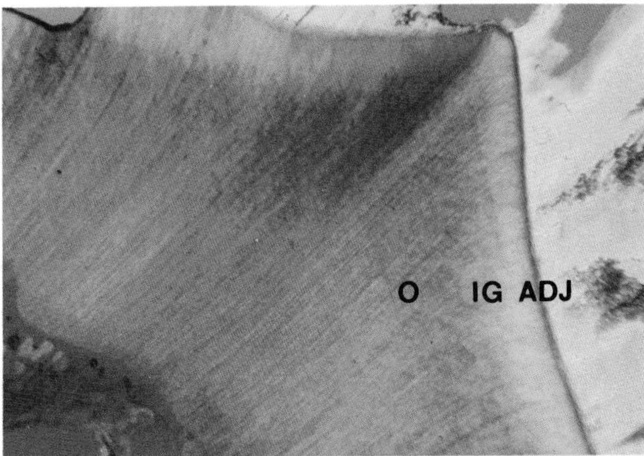

Figure 8.16

Longitudinal ground section viewed by polarized light microscopy. Contour lines of Owen (*O*) follow the outer contour of the dentin (*ADJ*) and run uninterruptedly through the interglobular zone (*IG*).

of Owen do not represent incremental deposition of dentin but only indicate phases of mineralization. They are visible under low-power magnification and they seem to follow the outer contour of the dentin. According to the original description of Owen in 1840, these lines result from the "occasional short bending of the tubules which are found along a line parallel with the outer contour of the crown."

Metabolic changes during the neonatal period are recorded in the dentin as heavy and accentuated lines that follow the same pattern as the contour lines of Owen. They represent hypocalcified bands separating the prenatal and the postnatal dentin, and have been referred to as the *neonatal lines* (Fig. 8.17). It is thought that these lines are caused by an interruption of growth of the dentin because of the metabolic adjustment of the infant at birth. Although the growth of the dentin is slightly delayed, the direction of the tubules is not altered (Fig. 8.18). The teeth that may reveal these lines are the primary teeth, and the permanent maxillary and mandibular first molars since

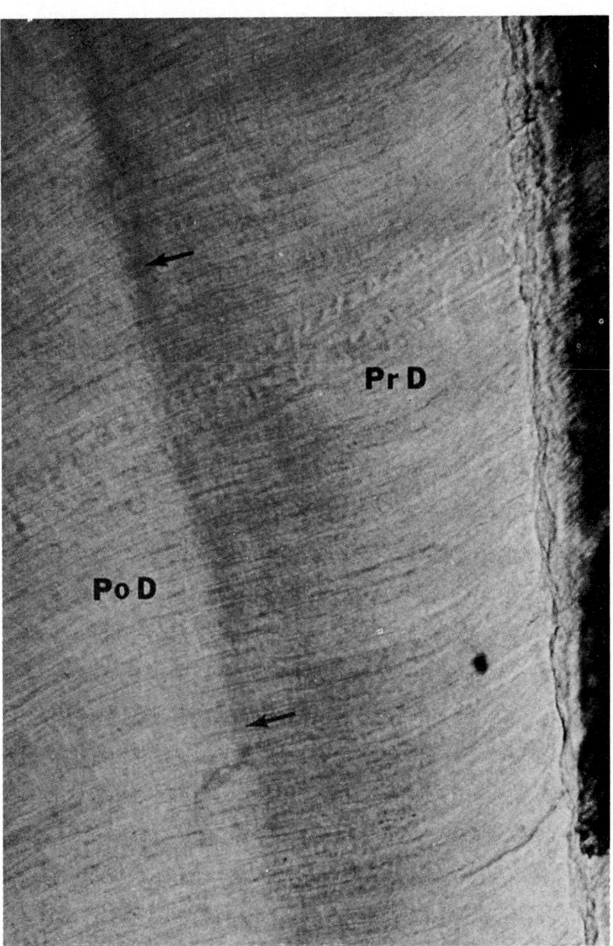

Figure 8.17

A longitudinal ground section of dentin showing the prenatal (*PrD*) and postnatal (*PoD*) dentine separated by neonatal line (*arrows*). Original magnification, 218.75 ×.

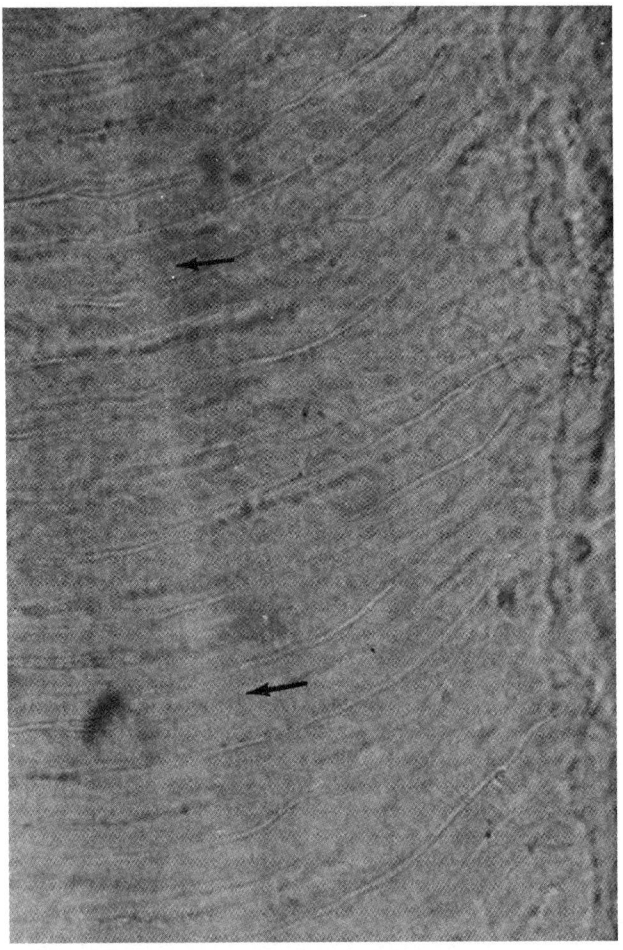

Figure 8.18

A higher magnification of Figure 8.17. Note that the direction of the dentinal tubules is not altered at the neonatal line (*arrows*). Original magnification, 70 ×.

their dentin is forming at birth. The other permanent teeth are not affected.

Interglobular Dentin

During the early stages of mineralization of the dentin, inorganic salts are precipitated in the organic matrix to form clusters of small, rounded globules called calcospherites or calcoglobules. These globules enlarge and coalesce to form a homogenous, incremental layer of calcified dentin. Failure of these globules to unite or fuse may result in the formation of irregular areas of uncalcified matrix known as the *interglobular dentin* (see Figs. 8.1, 8.3, and 8.11). It is also called the interglobular space, but this term is misleading because in actuality it is occupied by unmineralized organic substances. However, when dentin is prepared for histologic study, particularly in the preparation of undecalcified ground sections, these unmineralized areas become dehydrated and may leave spaces. The spaces may then be filled with debris because of grinding, cutting, or other laboratory procedures.

The interglobular dentin is usually found along the incremental lines of calcification. It occurs elsewhere in the dentin but the most common site is at the crown portion. In longitudinal ground section of the dentin under transmitted light, zones of interglobular dentin appear as dark, irregular bands near the outer surface of the dentin paralleling the contour lines of Owen (see Figs. 8.1 and 8.11).

Tomes' Granular Layer

In longitudinal ground section the dentin shows a layer of minute, irregular areas found immediately adjacent and parallel to the dentinocemental junction (Figs. 8.1 and 8.19). It appears granular when viewed under low power magnification and it is for this reason that Sir John Tomes called this the granular layer of dentin. The true nature of these layers is still not clear, although some believe that they are small groups of interglobular spaces caused by "disturbed mineralization of the dentin." They are not coincident with the incremental lines of von Ebner, however. With ordinary laboratory stain, the Tomes' granular layer is not demonstrable in decalcified section.

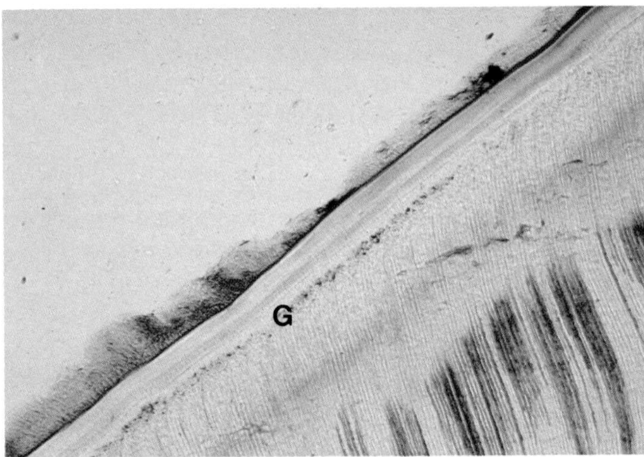

Figure 8.19

Longitudinal section through dentin showing granular layer of Tomes (G) just below the cemento-dentinal junction.

Predentinal Layer

In the early stages of dentinogenesis, before mineralization, an organic material is laid down. It consists mainly of collagenous fibers which are randomly oriented within a gelatinous, amorphous ground substance. This layer is known as the *predentinal layer* (Fig. 8.6). When mineralization commences, the interface between dentin and predentin is clearly demonstrated by regular hematoxylin and eosin stain. Although the rate of deposition of predentin diminishes during the later period of dentinogenesis it is still found in the mature human tooth.

Dentinal Junctions

At the earliest phase of tooth development, there appears to be a membrane between the ameloblastic and odontoblastic layers. Soon after mineralization commences, this membrane "disappears" and in its place can be seen the "interdigitation" of the enamel and dentinal matrices (Fig. 8.20). Under the electron microscope, the crystallites of enamel and dentin appear to be juxtaposed without the presence of a separating structure between them. The interface between enamel and dentin is called the *dentinoenamel junction* (see Fig. 8.5).

The junction between the calcified and uncalcified dentin is known as the *dentin-predentin junction* (Fig. 8.6). Electron microscope studies reveal no separating membrane in this junction.

Another dentinal junction is the one that separates the predentinal layer from the pulp tissue. This is called the *predentin-pulp junction* (Fig. 8.6). The junction is found to be composed of densely arranged collagenous fibers.

Between the calcified cementum and the dentin

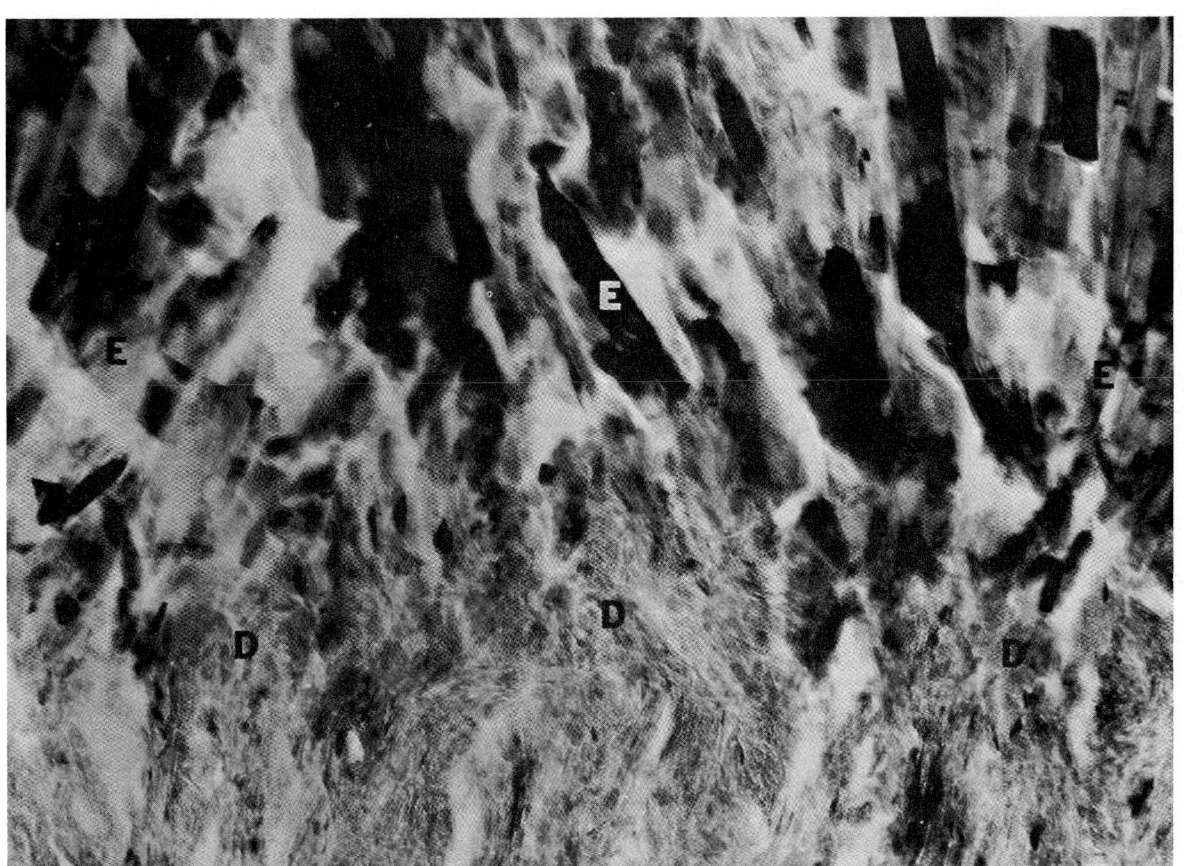

Figure 8.20

Juxtaposition of enamel (*E*) and dentinal (*D*) crystallites without evidence of separating membrane between them. Original magnification, 46,900 ×. (Reproduced from Johansen E. Ulstrastructure of dentine. In: Miles AEW, ed. Structural and Chemical Organization of Teeth. New York: Academic Press, 1967; by permission.)

of the root, a rather smooth boundary line is seen when this area is viewed under the light microscope. This line is known as the dentinocemental junction (Fig. 8.21). When examined under an electron microscope, this junction does not seem to demonstrate a distinct border or membrane, but instead the collagenous fibers of cementum and dentin appear to be in juxtaposition.

Physiological and Pathological Changes

Dentin formation is a continual process throughout the life of the tooth. In addition to *primary dentin,* other forms of dentin may be produced either normally or in response to a variety of stimuli, both physiologic and pathologic. The dentinal forms may be classified as (1) *secondary dentin,* (2) *dead tracts,* and (3) *sclerotic dentin.*

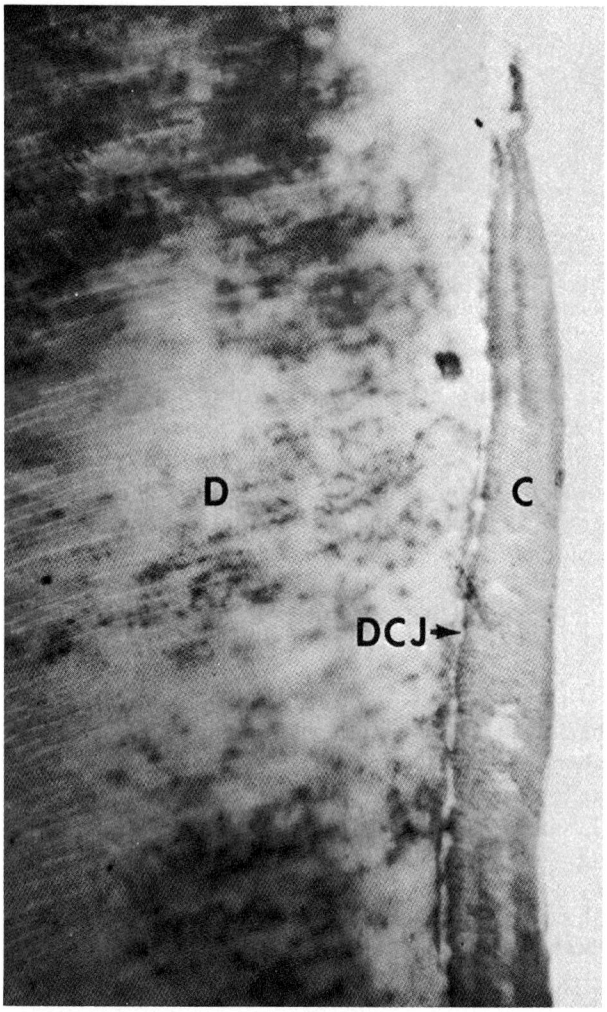

Figure 8.21

A longitudinal decalcified section of the dentin (*D*) and cementum (C). The interface between these two structures is called the dentinocemental junction (*DCJ*). Original magnification, 218.75 ×. (Reproduced from Johansen E. In Miles AEW, ed. Structural and Chemical Organization of Teeth, 1967, by permission of Academic Press.)

Secondary Dentin

This may be divided into two categories: (1) physiologic and (2) adventitious or reparative secondary dentin.

Physiologic secondary dentin is easily seen histologically as a regular and somewhat uniform layer of dentin around the pulp cavity. When examined under the light microscope, the dentinal tubules appear to take a different directional pattern, distinguishing them from the primary dentin (Fig. 8.22). The tubules are relatively the same in number and appear to be in continuity with the primary dentin. According to several investigators, this type of dentin has a slower rate of growth, which slowly decreases the size of the pulp cavity. This dentin is also distinguished from other forms of dentin since it is not found in conjunction with crown erosion, dental caries, or mechanical trauma.

Dentin which is formed in response to irritation is referred to as *adventitious* or *reparative secondary dentin.* It appears as a localized deposit on the wall of the pulp cavity, usually as a consequence of attrition, erosion, dental caries, and certain irritants (Figs. 8.23 and 8.24). Histologically the dentinal tubules of the reparative secondary dentin are sparsely distributed and are somewhat randomly oriented as compared with the regularly distributed dentinal tubules of primary dentin.

The reparative secondary dentin is also chemically different. The mucopolysaccharide content is far less than in primary dentin.

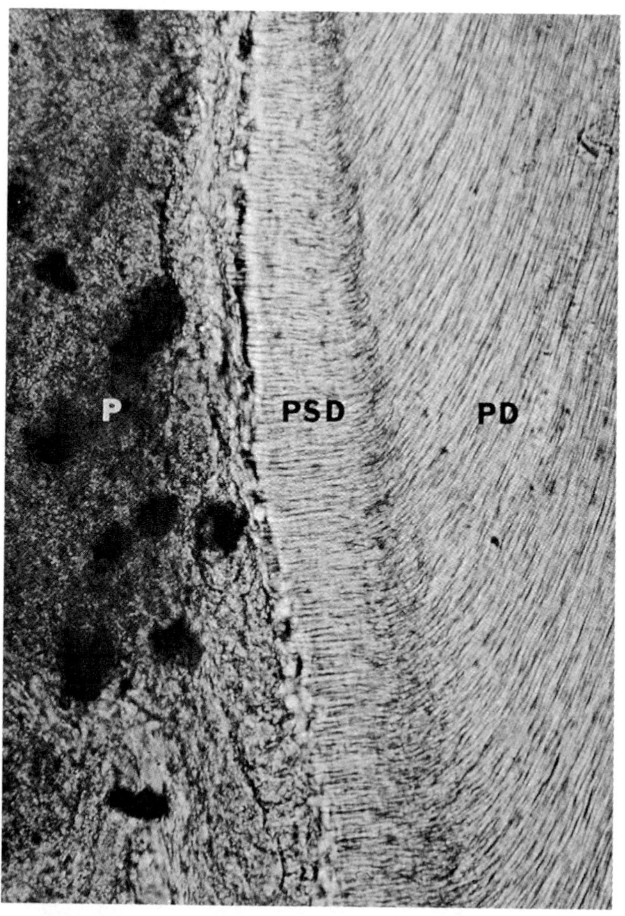

Figure 8.22

A longitudinal ground section with pulp tissue (*P*) showing the physiologic secondary dentin (*PSD*). Note that the direction of the dentinal tubules changes course as they approach the junction between the primary dentin (*PD*) and the physiologic secondary dentin. Original magnification, 187.50 ×.

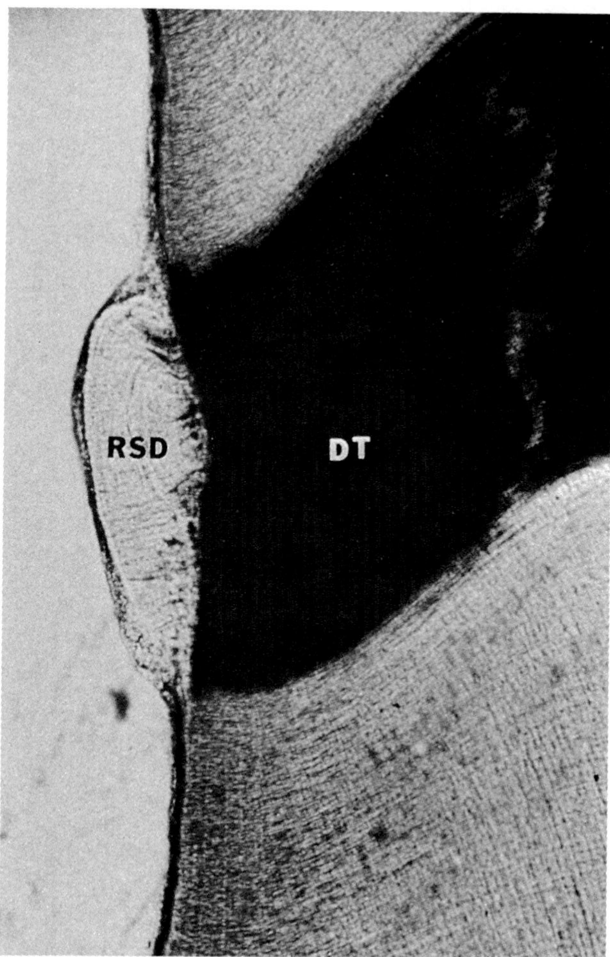

Figure 8.23

A longitudinal ground section showing reparative secondary dentin (*RSD*) on the pupal wall accompanied by exposed dentin and subsequent formation of dead tracts (*DT*). Original magnification, 25.1 ×.

Dead Tracts

A ground section of dentin, when viewed under transmitted light, may reveal dark zones that seem to follow the course of the dentinal tubules (Fig. 8.24). In some areas, they are cut short between the peripheral ends of the dentin. These areas are referred to as *dead tracts.* They are so-called because these tracts are believed to consist of groups of dead, coagulated cytoplasmic processes, or fatty, degenerated content of the dentinal tubules. When dentin is prepared for histologic examination, the mounting medium is unable to penetrate through the dead tracts, so that they are seen as opaque or dark areas under transmitted light. Although they are generally known to be associated with acute aggravation of the protoplasmic processes of the odontoblasts, dead tracts are also found in unerupted and in intact mature teeth. It is suggested, therefore, that dead tracts may also be caused by aging processes of the dentinal tissue.

Sclerotic Dentin (Translucent Dentin)

Like dead tracts, sclerotic dentin is a result of change in structural composition in the early formed primary dentin itself. It is seen in ground section as white or translucent areas when viewed under transmitted light (Fig. 8.25). Sclerotic dentin can occur anywhere in the dentinal structure, and can occur in more than one place. A closer histologic observation shows that these are areas of obliterated dentinal tubules in

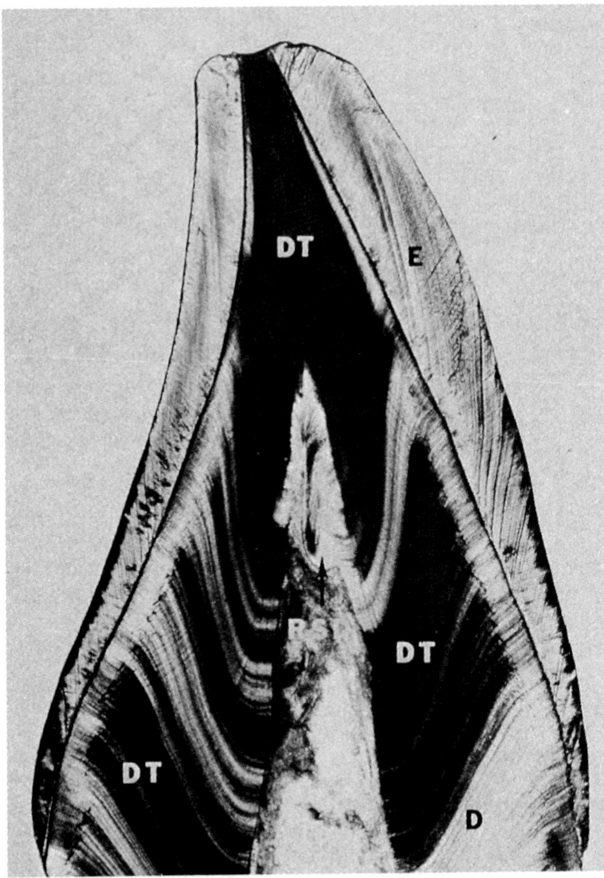

Figure 8.24
Dead tracts (*DT*) at the area of exposed dentin as well as in areas of unexposed portion of undecalcified section of dentin (*D*) and enamel (*E*). Note the reparative secondary dentin (*RSD*) at the area where the dentin has been exposed. Original magnification, 12 ×.

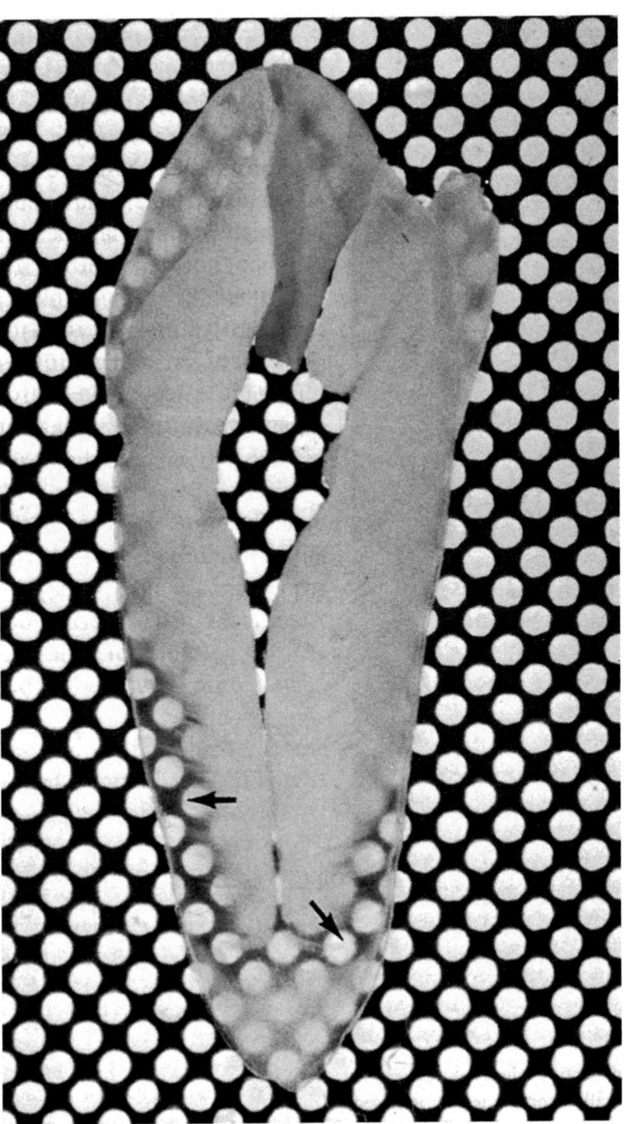

Figure 8.25
A ground section of a premolar tooth showing sclerotic dentin (*arrows*) at the root portion. Note the translucent effect of the sclerotic dentin as demonstrated by the grid underneath.

which the tubular content is now replaced by calcified material. Sclerotic dentin is more mineralized than normal dentinal tissue, and this has been confirmed by radiographic studies. According to several investigators, sclerosis of the dentinal tubules is considered an aging process, since it is usually observed in older teeth. On the other hand, it may result from external stimuli such as erosion or carious lesions.

Bonding Resins to Dentin

Although bonding restorative resins to enamel is a widely adopted practice, bonding these same resins to dentin remains a challenge. Dentin is anatomically and physiologically related to the pulp, and the biological integrity of this relationship must not be compromised. Several biocompatible approaches have been pursued with a view to establishing a chemical bridge between the dentin substrate and the resin. Binding sites such as the tissue calcium and/or the collagen matrix have been targeted. Early generation

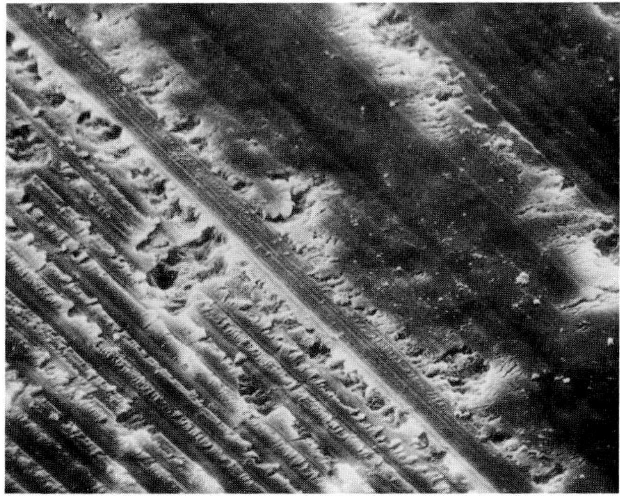

Figure 8.26
Scanning electron micrograph of a typical dentinal smear layer.

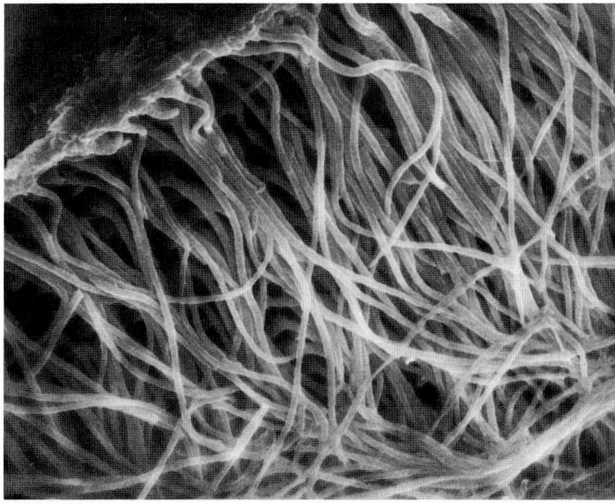

Figure 8.27
Demineralized preparation showing resin "strings" resulting from resin penetration into the dentinal tubules.

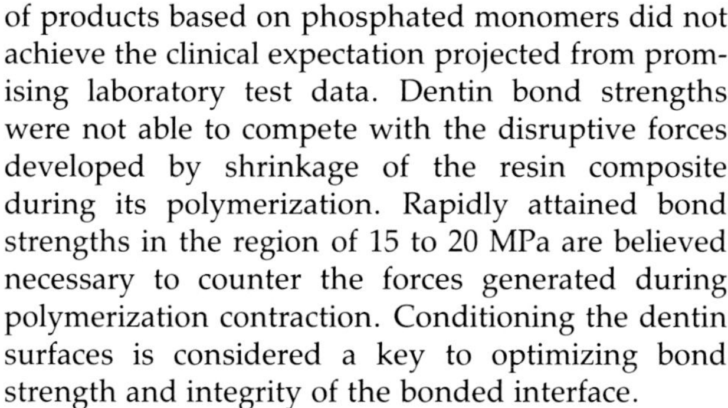

of products based on phosphated monomers did not achieve the clinical expectation projected from promising laboratory test data. Dentin bond strengths were not able to compete with the disruptive forces developed by shrinkage of the resin composite during its polymerization. Rapidly attained bond strengths in the region of 15 to 20 MPa are believed necessary to counter the forces generated during polymerization contraction. Conditioning the dentin surfaces is considered a key to optimizing bond strength and integrity of the bonded interface.

When dentin is cut and abraded, an altered surface morphology is created. This is known as the smear layer (Fig. 8.26). This tenacious layer consists of two zones in which particles of inorganic apatite are distributed. The outer zone is primarily degraded collagen and particles, while the inner zone shows disordered crystallite structure. The tubules are frequently occluded. The removal of the smear layer, which some believe to impart a protective function, is a source of much debate. To many the smear layer is a surface contaminant that should be modified or removed to facilitate resin interaction with unaltered dentin substrate. The latest generation of dentin bonding agents removes and/or modifies the smear layer. This facilitates permeation of resin into the dentinal tubules and the intertubular dentin (Fig. 8.27). Glutaraldehyde is added to some bonding agents to cross-link with collagen in the dentin. Hydroxyethyl methacrylate and phosphated monomers are still used for interaction with the calcium. Chemical bonding is significantly augmented by the micromechanical retention achieved through tissue permeation of the resin and the formation of what has been described as a hybrid layer. The phenomenon is similar to that achieved with enamel. The results from recent clinical trials with new formulations suggest a significant improvement over the early generation of products. Although dentin conditioning, a significant step with recent formulations, may result in an increase in dentinal fluid flow, its influence in dentin bonding requires further investigation.

Glass ionomer cements have been advocated as an alternative means of bonding restorative resins to dentin. The physical properties of these cements favor them as dentin substitutes, while resin composites complete the "sandwich" by replacing lost enamel.

Suggested Reading

Amprino R, Cammani F. Historadiographic and autoradiographic researches on hard dental tissues. Acta Anat 1956; 28:217–258.

Anderson DJ, Ronning GA. Dye diffusion in human dentine. Arch Oral Biol 1962; 7:505–512.

Arwill T. Some morphological aspects of the dentinal innervation. In: Anderson DJ, ed. Symposium on sensory mechanisms in dentine. New York: Pergamon Press, 1963:3–14.

Arwill T, Myberg N, Söremark R. Penetration of

radioactive isotopes through enamel and dentin. I. Diffusion of Na^{22} in fresh and coagulated dentinal tissues. J Dent Res 1965; 44:1299–1303.

Avery JK, Rapp R. An investigation of the mechanism of neural impulse transmission in human teeth. Oral Surg 1959; 12:190–198.

Awazawa Y. Electron microscope investigation of the dentin with particular regard to the nature of the area surrounding the odontoblast process. J Nihon Univ Sch Dent 1962; 5:31–54.

Battistone GC, Feldman MH, Reba RC. The manganese content of human enamel and dentine. Arch Oral Biol 1967; 12:1115–1122.

Benzer S. The development and morphology of physiological secondary dentine. J Dent Res 1948; 27:640–648.

Bergman G, Engfeldt B. Studies on mineralized dental tissue. VI. The distribution of mineral salts in the dentine with special reference to the dentinal tubules. Acta Odont Scand 1955; 13:1–7.

Bernick S. Difference in nerve distribution between erupted and non-erupted teeth. J Dent Res 1964; 43:406–411.

Bevelander G. The development and structure of the fiber system of dentin. Anat Rec 1941; 81:79–99.

Bevelander G, Benzer S. Morphology and incidence of secondary dentine in human teeth. J Am Dent Assoc 1943; 30:1075–1082.

Bevelander G, Nakahara H. The formation and mineralization of dentine (rat). Anat Rec 1966; 156(3):303–324.

Bhaskar SN. Orban's Oral Histology and Embryology. 10th ed. St. Louis: CV Mosby, 1985.

Blake GC. The peritubular translucent zones in human dentine. Br Dent J 1958; 104:57–67.

Bowen RI, Cobb EN, Rapson JE. Adhesive bonding of various materials of hard tooth tissue. J Dent Res 1982; 61:1070–1076.

Bradford EW. Interpretation of ground sections of dentine. Br Dent J 1951; 90:303–308.

Bradford, EW. Microanatomy and histochemistry of dentine. In: Miles AEW, ed. Structural and chemical organization of teeth. Vol II. New York: Academic Press, 1967:3–34.

Brännström M. Dentinal and pulp response. I. Application of reduced pressure to exposed dentine. Acta Odont Scand 1960; 18:1–15.

Brännström M. Dentinal and pulp response. II. Application of an air stream to exposed dentine—short observation period. Acta Odont Scand 1960; 18:17–28.

Brännström M. Dentinal and pulp response. III. Application of an air stream to exposed dentine—long observation period. Acta Odont Scand 1960; 18:235–252.

Brännström M. Dentinal and pulp response. VI. Some experiments with heat and pressure illustrating movement of odontoblasts into the dentinal tubules. Oral Surg 1962; 15:203–212.

Brännström M. Sensitivity of dentine. Oral Surg 1966; 21:517–526.

Brudevold F, Steadman L, Smith F. Inorganic and organic components of tooth structure. Ann NY Acad Sci 1960; 85:110–132.

Buonocore MG, Quigley J. Bonding of synthetic resin material to human dentin. J Am Dent Assoc 1958; 57:807–811.

Burnstone MS. The ground substance of abnormal dentin, secondary dentin and pulp calcification. J Dent Res 1953; 32:269–279.

Churchill HR. The sheath of Neumann (experimental proof of double staining in circumtubular areas of dentin). J Dent Res 1934; 14:243–250.

Davidson CL, de Gee AJ, Feilzer A. The competition between the composite-dentin bond strength and the polymerization contraction stress. J Dent Res 1984; 63:1396–1403.

Dirksen TR. The chemical composition of bone and tooth. Adv Fluorine Res 1965; 3:5–11.

Dirksen TR, Ikels KG. Quantitative determination of some constituent lipids in human dentin. J Dent Res 1964; 43:246–251.

Eastoe JE. Chemical organization of the organic matrix of dentine. In: Miles AEW, ed. Structural and chemical organization of teeth. Vol. II. New York: Academic Press, 1967:279–315.

Eick JD, Bowen RI, Erickson R, Cobb EN. TEM of the smear layer and the dentin adhesive interface. J Dent Res 1987; 66:268.

Eick JD, Wilko RA, Anderson CH, Sorensen SE. Scanning electron microscopy of cut tooth surfaces and identification of debris by use of the electron microprobe. J Dent Res 1970; 49:1359–1368.

Fearnhead RW. Histological evidence for the innervation of human dentine. J Anat 1957; 91:267–277.

Fearnhead RW. The neurohistology of human dentine. Proc R Soc Med 1961; 54:877–884.

Fearnhead RW. The histological demonstration of nerve fibers in human dentine. In: Anderson DJ, ed. Symposium on Sensory Mechanisms in Dentine. New York: Macmillan, 1963:15–26.

Fearnhead RW. Innervation of dental tissues. In: Miles AEW, ed. Structural and chemical organization of teeth. Vol II. New York: Academic Press, 1967:247–281.

Frank RM. Electron microscopy of undercalcified sections of human adult dentine. Arch Oral Biol 1959; 1:29–32.

Frank RM. Proceedings of the Third European Symposium on Calcified Tissue (Calcified Tissue, 1965). New York: Springer-Verlag, 1966.

Frank RM. Etude au microscope elèctronique de l'odontoblaste et du canalicule dentinaire humain. Arch Oral Biol 1966; 11(1):179–199.

Fusayama T, Okuse K, Hosoda H. Relationship between hardness, discoloration, and microbial invasion in carious dentin. J Dent Res 1966; 45:1003–1046.

Glimcher MJ. In: Calcification in biological systems. Publication No. 64. Washington, DC: American Association for the Advancement of Science, 1960:421–487.

Gwinnett AJ. The morphologic relationship between

resins and etched dentin. J Dent Res 1977; 56:1155–1160.

Gwinnett AJ. Aluminum oxalate for dentin bonding. An SEM study. Am J Dent 1988; 1:5–8.

Hampson EL, Atkinson AM. The relation between drugs used in root canal therapy and the permeability of dentine. Br Dent J 1964; 116:546–550.

Harting P. On the artificial production of some of the principal organic calcareous formations. Q J Micr Sci 1872; 20:118–123.

Harltes RF, Leaver AG. Citrate in mineralized tissue. I. Citrate in human dentine. Arch Oral Biol 1960; 1:297–303.

Herold RC, Kaye H. Mitochondria in odontoblastic processes. Nature (London), 1966; 210:108–109.

Hess WC, Lee CY. The isolation of chondroitin sulfuric acid from dentin. J Dent Res 1952; 31:793–797.

Irving JT. The sudanophil material at sites of calcification. Arch Oral Biol 1963; 8:735–745.

Jenkins GN. The physiology of the mouth. Oxford: Blackwell Scientific Publication, 1960.

Johansen E. Electron microscopic observation on sound human dentin. Arch Oral Biol 1962; 7:185–193.

Johansen E. Microstructure of enamel and dentin. J Dent Res 1964; 43:1007–1020.

Johansen E. Ultrastructure of dentine. In: Miles AEW, ed. Structural and Chemical Organization of Teeth. Vol II. New York: Academic Press, 1967:35–72.

Kaye H, Herold RC. Structure of human dentine. I. Phase contrast polarization, interference and bright field microscopic observations on the lateral branch system. Arch Oral Biol 1966; 11:355–368.

Kramer IRH. The distribution of collagen fibrils in the dentine matrix. Br Dent J 1951; 91:1–7.

Kramer IRH. Pulp changes of nonbacterial origin. Int Dent J 1959; 9:435–450.

Lehman ML. Tensile strength of human dentin. J Dent Res 1966; 46:197–201.

Marsland EA, Shovelton DS. The effect of cavity preparation on the human dental pulp. Br Dent J 1957; 102:213–222.

McLean JW, Prosser HJ, Wilson AD. The use of glass ionomer cements in bonding composte resins to dentin. Br Dent J 1985; 158:410–414.

Miller J. Micro-radiographic appearance of dentine. Br Dent J 1954; 97:7–9.

Munksgaard EC, Asmussen E. Bond strength between dentin and restorative resins mediated by mixtures of HEMA and gluteraldehyde. J Dent Res 1984; 63:1087–1089.

Nakabayashi N, Kajima K, Massuhara E. The promotion of adhesion by infiltration of monomers into tooth substrates. J Biomed Mater Res 1982; 16:265–273.

Owen R. Odontography text. London: H. Balliere, 1840/1845:460, 464.

Phillips RW. Skinner's Science of Dental Materials. 8th ed. Philadelphia: WB Saunders, 1982.

Piez KA, Likens RC. Calcification in biological systems. Publication No. 64. Washington, DC: American Association for the Advancement of Science. 1960:411–420.

Provenza DV, Seibel W. Oral histology: inheritance and development. 2nd ed. Philadelphia: Lea & Febiger, 1989.

Quigley MB, Starrs, JW, Zwarych PD. Demonstration of calcospherites in mature human dentin. J Dent Res 1965; 44:794–800.

Rapp R, Avery JK, Rector RA. A study of the distribution of nerves in the human tooth. J Can Dent Assoc 1957; 23:447–453.

Richardson A. Dead tracts in human teeth. Relation between incidence of tracts and age eruption state and degree of attrition. Br Dent J 1966; 121:560–563.

Rogers HJ. Concentration and distribution of polysaccharides in human cortical bone and the dentine of teeth. Nature (London) 1949;164:625–626.

Rowles SL. Chemistry of the mineral phase of dentine. In: Miles AEW, ed. Structural and Chemical Organization of Teeth. Vol. II. New York: Academic Press, 1967:201–246.

Rushton MA. Observation on fish's "dead tracts" in dentin. Br Dent J 1940; 68:11–13.

Schour I. The neonatal lines of the enamel and dentin in the human deciduous and first permanent molar. J Am Dent Assoc 1936; 23:1946–1955.

Schour I, ed. Noye's oral histology and embryology. 7th ed. Ann Arbor, MI: Books on Demand.

Schour I, Poncher HG. The rate of apposition of enamel and dentin as measured by the effects of acute fluorosis. Am J Dis Child 1937; 54:757–776.

Scott DB. The electron microscopy of enamel and dentin. Ann NY Acad Sci 1955; 60:575–584.

Scott DB, Wyckoff RWG. Electron microscopy of human dentine. J Dent Res 1950; 29:556–560.

Shroff FR, Williamson KI, Bertaud WS. Electron microscopic studies of dentin. Oral Surg 1954; 7:662–670.

Shroff FR, Williamson KI, Bertaud WS, Hall DM. Further electron microscope studies of dentin (the nature of the odontoblast process). Oral Surg 1956; 9:432–443.

Söremark R, Lundberg M. Analysis of concentrations of Cr, Ag, Fe, Co, Pt, and Rb in normal human dentine. Odont Rev Lund 1964; 15:285–289.

Söremark R, Samsahl K. Gamma-ray spectrometric analysis of elements in normal human dentin. J Dent Res 1962; 41:603–606.

Stack M. The chemical nature of the organic matrix of bone dentine and enamel. Ann NY Acad Sci 1955; 60:585–595.

Stanford JW, Poffenbarger GC, Kumpula JW, Sweeney WT. Determination of some compressive properties of human enamel and dentin. J Am Dent Assoc 1958; 57:487–495.

Stevenson TS. Fluid movement in human dentine. Arch Oral Biol 1965; 10:934–944.

Suzuki M, Gwinnett AJ, Jordan RE. Relationship between composite resin and the dentin treated with dentin bonding agent. J Dent Res 1986; 65:764.

Symons NBB. A histochemical study of the intertubular and peritubular matrices in normal human dentine. Arch Oral Biol 1961; 5:241–249.

Symons NBB. The microanatomy and histochemistry of

dentinogenesis. In: Miles AEW, ed. Structural and chemical organization of teeth. Vol I. New York: Academic Press, 1967:285–318.

Takuma S. Electron microscopy of the structure around the dentinal tubule. J Dent Res 1960; 39:973–981.

Takuma S. Ultrastructure of dentinogenesis, In: Miles AEW, ed. Structural and chemical organization of teeth. Vol I. New York: Academic Press, 1967:325–370.

Takuma S, Eda S. Structure and development of the peritubular matrix in dentin. J Dent Res 1966;45:683–692.

Takuma S, Kurahashi Y, Yoshioka N, Yamaguchi A. Some consideration of the microstructure of dental tissue, revealed by the electron microscope. Oral Surg 1956; 9:328–343.

Tao L, Pashley DJ. Effect of pulpal pressure on dentin bond strength. J Dent Res 1988; 67:285.

White AA, Hess WC. Phosphatase, peroxidase and oxidase activity of dentin and bone. J Dent Res 1956; 35:276–285.

Wislocki GB, Singer M, Waldo CM. Some histochemical reactions of mucopolysaccharides, glycogen, lipids, and other substances in teeth. Anat Rec 1948; 101:487–513.

Wislocki GB, Sognnaes RF. Histochemical reactions of normal teeth. Am J Anat 1950; 87:239–275.

Wyckoff RWG, Croissant O. Microradiography of dentine using characteristic x-rays. Biochem Biophys Acta 1963; 66:137–143.

Yoon SH, Brudevold F, Gardner DE, Smith FA. Distribution of fluorine in the teeth and fluorine level in water. J Dent Res 1960; 39:845–856.

9

The Dental Pulp

The dental pulp is the embryologic organ for tooth development. Once the tooth has formed, the pulp becomes a physiologic organ encased in hard tooth structure. The dental pulp occupies the central portion (pulp cavity) of the tooth and is surrounded by dentin (Fig. 9.1). It is in this cavity that virtually all of the soft tissues of the tooth are housed. Although the cells within the cavity can be regarded as mesenchymal or connective tissue elements serving to give bulk to the inner regions of the tooth, they in fact perform a number of other vital functions. The organization of the pulpal cells into layers reflects, to some extent, this functional diversity.

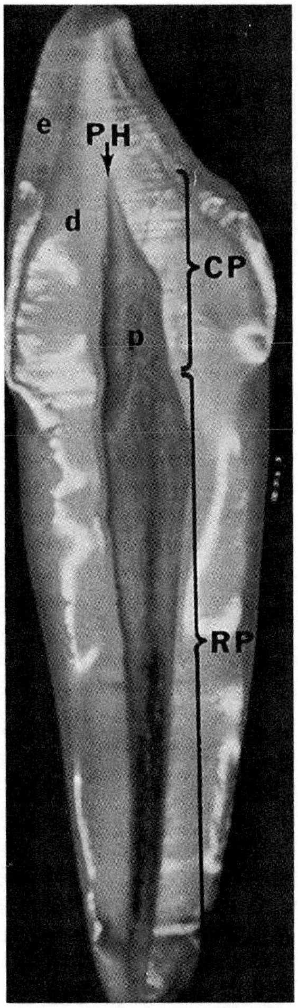

During the developmental period of the tooth, the pulp mesenchyme provides cells that are capable of producing dentin. The production of dentin is not limited to the developmental period but continues for the life of the tooth. In the adult condition, however, this dentinogenic activity proceeds gradually to produce what is called physiologic secondary dentin. There is, in addition, a dentinogenic process, which is intermittent and occurs only when the exterior surface of the primary dentin is traumatized, unduly irritated, or in any way injured. This process produces dentin as a reparative response to the irritation or destruction of primary dentin (Fig. 9.2). The laying down of this dentin (reparative dentin) is limited to the region under assault, thus demonstrating a conservative biologic economy.

Because of the presence of dentinal tubules, the pulp responds to dentinal irritation. In the event of bacterial invasion, this defense mechanism of the pulp is complemented by defense cells such as macrophages, lymphocytes, and fibrocytes, which are thereby induced into activity. Such a defense system

Figure 9.1

Ground section of a central incisor illustrating the coronal (*CP*) and radicular (*RP*) portions of the pulp. This section also shows the pulp horn (*PH*). Pulp (*p*); enamel (*e*); dentin (*d*).

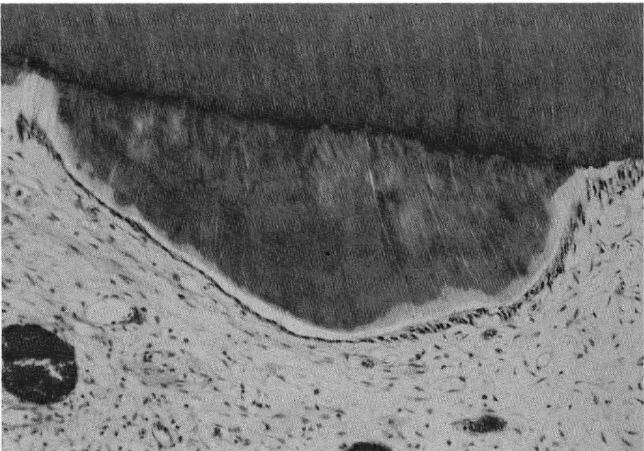

Figure 9.2

Reparative dentin. Note the line between the dentin and the reparative dentin called the calciotraumatic line. The dentin has an amorphous pattern with fewer irregular odontoblastic tubules.

is maintained in readiness, so to speak, by a very rich vascular supply that serves the entire pulpal region.

When the stimulus is weak, the response by the pulpal system is weak and the interaction goes unnoticed. When, on the other hand, the stimulus is great, the reaction is marked and the individual is well aware of the fact, i.e., the tooth aches! This is because the pulp houses an extensive nerve supply with only one function—to receive and transmit pain stimuli. In a sense it can be considered as part of the defense system, since it serves to bring to consciousness the threatened condition of the tooth. The root canal is essentially a blind sac that communicates directly with the supporting alveolar bone at the root apex. Once the pulp tissue degenerates, it fuels an apical inflammatory response. Unless the source is removed by either extraction or endodontic therapy, the cells in the bone and apical periodontal ligament erect a barricade against the insult; the result is apical periodontitis.

To further understand how these developmental, protective, sensory, and nutritive functions are carried out, it is necessary to consider in detail the morphologic and physiologic processes of the pulp.

General Description

The inner aspect of the dentin forms the boundaries of the pulp cavity. Within the pulp cavity lies the mass of the cellular components of the tooth, most of which consist of a variety of connective tissue elements. Anatomically the pulp is divided into two areas. The part of the pulp that lies in the crown portion of the tooth is called the *coronal pulp;* this includes the pulpal horns which project toward the cusp tips and incisal edges. The other portion of the pulp is more apically located and is referred to as the *radicular* (or root) *pulp* areas. The surface contours of the coronal or radicular regions of the pulp follow the contours of the overlying layers of dentin. Thus, the interior surface of the pulp cavity more or less follows the contours of the exterior surface of the tooth (Fig. 9.3).

The radicular pulp is continuous with tissues of the periapical area via an apical foramen. This foramen provides a patent channel through which blood and lymph vessels, nerves, and connective tissue elements gain access to the interior regions of the tooth. The apical foramen is often situated somewhat eccentrically rather than at the root apex, which is more centrally located (Figs. 9.3 and 9.4). The eccentric position is more clearly seen in cross-sections through the apical zone. The apical foramen is not the only means by which the pulp communicates with the periradicular connective tissues. Perforations that permit access to the periodontal tissue lying outside the chamber may be found along the radicular or root canal. These accessory or lateral canals may communicate with the periodontal ligament at any level of the root, although they are most frequently found in the apical third of the root. This fact is of great clinical significance. The lateral canals are filled with tissue elements similar to those found in the central or main root canal (Fig. 9.5).

Presumably lateral canals are created as a result of a defect in the formation of Hertwig's epithelial root sheath. These result from the failure of odontoblasts to differentiate and produce dentin. As a re-

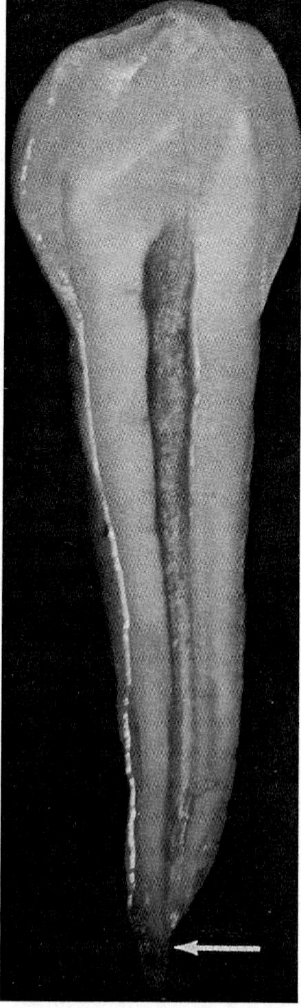

Figure 9.3

Ground section of a tooth with apical foramen (*arrow*) eccentrically positioned.

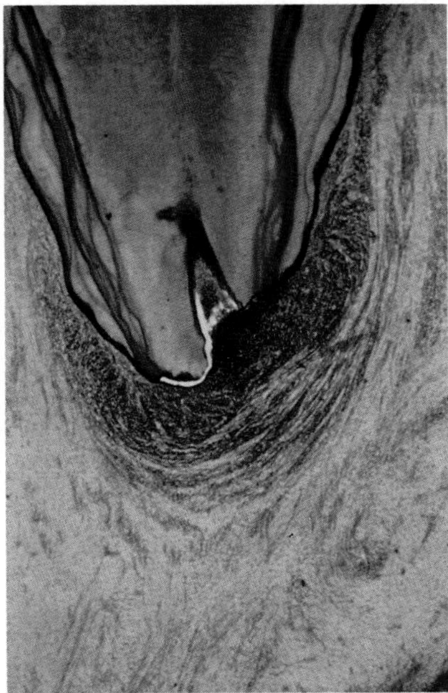

Figure 9.4
Eccentrically located apical foramen.

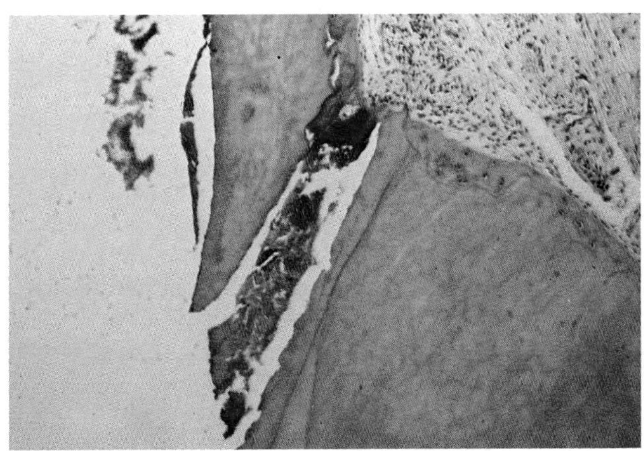

Figure 9.5
High magnification of a lateral canal. Note necrotic remains of pulp tissue. The periodontal ligament has produced a calcified barrier in an attempt to seal off the canal. (Courtesy of Drs. I. B. Bender and Samuel Seltzer, Albert Einstein Medical Center, Philadelphia, PA.)

sult, the tip becomes continuous with the periodontium. Exactly why such loci are exempt from odontoblastic differentiation is not clear at present, although there is the suggestion that local factors inhibit odontoblastic differentiation.

During development of the root, the central canal narrows by elongation and apposition of dentin. In relatively young teeth, in which the apical foramen is not yet fully formed, the apical orifice is rather wide. With increasing age and exposure of the tooth to physiologic functioning, secondary dentin decreases the diameter of the coronal and radicular cavities. In addition, a layer of cementum of varying length may cover the dentin along the apical orifice into the radicular region of the central canal.

The Odontoblastic Layer

The pulp chamber is lined by a layer of cells known as *odontoblasts.* Depending upon their location and degree of differentiation, the shape and size of odontoblasts vary. Those cells in the area lining the pulp horns are rather tall columnar cells, possessing round or ovoid nuclei that are basally located (Fig. 9.6). In areas lateral and cervical to the horns, fewer numbers of odontoblasts provide more space, the cells are somewhat shorter or cuboidal in shape, and they possess more centrally located nuclei. In the apical regions the cells are cuboid to squamoid, with the latter nearer the apical foramen. The nuclei of these cells range from ovoid to round and are highly chromophilic. The tallest of these cells are believed to be the most differentiated, whereas the shortest are least. This is reflected in the amount of dentin adjacent to such cells, indicating the extent of their secretory activity.

Seen through the electron microscope, the mature cytoplasm of the odontoblast possesses an extensive system of tubular structures known as rough endoplasmic reticulum, mitochondria, and ribonucleoprotein particles, which are interspersed throughout the cell. Dense bodies of various sizes are also observed. The Golgi apparatus is responsible for packaging and secreting collagen for the formation of dentin and eventually the predentin layer. The cell is enclosed by a plasma membrane with lateral surfaces showing some degree of interdigitation. Relatively little intercellular space can be seen between adjacent cells.

Immature odontoblasts, which arise from undifferentiated pulpal cells close to either the dentinoenamel junction or the original basement lamina, possess fewer cytoplasmic organelles. These increase in number, however, in conjunction with elongation of the cell. In this instance, the plasma membrane undergoes invaginations, particularly at the cell sur-

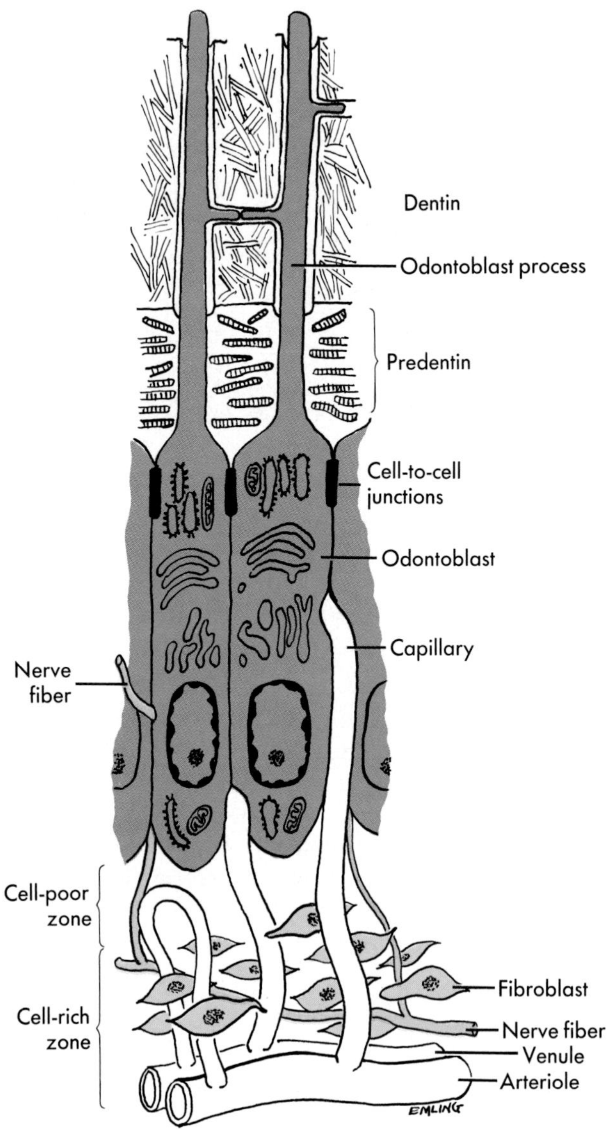

Figure 9.6

Diagrammatic representation of the odontoblast layer and subodontoblastic region of the pulp. (From Trowbridge HO. Pulp structure and function. In: Cohn S, Burns R, eds. Pathways of the Pulp. 5th ed. St Louis: Mosby–Year Book, 1991; by permission.)

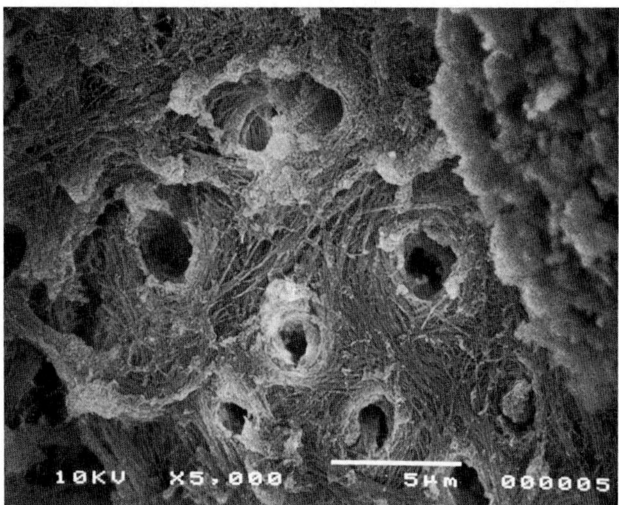

Figure 9.7

High-power scanning electron micrograph of the odontoblastic tubules in dentin that are normally occupied by the odontoblastic process. Note the large number of collagen fibers.

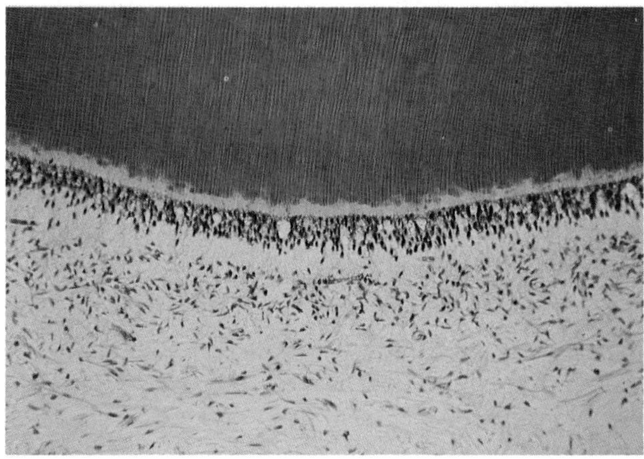

Figure 9.8

Morphologic zones of the mature pulp. From top to bottom, calcified dentin, predentin (pink), Palisaded columnar odontoblasts, "cell-free" zone, "cell-rich" zone, pulp proper. (From Trowbridge HO. Pulp structure and function. In: Cohn S, Burns R, eds. Pathways of the Pulp. 5th ed. St Louis: Mosby–Year Book, 1991; by permission.)

face facing the basal lamina. Perhaps the most notable of all changes that occur during differentiation is the migration of the nucleus from a central zone to the basal area (toward the pulpal region). Despite this translocation, the organelles appear to remain concentrated in the central regions. Concomitant alterations in cell shape involve the slender extension of the odontoblast processes (Tomes') into the distal regions (Fig. 9.7).

Subodontoblastic Layer of the Zone of Weil

Immediately adjacent to the odontoblastic layer is a relatively cell-free space called the *zone of Weil*, or the *subodontoblastic layer* (Fig. 9.8). Collagenous and unmyelinated nerve fibers as well as blood vessels are the main types of fibers found in this zone. Both the nerve fibers and blood vessels appear to branch out and penetrate the odontoblastic layer. Fibers coursing through this area are not readily seen in routine hematoxylin and eosin–stained preparations, but are quite evident when the sections are stained by silver-staining procedures. Narrowing of this zone occurs during periods of high activity such as dentin formation.

The Cell-Rich Zone

Deeper into the pulp chamber, immediately apposed to the cell-free layer, lies a densely populated cell layer of fibroblasts, macrophages, and lymphocytes. This represents nature's first line of defense against any insult to the dentin or pulp. However, this layer is not uniformly populated, since the coronal regions are more densely packed than is the radicular region; thus, the line of demarcation between the zone of Weil and the cell-rich layer is more pronounced in the coronal region. Nevertheless, the number of cells in the coronal regions of the cell-rich zone can and does vary. For instance, the cell-rich area in young teeth is not as highly populated as in older teeth. Disease may also cause variations in the cell population of this area. To varying degrees these cells are subject to endogenous and exogenous stimuli and frequently respond by further differentiation, growth, migration, and changes in shape. By contrast, the vascular and neural elements, which are also present in this zone, maintain their basic topographic and morphologic patterns (Figs. 9.9 and 9.10).

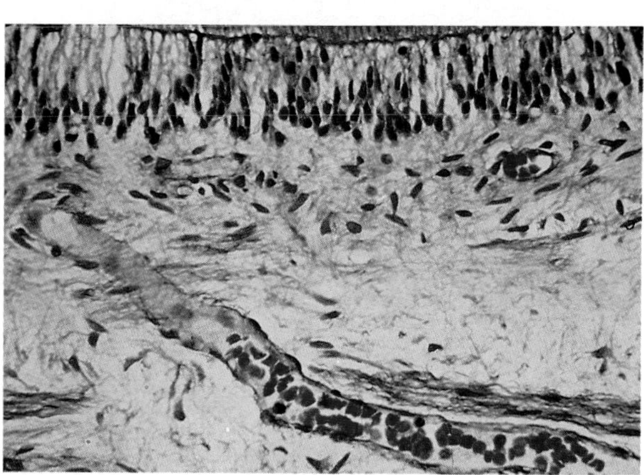

Figure 9.9
Arteriole ending as a capillary in the cell-rich zone.

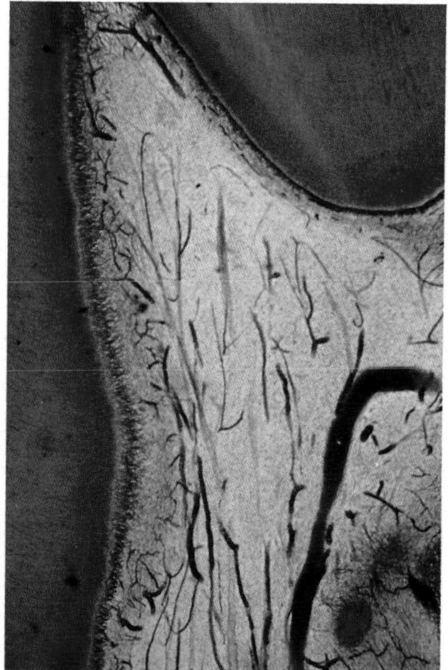

Figure 9.10
Nerve endings branching out beneath the cell-rich zone as the plexus of single nerve axons known as the plexus of Raschkow.

Central Pulp Region

The central pulp is bounded by the cell-rich layer and constitutes the innermost mass of cells. There appears to be no essential difference between the central pulp region and the surrounding cell-rich layer except that the latter is more densely populated.

Blood Vessels and Lymphatic Channels

The dental pulp possesses an extremely rich vascular supply, derived from branches of the dental arteries. The blood supply of the tooth may enter the apical foramen in either a single arteriole vessel or two or more branches (Fig. 9.11). The periodontal artery, which is also a branch of the dental artery, can subdivide and send smaller branches into the lateral root canals or it may enter the apical foramen with the pulpal artery. Shortly after these vessels enter the pulp cavity they establish a rich vascular network called a capillary plexus. This plexus is formed at the peripheral area of the pulp near the base of the odontoblastic layer. However, some of the capillary loops may extend beyond this layer and establish a close communication with the odontoblastic layer (Figs. 9.9 and 9.12). The location of this vascular plexus is important for supplying nutrient substances to the dentinal tissue (Fig. 9.13). From the capillary plexus, the blood is transported to the veins via small channels known as venules, and finally leaves the pulp canal of the tooth through the apical foramen.

Unmyelinated nerve fibers accompany most of the distributing arteries and arterioles. Therefore, it is believed that a vasomotor regulatory mechanism permits variation in the volume of blood that may enter these vessels.

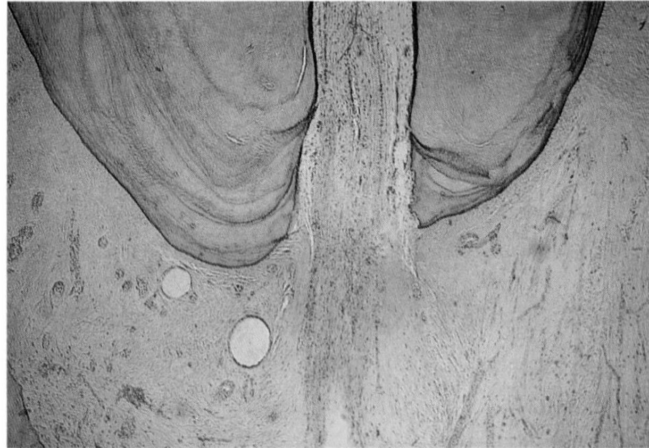

Figure 9.11
Neural, vascular and connective tissue elements entering the apical foramen. Notice the intimacy of tooth, connective tissue, and bone.

There is evidence that lymphatic channels are present in the pulp, although the course and distribution of these channels have not been clearly established.

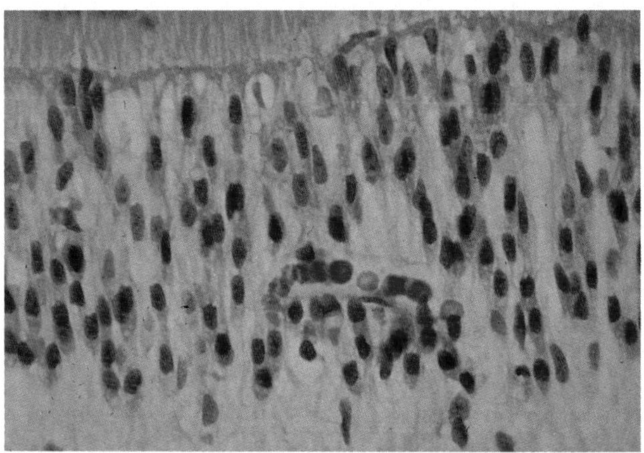

Figure 9.12
A capillary loop passing among the cells of the odontoblastic layer. (Courtesy of Dr. H. O. Trowbridge.)

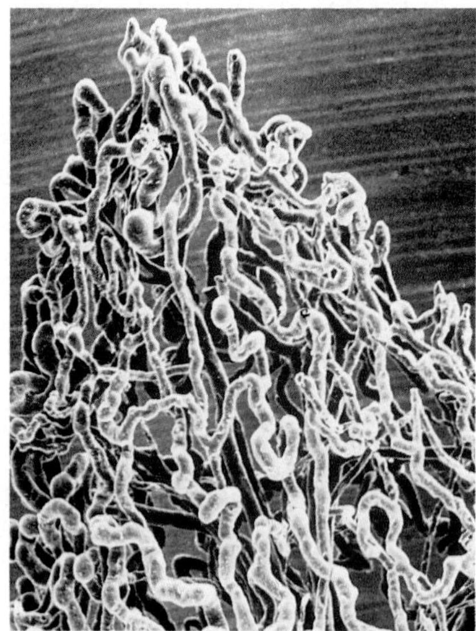

Figure 9.13
Scanning electron micrograph of the terminal capillary network in the pulp horn. (Courtesy of Dr. Yoshiaki Kishi, Kanagawa Dental College, Inaoka, Yokosuka, Japan.)

Innervations

Myelinated and unmyelinated nerve fibers accompany most of the vascular vessels that enter the root canal. The myelinated nerve fibers are believed to be sensory in nature. These nerves may take a straight course toward the coronal portion of the pulp, where they branch, and from a network of nervous tissue. Other myelinated nerve fibers may branch out shortly after they gain entrance to the pulp canal. These arborizations in the coronal and radicular pulp become more abundant with interlacing fibers as they approach the basal cell-free layer of Weil. This is known as the plexus of Raschkow (see Fig. 9.10). From this zone terminal branches are given off, and they pass between and around the odontoblast cells, forming ramifications at the odontoblast layer (Fig. 9.14). There is evidence that the terminal branches may also accompany some of the odontoblast processes toward the predentinal area.

In the pulp the myelinated nerve continues its course until the main trunk starts to divide into smaller branches and the myelin sheath disappears. The outermost sheath (sheath of Schwann) can still be recognized but may disappear at the most terminal branches of the nerve. These A delta and C nerve fibers are considered responsible for the sensitivity of the pulp and dentin and are found at the subodontoblastic layer, the odontoblast layer, and even in the predentinal layer.

The nerve fibers that are unmyelinated when entering the pulp cavity are believed to belong to the sympathetic nervous system, which controls the smooth muscle of the blood vessels. They accompany the blood supply of the pulp, terminating in the smooth muscle of the blood vessels as "knotted twig-like processes."

There is still some question as to whether these nerves extend into the calcified dentinal tissue. This is discussed in detail in Chapter 8.

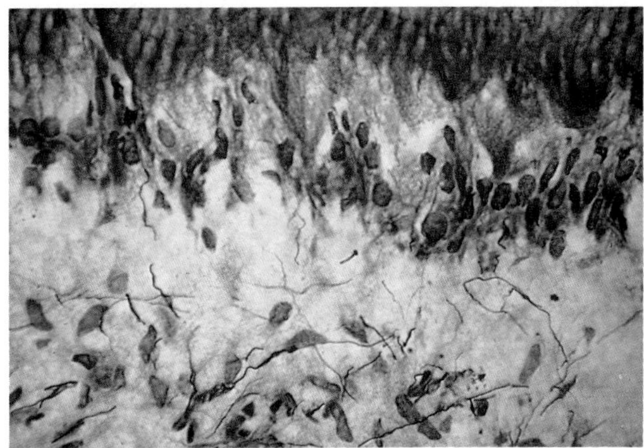

Figure 9.14
Nerve fibers in the subodontoblastic area. Fibers can be traced to the odontoblastic cell layer.

Functions of the Pulp

The pulp tissue performs several functions. It is formative, nutritive, sensory, and defensive.

Formative

A primary function of the pulp is to form dentin (Fig. 9.15). This activity begins at the earliest period of dentinogenesis, when the peripheral mesenchymal cells become differentiated into odontoblast cells. This function of the pulp continues throughout tooth development. Even after tooth maturation, the pulp tissue still forms physiologic secondary dentin. The pulp, being capable of reacting to physical or chemical insults, may also form calcified tissue known as reparative secondary dentin. This may be considered as a protective shield that prevents further destruction of the pulp. A detailed description of the different types of dentin has been presented in Chapter 8.

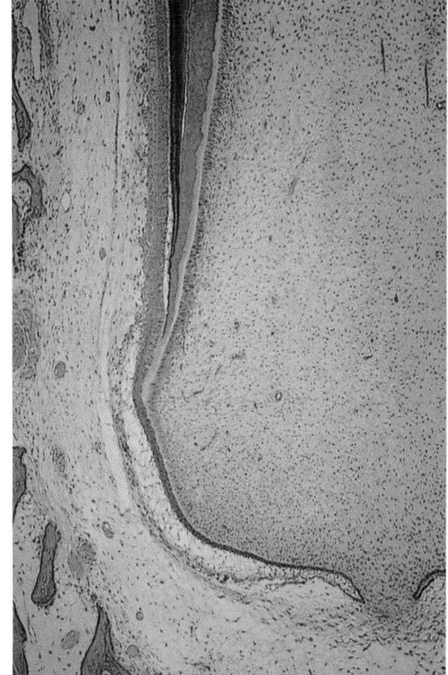

Figure 9.15
Early Hertwig's epithelial root sheath developing the formation of the root.

Nutritive

In the adult tooth the pulp keeps the organic components of the surrounding mineralized tissue supplied with moisture and nutrients. The rich vascular network, especially the peripheral capillary plexus, may afford a source of nutrition to the odontoblast cells and to their cytoplasmic extensions enclosed within the dentin. It has been speculated that these processes may supply various ions and molecules to the organic components of the dentin. The continued nutrition to the odontoblast cells and the pulp tissue maintains the vitality of the teeth.

Response to Injury

The dental pulp responds to injury by manifesting all the classic signs of inflammation: dilation of the blood vessels, followed by transudation of tissue fluids and extravascular migration of leukocytes within the pulp cavity. Because of the rigid, confined structure of the pulp cavity, the presence of increased, extravascular exudates bring about an increase of pressure on nerve and nerve endings, resulting in pain. After mild stimulation of brief duration the pulp tissue usually recovers, leaving little sign of the reactive process. Chronic stimulation, such as slowly progressing caries, causes the pulp tissue to react in a protective manner by laying down calcified material on primary or secondary dentin. This is the reparative dentin (Figs. 9.2 and 9.16). Under continuous severe stimulation, inflammatory processes continue, causing progressive dying of cells and local necrosis leading to the subsequent death of the pulp.

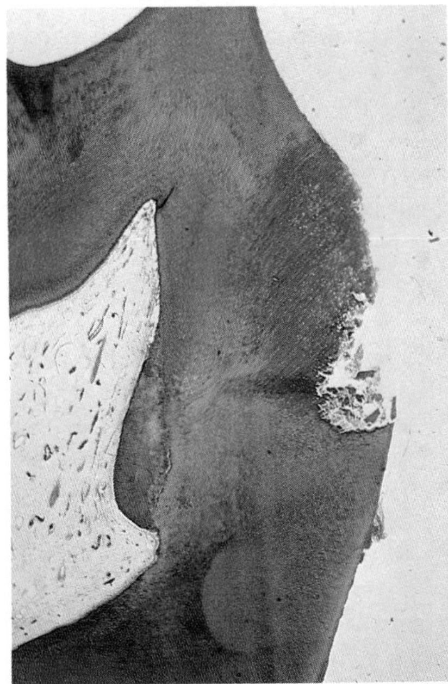

Figure 9.16
Reparative dentin deposited in response to a carious lesion in the dentin. (From Trowbridge HO. J Endodont 1981;7:52; by permission.)

Pulp Calcification

One might imagine that calcification in the pulp represents a pathologic change, but this phenomenon seems to occur often in healthy teeth, both erupted and unerupted. From a statistical standpoint, a great majority of teeth examined show calcification in the pulp.

Calcification in the dental pulp may be classified into two main categories: pulp stones and diffuse calcification. Pulp stones are usually found in the coronal pulp, whereas diffuse calcifications occur in the radicular portion of the pulp.

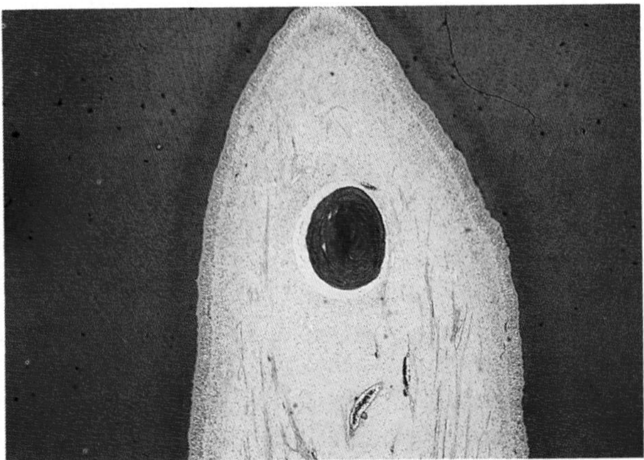

Figure 9.17
Pulp stone with a smooth surface and concentric laminations in the pulp of a newly erupted premolar extracted in the course of orthodontic movement (From Trowbridge HO. Pulp structure and function. In: Cohn S, Burns R, eds. Pathways of the Pulp. St Louis: Mosby–Year Book, 1991; by permission.)

Pulp Stones

Pulp stones occur usually in the coronal portion of the pulp and have a somewhat rounded outline with concentric lamellation (Fig. 9.17). Because they vary in microscopic structure, pulp stones are divided into those that are smooth with concentric laminations and those that have no particular shape.

Pulp stones that are found at the coronal portion of the pulp are atubular and have a concentric lamellar arrangement. According to some authors these pulp stones are the result of a formation of reticular fibers around a nucleus of degenerated cells in the pulp. Calcium salts are subsequently deposited in an attempt to "wall off" these degenerated cells. The pulp stones may increase in size and fuse with one another, or they may become adherent to or incorporated into the dentinal tissues. In some instances they can occupy the entire pulpal chamber and make root canal access very difficult (Fig. 9.18). It is thought that calcifications can occur secondary to a vascular accident that the pulp stones form as an attempt to seal an injured arteriole (Fig. 9.19).

Denticles are pulp stones that have a morphologic and histologic pattern similar to dentin, since they too are composed of a calcified matrix, with dentinal tubules and odontoblast processes. They form around epithelial remnant cells of Hertwig's root sheath. The tubules, however, are very scarce and irregular, so that they more closely resemble reparative secondary dentin than they do primary dentin. A true denticle may be "attached" to the wall of the pulp cavity or it may be "free" within the pulp tissue, usually found near the root apex. It should be clearly understood, however, that although some denticles may be truly free, an alteration in the direction of sectioning may show that a denticle is actually attached rather than free. Only serial sectioning throughout the entire area would show the true nature of the denticle.

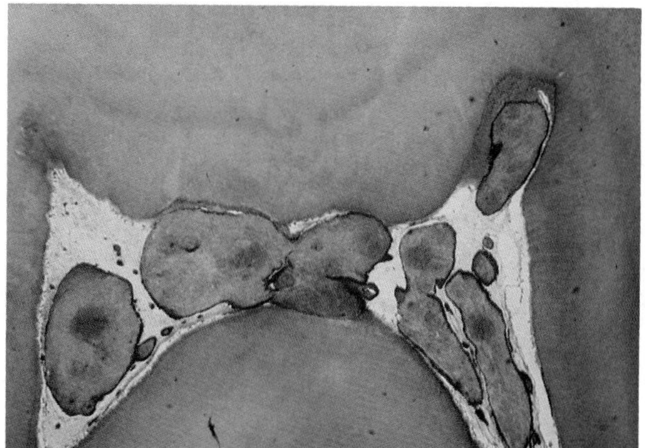

Figure 9.18

Pulp stones occupying much of the root canal chamber. (From Trowbridge HO. Pulp structure and function. In: Cohn S, Burns R, eds. Pathways of the Pulp. 5th ed. St Louis: Mosby–Year Book, 1991; by permission.)

Diffuse Calcification

Diffuse calcification in the pulp occurs in the root portion of the tooth. This calcification increases with age. The morphologic structure resembles that of calcified bodies that are usually found in the site where degenerative processes are taking place. In the dental pulp they appear as multiple, calcified bodies and are

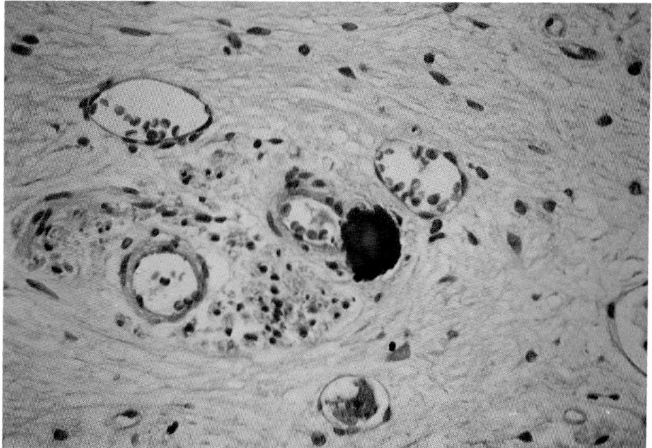

Figure 9.19

Pulp stone associated with the periphery of an arteriole.

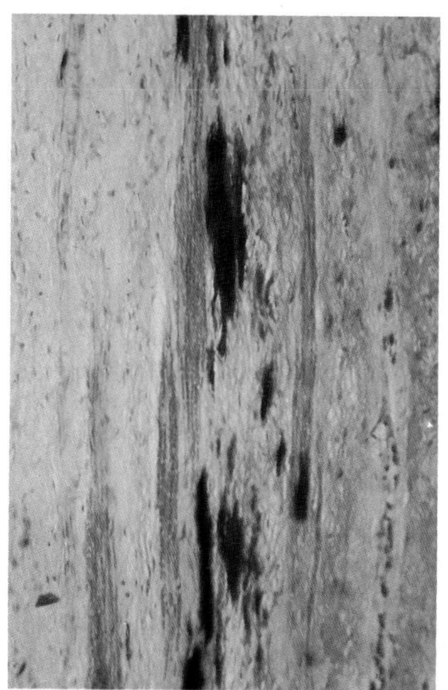

Figure 9.20

Diffuse calcification in a radicular pulp. The calcification appears to be associated with nerve trunks. (From Trowbridge HO. Pulp structure and function. In: Cohn S, Burns R, eds. Pathways of the Pulp. 5th ed. St Louis: Mosby–Year Book, 1991; by permission.)

distributed along the long axis of the pulp, paralleling some of the blood vessels and nerves. Subsequently some of these calcified deposits become enlarged and fuse with the neighboring bodies, forming one large mass. They appear amorphous and do not seem to demonstrate concentric, incremental lines (Fig. 9.20). Decreased blood supply and innervation, associated with age changes, are associated with these calcific changes.

These calcified bodies are clinically significant, since they complicate endodontic treatment. Since they may impinge upon nerves in the pulp, they are often mentioned as causative factors of pain that varies from trifacial neuralgia to pulpal neuralgia. However, this view is not commonly accepted; therefore, caution should be exercised in condemning a tooth simply because calcification is seen radiographically.

The question of why these calcified deposits occur in the pulp is as yet not clear. The consensus of opinion is that they are the result of degenerative or retrogressive changes in the pulp, since they are often found in aged teeth. Some believe that they are the products of pathologic changes; others claim that it is a protective mechanism against physical or chemical injuries. In any case, pulp calcification remains an unsolved phenomenon.

Age Changes

Because of the continued synthesis of secondary and the possible pulpal reactions to external irritants, the size of the root canals and pulp chambers decreases with age. For example, as a tooth wears during normal occlusal function, or through retrograde wear, the amount of secondary dentin synthesized usually equals the tooth structure lost. This phenomenon protects the dental pulp from exposure. Additional changes that relate to age include a decreased cellular component, decreased ground substance, and increased collagen fiber content. The odontoblasts eventually decrease in size and number, and dead tracts (odontoblastic tubules not occupied by the odontoblast) may form as a response to previous injury. Some teeth that have undergone extensive restorative and periodontal treatment demonstrate these age changes regardless of the individual's chronologic age.

Suggested Reading

Baumann E, Rossman SR. Clinical, roentgenologic and histopathologic findings in teeth with apical radiolucent areas. Oral Surg 1956;9:1330.

Bender IB, Seltzer S. The effect of periodontal disease on the dental pulp, Oral Surg 1972;33:458.

Bergenholtz G, Lindhe J. Effect of soluble plaque factors on inflammatory reactions in the dental pulp. Scand J Dent Res 1975;83:153.

Fuss Z, Trowbridge H, Bender IB, Rickoff BD, Sorin S. Assessment of reliability of electric and thermal pulp testing procedures. J Endodont 1986;12:301.

Rossman LE, Rossman SR. Endodontic surgery: diagnosis, considerations and technique. Comp Conti Ed 1981;II:18.

Rossman LE, Rossman SR, Garber DA. The endodontic-periodontic fistula. Oral Surg 1982;53:78.

Rossman LE. Interrelationship of endodontics and periodontics. In: Genco R, Coldman H, Cohen DW, eds. Contemporary periodontics. St. Louis: CV Mosby, 1990.

Rubach WC, Mitchell DF. Periodontal disease, accessory canals and pulp pathosis. J Periodontol 1965;36:34.

Seltzer S, Bender IB. The dental pulp. In: The pulp as connective tissue. 3rd ed. Philadelphia: JB Lippincott, 1984:78.

Seltzer S, Bender IB, Nazimov H, Sinai I. Pulpitis induced interradicular periodontal changes in experimental animals, J Periodont 1967;38:124.

Seltzer S, Bender IB, Ziontz M. The interrelationship of pulp and periodontal disease. Oral Surg 1963;16:1474.

Trowbridge HO. Review of dental pain—histology and physiology. J Endodont 1986;12:445.

Trowbridge HO. Pulp structure and function. In: Cohen S, Burns R, eds. Pathways of the pulp. 4th ed. St. Louis: CV Mosby, 1987:293.

Trowbridge HO, Enling RG. Inflammation: a review of the process. 3rd ed. Chicago: Quintessence Books, 1989.

10

The Periodontium

Studies conducted in population groups with fluoridated water supply have shown that the prevalence of dental caries in the adult has declined substantially and that more teeth are being retained in the same population. Such a decline in tooth loss can be attributed not only to the fluoridation of water, but also to better patient oral hygiene education and improvement in restorative dental materials.

In contrast, only 15 percent of the population is free from signs of periodontal disease. Loss of the attachment apparatus is now the primary cause of tooth loss in adults. Therefore, retention of the periodontium remains the most significant factor in the longevity of the dentition and a prime objective in dental procedures.

The periodontium (*peri*, "around"; *odont-*, "tooth"; Latin) is a dynamic and functional system and consists of those tissues that hold and support the teeth in the jaws. An understanding of the anatomy and physiology of the normal periodontium helps the practitioner to recognize abnormal findings and to preserve the normal function of periodontal attachment, thus helping patients to enjoy the natural dentition during their entire lifetime.

The mucous membrane covering the oral cavity can be classified as either masticatory mucosa or lining mucosa. The masticatory mucosa is a very dense, tightly fixed covering in the mouth that appears to be well designed to withstand the vigorous frictional activity of food preparation. The epithelial covering is thick and keratinized, and the underlying submucosa is composed of dense collagenous fibers. The gingiva, hard palate, and dorsum of the tongue make up the masticatory mucosa.

Lining mucosa covers the remainder of the oral soft tissues that are not covered by masticatory mucosa. Lining mucosa is a thin, freely movable tissue that tears and injures easily. The overlying epithelium is thin and nonkeratinized, while the submucosa is composed mostly of loose connective tissues with muscle and elastic fibers. A summary of the location, constituents, and appearance of both masticatory and lining mucosa appears in Table 10.1.

The gingival unit consists of epithelial attachment and gingiva. Gingival tissue covers the tooth and alveolar bone, and its function appears to be different from that of the attachment apparatus. The attachment apparatus includes the three supporting structures of periodontal ligament, alveolar process, and cementum (Table 10.2).

Table 10.2
The Subdivision of the Periodontium

- Gingival unit
  - Epithelial attachment
  - Gingiva
- Attachment apparatus
  - Cementum
  - Periodontal ligament
  - Bone

Table 10.1
Characteristics of Masticatory and Lining Mucosa

Characteristics	Masticatory Mucosa	Lining Mucosa
Location	Attached gingiva Hard palate Dorsum of the tongue	Similar to oral mucosa
Surface color	Light pink (possible melanotic pigmentation)	Bright red (possible melanotic pigmentation)
Surface texture	Stipple (orange peel)	Smooth surface
Elasticity	Tightly bound down	Very movable and elastic
Epithelium keratinization	Keratinized	Nonkeratinized
Rete peg formation	Present	Absent
Thickness	Thick layer	Thin layer
Fiber	Collagenous fiber	Collagenous and elastic fiber

Gingival Unit

The gingiva is masticatory mucosa that covers the tooth and underlying attachment apparatus. It encircles the neck of erupted teeth and firmly attaches to tooth and alveolar bone. The function of the gingiva is to adapt closely to the tooth and bone surfaces, thus sustaining the gingiva against the forces placed on it during mastication and protect the epithelial seal around the tooth from displacement (Figs. 10.1 and 10.2).

On clinical examination gingiva appears light pink in color, with a stippled surface and firm consistency, which gives the appearance of an orange peel. The coronal part of the gingiva rests on tooth and forms a scalloped configuration in the buccal and lingual aspects of the teeth, with both lateral sides placed higher at mesial and distal lineangle of tooth than the midcrown portion. It also occupies the entire space between the teeth below the contact area. The coronal part of the gingiva is called *marginal gingiva* and is placed loosely on the teeth. The marginal gingiva can be carefully pulled away from tooth in order to examine the gingival sulcus. The term *free gingiva* has been used widely in the past to describe the marginal gingiva that is not attached to the tooth. This term is no longer being used because there is little or no sulcus in the healthy gingiva.

Gingiva extends from the *gingival margin* to the mucogingival junction. The alveolar mucosa, which is lining mucosa, is found apical to the mucogingival junction and is continuous with the mucous membrane of the cheek, lip, and floor of the oral cavity. The gingiva ranges in width between 1 and 9 mm. In the interdental area, the gingiva is known as the *gingival papilla* (Fig. 10.3).

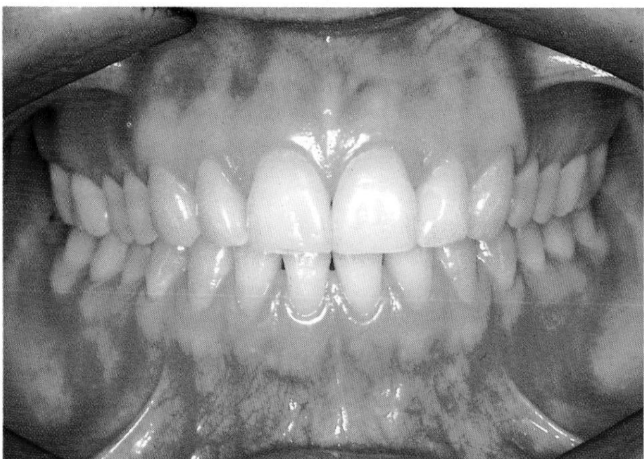

Figure 10.2

The clinically healthy tissue and dentition of an adult 42 years of age. Note the early recession in the lower anterior area.

In fully erupted human teeth the gingival margin is rounded and is located on the enamel about 0.5 to 2.0 mm coronal to the cementoenamel junction. The margin of the gingiva follows a wavy course around the tooth, and its form is influenced by the curvature of the cervical line of the tooth (Fig. 10.3).

The *gingival sulcus* is the space between the marginal gingiva and the tooth. It is bordered on one side

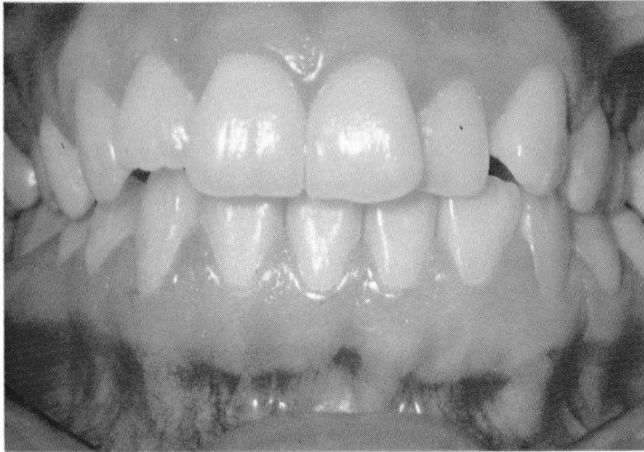

Figure 10.1

The clinically healthy gingival tissue and dentition of a young adult 18 years of age.

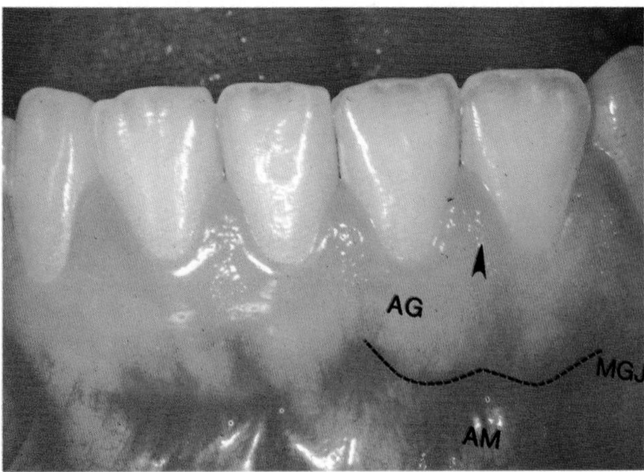

Figure 10.3

The anatomy of the normal gingival unit: *arrow*, interdental papilla; *MGJ*, mucogingival junction; *AG*, attached gingiva; *AM*, alveolar mucosa.

by the tooth surface and on the other by the epithelium lining the sulcus and covering the gingiva. The depth of the healthy gingival sulcus rarely exceeds 2.5 mm.

The *gingival papilla* is the interdental extension of the marginal gingiva, and its structure is determined by the contact areas of adjacent teeth, the course of the cementoenamel junction, and the proximity of the adjacent teeth. The shape of the gingival papilla is pyramidal in a mesiodistal direction, but buccolingually its structure varies according to the shape of the crowns of the teeth as well as the contact area and embrasure form. The *interdental papilla* may take the form of a concavity (*col*) in its mid-area in a labiolingual dimension. If the deciduous teeth separate, the col may disappear as the papilla rounds over, and a new col may reappear when the permanent teeth erupt. The interdental papilla seems to be rounder and flatter in the premolar and molar region than in the anterior portions of the mouth.

The *gingival groove* is a shallow groove that runs parallel to the margin of the gingiva. Less than half of all normal gingiva exhibits a gingival groove, and this groove also may be present in areas with inflammatory changes. Therefore, the gingival groove should not be used as a criterion for normal gingiva even though the groove, when present, roughly corresponds to the base of the gingival sulcus.

The sulcular aspect of gingiva facing the tooth is lined with a thin, nonkeratinized epithelium, whereas the outer surface of the gingiva is covered with keratinized epithelium. The gingival epithelium is derived from the ectoderm and is stratified squamous epithelium. It consists of the *oral epithelium, sulcular epithelium,* and *junctional epithelium* (Fig. 10.4).

The oral epithelium is keratinized stratified squamous epithelium and consists of a stratum basale, stratum spinosum, stratum granulosum, and stratum corneum, with a distinct stratum spinosum layer. The oral epithelium contains prominent rete pegs (Figs. 10.5 and 10.6).

The *lamina propria,* which connects the oral epithelium to the connective tissue, contains nonfibrillar collagen of types IV and VII. In addition, specific glycoprotein laminin, a product of epithelial cells, has been demonstrated in abundance in lamina propria. The epithelial cells attach tightly to each other by a structure called the *desmosome.* Cells of oral epithelium contain tonofibrils (a keratin precursor), which increase between the basal layer and the desquamating surface. The turnover time of cells in gingival epithelium is apparently 14 days.

The sulcular epithelium is nonkeratinized stratified squamous epithelium that lines the gingival sul-

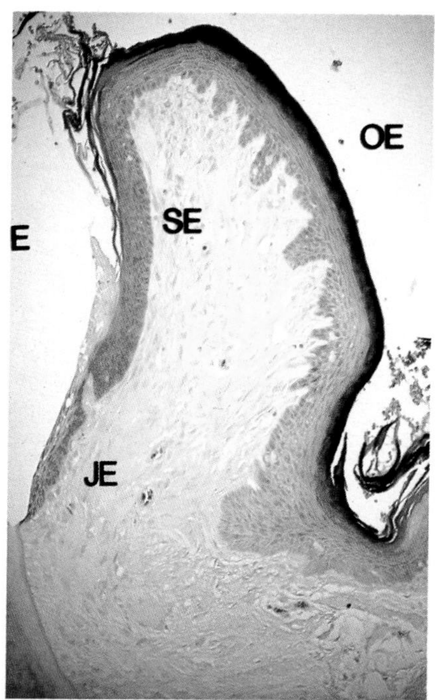

Figure 10.4

Histological section of gingival tissue: *OE,* oral epithelium with the keratinized surface extending from vestibule to the sulcular epithelium; *SE,* sulcular epithelium; *JE,* junctional epithelium.

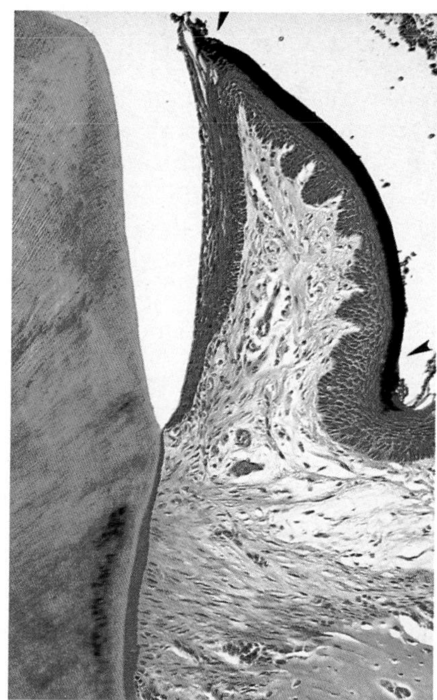

Figure 10.5

Histologic section of gingiva. Note the presence of keratinized layer between the two arrows covering the oral epithelium.

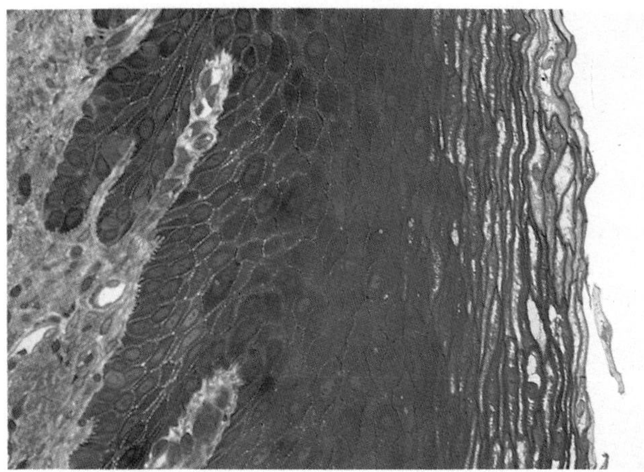

Figure 10.6
Higher magnification of oral epithelium. Note the superficial layer of the keratin and prominent rete pegs. (Courtesy of Dr. M. A. Listgarten.)

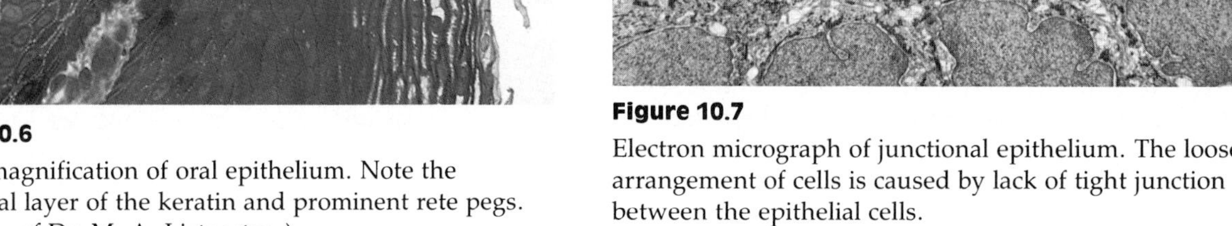

Figure 10.7
Electron micrograph of junctional epithelium. The loose arrangement of cells is caused by lack of tight junction between the epithelial cells.

cus. It lies between oral epithelium at the gingival margin coronally and junctional epithelium apically.

The junctional epithelium shapes the floor of the gingival sulcus and extends apically on the tooth surface to form the attachment seal around the tooth. It is nonkeratinized stratified squamous epithelium. Histologically, junctional epithelium presents unique features different from oral and sulcular epithelium. It is the only epithelium in the body to possess two basal lamina: one attaches the epithelium to the gingival connective tissue (external basal lamina), and the other attaches to the tooth structure (internal basal lamina). Junctional epithelium lacks rete pegs. Unlike oral and sulcular epithelium, which are impermeable, the junctional epithelium is permeable to migrating cells and fluids. This feature could be explained by the presence of significantly fewer intracellular junctions, like the desmosome in this tissue (Fig. 10.7).

The attached gingiva is firmly attached to the cementum and bone by the dense network of collagenous fibers. The width of attached gingiva varies from mouth to mouth and also in different areas in the same mouth. Generally, more attached gingiva is found in the maxilla than in the mandible, and the buccal surface of the mandibular first premolar seems to exhibit the narrowest zone of gingiva in the healthy adult periodontium. The hard palate is completely covered with masticatory mucosa. Variations in gingival color may be correlated with the thickness of gingiva, the degree of keratinization of gingival epithelium, the vascularity of the connective tissue, and the presence of pigment in gingival tissue (Fig. 10.8).

The alveolar mucosa is sharply delineated from the attached gingiva by the mucogingival junction and continues to the vestibular fornix. This tissue is rather thin, soft, loosely attached to the underlying bone, and of a deeper red color than the attached gingiva. Muscle attachments are noted in the alveolar mucosa, and frequently these freni are inserted close to the gingival margin or the tip of the interdental papilla. These bands of muscle fibers are covered by alveolar mucosa, not attached gingiva. The alveolar mucosa exhibits a thinner epithelial covering that tends not to keratinize, nor does it have any projections into the subadjacent connective tissue. The underlying submucosa contains loosely arranged colla-

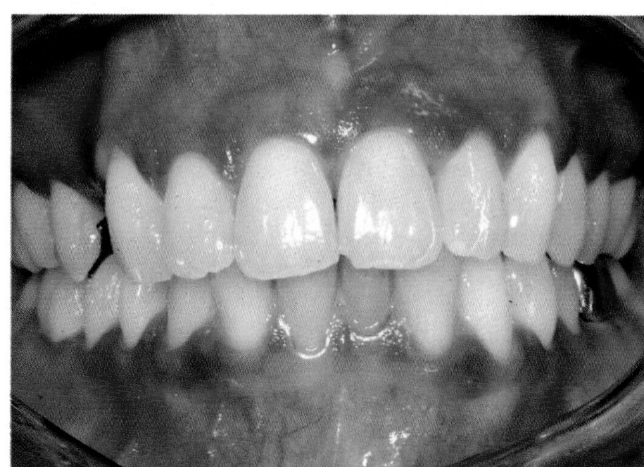

Figure 10.8
The clinical appearance of pigmented gingiva.

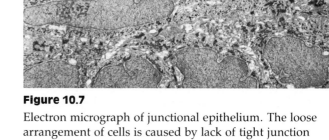

gen fibers, elastic tissue, fat, and muscle tissue (see Figs. 10.1 to 10.3).

The largest part of the gingiva by volume is made up of collagenous fibers elaborated by the principal connective tissue cell, the fibroblast. These fibers consist of coarse collagenous fibers embedded in the cementum known as *Sharpey's fibers,* and they extend toward the papillary area of the gingiva; their endings are traced to the subadjacent area of the covering epithelium. The fiber bundles pass outward from the cementum in groups consisting of a meshwork of small bundles, the fibers of which interlace with one another (Fig. 10.9).

In the buccolingual aspect, starting subjacent to the epithelial attachment, connective tissue fibers embedded in the cementum pass out at right angles to its surface for a short distance and then bend occlusally, extending into the gingiva and terminating in the papillary layer of the gingival epithelium. The fibers subjacent to those just described arise from the cementum and pass across the gingiva. Still further apically the fibers arise from the cementum, pass at right angles to the tooth directly over the alveolar crest, and incline apically between the outer periosteum of the alveolar process and the epithelial covering of the attached gingiva. These latter fibers join with small fibers arising from the outer periosteum and on the other side with fibers running into the papillary layer of the epithelium (Fig. 10.10). These bundles form distinct groups tending to hold the gingiva firmly against the tooth and to keep the attached gingiva closely adapted to the underlying bone and tooth.

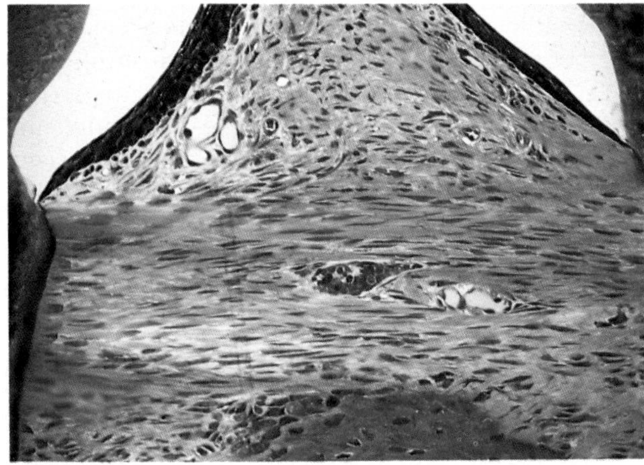

Figure 10.9

Mesiodistal section of gingival tissue. Note the cellularity and arrangement of the collagen fibers coronal to the crest of the bone.

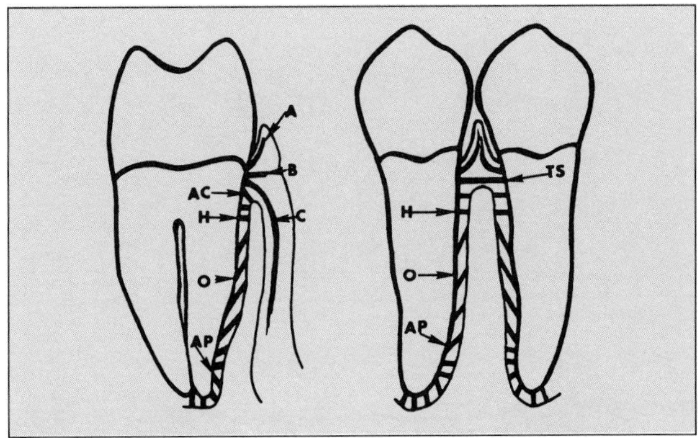

Figure 10.10

Principal fiber group of the gingival unit and attachment apparatus. Groups A, B, C, AC, and TC are gingival fibers and H, O, and AP belong to periodontal fiber. *A, B,* and *C,* dentogingival; *TS,* transseptal; *AC,* alveolar crest; *H,* horizontal; *O,* oblique; *AP,* apical fibers.

On the proximal side, the connective tissue fibers arise from the cementum at a higher level than those on the buccal and lingual aspects, since cementum extends more occlusally on the proximal surface than on the buccal or lingual aspects. (The curvature of the cementoenamel junction of the tooth must be considered.) The group adjacent to the epithelial attachment passes occlusally, traveling parallel to the sulcular epithelium, and terminates in the papillary layer of the covering epithelium of the gingiva. The next adjacent group of fibers also passes occlusally and seemingly makes up the framework for the interproximal gingiva. Directly subjacent to these, the fibers travel across the interproximal space over the alveolar crest and are attached to the adjacent tooth. Thus, these bundles form a distinct group that binds one tooth to another (the transseptal fibers). When labiolingual sections directly above the alveolar crest are studied, cross-sections of these fibers are apparent (Fig. 10.10).

Circular bands of connective tissue fibers surround the teeth and form a band tying the teeth together (Fig. 10.11). In the peak areas the fibers run crosswise to the gingival fibers, and in the interdental area they lie over the transseptal fibers perpendicular to them. Melcher described an interpapillary ligament as a narrow bundle of densely packed collagen fibers that connects the buccal and lingual peaks extending into the lamina propria beneath the outer epithelium. Below these fiber bundles collagen fibers turn mesially and distally, a part of the circular group. In addition to these fibers, the alveolar gingival group extending from the alveolar crest to the lamina propria has been described.

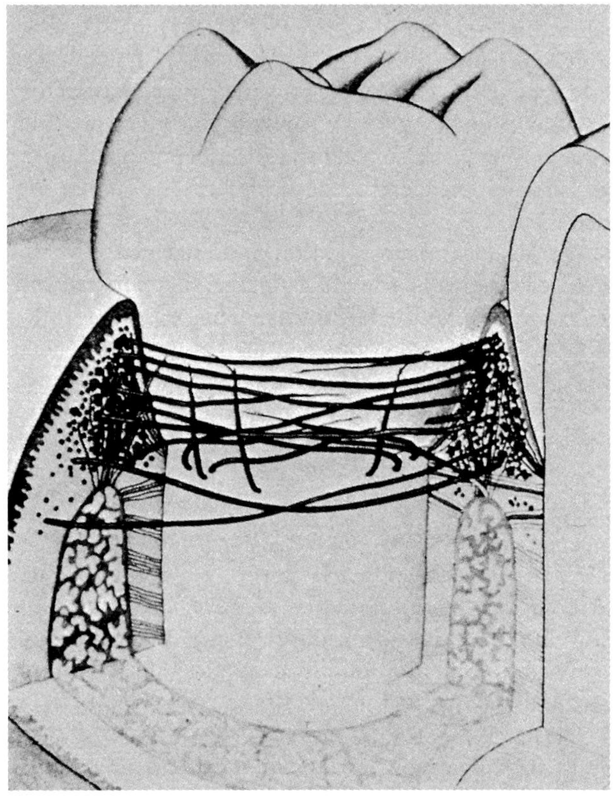

Figure 10.11

Drawing showing the circular fibers on the buccal surface of the gingival unit. (Reproduced from Anrim SS, Hagerman DA. The connective tissue fibers of the marginal gingiva. J Am Dent Assoc 1953; 47:271. Copyright by the American Dental Association.)

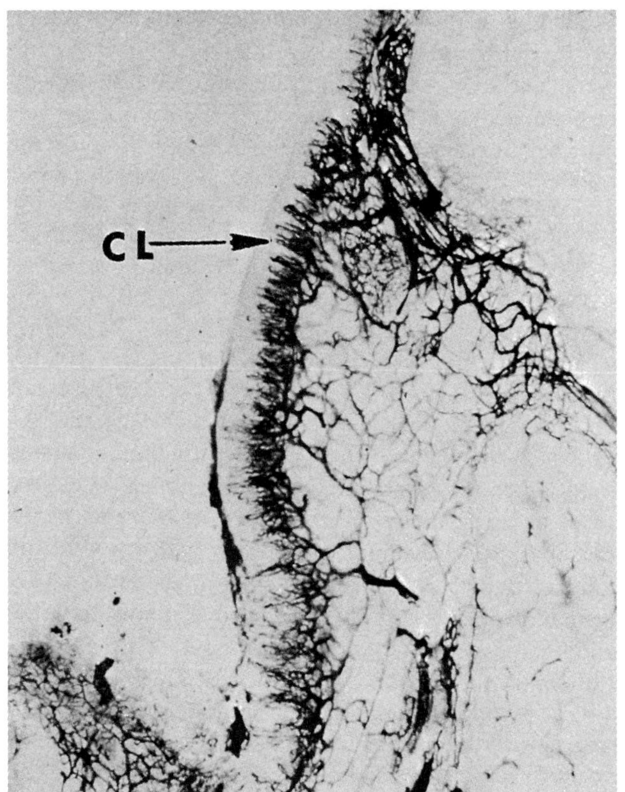

Figure 10.12

A buccolingual section through the incisor of a monkey perfused with refined India ink. Note the capillary loops (*CL*) in the connective tissue papillae. The rich blood supply in the gingival wall of the sulcus is evident. Magnification, 50×.

The fibers subjacent to the epithelial attachment act as a barrier against apical migration of this tissue, preventing subsequent recessions. Thus, the gingival fibers not only sustain the forces placed on the gingiva, but also inhibit apical migration of the epithelial attachment (see Fig. 10.10).

The blood supply of the gingival tissues is derived mainly from supraperiosteal vessels originating from the lingual, mental, buccinator, and palatine arteries. Anastomoses with the blood vessels of the periodontal ligament and the interdental septa can be traced. The gingiva are rich in capillary loops, which are noted in the connective tissue papillae below the basement membrane of the epithelial covering (Fig. 10.12).

Microscopic examination of clinically healthy gingiva discloses the presence of small numbers of lymphocytes and plasma cells in the connective tissue subjacent to the sulcular epithelium. Inflammatory cells have also been described in the epithelium.

Attachment Apparatus

The tooth is attached to the alveolus by numerous bundles of collagenous tissue (*principal fibers*) arranged in groups (Fig. 10.10). Between the groups there is loose connective tissue together with blood vessels, lymph vessels, and nerves. The principal fibers function as the investing and supporting mechanism for the tooth and are called the periodontal ligament. The attachment apparatus comprises the cementum, the periodontal ligament, and the alveolar bone. The periodontal ligament is the tissue that surrounds the roots of the tooth and attaches it to bony alveolus. Cementum is the hard, bone-like tissue covering the anatomic roots of the teeth. The alveolar bone is a plate of compact bone tissue and is radiographically termed lamina dura.

The function of the attachment apparatus is supportive, but there are also formative, nutritive, and sensory aspects. The supporting function consists of maintaining and retaining the tooth. The formative function is necessary for the replacement of tissue: cementum, periodontal ligament, and alveolar bone. Three specialized cells are associated with this function: cementoblasts, fibroblasts, and osteoblasts. The nutritive and sensory functions are fulfilled by the blood vessels and nerves, respectively. Thus, the attachment apparatus serves as a suspensory mechanism for the tooth, as a pericementum for the maintenance of the root covering, and as periosteum for the alveolar bone (Figs. 10.13 to 10.15).

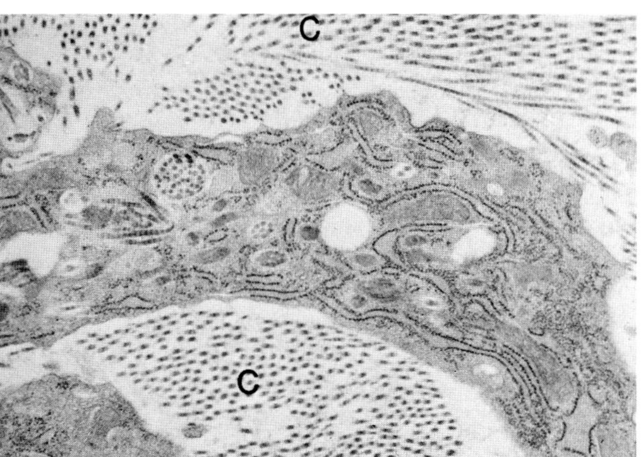

Figure 10.14

Electron micrograph of PDL fibroblast and surrounding newly formed collagen fiber.

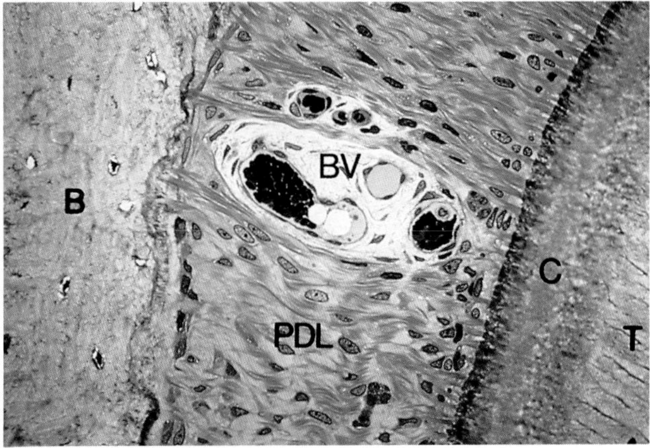

Figure 10.13

An occlusal cross section of periodontal ligament: *B,* bone; *PDL,* periodontal ligament; *BV,* blood vessel; *C,* cementum; *T,* tooth.

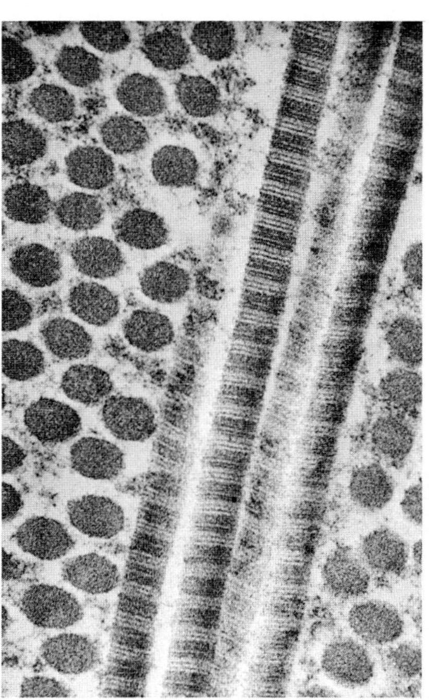

Figure 10.15

High power electron micrograph of collagen fiber in longitudinal and transverse direction.

Cementum

Cementum is the calcified connective tissue covering the entire anatomic root of the teeth from cementoenamel junction to the apex. It serves as calcified biological glue, thus anchoring the periodontal ligament fibers to the root. It is of mesodermal origin from dental follicle and, after tooth eruption, appears to be differentiated from adjacent periodontal ligament cells.

Cementum is thinnest at the cementoenamel junction, measuring 15 to 60 microns, and increasing in thickness, i.e., 150 to 200 microns toward the root tip. Histologically it is divided into two groups of *acellular* and *cellular cementum* according to the presence or absence of cellular element. Acellular cementum covers the coronal two-thirds of the roots and lacks the embedded cells. The cellular cementum contains cells embedded in the calcified matrix of cementum and can be found in the apical third of the roots and within furcation areas.

Cementum is made of organic and inorganic matrix. The organic part contains type I collagen and proteoglycan ground substance that makes up 45 to 50 percent of cementum. The remaining 50 to 55 percent consists of crystal of hydroxyapatite and water. Its degree of hardness is less than that of dentin, but it is more calcified than bone. Cementum is permeable to fluids and dyes. Electron microscopic studies of demineralized cementum revealed the presence of principal fibers of periodontal ligament that run in bundles in a more or less perpendicular direction to the tooth surface. These fibers are continuous with periodontal fibers and embedded in the cementum and later mineralized and forms the *Sharpey's fibers* (Figs. 10.16 to 10.18). A meshwork of loosely packed collagen fiber parallel to the root surface and surrounding the periodontal fibers is called *indifferent cementum fibrils.* These fibrils are surrounded by the ground substance and form the organic matrix that

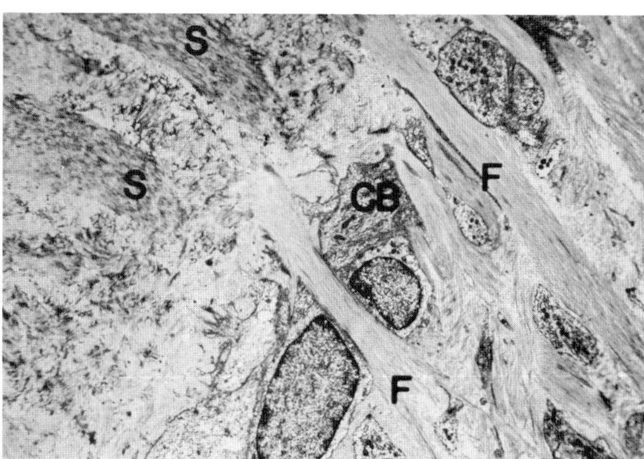

Figure 10.17

Electron micrograph of cementum: *S*, Sharpey's fibers; *F*, principal fibers; *CB*, cementoblasts. (Courtesy of Dr. M. A. Listgarten.)

becomes mineralized as cementum. Collagen fibrils, which are part of the mineralized cementum, extend from the cementum surface and are continuous with the collagen fibril of surrounding, nonmineralized periodontal connective tissue.

Unlike bone, cementum exhibits little turnover and grows by apposition. This is reflected by the presence of *appositional lines* in both cellular and acel-

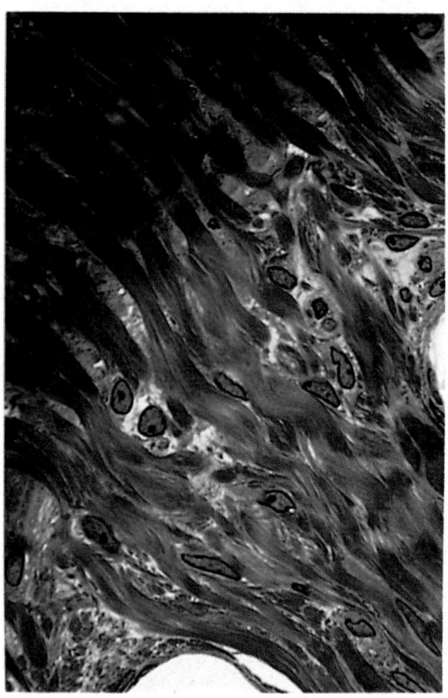

Figure 10.16

Histologic section of the rat periodontium. Note the attachment of the fibers to the cementum.

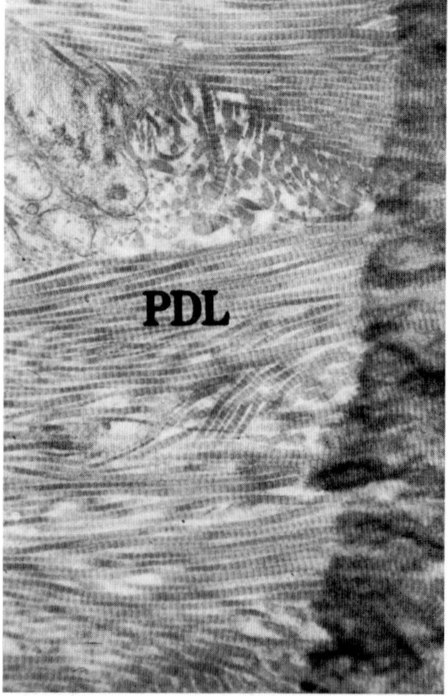

Figure 10.18

Higher-magnification electron micrograph of inserted collagen PDL fibers in the cementum.

lular cementum. *Cementoblasts* synthesize both collagen fibrils and ground substance. These cells, like their bone counterparts, also participate in the calcification process. During rapid cementum formation, cementoblasts can become embedded in cementum and form *cementocyte.* Cementum may become resorbed in some instances; the cell responsible for cementum resorption is called the *cementoclast,* a giant cell with features similar to the osteoclast.

The structure of cementum and the cellular mechanism that regulates cementum formation is poorly understood, primarily owing to the difficulty of obtaining a sufficient quantity of this tissue. In recent years much attention has been given to studying in more detail the composition and development of cementum, partly because of the significance of cementum in regenerating diseased periodontal tissue.

Alveolar Process

The tissue elements of the alveolar process are no different from those of bone elsewhere. The alveolar bone portion of the alveolar process lines the sockets into which the roots of the teeth fit. It is thin, compact bone that is pierced by many small openings through which blood vessels, lymphatics, and nerve fibers pass. The alveolar bone fuses with the cortical plates of the labial and lingual sides at the crest of the alveolar process. The alveolar bone contains the embedded ends of the connective tissue fibers of the periodontal membrane (Sharpey's fibers). The cancellous portion of the process occupies the area between the cortical plates and the alveolar bone, and is called "supporting bone." It is continuous with the *spongiosa* of the body of the jaws. The spongiosa occupies most of the interdental septum but a relatively small portion of the labial or lingual plates. In these, the incisal region has less spongiosa than the incisal region of the molar areas. The architectural arrangement of the trabeculae and their character are related to the demands of function (Figs. 10.19 to 10.21).

Bone tissue is continually undergoing change. Characteristically, bone apposition and resorption occur. In the alveolar bone, adjacent lamellae can be distinguished by so-called cementing lines. When a bony surface is inactive for a period of time, a baso-

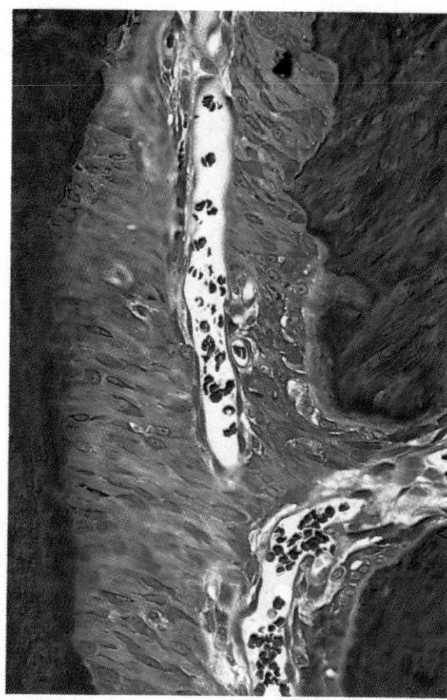

Figure 10.19

Histologic section of the rat periodontal ligament. Note the rich vascularity of the periodontal ligament.

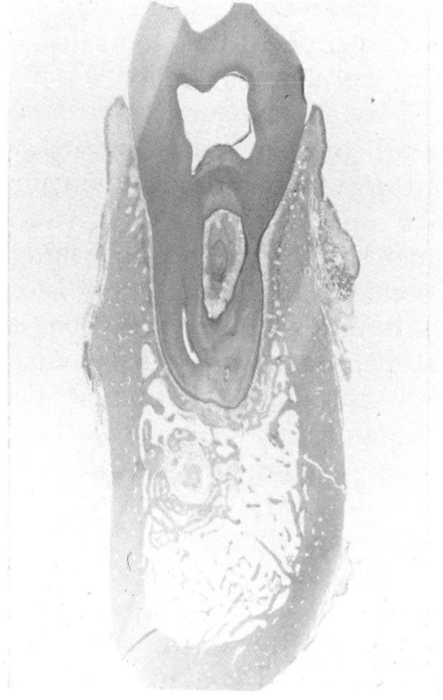

Figure 10.20

A buccolingual section through a human mandibular molar and the periodontium. Note the bone proper surrounding the root as thin cortical bone and the supporting bone holding both bone proper and the root.

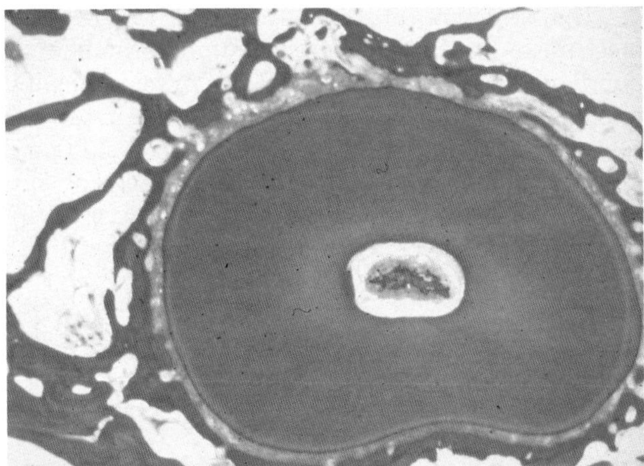

Figure 10.21

Cross section of tooth and bone. Note the cortical bone proper and the supporting cancellous bone.

philic line forms. These lines are seen over sections where apposition or resorptive phases have occurred and thus reveal the changes that have previously taken place.

Thus, bone is a relatively active tissue, and comparison of it to cementum discloses an unlike activity. This can be seen easily microscopically in tissues of adult persons. Very little apposition of cementum is seen, whereas a definite remodeling of the alveolar bone is apparent. This observation is of great significance since the periodontal ligament unites these tissues. It can be reasoned, therefore, that there is a need for some mechanisms to allow for an independence of these two hard tissues.

Bone is a highly specialized mesoblastic tissue consisting of organic matrix and inorganic matter. The matrix is composed of a groundwork of osteocytes and intercellular substance. The inorganic portion consists chiefly of calcium, phosphate, and carbonate in the form of apatite crystals. Bone is first laid down as an open framework of spongy bone, some of which becomes compact later on. The spaces in the spongiosa are termed marrow spaces. Under normal conditions bone is constantly subject to coincident tissue growth and resorption, which are finely coordinated. Microscopically bone surfaces may exhibit areas of bone apposition, areas where bone is undergoing resorption, and other areas where the status quo is being maintained. Under normal conditions the last predominates (Figs. 10.22 to 10.30).

Ritchey and Orban pointed out that in the absence of periodontal disease the configurations of the crest of the interdental alveolar septa are determined by the relative positions of the adjacent cementoenamel junctions and also that the width of the interdental alveolar bone is determined by the tooth form present. Relatively flat proximal tooth surfaces call for narrow septa, whereas in the presence of extremely convex tooth surfaces, wide interdental septa with flat crests are found.

Alveolar and Supporting Bone

Alveolar bone is bone that is deposited next to the periodontal ligament and is itself supported by bone. One or more large arteries, veins, and nerve bundles are longitudinally situated in the interradicular bony process, and branches from them enter the periodontal ligament through the many openings in the cribriform plates.

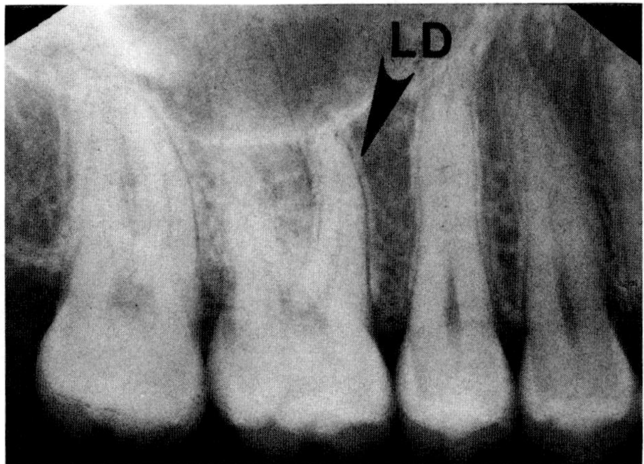

Figure 10.22

Radiograph of maxillary molar premolar area: *LD,* lamina dura, a radiopaque line surrounding the root.

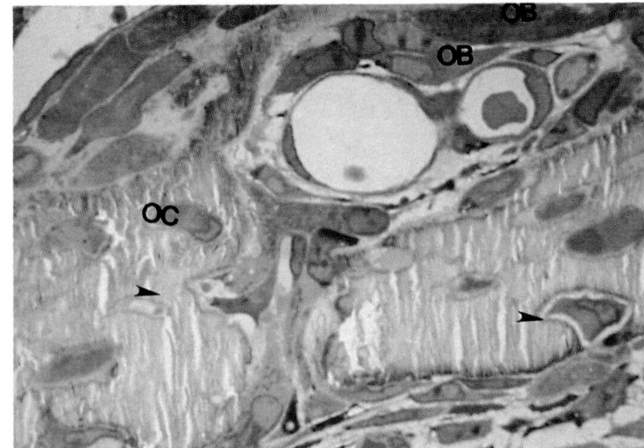

Figure 10.23

Histologic section of human bone. *OB,* osteoblast covering the bone surface; *OC,* embedded osteocyte in bone matrix; arrows point to the newly embedded osteocytes.

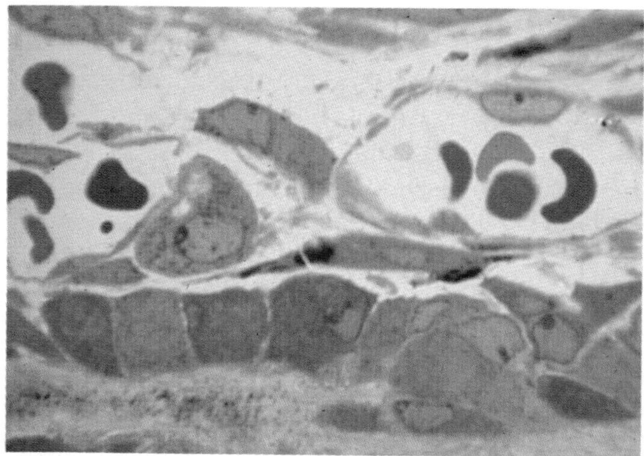

Figure 10.24

Histologic section of newly formed bone. Note the active osteoblasts lining the newly formed osteoid.

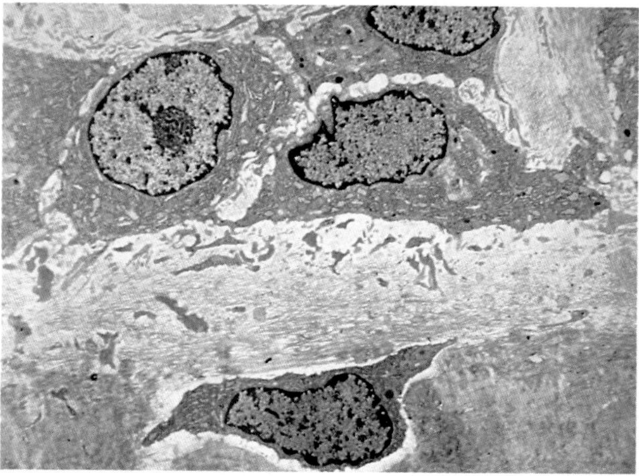

Figure 10.25

Electron micrograph of osteoblasts. Note the presence of osteocyte enclosed in the osteoid.

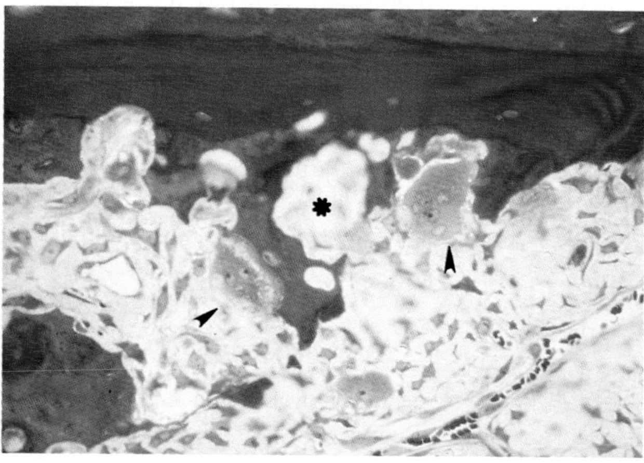

Figure 10.26

Histologic section of the bone resorbing site: osteoclast (*arrows*); howship lacunae (*).

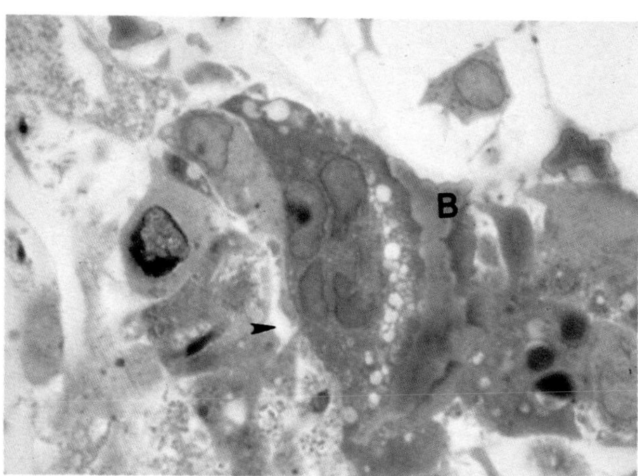

Figure 10.27

Bone undergoing resorption by a giant multinucleated osteoclast (*arrow*); note the presence of vasculated region of active resorption adjacent to bone (*B*).

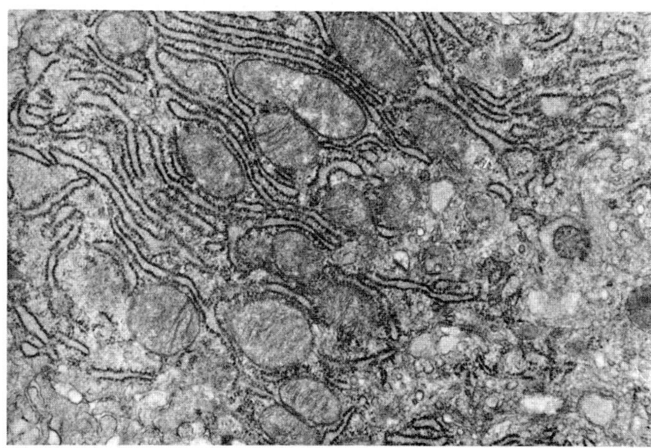

Figure 10.28

High power electron micrograph of ruffled border, the resorbing apparatus of osteoclast.

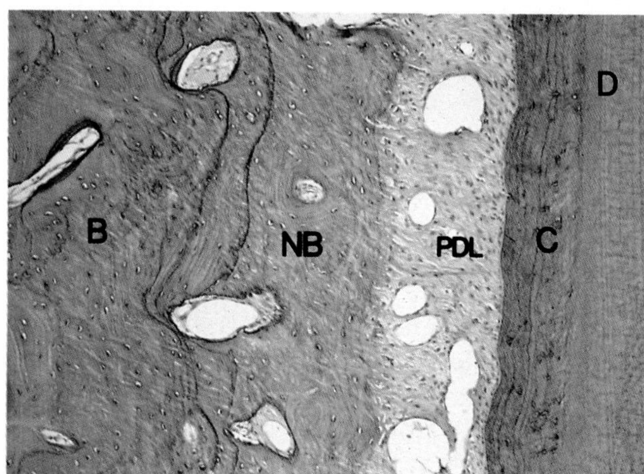

Figure 10.29

Histologic section of the apposition side of alveolus: *B*, bone; *NB*, new bone; *PDL*, periodontal ligament; *C*, cementum; *D*, dentin.

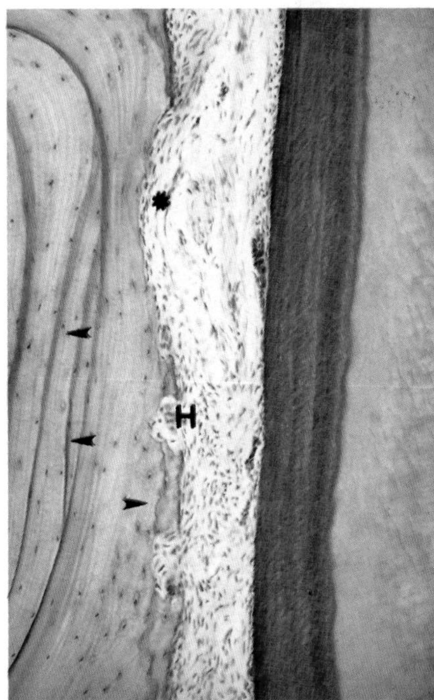

Figure 10.30
Histologic section of resorptive side of alveolus: *H*, howship lacunae; *, inacctive resorbing site; *arrow*, apposition lines.

Relationship of Alveolar and Supporting Bone to Function

The bone housing the tooth is dependent upon the function exerted on the tooth to maintain its structure. The changes in the supporting bone and in the periodontal ligament when the occlusal stress to the teeth is withdrawn, as when antagonists are lost, attest to the dependence of these tissues to functional stimulation. In fact, after longstanding loss of function, changes in the alveolar bone may also be noted. In jaws in which the teeth are subjected to intense occlusal stress, it is usual to find the spongy or supporting bone to be composed of thicker and more numerous trabeculae. Although bone tissue is subject to function for the maintenance and arrangement of the trabeculae, there are other factors that may be involved, should a disease process be present, which will interfere with the normal balanced process of anabolism and catabolism characteristic of bone tissue (Fig. 10.20).

Where numerous bundles of collagen fibers become incorporated in the bone, the term *bundle bone* is applied. The alveolar bone adjacent to the periodontal ligament contains numerous fibers, the anchorage portion of the collagen fibers of the peridontal ligament. These are referred to as Sharpey's fibers. This bone has an apparent lamellation produced by incremental lines parallel to the surface but with no relation to changes in fibril direction as in lamellar bone. Bundle bone forms the immediate bone attachment of the periodontal ligament.

Periodontal Ligament

The fibers of the periodontal ligament proper, attaching the tooth to the alveolar housing, are arranged in four groups: (1) the alveolar crestal group, extending from the cervical area of the tooth to the alveolar crest; (2) the horizontal group, running perpendicularly from the tooth to the alveolar bone; (3) the oblique group, obliquely situated with insertions in the cementum, and extending more apically in the alveolus (approximately two-thirds of the fibers fall into this group); and (4) the apical group, radiating apically from tooth to bone. In multirooted teeth a group of interradicular fibers are observed. The arrangement of the groups of the fiber bundles is designed to sustain the tooth against forces to which it is subjected. The structure of the periodontal ligament, however, continuously changes as a result of the functional requirements (Figs. 10.31 and 10.32).

The main portion of the periodontal ligament is composed of bundles of white, collagenous, connective tissue fibers that extend from the cementum to the alveolar bone. High-power inspection reveals that a few collagen fibers emerge from the cementum in what appears to be (under low-power magnification) a single strand from a single location. These fibers may be termed a bundle. These bundles are gathered together into a group. Although under low-power observation these bundles seemingly run across without interruption, close observation reveals that single fibers do not span the entire distance, but that there is an interweaving mechanism. The cellular element of the periodontal ligament is composed of typical long, slender, and spindle-shaped fibroblasts with oval-shaped nuclei. These are found in alignment with the collagen fibers. The fibers are arranged

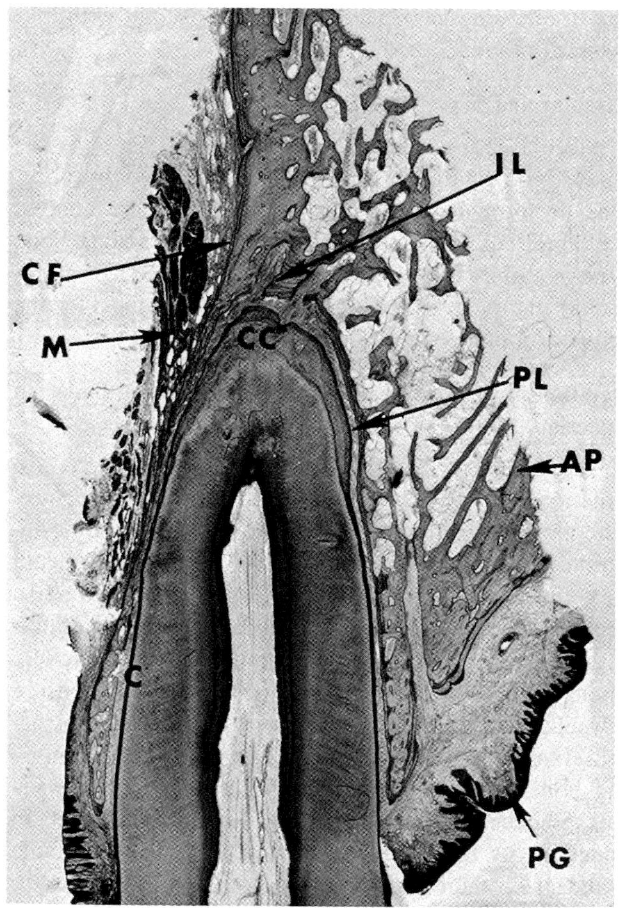

Figure 10.31

A labiolingual section of a maillary canine from a person 45 years old. Note palatal gingiva (*PG*); alveolar process (*AP*); periodontal ligament (*PL*); canine fossa (*CF*); muscle (*M*); incremental lines in alveolar bone (*IL*); acellular cementum (*C*); cellular cementum (*CC*). Magnification 4×.

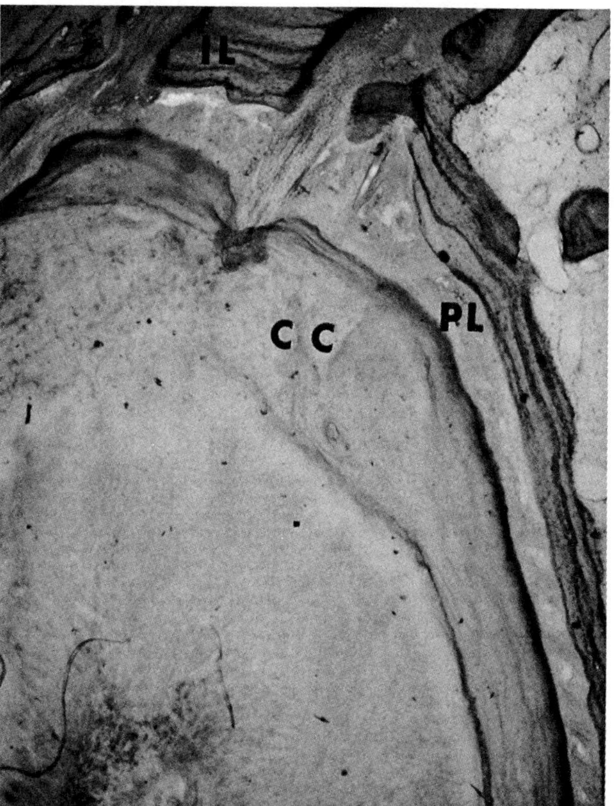

Figure 10.32

High-power magnification of specimen in Fig. 10.31. Note cellular cementum in apex of tooth (*CC*); periodontal ligament (*PL*); incremental lines in alveolar bone (*IL*). Magnification 48×.

in groups between which are found round or oval spaces containing blood and lymph vessels and nerves. These are surrounded by loose connective tissue.

The blood vessels found in the periodontal ligament arise mainly from the bone marrow of the supporting bone through lateral perforations of the alveolar bone and extend from the periapical vessels. They form an elaborate anastomosing network (Figs. 10.33 and 10.34). These vessels are supplied by their

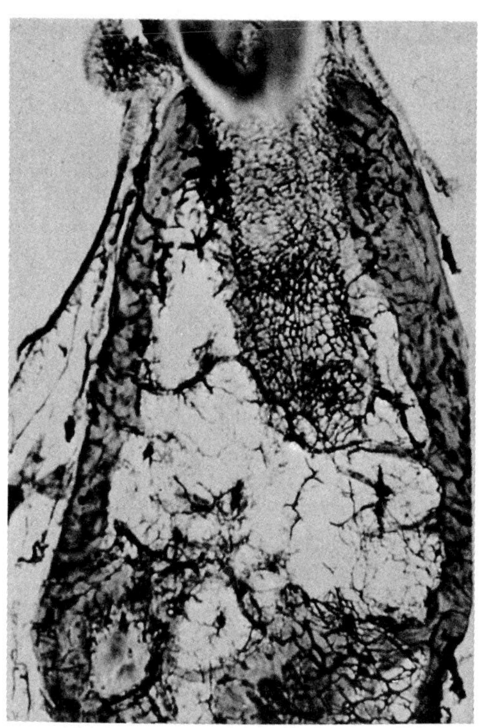

Figure 10.33

A buccolingual section through the premolar of a monkey perfused with refined India ink. The numerous vessels of the periodontal ligament surrounding the root are filled with ink.

own sympathetic nervous system. The lymphatics form a complicated pattern. The nerves are both myelinated and naked. Their endings have been described as knob-like swellings, rings, or loops around fiber bundles, and free endings between fibers. They are proprioceptive, and the sense of localization is imparted through them.

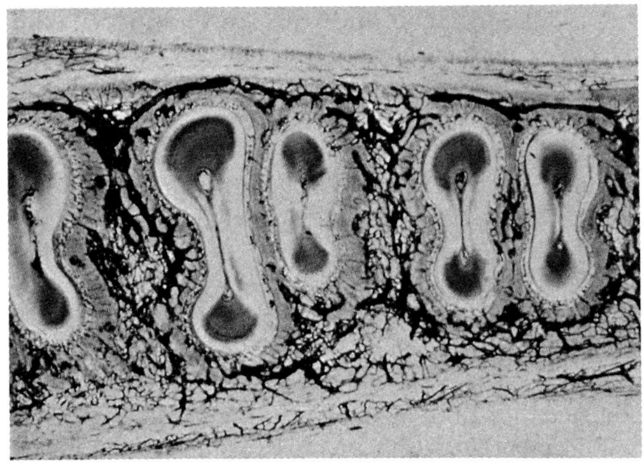

Figure 10.34

A horizontal section through the posterior region of a perfused monkey. Note the rich vascular plexus behind the alveolar bone in the marrow spaces passing through the perforations in the alveolar bone into the periodontal ligament.

Mesial Movement of the Teeth

Because of slight buccolingual movement of the teeth normally possible in the masticatory process, the contact areas between the teeth show progressive abrasion with age. As a result of this wear, the mesiodistal width of the teeth becomes narrower. It has been estimated that this interproximal abrasion causes the loss of 1 cm in the anteroposterior length of the total tooth by the age of 40. Thus, in order to maintain a protective contact relation for the gingival tissue and also to preserve proximal contact for support against external forces, the teeth move mesially. With the wearing of the cusps of the teeth, this compensatory migration of the teeth actually proceeds in a mesioocclusal direction.

Physiology of the Epithelial Attachment

The epithelial attachment is situated on the tooth surface during the eruptive phase of the tooth. Most investigators have demonstrated that when the base of sulcus reaches the cementoenamel junction, epithelial proliferation onto the cementum has occurred. The prevalent theory proposed by Gottlieb states that, with increasing age, the epithelial attachment proliferates apically from the enamel until it is entirely on the cementum and continues to do so throughout life. In recent years this theory has been challenged, and many investigators believe that such recession onto the cementum is pathologic in nature.

The observation that when the base of the sulcus is situated at the cementoenamel junction, the epithelial attachment is on the cementum, brings up the following questions. "Where should the base of the sulcus normally be located in adult life?" "Should it be situated at the enamel surface, the base of the epithelial attachment lying at the cementoenamel junction?" "If so, is any further recession physiological?" "Thus, clinically, should the gingival margin be located on the tooth surface directly apical to the greatest contours?"

Gottlieb divided eruption into four stages. In the first stage the deepest point of the epithelial attachment is at the cementoenamel junction. In the second stage the deepest point of the attachment is on the cementum. However, the bottom of the crevice is still on the surface of the enamel. The clinical crown is still smaller than the anatomic crown. In the third stage the bottom of the gingival crevice is at the cementoenamel junction, and the deepest point of epithelial attachment is still farther along the cementum. The anatomic and clinical crowns are identical. In the fourth stage both the bottom of the gingival crevice and the deepest point of the epithelial attachment are below the cementoenamel junction. The clinical crown is larger than the anatomic crown.

Thus, Gottlieb believed that gingival recession was the result of a normal physiological process to be found in elderly people. This process he termed passive eruption and described it as an atrophy of the gingival margin associated with the apical proliferation of the epithelial attachment alongside the cementum. He believed that the rate of the recession varies not only from person to person but also from one tooth to another in the same mouth.

Recent studies of this problem indicate that passive eruption or the apical shift of the dentogingival junction is not a physiological process. Migration of the sulcular epithelium beyond the cementoenamel junction is possible only after destruction of the most coronal group of Sharpey's fibers. Dissolution of these fibers and apical recession of the gingival margin should be considered pathological at any age.

Physiological Forces Influencing the Dentition

Various forces of physiological phenomena influence the fully developed dentition. Some are the forces developed by the muscles of mastication; others originate from facial muscles; others originate from the tongue. Thus there is a functional equilibrium, all of the forces acting upon the masticatory apparatus, for example, the force of the lips counteracting that of the tongue, and the force of the cheeks also equalizing that of the tongue.

Tooth Suspension

The transmission of masticatory forces to the supporting structures of the tooth is the function of the attachment apparatus. Three factors operate: (1) the principal fiber apparatus of the periodontal ligament; (2) the shape and size of the root of the tooth; and (3) the fluid content of the periodontal ligament.

Gottlieb believed that the number of fiber bundles of the periodontal ligament per unit area and the square area of the root surface were most important since the fiber apparatus sustained the masticatory force. On the other hand, Boyle described the mechanism of tooth suspension as hydraulic pressure on the walls of the alveolus. Escape of fluid by means of vascular channels communicating with the bone marrow spaces allows for a gradual extension of the periodontal fibers when the full force of occlusion is ultimately transmitted as tension to the alveolar bone. He further stated that further efficiency in the absorption of occlusal forces is secured by the spiral form of the teeth themselves and the resiliency of the dentin of which they are composed, showing the cross-sectional form of the tooth root to be efficiently designed to resist forces tending to flatten the arc of longitudinal curvature of the tooth. He explained that the form also offers efficiently shaped surfaces for the transmission of pressures on the labial and mesial sides, which furnish maximal surface for attachment of the periodontal fibers on the lingual and distal sides.

Churchill also had indicated that a hydraulic mechanism, operating via the fluid content of the blood of the periodontal ligament, acted as a means for absorbing force on the tooth.

Suggested Reading

Ainamo J, Talari A. The increase with age of the width of attached gingiva. J Periodont Res 1976; 11:182–188.

Armitage GC, Svanberg GK, Loe H. Microscopic evaluation of clinical measurements of connective tissue attachment levels. J Clin Periodontol 1977; 4:173–190.

Bartold PM. Proteoglycans of the periodontium: structure, role and function. J Periodont Res 1987; 22:432–444.

Beertsen W. Collagen phagocytosis by fibroblasts in the periodontal ligament of the mouse molar during the initial phase of hypofunction. J Dent Res 1987; 66:1708–1712.

Beertsen W, Everts V. Collagen degradation in the gingiva of the mouse incisor: epithelium-connective tissue interactions. J Periodont Res 1981; 16:524–541.

Bosshardt D, Luder HU, Schroeder HE. Rate and growth pattern of cementum apposition as compared to dentine and root formation in a fluorochrome-labelled monkey (*Macaca fascicularis*). J Biol Buccale 1989; 17:3–13.

Cho M-I, Garant PR. Ultrastructural evidence of directed cell migration during initial cementoblast differentiation in root formation. J Periodont Res 1988; 23:268–276.

Freeman E, Ten Cate AR, Dickinson J. Development of a gomphosis by tooth germ implants in the parietal bone of the mouse. Arch Oral Biol 1975; 20:139–140.

Fullmer HM, Sheetz JH, Narkates AJ. Oxytalan connective tissue fibers: a review. J Oral Path 1975; 3:291–316.

Garant PR. Collagen resorption by fibroblasts: a theory of fibroblastic maintenance of the periodontal ligament. J Periodontol 1976; 47:380–390.

Glavind L, Zander HA. Dynamics of dental epithelium during tooth eruption. J Dent Res 1970; 49:549–555.

Gothlin G, Ericsson, JLE. The osteoclast: review of ultrastructure, origin and structure-function relationship. Clin Orthop 1976; 120:201–231.

Gould TRL, Brunette DM, Westbury L. The attachment mechanism of epithelial cells to titanium *in vitro*. J Periodont Res 1981; 16:611–616.

Grant D, Bernick S. The formation of the periodontal ligament. J Periodontol 1972; 43:17–25.

Grant D, Bernick S, Levy BM, Dreizen S. A comparative study of periodontal ligament development in teeth with and without predecessors in marmosets. J Periodontol 1972; 43:162–169.

Grant DA, Stern IB, Listgarten MA. Periodontics. 6th ed. St. Louis: CV Mosby, 1987.

Grossman ES, Austin JC. A quantitative electron microscope study of desmosomes and hemidesmosomes in vervet monkey oral mucosa. J Periodontol Res 1983; 18:580–586.

Hashimoto S, Yamamura T, Shimono M. Morphometric analysis of the intercellular space and desmosomes of rat junctional epithelium. J Periodont Res 1986; 21:510–520.

Hassell TM, Stanek EJ III. Evidence that healthy human gingiva contains functionally heterogeneous fibroblast subpopulations. Arch Oral Biol 1983; 28:617–626.

Heritier M. Experimental induction of cementogenesis on the enamel of transplanted tooth germs. Arch Oral Biol 1982; 27:87–98.

Karring T, Lang NP, Loe H. The role of gingival connective tissue in determining epithelial differentiation. J Periodont Res 1975; 10:1–11.

Listgarten MA. Normal development, structure, physiology and repair of gingival epithelium. Oral Sci Rev 1972; 1:3–67.

Listgarten MA. Structure of surface coatings on teeth: a review. J. Periodontol 1976; 47:139–147.

Lozdan J, Squier CA. The histology of the mucogingival junction. J Periodont Res 1969; 4:83–93.

Massoth DL, Dale BA. Immunohistochemical study of structural proteins in developing junctional epithelium. J Periodontol 1986; 57:756–763.

McDougall WA. Penetration pathways of a topically applied foreign protein into rat gingiva. J Periodont Res 1971; 6:89–99.

McDougall WA. The effect of topical antigen on the gingiva of sensitized rabbits. J Periodont Res 1974; 9:153–164.

Moll R, Franke WW, Schiller DL, Geiger B, Krepler R. The catalog of human cytokeratins: patterns of expression in normal epithelia, tumors and cultured cells. Cell 1982; 31:11–24.

Prockop DJ, Kivirikko KI, Tuderman L, Guzman NA. The biosynthesis of collagen and its disorders. N Engl J Med 1979; 301:13.

Rifkin BR, Brand JS, Cushing JE, Coleman SJ, Sanavi F. Fine structure of fetal rat calvarium: provisional identification of preosteoclasts. Calcif Tissue Int 1980; 31:21–28.

Roberts WE, Wood HB, Chambers DW, Burk DT. Vascularly oriented differentiation gradient of osteoblast precursor cells in rat periodontal ligament: implications for osteoblast histogenesis and periodontal bone loss. J Periodont Res 1987; 22: 461–467.

Rose ST, App GR. A clinical study of the development of the attached gingiva along the facial aspect of the maxillary and mandibular anterior teeth in the deciduous, transitional and permanent dentitions. J Periodontol 1973; 44:131–139.

Schroeder HE. Gingival tissues. In Cohen B, Kramer IRH, eds. Scientific foundations of dentistry. London: William Heinemann, 1976:426–439.

Schroeder HE, Scherle WF. Cemento-enamel junction revisited. J Periodont Res 1988; 23:53–59.

Selvig KA. The fine structure of human cementum. Acta Odont Scand 1965; 23:423–441.

Selvig KA, Hals E. Periodontally diseased cementum studied by correlated microradiography, electron probe analysis and electron microscopy. J Periodont Res 1977; 12:419–429.

Silness J, Gustavsen F, Fejerskov O, Karring T, Loe H. Cellular, afibrillar coronal cementum in human teeth. J Periodont Res 1976; 11:331–338.

Smith RG. A longitudinal study into the depth of the clinical gingival sulcus of human canine teeth during and after eruption. J Periodont Res 1982; 17:427–433.

Somjen D, Binderman I, Berger E, Harell A. Bone remodelling induced by physical stress is prostaglandin E_2 mediated. Biochim Biophys Acta 1980; 627:91–100.

Squier CA. Keratinization of the sulcular epithelium—a pointless pursuit? J Periodontol Res 1981; 52:426–429.

Squier CA, Collins P. The relationship between soft tissue attachment, epithelium downgrowth and surface porosity. J Periodont Res 1981; 16:434–440.

Stanley JR, Woodley DT, Katz SI, Martin GR. Structure and function of basement membrane. J Invest Dermatol 1982; 79:69s–72s.

Ten Cate AR, Mills C. The development of the periodontium: the origin of alveolar bone. Anat Rec 1972; 173:69–78.

Ten Cate AR. Formation of supporting bone in association with periodontal ligament organization in the mouse. Arch Oral Biol 1975; 20:137–138.

Tennebaum H, Tennebaum M. A clinical study of the width of the attached gingiva in the deciduous, transitional and permanent dentitions. J Clin Periodontol 1986; 13:270–275.

Van Steenberghe D. The structure and function of periodontal innervation: a review of the literature. J Periodont Res 1979; 14:185–203.

Wennstrom JL. Lack of association between width of attached gingiva and development of soft tissue recession. A 5-year longitudinal study. J Clin Periodontol 1987; 14:181–184.

Willis RD, DiCosimo CJ. The absence of proprioceptive nerve endings in the human periodontal ligament: the role of periodontal mechanoreceptors in the reflex control of mastication. Oral Surg 1979; 48:108–115.

Zwarych PD, Quigley MB. The intermediate plexus of the periodontal ligament: history and further observations. J Dent Res 1965; 44:383–391.

Part Three

The Masticatory System

Introduction

The Masticatory System and Its Relation to Other Functional Units

The shape and organization of living organic structures can only be fully understood when assessed in connection with the functions in which they are involved. It is obvious that the morphology of each individual tooth is of great clinical significance. A single tooth by itself, however, cannot perform the necessary masticatory and occlusal functions. It is only when the individual teeth are anatomically and physiologically in the proper relationship to each other to join what is called the "dentition" that they can function as an essential component of the masticatory system.

The masticatory system as a whole forms a functional unit, which consists of the dentition, the periodontium, the jaws, the temporomandibular joints, the muscles involved in moving the mandible, the lip-cheek-tongue system, the salivary system, and the neuromuscular and nutritive (vascular) mechanisms involved in the maintenance of proper function. In this chapter we shall consider primarily the correlation between form and function in the masticatory system, especially with respect to features involving the morphology of the dentition. The description is based upon examination of young adult masticatory systems, with no attempt to present the numerous normal biological variations that occur within this population. The systematic anatomy of the cranium and the whole masticatory system as well as its physiology have been treated thoroughly in many texts. Therefore, no attempt has been made to repeat the description of anatomic or physiologic details unless they are pertinent to the understanding of function.

The head houses and protects a number of anatomic structures which are necessary for the maintenance of life and/or well-being of the individual. A single structure may serve one or more functional units. For example, the eye is solely committed to the visual system, while the tongue participates in the speech, masticatory, and respiratory systems. As is seen, the masticatory system is but one of several functional units that use anatomic structures in common with other systems.

The masticatory system is described in three sections: (1) the temporomandibular joint and mandibular function, (2) the dentition: its alignment and articulation, and (3) the self-protective features of the dentition.

12

The Temporomandibular Joint and Mandibular Function

Principles of Mandibular Function

Energy

Energy is necessary to hold, cut off, and comminute most kinds of food and to transport the bolus of food. It is also required to lift the mandible in swallowing movements and to perform such parafunctional activities as holding foreign bodies and bruxing or clenching the teeth. The energy needed for such tasks is provided primarily by the jaw muscles and by the muscles of the lip-cheek-tongue system. Energy is further necessary to provide transport of the bolus of food from the mouth into and through the esophagus.

The expenditure of energy results in *motion, change of form,* and *release of force. Motion,* such as shifts of the mandible from one position to another without tooth contact, and *change of form* of a muscular body like the tongue in deglutition, can be carried out by a pattern of muscle contractions alone. However, when strength is needed, as in the crushing of hard food or in locomotion, transmission and transformation of muscular energy into *force* is necessary. This is accomplished by means of joints and levers topographically related in such a way that an optimal effect can be obtained.

Jaw Biomechanics

In any case where two bones are connected by means of a movable joint one of the bones must be fixed in order for movement of the other to occur relative to it. Two bones connected by a movable joint can either move toward each other or away from each other. The movement is initiated and effected by muscles. Those muscles that bring one bone closer to the other are called *flexors;* those that move them apart are called *extensors.* Movement is not unlimited, however. In all movable joint systems there are mechanical limits placed on movement. For example, in the upper extremities, the forearm and upper arm can be extended only to a point where the two limbs lie in approximately the same 180-degree plane. In flexion, however, the two limbs can be brought into contact with each other. The mechanical limit to movement of the arm is a bony one, whereas that limiting extension of the mandible upon the cranium (opening of the jaws) is primarily ligamental.

In the case of either flexion or extension, one arm of the leverage system must be stabilized (or fixed) while the forces exerted by muscles move the other part (see Fig. 12.1). In the arm the upper portion is habitually fixed upon the pectoral girdle while the lower part moves away from or toward it. In the case of the skull, the cranium is fixed and the mandible is movable. The action of flexor and extensor muscles is complementary in that the highly coordinated action of each is essential for steady movement. If a movable bone is to be fixed in a given position, the reciprocal action of the antagonist muscles is required. The horizontal movable arm is a lever of Class 3, and since point *X* travels a greater distance than point *Y,* less force is delivered at point *X* than point *Y.* In other words, the greater the distance from the fulcrum of the Class 3 lever, the less will be the force delivered for a given amount of movement of the lever arm.

Leverage and Forces—Fundamental Architecture of the Mandible and the Cranium

There are two major osseous parts functioning in the masticatory system: the cranium and the mandible. The *cranium* is the static part. It consists of relatively thin, curved, continuous walls with bony buttresses that appear to be placed in the tracks of maximal support and force transduction. The "hemispherical" shape of the neurocranium and the compartmentalized cell-like structure of the attached viscerocranium make the total cranium very rigid and resistant to deformation or fracture. Forces transmitted to the upper dental arch by means of occlusal activity tend to follow the tracts of support until they fade and dissi-

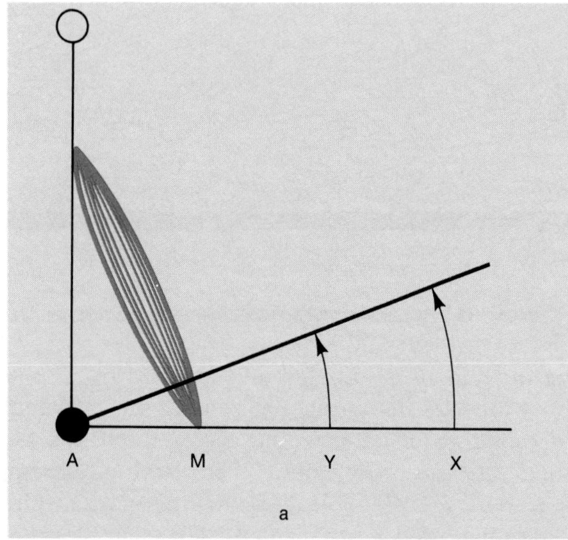

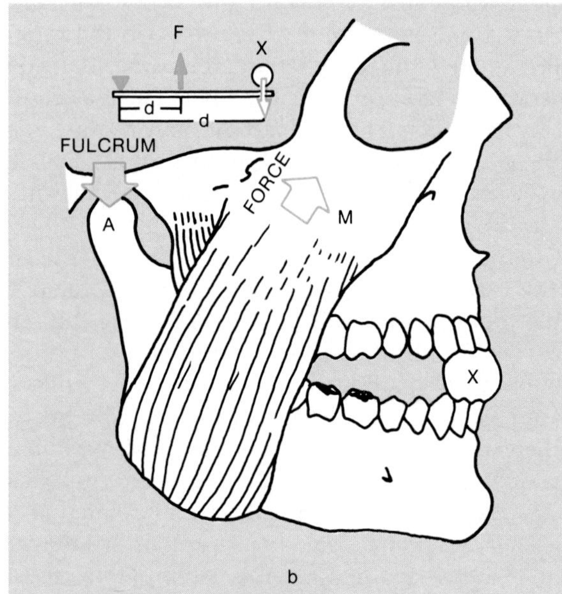

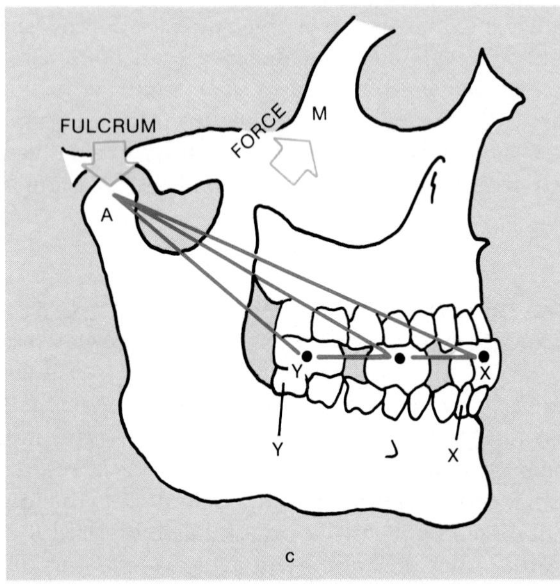

pate. The single-rooted teeth in the anterior part of the dental arch and the buccal roots of the molar teeth apparently lead the forces primarily along the outer walls of the facial cranium and the cranial vault. The palatal roots lead the forces primarily along inner walls and the hard palate (Fig. 12.2). All of the roots are placed in an oblique direction. The upper dental arch represents the relatively stable part of the functioning system like an anvil that is being hit by the hammer.

The *mandible* is the mobile part of the system and its primary purpose is to carry and move the lower dental arch. Leverage and force transmission are the most obvious functions of this heavy, thick-walled, horseshoe-shaped bone. The central part of the mandible is situated around the mandibular canal and protects essential structures such as the mandibular nerve and the corresponding vessels. The entrance to the canal (mandibular foramen) is located at the zone of minimal mandibular movement during habitual opening. By its location it affords protection to the large nerves and vessels against excessive torque during mandibular function (Fig. 12.3). The right and left central parts are united rigidly at the chin (Fig. 12.3). To these united parts of the mandible are attached the articular, muscular, and alveolar processes. The articular processes, along with the mandibular condyles,

Figure 12.1

a, Application of muscular force at point *M* causes motion around the joint *A*. If the vertical arm is stabilized, and therefore steady, the horizontal arm moves upward. Because of the arrangement of the joint and the insertion of the muscle in *M,* point *X* moves over a greater distance than point *Y*. The force delivered by the horizontal arm at point *Y* is greater than that at point *X*. *b* and *c,* diagrammatic representation of the jaw lever system using the symbols from *a*. Drawn with modification from Silverman, 1961.*

* In the case of the jaw, these figures assume that the articulation functions as a true hinge, which is only true for some functions. Once the mandible moves from this position, e.g., during unilateral biting, it is more correct to consider the mandible as a loaded beam, supported by the bite point and the two condylar heads. Under these conditions, static mechanics become a more appropriate method for analyzing the forces involved, and suggest that forces on the condylar heads may be asymmetrical. Consequently, in unilateral molar biting, it is thought that compressive forces through the working-side articulation are considerably less than those through the nonworking side. During dynamic movements such as those that occur during chewing, force relationships become more complex, since they involve length changes in the muscles and are affected by the velocity of movement.

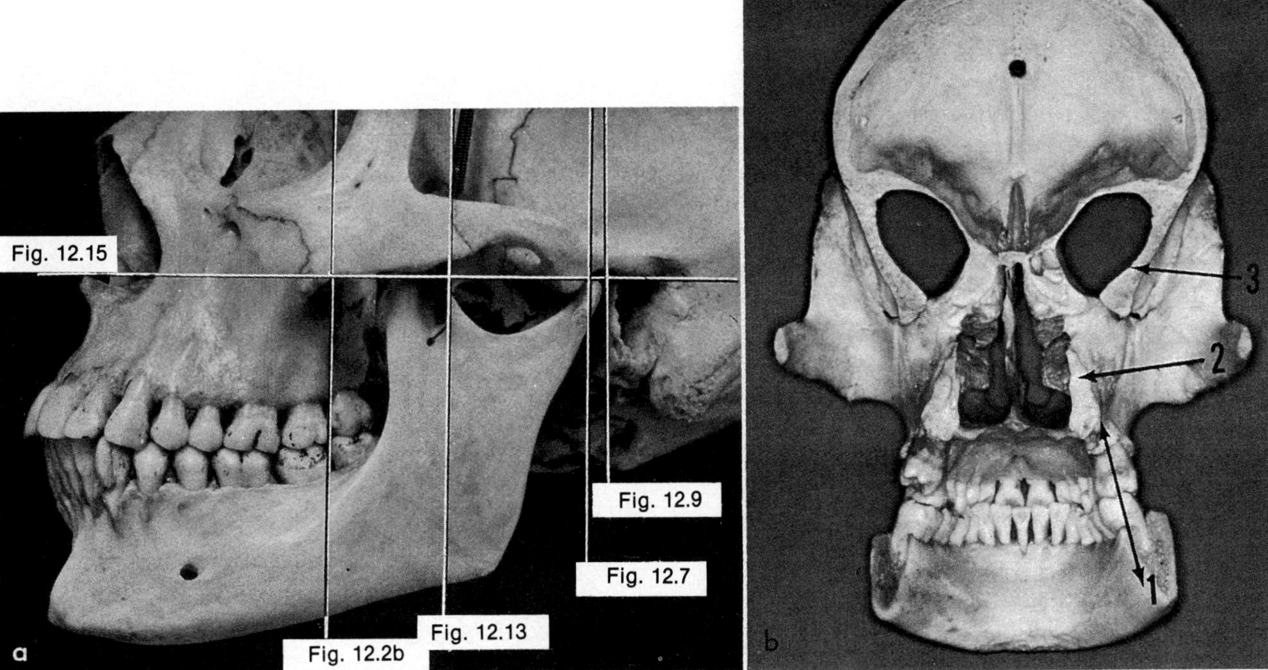

Figure 12.2

a, This plate is to be used to orient the viewer to the plane of the sections of Figures 12.2*b*, 12.7, 12.9, 12.13, and 12.15. *b*, Coronal section through a cranium, frontal part, seen from behind. Note that the general directions of the molars are converging upward medially (*1*). Note also the two flying buttresses, the palatal vault (*2*), and the cranial vault (*3*).

are discussed later. Their purpose is to support and stabilize the posterior part of the mandible during functional movements. The larger muscular processes (the coronoid processes and the angles of the mandible) serve as insertion areas for the powerful temporal, medial pterygoid, and masseter muscles. Many other somewhat less marked bony sites of muscle insertions are also found on the mandible. Among these are the pterygoid fovea below the condyle (for insertion of the lateral pterygoid muscle), the digastric fossae and the mental spines (for insertion of the digastric, genioglossal, and geniohyoid muscles), and the mylohyoid lines (for insertion for the mylohyoid muscle).

The alveolar process carries the dental arch. Unlike the other processes of the mandible, the alveolar process is formed along with the development of teeth and will disappear if the teeth are lost. The arch of the alveolar process is somewhat more constricted in the molar region than that of the mandibular corpus (Fig. 12.4). This permits the mandibular molar teeth to come into full occlusion with the opposing teeth, and still provide sufficient space for those structures which normally reside under the so-called molar shelf, such as the base of the tongue, the suprahyoid muscles, and the salivary glands (Fig. 12.4).

The apices of the molar root are related to the shape of the shelf and are placed buccal to the crowns

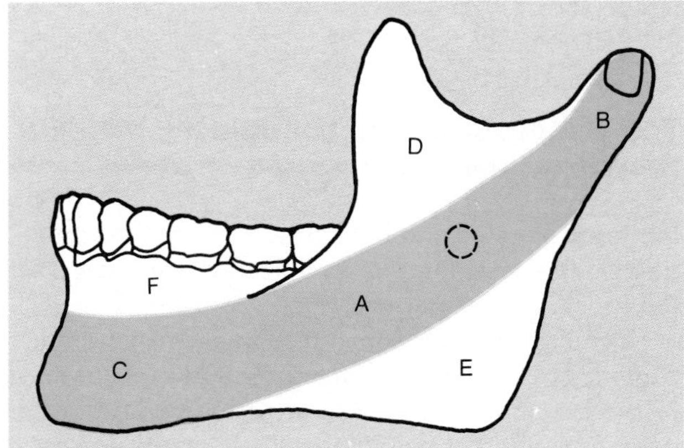

Figure 12.3

Functional zones of the mandible: *A*, protection of nerves and vessels; *B*, articular process; *C*, connection of the two mandibular halves; *D* and *E*, muscular processes; *F*, dental (alveolar) process

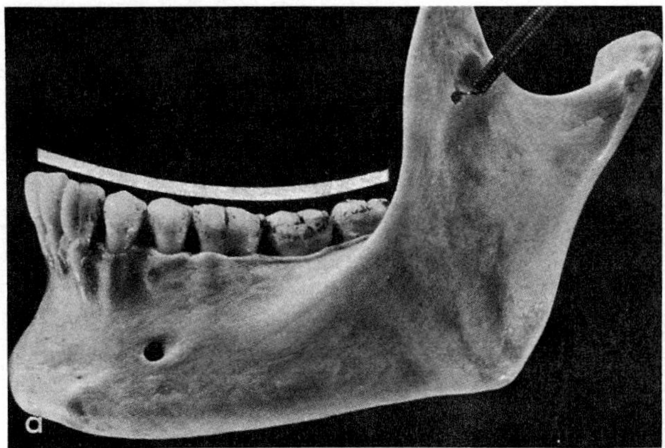

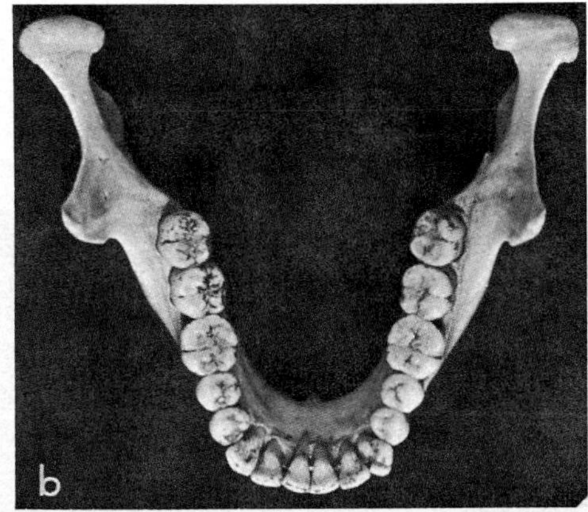

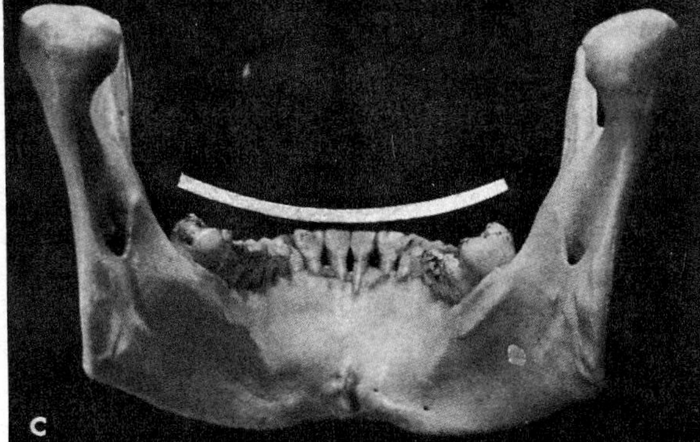

Figure 12.4
The mandible seen from the side (*a*), from above (*b*), and from behind (*c*). Note the occlusal curve and the molar shelf and the processes mentioned in Fig. 12.20.

so that the long axes of the teeth almost resemble the direction of an upward-inward swing of the mandible in chewing (see Fig. 12.2*b*).

The functional implications of the horizontal and the vertical bends of the mandibular bone not only require that both sides function simultaneously, but also that adequate room for both the tongue and its associated structures as well as for the passage lines of air, food, blood supply to the brain, and so on, be maintained. It also provides the mandible with a certain measurable elasticity. In wide opening movements when both lateral pterygoid muscles are most active, the mandibular and thus also the dental arch is narrowed. The deformation amounts to around 0.05 to 0.10 mm in the molar region (Osborne, 1961). The elasticity of the mandible, like that of the long tubular bones, probably provides a buffer effect against the action of sudden external or muscular forces.

The Temporomandibular Joints—Movable Stabilizers

Joints are situated and built so as to permit the movements, leverage, and/or stabilization necessary for the function to be performed.

People who for some reason lack mandibular condyles can move their mandible and execute most of the jaw movements to be described. However, if precise or forceful mandibular movements are to be performed, the mandible must be stabilized by means of joints. Equalized stabilization without excessive muscular work, and the ability to perform almost identical movement of the right and left side of the jaw, as in symmetrical jaw movements, call for two joints. The joints are arranged bilaterally at each end of the mandible, and are capable of being moved in a well-coordinated, asymmetrical fashion. People with only one functioning temporomandibular joint can still perform most mandibular movements. But in such persons the jaw muscles have to stabilize the mandible in an attempt to substitute for the missing joint. This sometimes leads to a disharmonious function.

Since the mandible can perform opening-closing, protrusive-retrusive, lateral movements, and combinations thereof, each joint must be capable of both *rotatory* and *translatory* movements. In *sym-*

metrical movements (opening-closing or protrusive-retrusive movements), the two joints perform almost identical movements simultaneously. In *asymmetrical* movements (lateral and lateral protrusive movements) the two joints still function simultaneously, but the rotatory and translatory movements are not in phase; in other words, they are performed at different times and in different combinations and magnitudes at the two sides.

The location and the shape of the temporomandibular joints comply with this rather complicated functional scheme. As in other mammals that can perform horizontal jaw movements, the joints are situated above and behind the dental arches, on the right and left border of the cranial base, and somewhat in front of the cervical spine.

If the two joints had to perform only identical and simultaneous movements, the articular surfaces on the cranial and mandibular sides could have direct contact with, and fit exactly against, each other. However, when asymmetrical movements are carried out, the movements of the *working* (ipsilateral) condyle are small and take place "on the spot," whereas the nonworking (contralateral) condyle usually performs more pronounced movements while shifting its place in the articular compartment. When, for example, a mandibular movement to the left is performed, the left condyle (working condyle) may move slightly, sliding laterally, turning to the left, and rotating forward. At the same time the right condyle (nonworking condyle) moves anteriorly downward and medially, and also rotates at the same time. In movements to the right the roles of the condyles are reversed. Thus, in order that there be no interference with the movements of the bony parts of the joints, they must not fit tightly to each other. It is, therefore, characteristic of the temporomandibular joints that the articular surfaces are incongruous and that the necessary articular contact and stabilization in any position are established by a flexible articular disc of fibrous tissue, the meniscus, which fits in between the mandibular condyle and the glenoid fossa.

The Mandibular Condyle

The ascending ramus of the mandible extends upward to form two processes—a coronoid process anteriorly, and a condylar process posteriorly. The latter terminates in an oblong condyle, 15 to 20 mm in mediolateral and 8 to 10 mm in anteroposterior dimensions. The posterior aspect is rounded and convex, whereas the anteroinferior aspect is concave (fovea pterygoidea). Medially and laterally the condyle terminates in somewhat pointed areas, the poles. Although the lateral pole is only slightly prominent, the medial pole extends well beyond the neck of the condyle and is positioned more posteriorly (Fig. 12.4*b*). A line drawn through the two poles of the condyle will extend in a rather horizontal direction medially and posteriorly toward the anterior border of the foramen magnum, where it meets the corresponding line from the other side. These lines are approximately parallel with lines that connect the corresponding buccal and lingual cusps of the premolar and molar teeth.

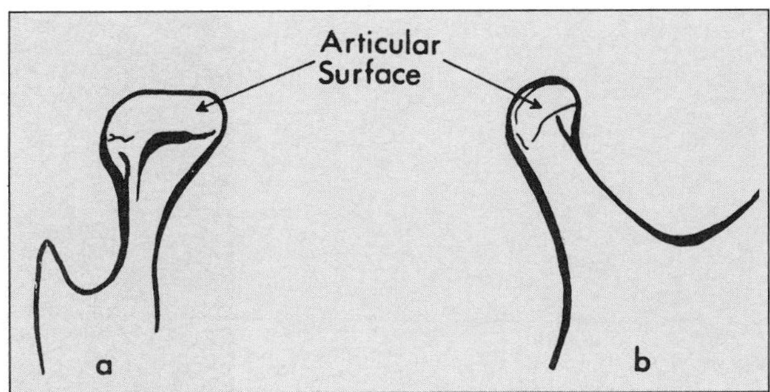

Figure 12.5
Sketch of a right condyle as seen from the front (*a*) and the right side (*b*). Note the articular surface.

The articular surface of the condyle resembles to a certain degree a date stone. It is slightly convex anteroposteriorly, and mediolaterally it is either rather straight or somewhat convex. Sometimes it has a shorter lateral and longer medial part separated by a short, rounded ridge or, occasionally, by a shallow groove. The articular surface is directed forward and upward, and its posterior margin is usually the most superior point on the mandible. The articular surfaces of both the condyle and fossa are covered with an avascular fibrous tissue containing a small number of cartilage cells (Fig. 12.5). This is the only movable joint with articular surfaces not covered by hyaline cartilage, apparently indicating that the temporomandibular joints are not static weight-bearing structures. Instead, they are adapted to shifting vectors of force, such as in chewing. Throughout life the shape of the condyle may undergo changes, some of which are related to changes in mandibular function and occlusion.

The Cranial Articular Surface

The cranial articular surface of the joint is situated on the inferior side of the temporal bone just anterior to the tympanic bone and posterior to the root of the zygomatic process (Fig. 12.6). It consists of a posterior depression (the articular, or glenoid, fossa) and an anterior eminence (the articular tubercle or gle-

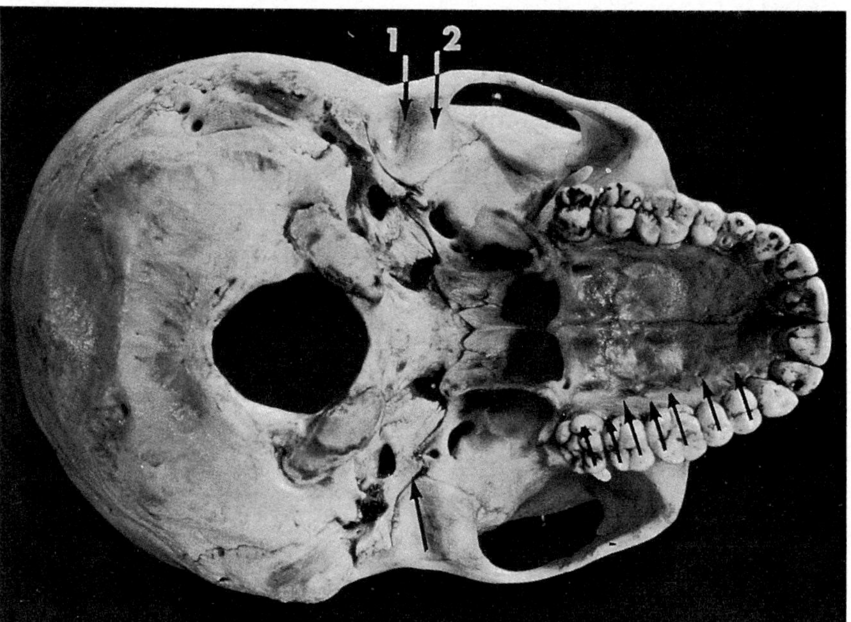

Figure 12.6

Inferior view of the cranium. Note the upper dental arch, the bony palate, the external cranial base, the right and the left fossa mandibularis (*1*) and the tuberculum articulare (*2*). Also note the coincidence between the mediolateral direction of the fossae and lines connecting the buccal and the corresponding lingual cusps of premolars and molars of the same side (*arrows*).

noid eminence). The articular fossa is a vault, concave in both the mediolateral and anteroposterior directions. It is oblong mediolaterally and the direction of its long axis resembles that of the condyle. The roof of the fossa is very thin, indicating that the role of this part of the joint is rather passive. The deeper part of the fossa apparently acts more or less as a bed for the thicker posterior part of the articular disc when it is resting in its most posterior position. The articular surface proper is the posterior and inferior part of the articular eminence, which is a roll of bone, more or less steep in its posterior slope, with an anteroposterior curvature of variable constricture. The transition from the articular eminence to the infratemporal surface of the cranial base is gradual.

It has already been pointed out that the cranial and mandibular surfaces of the joints are not congruent. They do not touch each other even when the teeth are in intercuspal contact. The distance from the articular surface of the condyle to the opposing cranial surface is greater medially than laterally. The space between these two surfaces is filled by the articular disc (Fig. 12.7).

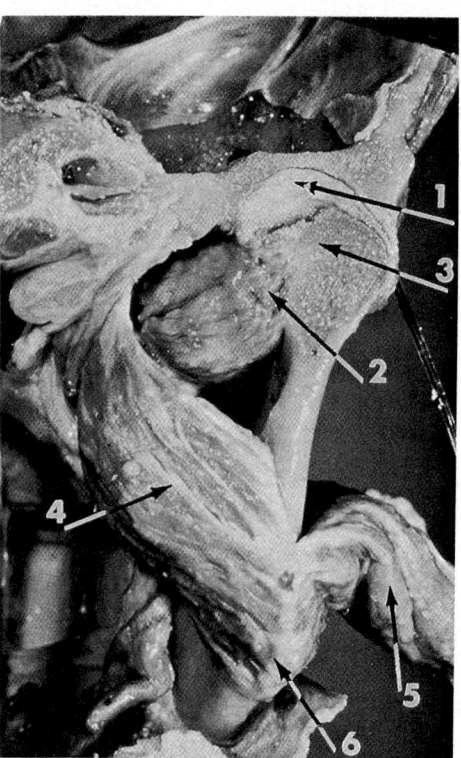

Figure 12.7

The right temporomandibular joint from behind. The joint is opened by a vertical pole-to-pole section of the condyle. Note the position of the disc (*1*). The disc is thicker medially than laterally. Also note the inferior part of the lateral pterygoid muscle (2) inserting on the condyle (*3*). The medial pterygoid (*4*) and the masseter muscles (*5*) form a muscular sling around the angle of the mandible (*6*). (Courtesy of Dr. P. A. Knutsen.)

The Articular Disc

The most important functional demand placed upon the articular disc is that it must change its position and its shape in such a way that it can fill the space between the bony articular surfaces and stabilize the posterior part of the mandible during any phase of mandibular movement.

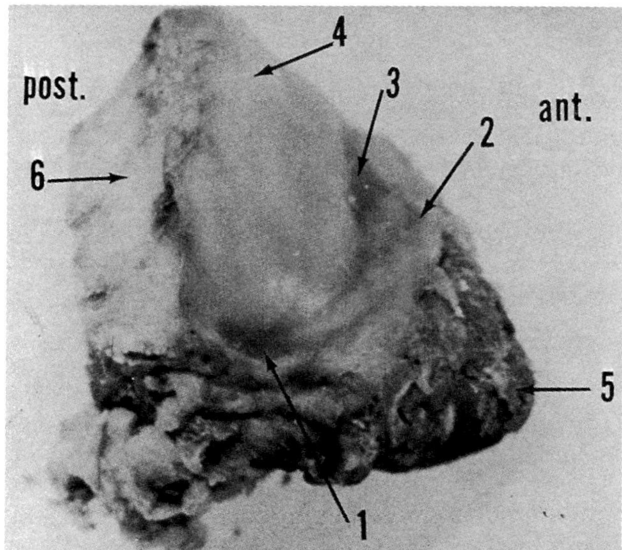

Figure 12.8

A right articular disc seen from the right side and somewhat from above and behind. Note the shiny rectangular disc with the downward bending triangular lateral flap (*1*). There is an anterior band (*2*), an intermediate zone (*3*), and a posterior band (*4*). Anteriorly (ant.), parts of the lateral pterygoid muscle (*5*), and posteriorly (post.), parts of the bilaminar zone (*6*) are seen.

Seen from above, the disc is oval or somewhat rectangular in shape with triangular flaps extending medially and laterally. These flaps are bent downward and attached by their tips to the condyle just below its lateral and medial poles (Figs. 12.7 and 12.8).

The posterior half of the disc is rather thick (posterior band). A thinner, flexible central portion, the intermediate zone, extends between the flaps; anterior to it, the disc is somewhat thicker although not as thick as in the posterior part (the anterior band) (Fig. 12.8). The disc is, as a whole, thicker medially than laterally in conformity with the configuration of the space between the bony articular surfaces.

The attachment of the disc to the condyle below the lateral and medial poles is such that it can move or slide passively forward or backward over the condyle like a bonnet can be pushed back and forth over the head. In addition, because of the relatively long flaps, the disc is able to twist slightly on top of the condyle. Such micromovements are necessary if the disc is to be able to slide between and contact the temporal and mandibular articular surfaces evenly in any position. The surfaces of the disc are very smooth, minimizing the amount of friction between the disc and the articular surfaces. Because the disc consists of fibrous tissue it is somewhat flexible. Flexibility is further enhanced by the shape of the disc itself. If the disc, in its anteroposterior movement, had to slide around a cylinder it would not be necessary for it to change its shape. However, since the shape of the articular eminence only roughly resembles a cylinder and the disc is somewhat twisted in asymmetrical movements of the mandible, it is mechanically essential that the disc be able to change its shape slightly. It can, in fact, do this because the thinner intermediate zone, which runs from flap to flap, permits the disc to become flatter, more curved, or even twisted as necessary to fill the articular space.

The Joint Capsule

The capsule surrounding the joint is like a rather loose cuff, wide at the cranial base and tapering toward the mandibular neck (Fig. 12.9). Fibers from the anterior and posterior edges of the disc mingle with fibers from the capsule; thus, upper and lower compartments of the joint are formed (Fig. 12.10). It is

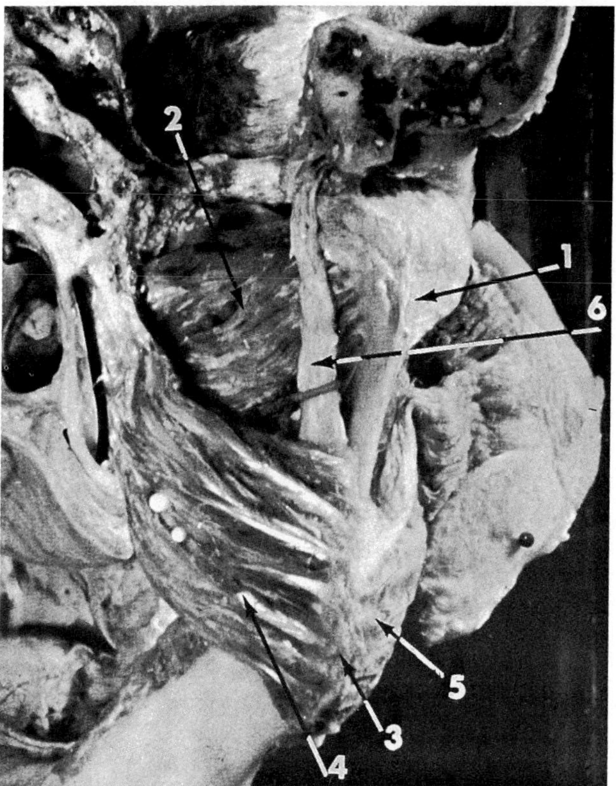

Figure 12.9

A right temporomandibular joint with joint capsule (*1*) from behind. Note the lateral pterygoid muscle (*2*) and the muscle sling around the angle of the mandible (*3*) composed of the medial pterygoid (*4*) and masseter (*5*) muscles downward on the medial side of the joint and the lateral pterygoid (*2*). (Courtesy of Dr. P. A. Knutsen.)

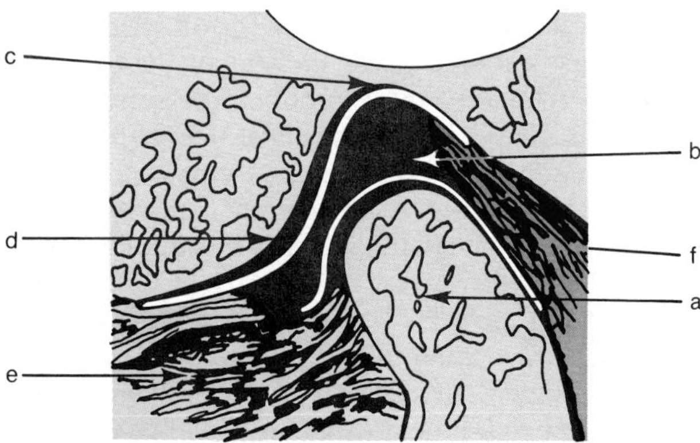

Figure 12.10

Sketch of the temporomandibular joint structures as seen in an almost sagittal section: *a*, condyle; *b*, disc; *c*, mandibular fossa, *d*, tuberculum articulare; *e*, lateral pterygoid; *f*, bilaminar zone. The white lines on either side of the disc represent the upper and lower compartments.

important to realize that only the edges of the medial and lateral flaps are attached to the capsular cuff so that the upper compartment has a recess medially and laterally corresponding to the flaps (see Fig. 12.7); otherwise the micromovements of the disc would be limited or not possible. The upper compartment extends forward below the eminence so that the disc can slide into this area and support the condyle in the extreme opening position. The condyle, in extreme opening, is situated inferiorly and at times slightly anteriorly to the most inferior part of the eminence. At the same time the condyle rotates forward on the inferior side of the disc, so that the disc seems to slide backward over the condyle like a bonnet being pushed back onto the neck. To permit this, the lower compartment has to extend considerably downward on the posterior side of the condyle. The disc is attached at its posterior border to a layer of highly vascular, cushion-like loose connective tissue that is covered with synovial membrane on both the superior and inferior sides. This tissue is collectively referred to as the *bilaminar zone* (Rees, 1954). Being attached, it follows the moving disc, filling the empty space which would otherwise be created by the moving condyle.

It should be realized that the excursions of both condyle and disc are very short in most of the usual mandibular movements. Only in extreme opening, lateral, or protrusive movements of the mandible do the condyle and disc make pronounced excursions. In such situations the movements of the disc may not necessarily be in phase with those of the condyle. For example, in the case of a steep articular eminence, the condyle moves in the opening movement by first rotating and sliding slightly anteriorly on the inferior side of the disc. Then, at the point where the capsular and temporomandibular ligaments are taut, the condyle starts sliding forward, and the disc is drawn out of its bed forward between the eminence and the condyle.

The movements of the disc within the articular space are generally passive, i.e., not caused by direct muscular activity. All the articulating surfaces of the joint, including those of the disc, are very smooth, are lubricated by synovial fluid, and show inclined planes of varying steepness. The shape of the space between the cranial and the mandibular surfaces of the joint is changed as soon as the condyle is moved. Because of the slippery surfaces and its flexibility the disc will passively shift into that site where it fits the best, i.e., where it has maximum contact with the articular surfaces of the joint and where it can offer the best support for the condyle.

In those positions or movements where muscular stabilization of the mandible is needed, e.g., when biting on a nut or when only a few anterior teeth contact as is sometimes seen in brushing the teeth, it may be necessary for the disc to be held or stabilized in position somewhat forward on the posterior slope of the articular eminence. This is accomplished by contraction of the upper portion of the lateral pterygoid muscle, which is attached to the anterior part of the joint capsule and to the articular disc. Upon relaxation of the upper lateral pterygoid muscle the disc can again slide passively in the articular compartment, and take the position where it fits the best. This probably accounts for the fact that there are no other muscles attached to the articular disc.

When the disc is stabilized in the posterior part of the articular fossa, the condyle can slide a little laterally on its lower slippery surface. When this happens as part of a lateral mandibular glide, the movement component is known as the *Bennett movement*.

To summarize, in movement of the mandible the disc moves passively and freely into the momentary space between the temporal and mandibular surfaces of the joint. Only when the disc stabilizes the mandible does it need support by a forward pull of the upper lateral pterygoid muscle. Although some fibers of the superior lateral pterygoid muscle insert into the disc, most fuse with those of the inferior head and insert into the fovea of the condylar neck. The anterior part of the disc is considered to be attached to the top of the superior lateral pterygoid, much like a foot resting on the pavement, and may have connective tissue attachments binding muscle to disc. It is reasonable to postulate that activity in the superior lateral pterygoid may be responsible for stabilizing

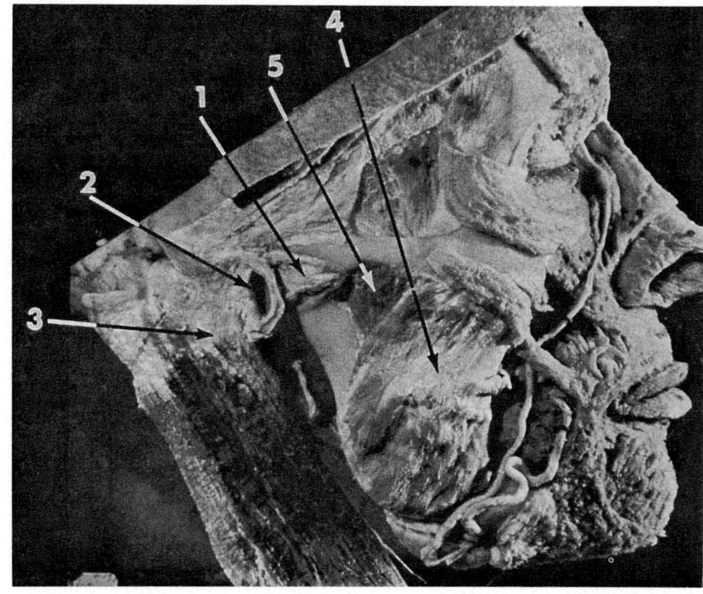

Figure 12.11

Skull from the side. Note the joint capsule (*1*) just in front of the external acoustic meatus (*2*). Behind this opening is the insertion of the sternocleidomastoid muscle (*3*). Note the direction of the masseter muscle (outer layer) (*4*). Just in front of the temporomandibular joint a small triangle of the upper dorsal part of the medial layer of the masseter muscle is seen (*5*). (Courtesy of Dr. P. A. Knutsen.)

the articular disc. The disc is spacefilling, stabilizing, and able to perform micromovements.

The Capsular Ligaments

The joint capsules are reinforced laterally and medially by means of fibrous strands. The lateral reinforcement is the stronger and thicker and takes the character of a ligament (the temporomandibular ligament). It is fan-shaped, broad on the zygomatic arch, and narrow in its insertion on the neck of the mandible (Fig. 12.11). When the mandible is retruded, the anterior part of the ligament is drawn taut and so are the more horizontal fibers in the medial capsular wall (Aarstad, 1954). The condyles are thus prevented from being displaced further backward than the taut ligaments allow. During the initial phase of an opening movement the anterior part of the ligament first becomes taut because its point of insertion on the neck of the mandible is swinging backward. When it is taut the neck cannot move further back, and thus the condyle has to move forward and downward, sliding on the disc and the articular eminence. This is the reason for the forward bend of the lower part of the retruded opening border movement (see Fig. 12.18*b*). In the meantime, the tension passes over the ligament to the posterior fibers as well, and the mandibular point of insertion of the ligament thus acts as a sling for some of the swinging movements of the mandible.

The capsular ligaments also prevent the condyle from performing excessive lateral movements. Further, the joint capsules and the capsular ligaments play an important role in the nervous coordination of the movements, postures, and positioning of the mandible, containing as they do numerous sites of proprioceptors.

The Jaw Muscles

Any single action of the mandible is the product of the closely integrated and highly coordinated performance of several jaw muscles.* It should also be realized that coordinated efforts on the part of the postcervical muscles are necessary to stabilize the cranium against mandibular movements. Muscles can be part of several movement patterns, and any single muscle can participate in several different activities. This is the case, for example, when homologous muscles on either side are synergists in a symmetrical movement, and antagonists in an asymmetrical movement (see Fig. 12.19). None of the jaw muscles is arranged in the line of movement. All are at oblique angles to the resulting force or movement.

In the masticatory system muscles are needed to (1) elevate the mandible as in closing movements, (2) depress the mandible as in opening movements, (3) protrude the mandible, (4) retrude the mandible, and (5) perform lateral movements. But one should never forget that the real movements are always complex patterns in which many of the single movements are combined and that a classification like the above is oversimplified.

*By "jaw muscles" we mean all muscles that arise from or insert in the mandible and that contribute to the movement of the mandible.

The Elevator Muscles

The elevator muscles include the two masseter muscles, the two medial (internal) pterygoid muscles, and the two temporal muscles (especially their anterior parts). The masseter and medial pterygoid muscles form sling in which the gonial angle of the mandible rests. Both muscles exert similar forces upon the mandible, the former inserting on the external surface of the angle, the latter on the internal. Acting synergistically, as they must, they are the primary closing muscles, and hence effect lateral stabilization of the mandible. The direction of the fibers of both muscles is roughly perpendicular to the occlusal plane when the mandible is open.

If a transverse line were constructed passing through the two mandibular foramina it would describe an axis about which the mandible rotates during *habitual* opening and closing movements. In other words, the portion of the ramus in the immediate area of the foramen is that part of the mandible that moves the least. The transverse axis also passes through the approximate center of the masseter and medial pterygoid muscles. For this reason the change in length of the muscles is minimal during opening and closing activities of the mandible. The masseter muscle is described as multipennate, broad in cross-section, with limited possibilities for elongation, but great potential for powerful contraction. The masseter has several overlapping layers in its posterior, superficial part, but can be broadly described as being composed primarily of deep and superficial parts, each with strong phylogenetic links. The fibers of the outer layer run downward and backward from their origin on the zygomatic arch. Those of the inner layer are more vertically directed (Fig. 12.12). The two layers have the capacity to act at different degrees of mandibular opening, depending upon which layer is fully or partially activated. This in turn, is correlated with the degree of mandibular opening. Since this process occurs in a continuous gradient, a smooth mandibular movement results.

The medial pterygoid muscle is also multipennate. Like the masseter, this is a quadrate-shaped muscle, although it has a smaller cross-sectional area. This implies that it produces less force than the masseter. The multiplicity of its fiber directions and its pronounced anterior and lateromedial lines of action make this muscle particularly suited to actions such as the power-stroke of mastication, which requires a strong, medially directed component of force on the mandible. Together, the medial pterygoid muscles and the temporal muscles are responsible for postural movements and the maintenance of jaw posture. Working as a unit, the two medial pterygoids have a considerable influence on jaw movement in the horizontal plane. Acting together they effect protrusion and elevation; acting unilaterally they produce lateral movement with a strong elevating component.

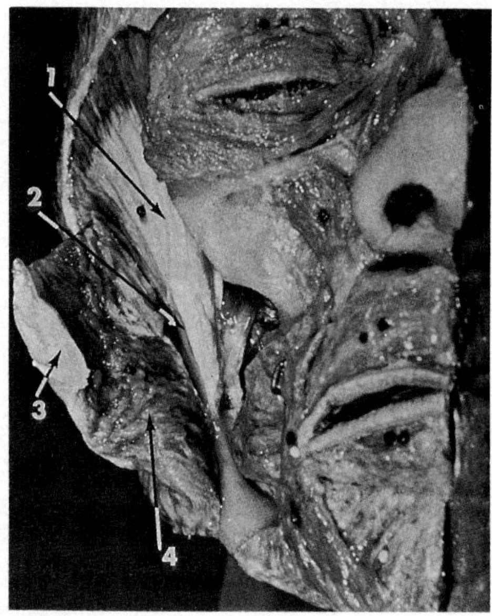

Figure 12.12

The white tendon of the temporal muscle (*1*) inserts on the coronoid process of the mandible (*2*). The zygomatic bone is cut and turned laterally to make the tendon visible (*3*). Note the medial side of the masseter muscle (*4*). (Courtesy of Dr. P. A. Knutsen.)

The temporal muscle is fan-shaped. Functionally it acts like two muscles: the anterior part as an elevator muscle and the posterior part as a retruding muscle. If the muscular activity runs over the entire muscle from the anterior to the posterior fibers, the resultant direction of traction will mimic the upward swing described by the coronoid process of the mandible during mandibular closure. Therefore, if the activity of the temporal muscle spreads from anterior to posterior, an even pull in the closing motion will result.

The temporal muscle is bipennate. An *inner layer* of muscle fibers converges vertically down the lateral wall of the cranium to a central blade-like tendon, which inserts on the coronoid process and along the anterior edge of the ascending ramus. The *outer layer* descends in a more medial direction arising from the temporal fascia (Fig. 12.13). The action of the anterior part of the muscle results in an upward pull that can direct the mandibular teeth into maximal occlusal contact. As this muscle has comparatively long fibers

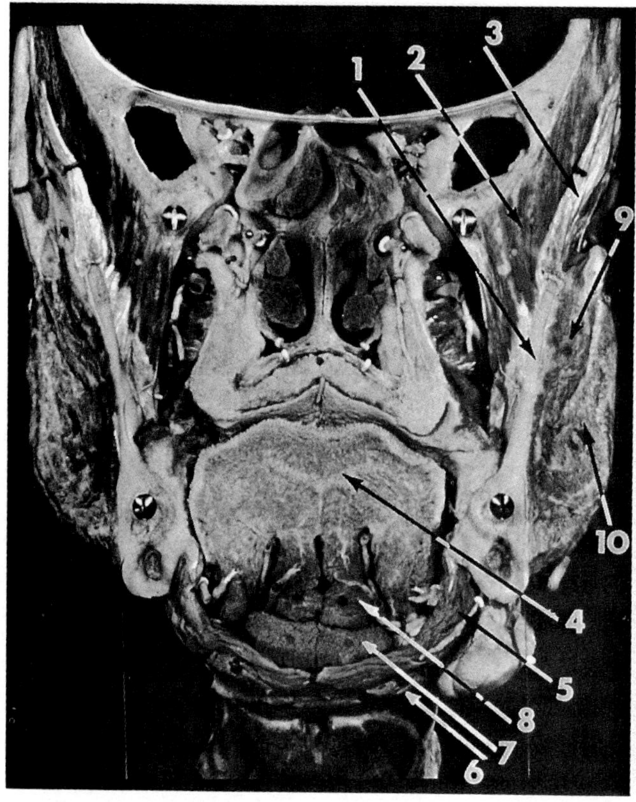

Figure 12.13

Coronal section of the head through the coronoid processes (*1*). Note the direction of the fibers (*2*) and the central fibrous blades (*3*) of the temporalis muscles. Also the tongue (*4*) and the suprahyoidal muscles. The mylohyoid muscle is forming the floor of the mouth (*5*). On the inferior side are flat anterior bellies, of the digastric muscle (*6*). On the superior side are the geniohyoid (*7*) and the genioglossus muscles (*8*). On the lateral side of the ascending rami sections through the masseter muscles (*9*) the parotid gland (*10*) can be observed. (Courtesy of Dr. P. A. Knutsen.)

it can also be active as an elevator when the person is biting a large bolus of food.

All the jaw closing muscles are supplied with muscle spindles and are presumed to have tendon organs as well. This contrasts with the jaw opening muscles, including the lateral pterygoid muscles, which for practical purposes are virtually devoid of spindles. Aside from the fact that the elevator muscles all demonstrate stretch reflexes that result in jaw closing, the presence of muscle spindles, with the gamma motor innervation that accompanies them, provides the jaw elevator muscles with a control system that is well suited for the maintenance of jaw posture and the generation of finely graded bite forces.

The Protruder and Retruder Muscles

The lateral (external) pterygoid muscle consists of a small upper and a large lower head (Fig. 12.14). The lower head arises from the lateral lamina of the pterygoid process and inserts in the pterygoid fovea on the neck of the mandible. Its orientation (at approximately right angles to the condylar head) is such that it effects at once a downward, forward, and medial movement of the condyle (Fig. 12.15).

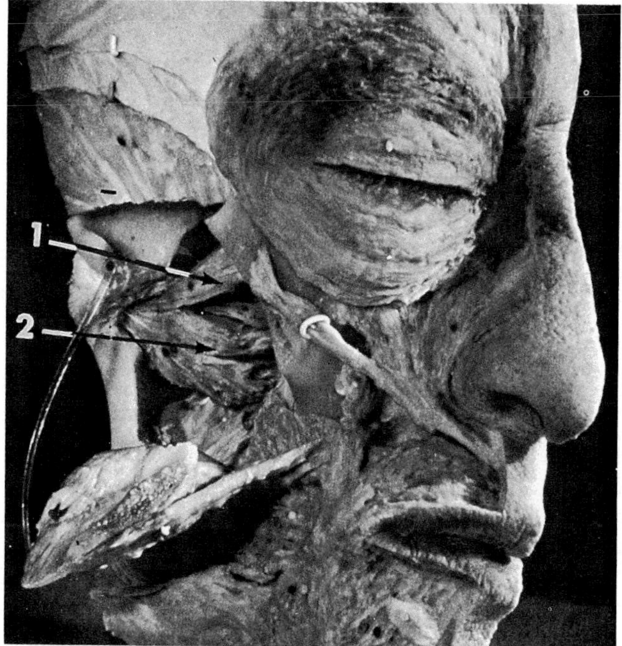

Figure 12.14

The upper (*1*) and lower heads (*2*) of the lateral pterygoid muscle. (Courtesy of Dr. P. A. Knutsen.)

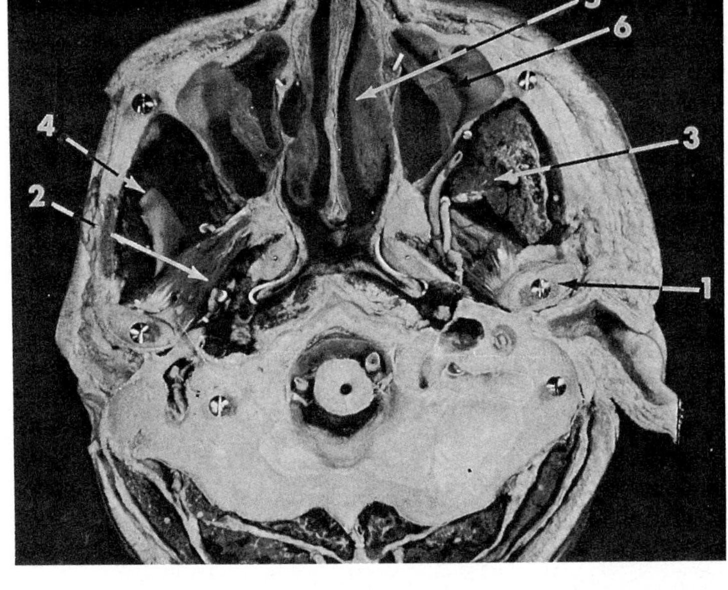

Figure 12.15

Horizontal section of the head through the condyles (*1*). Note the condylar heads (marked by screw heads). The lateral pterygoid muscles (*2*) are directed forward medially and backward laterally and insert on the medial anterior side of the condyles. On the right side a horizontal cut through the temporal muscle is seen (*3*). On the left side the coronoid process is visible (*4*). Note also the nasal cavity (*5*) and the maxillary sinus (*6*) on both sides. (Courtesy of Dr. P. A. Knutsen.)

The upper head may be, as mentioned earlier, a stabilizer of the articular disc in protrusive or lateral positions of the mandible. The combined pull of the right and left muscles will move the condyles in an anterior direction. Thus, simultaneous action of both lateral pterygoid muscles and the elevator muscles results in protrusion of the mandible. Simultaneous action of the posterior temporal elevator muscles results in retrusion of the mandible (Figs. 12.16 and 12.19).

The Depressor Muscles

These muscles are active in mandibular opening. Functionally they comprise the lateral pterygoid and digastric muscles as well as other suprahyoid muscles. The combined forward pull of the two lateral pterygoid muscles and the backward-downward pull of the anterior bellies of the two digastric and other suprahyoid muscles rotate the mandible around a movable "axis," which passes through an area around the mandibular foramina during "free" opening and clos-

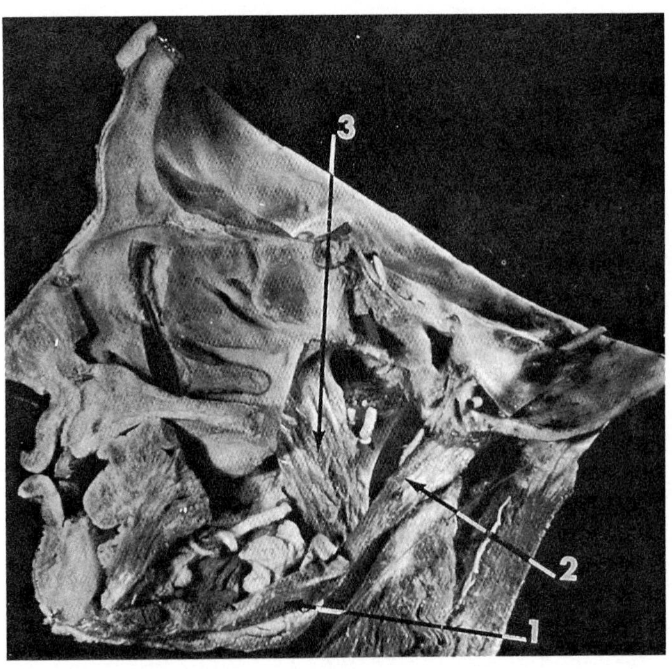

Figure 12.16

Sagittal section of the head showing the anterior (*1*) and the posterior belly (*2*) of digastric muscle. Note also the medial pterygoid muscle (*3*). (Courtesy of Dr. P. A. Knutsen.)

ing movements (Fig. 12.16). If, however, the posterior temporal muscles and the posterior bellies of the digastric muscles act concomitantly as retractors, the pull of the suprahyoid muscles causes a retruded opening movement, provided that the infrahyoid muscles stabilize the hyoid bone (Fig. 12.16).

Muscles That Cause Lateral Movements

Lateral "border" movements are produced by the combined action of the elevator, the retruder on the working side (posterior temporal), and the contralateral protruder (lateral pterygoid) of the nonworking side. Lateral movements combined with protrusion (*lateral protrusive* movements) require an even more complex pattern of muscular activity. An oblique shift of the mandible to a right lateral protrusive contact position is caused when elevator muscles, in conjunction with protruders of the left side, and to a certain degree of the right, act as the prime movers. At the same time the depressors and retruders of the left side, and to a more pronounced degree, those of the right side, hold back or stabilize the moving mandible. It should be noted that the protruders and retruders are grossly parallel and that their anteroposterior direction is not sagittal but oblique from medial to lateral so that they have an optimal direction of action in the unilateral action of the lateral swing. In Figure 12.19 it can easily be seen that the protruders and retruders have to be prime movers and stabilizers respectively in all combined lateral movements, be they border movements or intermediate movements.

In summarizing, several of the jaw muscles have two components, e.g., the masseter, temporal, lateral pterygoid, and digastric muscles. Besides having specific functions they have slightly different directions of contraction so that they can always act optimally no matter what the conditions. Acting in concert the various components of these muscles produce smooth, coordinated movements.

Neuromuscular Control of the Jaw Muscles

Collectively, the jaw muscles are responsible for complex movements of the mandible and for the generation of high bite forces between the teeth. Adequate control of both functions requires a comprehensive and sensitive system for signalling relevant information from the periphery. This information is used to modulate ongoing functions, and contributes to memory and learning. A very precise method for regulating muscle contraction is also required. Many muscles are involved, and each has a unique line of action. Theoretically they can be activated in various combinations, and if multipennate or layered, single muscles can be activated differentially.

There are many sources of feedback from peripheral mechanoreceptors. The most important of these include the mucosal, gingival, periodontal, periosteal, sutural, and articular receptors, as well as the specialized endings within the jaw-closing muscles, namely the muscle spindles and Golgi tendon organs. Information concerned with jaw movement is predominantly signalled by articular receptors, the majority of which are located in the posterolateral part of the capsule, and by receptors in the jaw muscles including the muscle spindles. Information about bite force is probably relayed by regional nerve endings around the teeth involved, e.g., by the gingival, periodontal, periosteal, and possibly by more distant sutural receptors, and by tension-sensing tendon organs in the muscles responsible for generating the bite force. All these mechanoreceptor fields contain endings variously able to signal the magnitude, rate of change, and direction of the stimulus concerned, whether this be movement or force.

Peripheral information is relayed by the trigeminal afferent system to the trigeminal nuclei in the brain stem. From here it travels along thalamocortical paths to be used in the perception of jaw position, jaw movement, and tooth force. The brain stem nuclei, however, are also responsible for segmental reflexes and for a significant amount of sensorimotor integration.

The two primary brain stem reflexes are the jaw-closing reflex and the jaw-opening reflex. The jaw-closing reflex is a simple stretch reflex mediated by the muscle spindles in the jaw-closing muscles. It is relayed by the mesencephalic trigeminal nucleus and is monosynaptic. It is evoked by transient, downward movement of the mandible, e.g., by a menton tap. Its primary function seems to be to provide postural stiffness to the lower jaw during whole-head movements of the kind that occur during locomotion. The jaw-opening reflex is equivalent to the flexion-withdrawal reflex of the limbs. It is mediated via the main sensory and spinal trigeminal nuclei and is polysynaptic. It is evoked by intraoral and perioral mechanical and noxious stimulation, and results in rapid, transient jaw opening. Consequently it is considered a protective or avoidance reflex. A lateral jaw reflex allied with the jaw-opening reflex has been reported in experimental animals, but not in man. Here, a sharp tap to the teeth results in horizontal jaw movement to the contralateral side.

A jaw-unloading reflex also occurs in man, but this is not considered to be a true brain stem reflex since it has a longer latency than the others. It is possibly mediated by muscle spindles as well as other receptor systems influenced by jaw unloading and may be transcortical. Whatever pathway is involved, it is considered to be a long loop. The reflex is evoked by sudden unloading of the jaw-closing muscles, for example when a nut that is being compressed between the teeth suddenly fractures. At this point, bite force ceases and the jaw closes rapidly. Tooth contact is prevented by inhibition of the jaw-closing muscles and, if necessary, by activation of the digastrics. For this reason the reflex is thought to be protective, and probably occurs frequently during the early stages of chewing.

The brain stem also contains an organized collection of neurons, which together form a pattern generator for rhythmic jaw movements of the kind seen in mastication. The rhythmic jaw muscle activity produced here in opposing muscle groups can be triggered by cortical, presumably voluntary drive, or by appropriate peripheral stimulation, e.g., regional intraoral pressure. Thus the brain stem provides an important substrate for the integration of motor and sensory drive.

Many areas above the level of the brain stem are involved in the control of coordinated jaw movement, and many are capable of modulating activity in the brain stem, including its reflexes. Specific regions of the sensorimotor cortex are associated with discrete oral regions and discrete patterns of jaw movement. In addition, recognizable chewing movements can be produced when many parts of the basal ganglia and limbic system are stimulated. Control of the jaw muscles is thought to involve extrapyramidal motor pathways and is exerted bilaterally at all levels in the central nervous system, a feature that is not surprising, given the unique nature of the mandible and the biomechanical need for simultaneous activation of bilateral muscle groups. In this regard the trigeminal motor system is distinctive.

The inherent capacity of the trigeminal motor system for rhythmicity and for patterned, stereotypic muscle contraction as a consequence of extrapyramidal and limbic activation is especially relevant to habitual, rhythmic activities like clenching and toothgrinding. These conditions, which involve extensive muscle use, occlusal wear, and in some cases, articular disorders, are currently thought to be behavioral responses to stress and anxiety.

Neuromuscular Activity upon Assumption of the Intercuspal Contacting Position

The closure of the mandible and the subsequent engagement of the dentition into the intercuspal contacting position involves several physiologic mechanisms. The activity itself can be divided into conscious effort, unconscious effort, and the more complex, all-encompassing, preconscious effort.

The conscious effort is that pattern of activity or behavior of which we are aware. This does not necessitate control. Control comes into play when there is awareness and the possibility of choosing in order to effect a change in the pattern.

The unconscious effort is that pattern of activity or behavior of which we are not aware. Reflexes are good examples. They are automatic and therefore are not under our control. Parafunctional activity (bruxism) is often an unconscious effort.

The preconscious effort lies between conscious and unconscious efforts and involves both aspects. It involves factors of which the individual typically is unaware, but he could become aware of some parts of the mechanism if he turned his attention to it. Mastication is an example of this pattern. Therefore, in this category we have some conscious awareness, some automated unconscious patterns, and varying levels of awareness between the two.

Let us now make a conscious effort to close the mandible and describe the mechanisms involved. The decision to close is made at the highest level of the central nervous system, the cerebral cortex, and the command is relayed down the extrapyramidal tract to the effector muscles, the elevators of the mandible. This conscious decision stimulates a volley of impulses that travel down the motor tracts to the myoneural junction of the effector muscles, the masseters, temporalis, and internal pterygoids.

In order to facilitate the activity of these muscles in elevating the mandible, the mandibular depressors (the infrahyoids and the inferior head of the external pterygoids) are inhibited in their contractile activity. The postcranial stabilizing muscles are also recruited to support the cranium in its postural relation for this activity. This preconscious activity, and quite possibly somewhat involving some unconscious process, gives some idea of the complexity of this seemingly simple physiologic activity.

As the mandible begins to elevate, the condyles begin to alter their spacial relations to the soft tissues, such as the ligaments, and to the joint cavities themselves. Ligaments contain no contractile protein, but still they can and do affect motion. When fibers of a ligament are distended, sensory end-organs lying in juxtaposition to these fibers fire when threshold is reached. Impulses are then relayed along sensory nerve fibers to motor nerves so that the appropriate muscle fibers can contract. This corrects the position of the articulating bone so that the fibers of the offended ligament will not continue to be stretched.

These off-course corrections continue until the inclined planes of the occlusal surfaces of the teeth engage contact and the mandible is further directed toward the position of maximum intercuspation. This new contact recruits the receptors of the periodontal ligament to add further neurologic refinement to the closing pattern.

When the end point (maximum intercuspation) is reached, the isotonic contraction phase of the muscles converts to the isometric contraction phase. Tension builds up in the connective tissue fibers of the tendons of these muscles until the sensory end-organs contained within the tendons, the Golgi tendon organs, reach threshold and exert an inhibitory influence on their respective contracting muscles. This decreases the tension and allows for withdrawal to ready the mechanisms for the next cycle. Concurrently and similarly, the receptors in the periodontal ligaments also fire and participate in the occlusal disengagement process.

All of these activities are monitored and encoded by the central nervous system through feedback mechanisms, thus facilitating a repetition of the activity if needed. If the process is repeated, it need not involve the higher centers as in the initial activity, and motor activity can be continued at a level closer to the effector mechanisms. This will be a more automated and less conscious (possibly unconscious) effort.

The muscle spindles enter the picture, refining the motor activity through the stretch reflex and allowing for less deviation or deflection and more precision in the closure. The occlusal contacts will be closer to the cuspal receiving areas than on the first closure. Special attention ought to be directed to the muscle spindle mechanisms and reflex activity for a clear understanding of muscle contraction.

The muscle spindles lie parallel to the skeletal muscle fibers and, through connective tissue attachments and feedback mechanisms, are capable of monitoring the length of these fibers. The stretch reflex facilitates repetitious movements and refines the motion with each subsequent closure. This activity is automatic and is an unconscious effort.

All of the neural end-organs, including the muscle spindles, the sensory endings in the articular capsules, and the periodontal ligament receptors, aid in sensing the mandible toward the end-point position of maximum intercuspation. This intricate network continually adjusts muscle fiber activity so that the occlusal slide into the end-point position is within the normal (nonpathologic) range. The assumption of this position in the final stage, therefore, is a tooth-guided event and is finalized by the contacting inclined planes of the teeth. The duration of this tooth-guided period has been measured as 3 to 5 msec for normal (nonpathologic) dentitions. In anterior protected occlusions this contact is on the anterior teeth. In group function occlusions the contact is on the posterior teeth on the working side in the lateral return glide and on the anterior teeth during retrusion.

Parafunctional activity (bruxism), such as clenching and grinding, overrides the protective reflexes. These reflexes are therefore suggestive and not obligatory. This is especially true of the periodontal ligament receptors. Their activity "suggests" at an unconscious level, the disengagement of the dentition.

During mastication the presence of the bolus adds another consideration to the final moments of contact. The bolus on the working side can cause a sagittal rotation of the mandible enabling the guiding cusps (the lingual of the lower and the buccal of the upper) to engage in contact prior to any other teeth. The bolus functions as a fulcrum during this motion. This maneuver is possible because of the presence of a space in the joint called the intraborder space. This space exists between the articulating members of the joints. When the tooth surfaces engage in contact, the joints are prevented from reaching extreme or border path relations. The sagittal rotation of the mandible continues, alternating sides until the bolus is reduced and the dentition can enter into the position of maximum intercuspation. As the bolus is reduced, sagittal rotation is gradually decreased and the final closures are similar to the sequence previously described without the presence of the bolus.

To summarize mandibular closure can be divided into the following phases:

1. Initial contraction of the elevator muscles and relaxation of the depressors, and stabilization by the postcranial stabilizers
2. Off-course muscular corrections stimulated by the ligamentous activity of the neuromuscular mechanisms and the muscle spindles
3. Tooth contact on inclined planes directing the mandible toward the position, and the recruitment and refinement by the periodontal ligament receptors
4. Continuation of the above until the end-point position is reached

Characteristics of the Mandibular Movements

The human head more or less resembles a sphere or globe that is balanced upon the vertebral column. If the mouth is opened maximally (the mandible being depressed) the head tilts backward slightly, as in a yawn. When the mouth closes, the head returns to its former position. Perhaps the opening of the mouth upsets the state of equilibrium so that the backward movement of the head is necessary to maintain balance. On the other hand, it may be related to the constriction of the prevertebral vessels and passages caused by maximum depression of the mandible. In such a case, the backward movement of the head may be necessary to free the passages.

Movements of the Mandible

Mandibular movements can be classified as: border, contact (or glide), and free. *Border movements* may be described as follows. If one were to plot the total number of positions of a single point on the mandible as the mandible produced all possible extreme movements, a three-dimensional figure would result. The surface of this figure would describe the maximum (or border) movements of the mandible relative to this one point. *Contact movements* are those during which the maxillary and mandibular teeth maintain contact; the movements are thus sliding or gliding ones. *Free movements* are those in which a given reference point fails to reach its border and wherein the teeth do not come into contact.

All possible movements of the mandible, when combined, form a characteristic pattern. According to Posselt (1957) this pattern, which is the so-called *envelope* of mandibular motion, can best be illustrated by recording the path (movement space) traced by a fixed point on the mandible, e.g., the contact point between the central incisors. Although this particular movement space has a pattern specific for the contact point, it must be realized that there is an infinity of points on the mandible, each of which has its own movement space that varies slightly around a central theme.

The movements of the mandible in opening and closing describe curved trajectories. Since the mandible is hinged behind and above the teeth, the molars follow a more horizontal path in closing than do the anterior teeth which have a more vertical movement (Fig. 12.17).

If the mandible is maximally retruded, it is able to perform a rotatory, hinge-like movement (terminal hinge movement) around an imaginary horizontal axis (the hinge axis), which passes through the joint region on both sides. Such a movement can generally be performed until the incisal edges of the front teeth are separated 20 to 25 mm (Fig. 12.18). By further opening and retruding the mandible the condyles translate forward and the incisal point describes a curve as shown in Figure 12.2*b*, until the incisal edges are separated 40 to 50 mm. The separation is, on average, larger in younger persons than in older (Sheppard, 1965). The posterior border movement from extreme opening to closing is often described as a diphasic curve, with the upper and lower arcs being of approximately the same length. The path of protruded maximum opening and closing movements is located 10 to 12 mm anterior to the aforementioned and is concave on its posterior aspect, but not segmented (Fig. 12.18).

The movements thus described are border movements. It is not possible to perform movements outside of the extreme lines that enclose the movement area as seen in the midsagittal plane (see Fig. 12.18). The border movements *can only be* performed with conscious effort or with guidance by another person. All habitual unconscious reflex movements fall within the envelope borders as seen in line δ in Fig. 12.18,

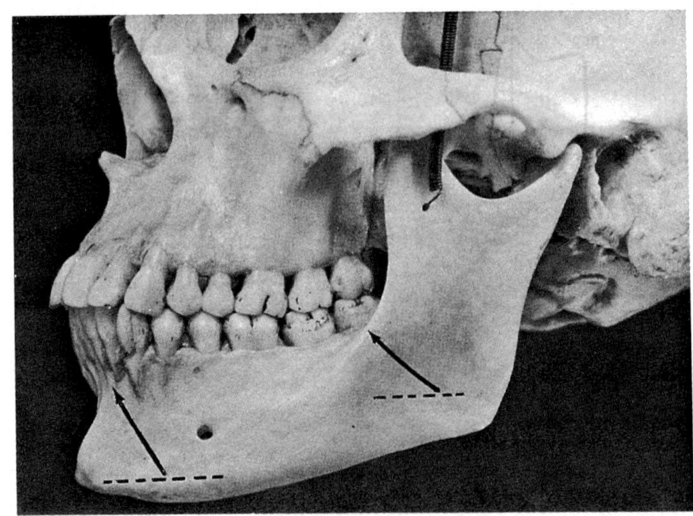

Figure 12.17

In a pure rotatory movement of the mandible around a transverse axis through the condylar region of either side, the swing (*arrows*) of the front teeth is more vertical than that of the molars. The movement of the front then resembles α in Figure 12.18*b*. Note the occlusal curve. The dental arches are in the intercuspal position.

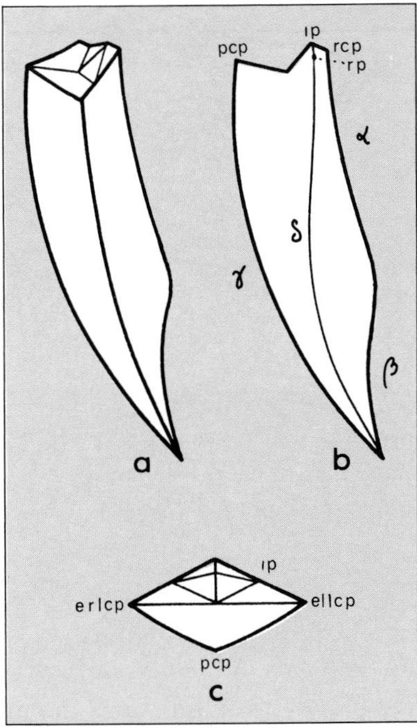

Figure 12.18

a, The envelope of motion of the contact point between the lower central incisors is seen from the left side. *b,* sagittal section of the envelope of motion. When the mandible performs symmetrical motions, the incisal point can only be moved in the midsagittal plane, i.e., it can be moved on and inside of the *thicker lines,* which represent the border movements. α, pure rotatory retruded opening movement; β, the condyles moving forward; γ, protruded closing movement; δ, a free closing movement which passes the rest "position" *rp,* and ends in the intercuspal position *ip. rcp,* retruded contact position; *pcp,* protruded contact position. *c,* the envelope of motion as seen from above. *erlcp,* extreme right lateral contact position; *ellcp,* extreme left lateral contact position; *ip,* intercuspal position; *pcp,* protruded contact position.

which indicates an habitual, free opening and closing movement. The closing end point of these movements in the normal, healthy masticatory system is the *intercuspal position.*

In the intercuspal position of the mandible there is maximal contact and coincidence between the upper and the lower occlusal surfaces. The intercuspal position is the most closed occlusal position and has been variously referred to as the position of *maximum intercuspation,* the *habitual position,* the *acquired position,* and *centric occlusion.* As the teeth meet at or near the end of a closing stroke, the many oblique facets on the cusps of the teeth tend to guide the mandible into its terminal, most closed position. However, in free, unconscious, closing movements and in chewing, the mandible is not guided into the intercuspal position by mechanical means. The guidance is furnished by acquired neuromuscular reflex patterns that direct the mandible into immediate, maximum contact or very close to it. The afferent impulses that originate on occlusal contact seem to facilitate the acquired reflex pattern, so that the position can be reached repeatedly and unconsciously, as is seen in short, fast chopping movements of the mandible. The same type of neuromuscular phenomena operate in walking.

The closing end point of the retruded border movement (the *terminal hinge movement,* Fig. 12.18) is the retruded contact position. In this position the upper and lower occlusal surfaces may contact at only one point or at several points, either clustered or scattered over the entire occlusal table. In 10 percent of persons with natural, healthy, and harmoniously functioning masticatory mechanisms (physiologic occlusion), the cranial end points of free habitual closing movements and of retruded closing movements coincide. In other words, the intercuspal position in this group occurs in the retruded contact position. In the remaining 90% of persons with a physiologic occlusion, the intercuspal position is located about 0.25 to 2.25 mm (1.25 ± 1 mm; Posselt, 1957) anterior to the retruded contact position (Fig. 12.18). Obviously, the *biological variation is rather marked.*

The lateral movements of the mandible are also somewhat curved as the mandible revolves around either the right condyle (Fig. 12.19, movements *a* and *d*) in a right lateral movement, or the left condyle (Fig. 12.19, movements *b* and *c*) in a left lateral movement. The side to which the mandible moves is referred to as the *working side,* and the condyle of that side as the *working condyle.* The small sliding lateral movement of the working condyle, commonly called the *Bennett movement,* has the effect of straightening the posterior curves (Fig. 12.19*a* and *d*), so that the result is an almost rhomboidal horizontal movement area (Fig. 12.19*a* to *d*). The sides of the rhombus represent border movements of the envelope of motion viewed from above. Natural, habitual movements or postures are to be found within the area of the rhombus.

In a lateral view the free movements of the mandible are curved or S-shaped. When performing free movements, the mandible is suspended in the jaw muscles, and it is therefore the coordination of all muscles participating in moving or stabilizing activities in a given course of motion that determines the single stroke of movement. Unlike border movements, which are reliably reproduced at will or under guidance, free movements may describe an infinite number of patterns that resemble but are not identical

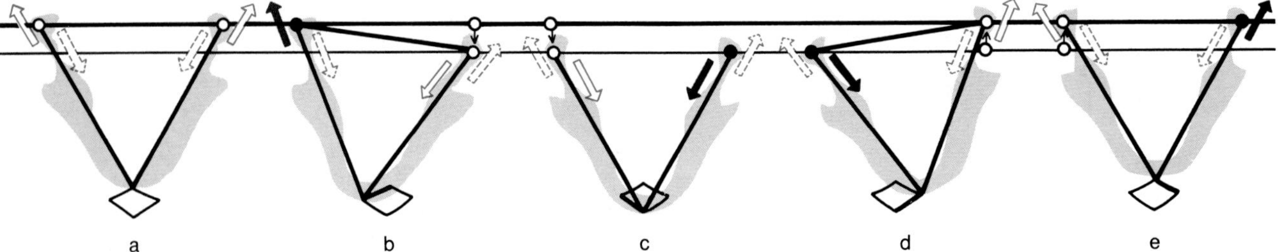

Figure 12.19

Sketches of a mandible performing movements along the borderlines of a horizontal section of the envelope of motion, *a*, retruded position. *b*, movement from the retruded to the extreme right lateral position, then (*c*) to the protruded and (*d*) to the extreme left lateral position and finally (*e*) back to the retruded position. ○, joint which "moves on the spot," the so called working condyle; ●, nonworking or moving condyle. The *arrows* represent the moving and stabilizing forces of protractor and retractor muscles. *Red arrows* represent stabilizing forces; *black arrows* represent forces that restrict the movement of a condyle.

to one another. What is more, no one free movement pattern can be precisely reproduced except purely by accident.

At an opening of 1 to 4 mm (2.5 ± 1.5 mm; Posselt, 1957) below the intercuspal position there is found a mandibular posture, where a relative muscular equilibrium exists—the *postural position* of the mandible. When the person is standing or sitting upright with the head in balance, the teeth separated, and the mandible suspended elastically, so to speak, in the musculature, the activity of the jaw muscles is at a minimum. The postural position is the beginning and the endpoint of most mandibular movements. As the mandible is suspended in the muscles, this posture, like other postures, is characterized by a certain variation even within the same person. The distance between the postural position and the intercuspal is termed the *freeway space*. Because of the nature of jaw suspension, the freeway space will have a greater dimension in the incisor region than in the molar region.

If chewing is observed in frontal aspect, the mandibular movement (the so-called *masticatory cycle*) usually describes a more or less pear-shaped figure (Fig. 12.20).

In reviewing the chief occlusal relations in the envelope of motion, it can be stated that (1) the *intercuspal position* is a "tooth-guided" position, since the mandible is guided to this position by the tooth contacts that appear to create the maximum mechanical stability for the mandible; (2) the *retruded contact position* is a "ligament-guided" position, since this is caused by the distention of the temporomandibular and capsular ligaments in the most superior posterior placement of the condyle; and (3) the *postural position* is a "muscle-guided" position, since the mandible is suspended in a position of equilibrium relative to the cranium by means of minimum coordinated muscle action (Figs. 12.19 to 12.21).

An implication of these complex possibilities of movement is that man, who is omnivorous, can handle any type of food between the teeth, be it meat or vegetables, soft or hard, tough or crisp, fibrous or stringy. In carnivores we find primarily vertical cutting or shearing movements and in ruminants mostly laterally directed, horizontal grinding movements of the mandible. Both can be performed in man, although not in such a specialized manner as in other mammals. The rodents perform small protrusive-

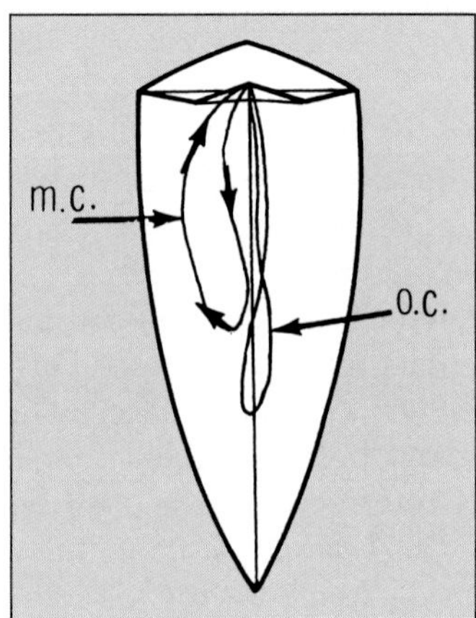

Figure 12.20

The envelope of motion as seen from behind. Two types of free movements are indicated as curved lines starting and ending in the intercuspal position: *right*, a simple opening-closing movement. (*o.c.*); *left*, a chewing stroke (*m.c.*).

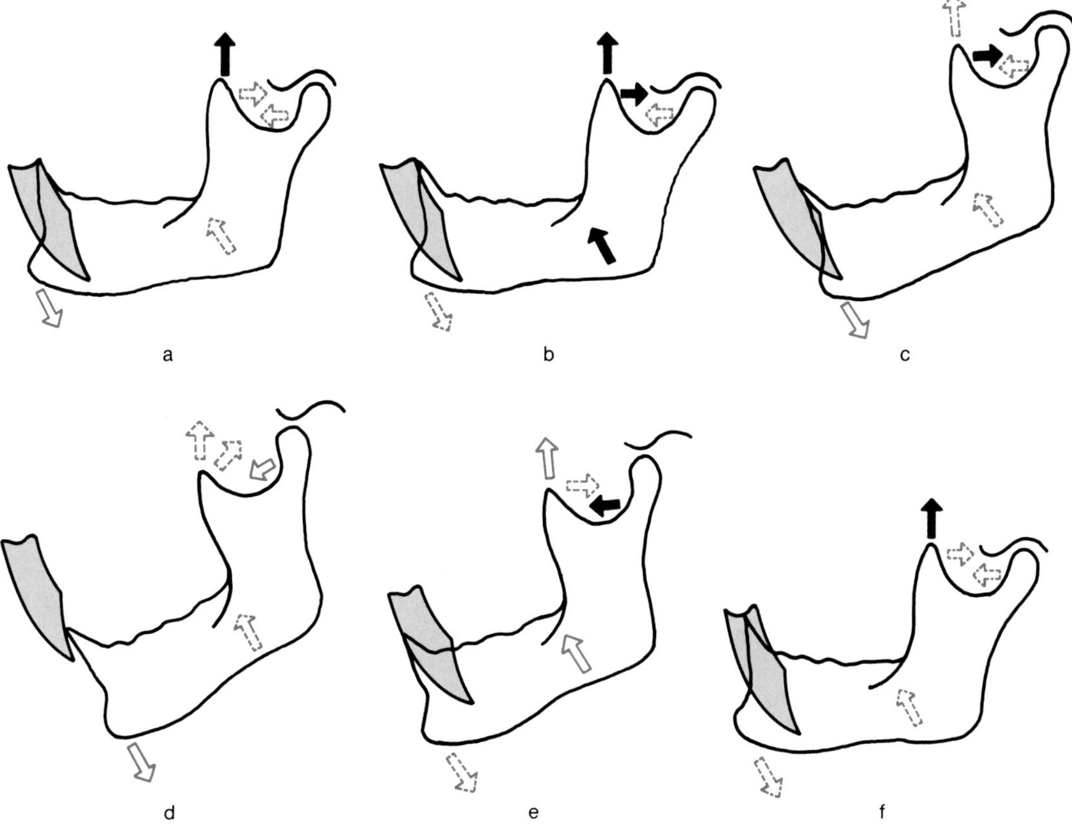

Figure 12.21

Sketches of the action of elevator, depressor, protractor, and retractor muscles in the performance of symmetrical opening and closing border movements as well as contact movements. *Black arrows,* forces that restrict a movement; *red arrows,* forces that cause a movement; *dotted arrows,* stabilizing forces. For explanation of positions, see Figure 12.19.

retrusive horizontal movements of the mandible while gnawing, and similar movements can also be performed in man, e.g., in nibbling corn on the cob. The architecture of the structures involved tends to produce chewing movements in harmony with the function.

Mastication

The mastication of food is an activity that is composed of a series of acquired neuromuscular reflexes. The masticatory performances vary with the consistency of food being ingested, the person's chewing habits, and his state of comfort relative to the component structures involved.

The act of mastication in terms of tough foods, intact dentition, and normal masticatory behavior can be divided into three stages (1) incision, (2) chewing, and (3) deglutition.

Incision

Incision is the function of grasping or biting off a portion of food that is of suitable size for chewing. During incision the mandible bites in a protrusive, or more frequently, a lateral protrusive position so that the anterior teeth, which present chisel-like cutting edges well designed for this purpose, can readily penetrate the food mass as the mandible is further closed in a retruded direction. It is believed that during incision in primates the anterior teeth serve as a tactile sensory organ for the testing of physical properties of food and that they must be able to perform this function free of posterior tooth contact. At the completion of the incisive bite the food rests upon the tongue so that it can then be directed to the posterior teeth for chewing.

Chewing

The chewing phase serves to reduce the particle size of the food and mix it sufficiently with saliva so that the consistency of the resultant bolus will allow the swallowing act to take place.

The trituration of food is carried out by the posterior teeth, which present occlusal tables with very efficient grinding surfaces (triangular ridges of the cusps) and escape sluiceways (the interproximal embrasure and developmental and supplemental grooves) that appear to enhance this function. In addition, since these teeth are located closer to the temporomandibular joint (the fulcrum point of the mandibular closure) their cutting efficiency is further enhanced by a reduction in the length of the effective lever arm of the third class lever system of jaw suspension (see Fig. 12.1).

Typically the human chewing cycle consists of several phases, including opening, fast closing, and slow closing. The sequence is completed in approximately 1 second. The opening movement is smooth, and the transition between fast and slow closing occurs when the bolus is engaged. Slow closing is associated with the power stroke of mastication, which includes movement into and through the intercuspal position. It is common for the mandible to dwell for about one-fifth of a second in the intercuspal position. Activity in the elevator muscles is strongest about 50 msec before full intercuspation occurs. When allowance is made for mechanical activation of the muscles and differences in timing between them, peak interocclusal forces occur just prior to and within the intercuspal position itself. These forces then dissipate as the jaw slides through tooth intercuspation to begin the next stroke. Owing to direction of the chewing stroke and the timing of the various muscle groups involved, interocclusal forces are constantly changing during mastication and are therefore never directed vertically along the long axes of the teeth.

The chewing of food is vertical and cyclic in nature. The number of strokes necessary to prepare a given food mass for swallowing varies from person to person, but seems to be consistent for each.

Evidence suggests that contact or near-contact does occur during chewing, especially during the terminal strokes of a chewing sequence. Here gliding contacts are found in the last millimeter or two as the teeth slide into the intercuspal position. The actual zones of contact depend upon the individual occlusion, but characteristically involve guiding inclines on the inner inclines of working-side teeth, typically on the canines, or on other teeth as well if they meet in group function. Nonworking-side contacts are also possible. Evidence seems to indicate that only a small portion of maximum biting force is used in the mastication of food.

After incision, when food is guided to the posterior teeth by the tongue, the first few strokes may occur with food being crushed on both sides of the mouth simultaneously. Very shortly thereafter, the food is placed on the preferred side with the major portion of the chewing act being unilateral. In studies of "primitive" and "civilized" peoples there was evidence that only the former used both sides of the mouth to an equal degree in chewing a given bolus (Beyron, 1964).

Because of the rotatory nature of the closing movements of the mandible, the interocclusal distance is larger in the anterior part of the mouth than in the posterior at a given degree of mouth opening. This difference in interocclusal distance is in accordance with the functional demands in incision and chewing. When a bulky bolus of food has just been cut off by the incisors it is first crushed in the premolar areas, where room can easily be provided without excessively opening the mandible. Later, after some chewing strokes have reduced the food particle size, the trituration proper takes place in the molar region, where the interocclusal distance is rather small in ordinary chewing.

During the chewing of food by the posterior teeth, the mandible opens and closes on the food with the preferred side in a vertically lateral or slightly protruded lateral position with a definite distal thrust as it attempts to return to the intercuspal position. The lip-cheek-tongue system gathers the comminuted food and saliva mixture and positions it on the occlusal tables of the lower posterior teeth after each stroke. Masticatory efficiency is apparently related to the number of posterior teeth present—what has been termed the "effective food platform area" (Yurkstas, 1954).

The chewing cycles cease when the bolus has reached a consistency suitable for swallowing, and again, this varies among different persons. It is at this time that the tendency for tooth contact may occur. The duration of the various phases of the masticatory cycle and its form are dependent upon the nature of the food bolus. The length of the cycle is greater for harder foods, and the lateral deviation of the mandible is wider. The transition between the chewing and swallowing phases of mastication depends upon the accumulation of saliva and appears to be independent of bolus particle size.

Deglutition

Masticatory swallowing begins as a voluntary muscular act and is completed involuntarily. The mechanics of swallowing require that the following acts take place: (1) the anterior portion of the mouth is sealed;

(2) the soft palate is raised; (3) the hyoid bone is raised to close off the trachea; (4) the posterior portion of the tongue is engaged in a piston-like thrust causing the bolus to be pushed into the oral pharynx; (5) the act of swallowing takes place.

In the fourth and fifth phases the mandible must be braced in order (1) to allow the posterior portion of the tongue, which originates from it, to thrust distally, and (2) to counteract the effect of the suprahyoid musculature which, in raising the hyoid bone simultaneously acts to depress the mandible. The bracing of the mandible is accomplished by means of either direct tooth contact or indirect (food intervening) tooth contact, both at or near the intercuspal position.

Several swallows are necessary to empty the mouth of a given food mass. After the bolus of food has passed into the pharynx the superior portion of the posterior walls presses forward to seal the pharynx and the esophageal phase of swallowing commences. The latter is accomplished by involuntary peristalsis that moves the bolus through the entire length of the digestive tract.

The act of swallowing is an innate neuromuscular reflex that is either present at birth or established shortly thereafter. This activity is considered to be very primitive and can be accomplished *despite* the presence of tremendous tissue destruction or loss of much of the masticatory structures through disease or injury (Silverman, 1961).

Empty mouth swallowing occurs frequently throughout the day, and is an important function that rids the mouth of saliva and helps to moisten the oral structures. The hourly rate of nonmasticatory swallowing is apparently related to the amount of salivary flow, and in most instances may be an involuntary reflex activity. The average is thought to be about 40 per hour during the wakeful hours, diminishing to a few per hour during sleep (Flanagan, 1963).

During typical empty mouth swallowing the mandible is braced in the intercuspal position to allow for proper stabilization.

Atypical swallowing or empty mouth swallowing without tooth contact may be classified as *retained infantile* or *adult* swallowing. Retained infantile swallowing is the form of deglutition that is related to the sucking reflex and is characterized by the tongue protruding forcefully between the strongly constricted lips. Adult atypical swallowing occurs with the tongue between some or all of the teeth while the jaw muscles are in a state of contraction during the bracing.

13

The Dentition: Its Alignment and Articulation

The Dental Arch and the Lip-Cheek-Tongue System

The lips and the cheeks externally, and the tongue internally, enclose a so-called neutral space that is occupied by the mandibular and maxillary dental arches (Fig. 13.1). The teeth are therefore in the midst of powerful opposing muscular forces. The powerful muscular structures are well coordinated and have the important function of collecting, placing, and keeping the food on the occlusal table during mastication. Because of their high degree of coordination, it is justifiable to regard them as one functioning entity: the lip-cheek-tongue system.

If the system is in balance, equal forces are directed against the teeth from both the lingual and the lip-cheek sides. The neutral space is, in other words, a space in which a *relative equilibrium of forces is normally maintained.* Imbalance of the internal and external forces in this system can result in malocclusion, that is, an abnormal alignment of the dental arches. An example of this imbalanced state is the case of tongue-thrusting, wherein there is abnormal forward thrust of the tongue against or between the anterior teeth during swallowing. This results in a greater outward directed force against the teeth than inward directed force and may cause protrusion of the anterior teeth. On the other hand, the imbalance of forces may occur in the opposite direction, as in mouth breathing, where the pressure of the lips on the teeth is not counteracted by the outward pressure of the tongue.

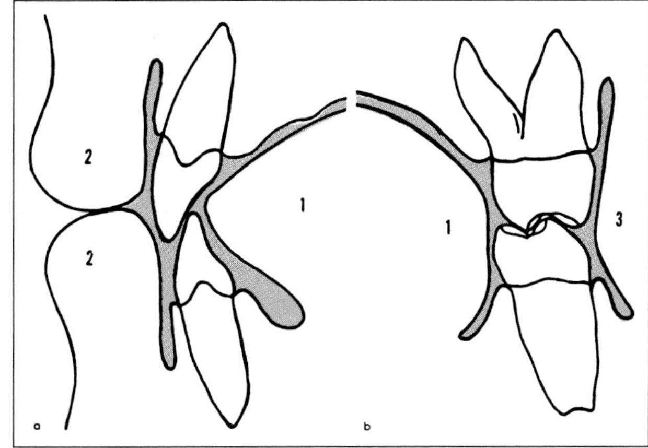

Figure 13.1

The lip-cheek-tongue system and the neutral space. *a,* anterior region of mouth. The neutral space is *shaded* and the tongue and lips conform to the cross-sectional forms of the teeth in occlusion, *1,* tongue; *2,* lip; *b,* posterior region of the mouth. The neutral space is *shaded. 1,* tongue; *3,* cheek.

In addition to the intermittent modeling pressure and aligning forces, the lip-cheek-tongue system, along with the intercuspation of the teeth, helps to prevent tooth deviations in a buccal or lingual direction. The general shape of the proximal surfaces of the teeth also helps to maintain the shape of the arch. The proximal surfaces of the teeth converge lingually, and their curvature decreases from the anterior to the molar region, resulting in comparatively flat proximal contact areas in the posterior teeth. The flat contact areas serve to stabilize the arch in a mesiodistal direction. There is a tendency toward mesial drift of the teeth in the dental arches, probably caused by upward-forward swing of the mandible.

The Axial Positioning of Teeth

Practically all teeth are aligned in their arches with varying degrees of inclination of their axial centers relative to a vertical line both in a mesiodistal and faciolingual direction.

In the hypothetically ideal state, the various axial inclinations of teeth will result in a continuity of tooth forms. Usually the cusp tips of the posterior teeth in alignment conform to a fairly even linear curve in the

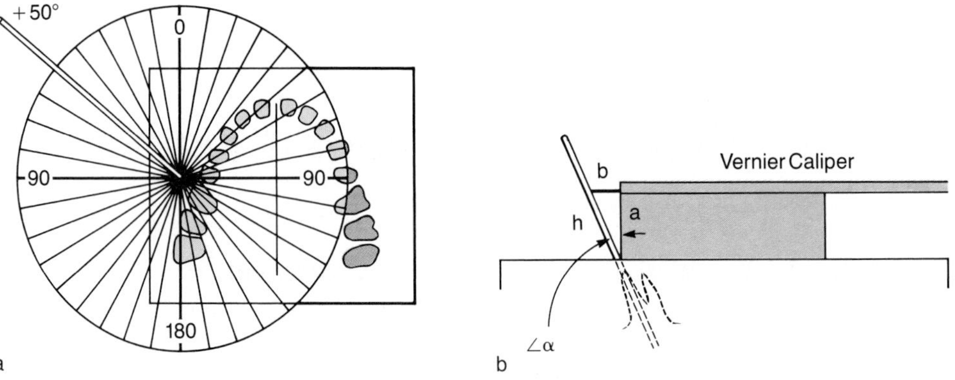

Figure 13.2

The technique for measuring inclincation and angulation as used by Dempster *et al. A,* inclination angle of root is measured on stone model of maxillary alveoli set in plate of plaster as shown. Wire placed axially in upper first molar root socket is measured by transparent protractor with its axis of symmetry parallel to midsagittal plane of palate. *B,* measurement of amount of angulation of wire relative to "plane of the alveolar margins." Using sliding depth gauge of Vernier caliper (*b*) and fixed height (*a*), angle (∠α) of right triangle completed by wire (*h*) may be determined trigonometrically. (Reproduced from Dempster *et al.*, 1963, copyright by the American Dental Association. Reprinted by permission of *The Journal of the American Dental Association.*)

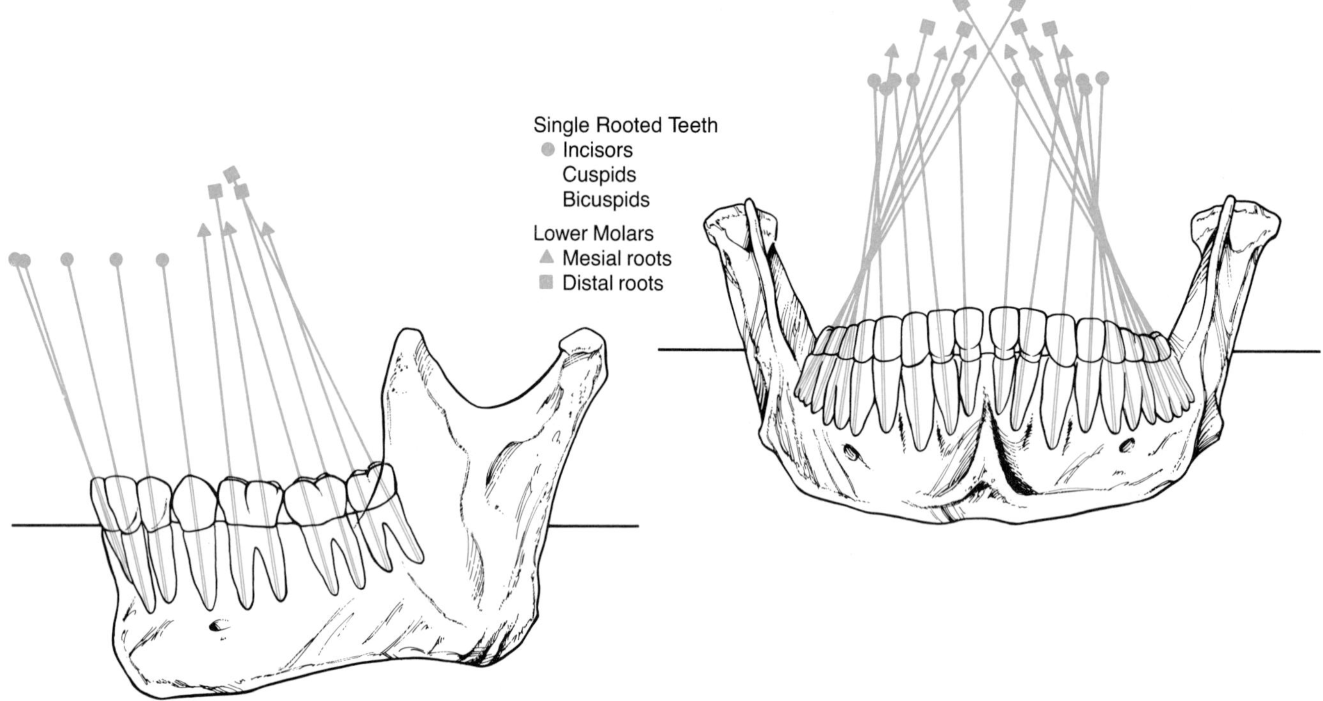

Figure 13.3

Complete orthographic projection of mandibular teeth as seen from anterior and lateral aspects showing arrangement of teeth relative to alveolar bone. Degree of obliquity of roots of right and left teeth of 11 jaws has been averaged. Root axes have been extended beyond crowns to emphasize angular pattern. (Reproduced from Dempster *et al.*, 1963, copyright by the American Dental Association. Reprinted by permission of *The Journal of the American Dental Association.*)

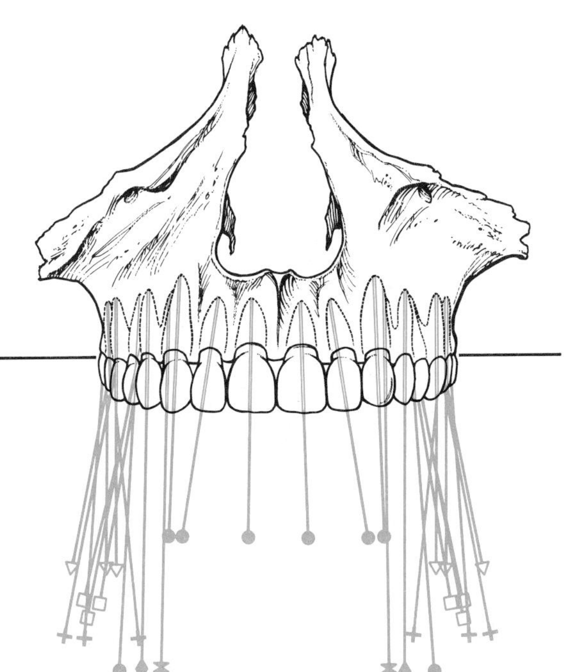

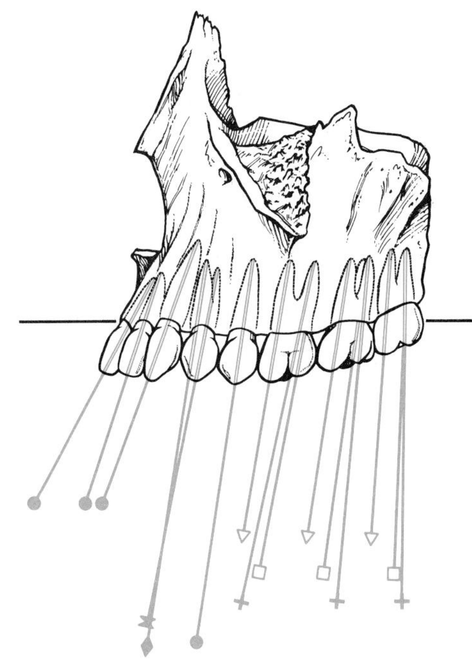

Figure 13.4

Composite illustration of maxilla and upper teeth as seen from anterior and lateral aspects showing average arrangement of teeth. Amount of slant shown by roots represents mean of combined right and left teeth of 11 jaws. Longitudinal axes of roots of teeth have been extended beyond crowns and are shown in orthographic projection. (Reproduced from Dempster *et al.*, 1963, copyright by the American Dental Association. Reprinted by permission of *The Journal of the American Dental Association.*)

anteroposterior direction (curve of Spee; see Fig. 12.4*a*). A transverse occlusal curve also exists for each right and left posterior tooth and like the curve of von Spee is concave above and convex below (transverse curve or curve of Wilson).

The long-held belief that the occlusal surfaces of the natural dentition are aligned three dimensionally on the surface of a sphere (Monson) has fallen into disrepute. Attempts to demonstrate the presence of the Monson spherical curve as a naturally occurring phenomenon have been unsuccessful. The teeth appear to align themselves upon two unrelated two-dimensional linear curves, an anteroposterior curve and a mediolateral curve.

The degree of axial root inclination from the vertical line perpendicular to the occlusal table varies for each tooth and to a greater or lesser degree for each class of teeth. Maxillary teeth seem to show the least statistical variation in root inclination. The mandibular central incisors and canines usually present the greatest variation (see Fig. 13.2 for method of taking measurements). (See Figs. 13.3 and 13.4 for the diagrammatic representation of tooth alignment.)

Maxillary Arch

With the exception of the third molars, the maxillary incisors demonstrate the greatest root angulation in the mouth (29 degrees). The premolars are usually aligned with their axial centers nearly perpendicular to the occlusal plane. The axial angulation of the maxillary molar rarely exceeds 15 degrees and all roots point palatally except for the distobuccal root of the maxillary first molar. The lingual roots of the molar usually have greater palatal inclination than do the buccal (see Table 13.1 and Fig. 13.4 for inclination and angulation of roots).

Mandibular Arch

The mandibular incisors and canines have the greatest deviation in root angulation. The root apices of the mandibular incisors are mesially directed and inclined to the lingual.

The mandibular premolars, like their maxillary counterparts, are also aligned with their centers near-

Table 13.1
Inclination and Angulation of Roots of Teeth in 11 Skulls

Root	Mean Inclination (degrees)	±AD*	Mean Angulation from Vertical (degrees)	±AD*	No. of Roots Measured†
Maxillary roots					
Third molar lingual	103	42	12.3	3.9	11
Third molar distobuccal	89	40	11.3	4.6	7
Third molar mesiobuccal	72	39	11.6	5.5	7
Second molar lingual	61	44	10.7	3.2	20
Second molar distobuccal	28	66	9.3	2.8	16
Second molar mesiobuccal	0	78	9.6	3.9	16
First molar lingual	45	30	13.0	4.9	22
First molar distobuccal	−28	35	13.0	4.6	22
First molar mesiobuccal	−2	46	10.4	3.9	22
Second bicuspid	19	36	8.6	3.6	22
First bicuspid lingual	8	20	10.4	3.4	12
First bicuspid buccal	3	22	9.6	3.2	12
Cuspid	6	14	20.6	3.2	22
Lateral incisor	16	6	29.0	3.4	22
Central incisor	2	5	29.0	4.1	22
Mandibular roots					
Third molar mesial	−53	15	32.6	4.5	10
Third molar distal	−51	16	38.5	8.0	9
Second molar mesial	−51	19	25.4	4.6	22
Second molar distal	−53	18	28.0	3.4	22
First molar mesial	−58	36	12.8	5.6	22
First molar distal	−58	23	16.8	4.0	22
Second bicuspid	−34	54	10.1	3.4	22
First bicuspid	14	35	9.8	3.9	22
Cuspid	13	27	14.6	6.4	22
Lateral incisor	17	10	21.2	6.4	22
Central incisor	2	15	19.3	7.5	22

*AD, average deviation

†Where the number is less than 22, fused roots, which have not been included in the table, or missing third molars will account for the discrepancy.

ly perpendicular to the occlusal plane. The mandibular first premolar, unlike the remaining lower posterior teeth, has a lingual tilt to the root apex. The mandibular premolars and molars appear to have the least variability in their degree of tilt. The mandibular molars are inclined with their root apices toward the buccal to a much greater extent than their maxillary counterparts are inclined palatally. The mandibular third molars usually exhibit the greatest root angulation in the mouth (see Table 13.1 and Fig. 13.3).

In demonstrating ideas about axial positioning of the teeth, subjective clinical averages are used (Table 13.2 and Fig. 13.5). Unfortunately, the sample was inadequate to establish clearcut parameters in the axial positioning of the roots. The accompanying illustrations (Figs. 13.6 to 13.19) were compiled by photographing duplicate teeth aligned as closely as possible with measurements suggested by Dempster *et al* (1963). The third molars are not shown because of their extreme variability in form, position, and eruption.

The Occlusal Surfaces

The general shape of the occlusal surfaces of the dental arches appears to be closely related to character-

Table 13.2
Suggested Axial Inclinations of Teeth for Study Purposes

Tooth	Angle of Mesiodistal Inclination of the Tooth Central Axis with a Vertical Line (degrees)	Angle of Faciolingual Inclination of the Tooth Central Axis with a Vertical Line (degrees)
Maxillary arch		
Central incisor	2*	28
Lateral incisor	7	26
Canine	17	16
First premolar (buccal root only)	9	5
Second premolar	5	6
First molar (palatal root only)	10	8
Second molar (palatal root only)	8	10
Mandibular arch		
Central incisor	2*	22
Lateral incisor	0	23
Canine	6	12
First premolar	6	9
Second premolar	9	9†
First molar (mesial root only)	10	20†
Second molar (mesial root only)	14	20†

By holding extracted teeth in the hand to conform to the measurements above as seen in the illustrations of Figure 13.3, the teeth are in a more favorable position to be examined for effects of tooth form and alignment.
*Inclination to distal.
†Inclination to lingual.

istics of the lateral contact and closing movements of the mandible. The mesiodistal cusp height (Fig. 13.5), which is an expression of the pointedness of the cusps, gradually decreases from the canines to the molars. Thus, in the anterior part of the mouth, teeth are found which have either chisel-shaped cutting edges or one or two comparatively high, pointed cusps. Large boli of food, which need coarse cutting or chopping, are treated with sharp-edged or pointed occlusal surfaces, which are able to crush the food without application of heavy forces. Since incisal edges and cusp tips have small surfaces, the cutting pressure is high, even when moderate closing forces are applied. In the molar region, the cusps, although shorter and blunter, are increased in number with consequent expansion of the platform area. Cuspal interferences during function are not likely to occur, even in small interocclusal working distances.

As previously stated, the path of the anterior teeth in the closing movement of the mandible is more vertical than is that of the molars. Anterior cusps that are high and steep, and posterior cusps that are low and flat are well suited for this arrangement. Because of the curve of Spee, the angle at which the teeth occlude is approximately the same in the anterior and posterior parts of the dental arch (Fig. 13.5). This factor may tend to permit the periodontium of different teeth to be equally loaded in occlusal contact.

Occlusal Contact

The occlusal surfaces of the dentition are characterized by cusps, grooves, and sulci. When unworn they are curved rather than straight or flat; therefore, when the upper and lower occlusal surfaces meet, they make contact on many points, or small contact areas. The character of occlusal contacts in the unworn dental arch are point-to-point, point-to-area, edge-to-edge, edge-to-area, *but not area-to-area.* This makes chewing easier to perform, since there are abundant food spill-ways on the occlusal table.

Even in dentitions showing natural, physiologic attrition one does not find area-to-area contact. Because of the different rates of attrition of enamel and dentin, caused by the difference in hardness of these two tissues, the surface remains irregular, so that only point or edge contacts occur. However, in bruxism the direct tooth-to-tooth contact may result in nonphysiologic area-to-area contacts.

The Arrangement of the Cusps

The cusps of the teeth appear to be arranged with special regard for the functional demands of stabilization of the mandible, and to permit mandibular contact movements without cuspal interferences.

Normally a tooth has contact with two teeth in the opposing arch. The only exceptions are the lower central incisors and the upper third molars. In the mandible a tooth is situated more mesially and lingually than its counterpart in the maxilla (Fig. 13.5). Accordingly, each mandibular tooth in the intercuspal position contacts two maxillary teeth—its class counter-

(*text continues on page 249*)

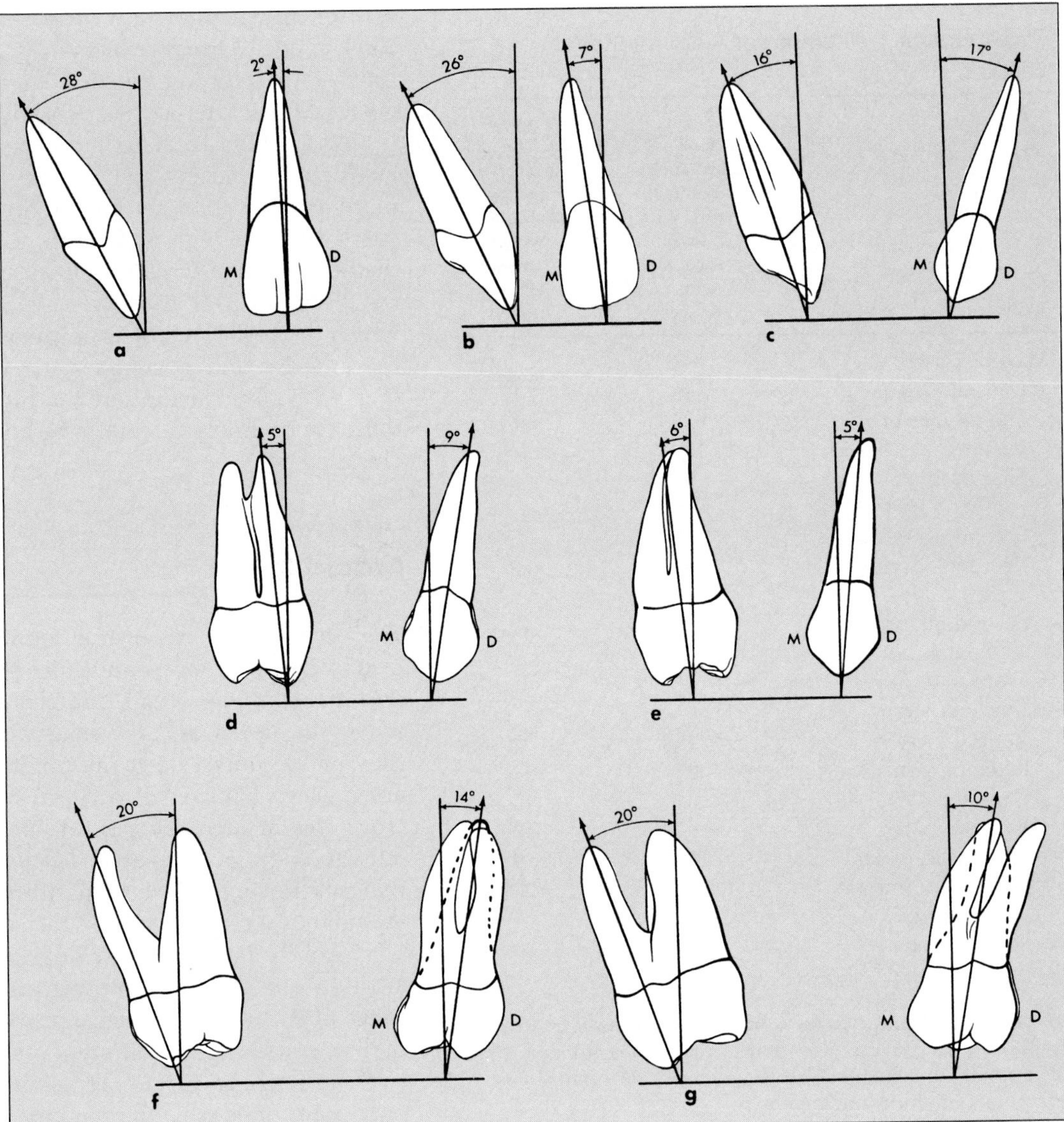

Figure 13.5

Diagrammatic presentations of the mesiodistal and faciolingual axial inclination angles with a vertical reference line. The tooth sizes are *not* proportional. Maxillary teeth (*a–g*). *a*, central incisors; *b*, lateral incisor; *c*, canine; *d*, first premolar; *e*, second premolar; *f*, first molar; *g*, second molar.

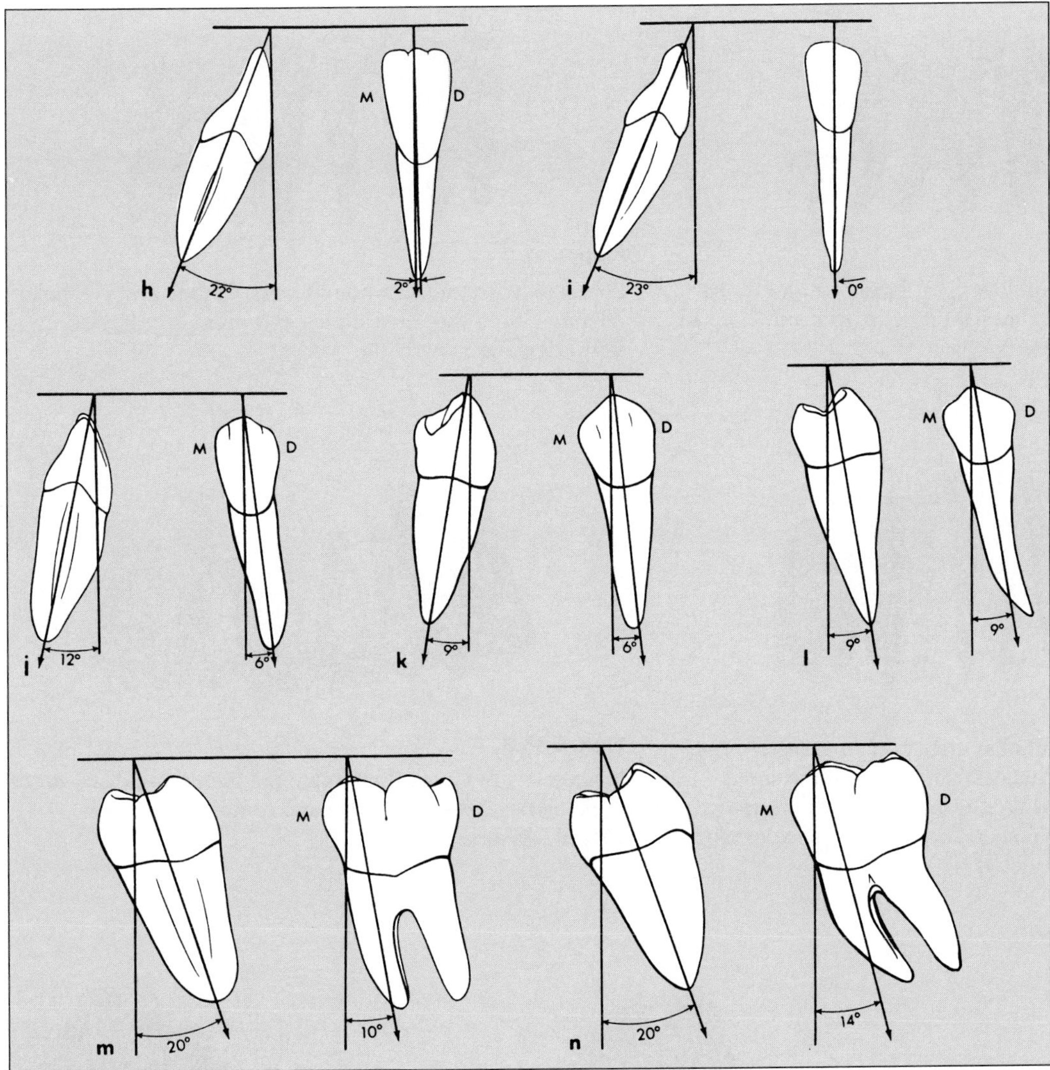

Figure 13.5, *cont'd.*

Mandibular teeth (*h–n*). *h*, central incisor; *i*, lateral incisor; *j*, canine; *k*, first premolar; *l*, second premolar; *m*, first molar; *n*, second molar.

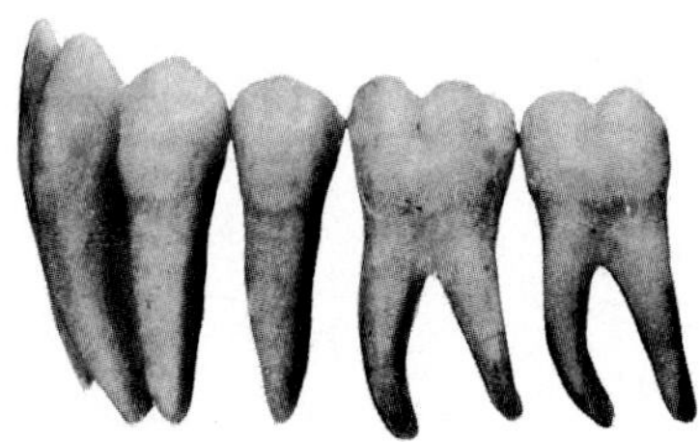

Figure 13.6
Buccal view of the mandibular arch. Premolar and molar relations; note increasing mesial tilt of crowns and front to back in the posterior teeth.

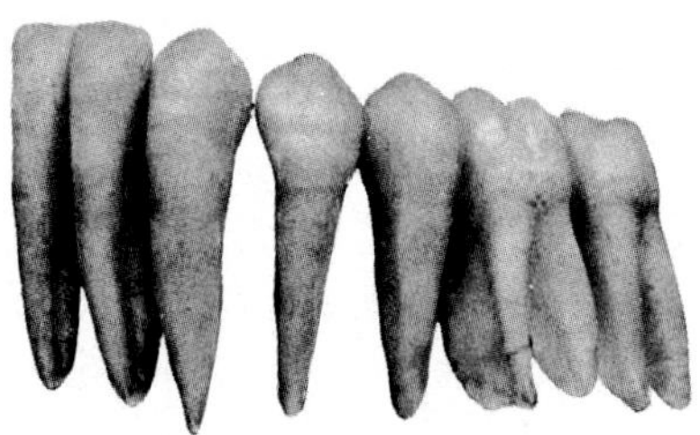

Figure 13.7
Buccal view of the mandibular arch. Canine and premolar relations: note that the canines and premolars have only slight deviations from the vertical.

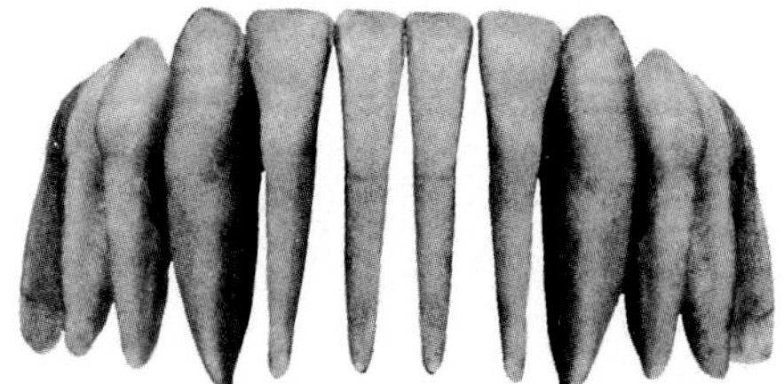

Figure 13.8
Buccal view of the mandibular arch. Incisor relations: note that the first premolar roots are aligned with the same lingual tilt to the apex as are the anterior teeth but that the second premolar exhibits a buccal tilt to the apex as seen in the mandibular molars.

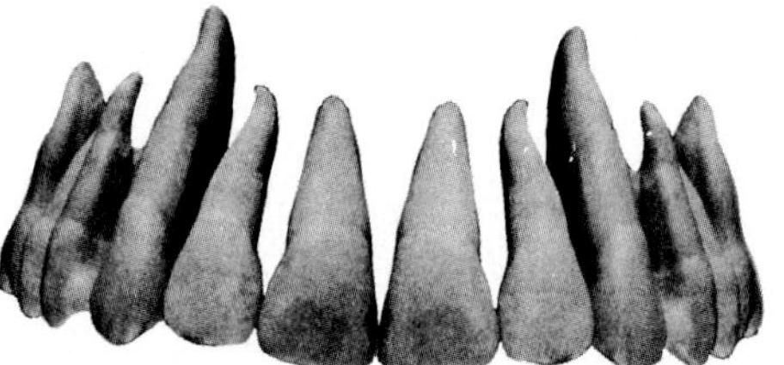

Figure 13.9
Labial view of upper arch. Note the increasing distal tilt of the crowns of the lateral incisors compared with the central incisors.

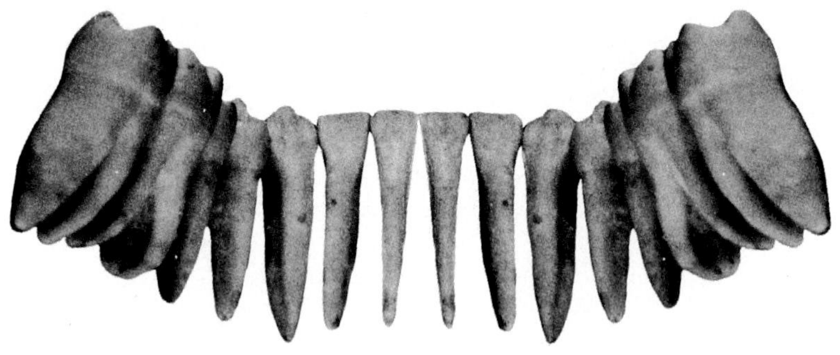

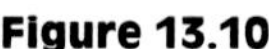

Figure 13.10
Lingual view of the lower arch. Note the severe lingual tilt of the molar crowns. The occlusal surfaces seem to conform to the convex side of a transverse curve.

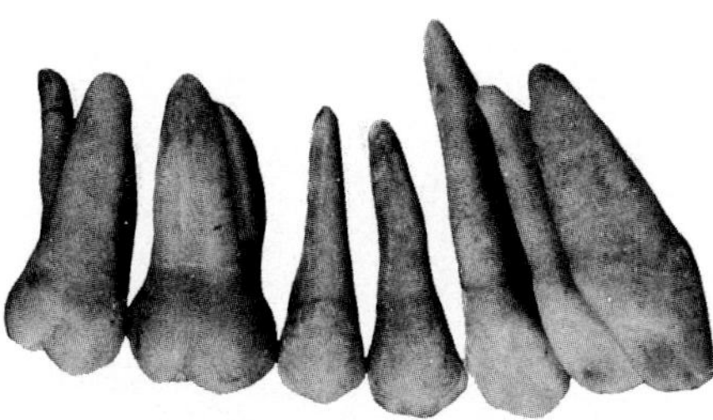

Figure 13.11

Lingual view of the maxillary arch. Molar area: note increasing mesial tilt of crowns of the posterior teeth from front to back.

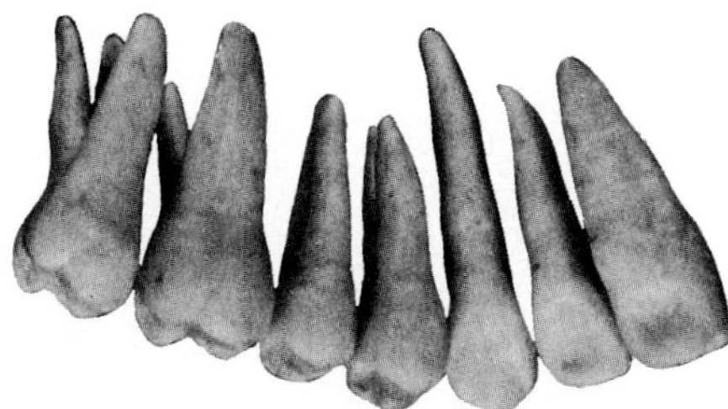

Figure 13.12

Lingual view of the maxillary arch. Canine-premolar area: note that the cementoenamel junctions of adjacent teeth are at the same levels. The occlusal surfaces align themselves against the concave portion of the curve of von Spee.

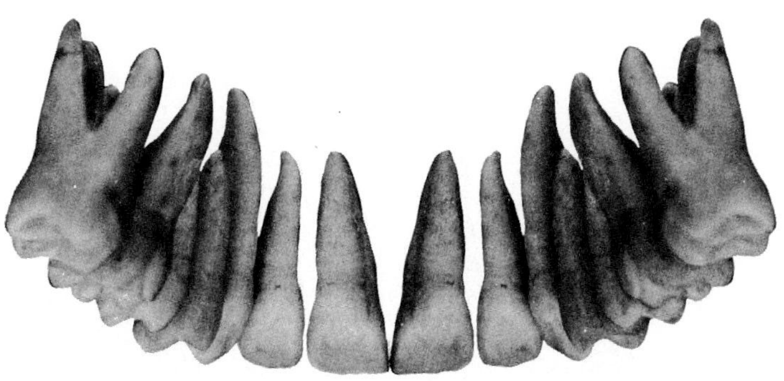

Figure 13.13

Lingual view of the maxillary arch. Incisor area: emphasized in this view is the severe buccal tilt of the molar crowns, which seem to conform to the concave surface of the transverse curve.

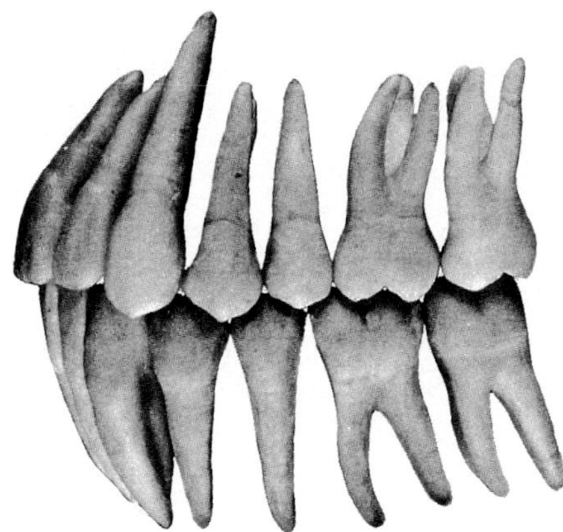

Figure 13.14

Buccal view of the teeth in the intercuspal position. Molar and premolar views demonstrating that the alignment of the roots of the teeth closely approximate the direction of mandibular closure so that the curvatures of the anterior roots are more vertically arranged than the curvatures of the molar roots which are more horizontal.

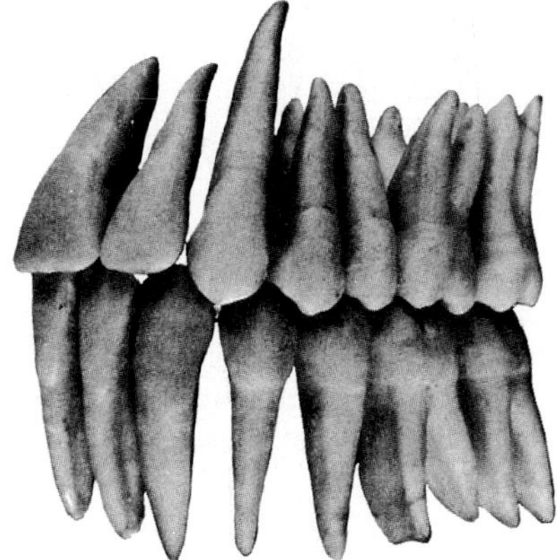

Figure 13.15

Buccal view of the teeth in the intercuspal position. Canine premolar area: the canines and especially the premolars demonstrate the least axial tilting of all the teeth.

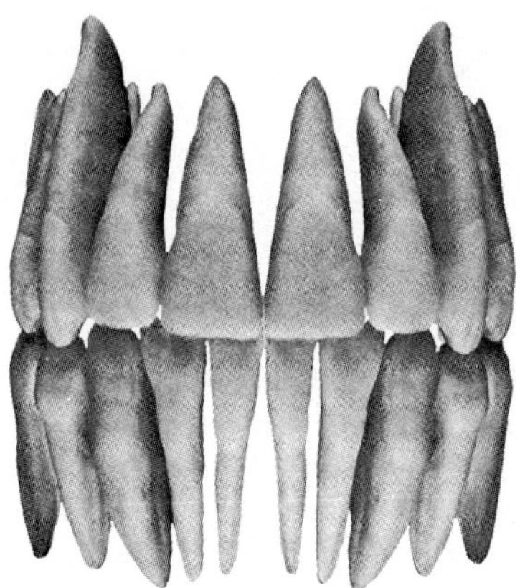

Figure 13.16

Buccal view of the teeth in the intercuspal position. Incisor area: note the vertical overlap (overbite) of the maxillary incisors. In most mouths, the opposing incisors do not contact in the intercuspal position.

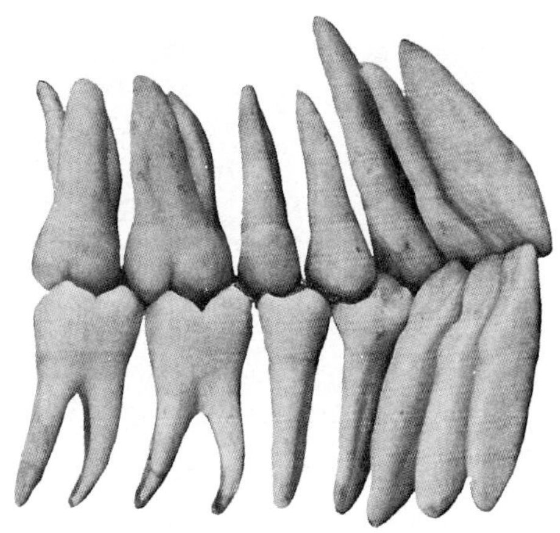

Figure 13.17

Lingual view of the teeth in the intercuspal position. Molar and premolar area: this view also emphasizes the vertical (overbite) and horizontal (overjet) relations of the anterior teeth.

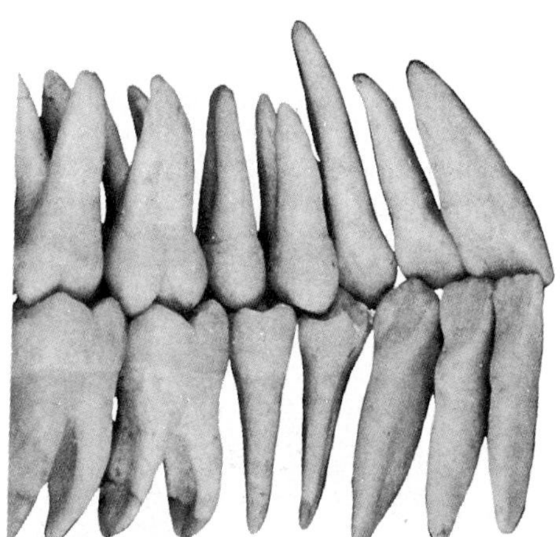

Figure 13.18

Lingual view of the teeth in the intercuspal position. Canine area: the relation of the maxillary canine to the mandibular canine and mandibular first premolar area seen in this view shows why these three teeth are thought of as a "functional entity" in the dentition.

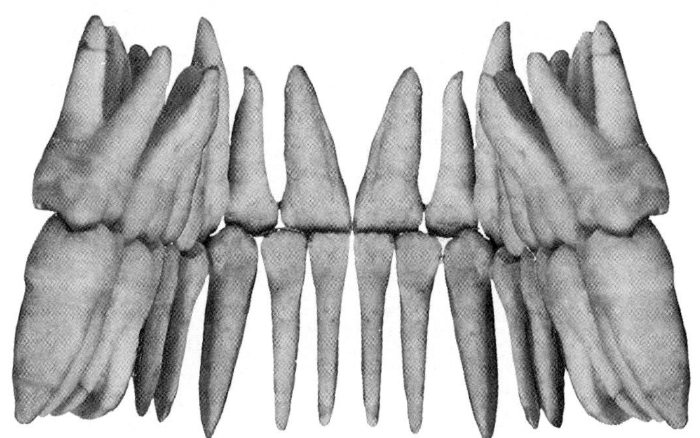

Figure 13.19

Lingual view of the teeth in the intercuspal position. Incisor view: the contrast of the maxilla and mandibular molars axial inclinations into the remaining dentition.

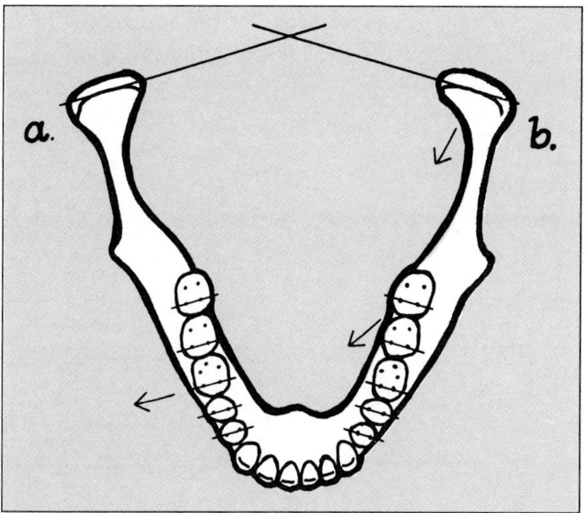

Figure 13.20

The general direction of the condyles and the connecting lines between the facial and the corresponding lingual cusps are grossly parallel and coincident with the lateral swing of the working condyle. *a,* working condyle; *b,* nonworking condyl. Lines through the poles of the condyles are parallel to the cusp connecting lines and meet in the region of the anterior boundary of the foramen magnum. The movement of the nonworking condyle is perpendicular to the condylor pole lines.

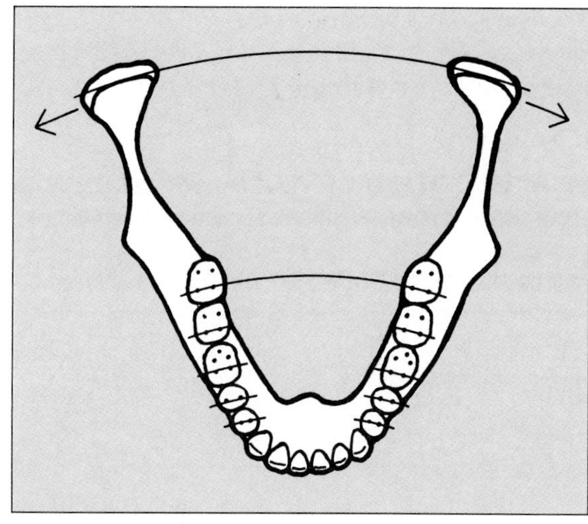

Figure 13.21

The so-called immediate Bennett shift in lateral jaw movement where the arrangement of cusps and condyles allows small lateral contact movements of the mandible. The rear part is larger than in the front as if the mandible would rotate around a vertical axis in the midline anterior of the arches.

part and the tooth immediately mesial to it. For example, the mandibular first molar makes contact with the maxillary first molar and second premolar.

The lingual cusps on the upper teeth and the buccal cusps on the lower teeth have contact on all sides (*supporting cusps*), whereas the buccal upper cusps and the lingual lower cusps make contact only on their occlusal sides (*guiding cusps*). This kind of interdigitation has the effect of stabilizing the mandible against the cranium when the teeth meet in simultaneous contact in the intercuspal position. The elevator muscles contract when the teeth are in full intercuspation; the mandible is completely locked and can move to another occlusal contact position or free movement only if there is some relaxation of the elevator muscles. It is worthwhile to note that contact between opposing anterior teeth is not necessary in order to achieve intercuspal stabilization. As a rule, the anterior teeth are slightly out of contact in the intercuspal position. Occlusal stabilization of the mandible can be achieved although the intercuspation does not demonstrate the so-called normal morphologic occlusal pattern described above and in the next section. In other words, mandibular stability can occur both with and without morphologically normal cusp relations.

The cusps are arranged in such a way that lateral contact movements can be made normally without cuspal interferences. Imaginary lines connecting the facial and the functionally corresponding lingual cusps (not necessarily on the same teeth) have a distal and lingual direction, forming angles of about 120 degrees with the corresponding lines from the other side. On each side the lines are nearly parallel with the direction of the working condyle (Figs. 13.20 and 13.21). The lateral movements of the mandible take a course approximately along the aforementioned lines, allowing the cusps to slide between each other in lateral contact movements. This does not mean that contact over the entire extent of the occlusal table takes place at that time. The so-called balanced articulation, characterized by even contact over the entire occlusal table in all contact movements, rarely if ever occurs in the natural dentition.

As a rule, few pairs of antagonists have occlusal contact during lateral mandibular glide. In the dentition with slight attrition the teeth involved are usually found in the canine region.

The following section is presented in "Atlas" format, in order to facilitate the visualization of the mechanics of tooth articulation. The text and illustrative material are presented concurrently side by side so that an "animated commentary" may be created (Figs. 13.22 to 13.41).

The Articulation of Teeth—Mechanics and Landmarks

The Nature of the Posterior Occlusal Surface

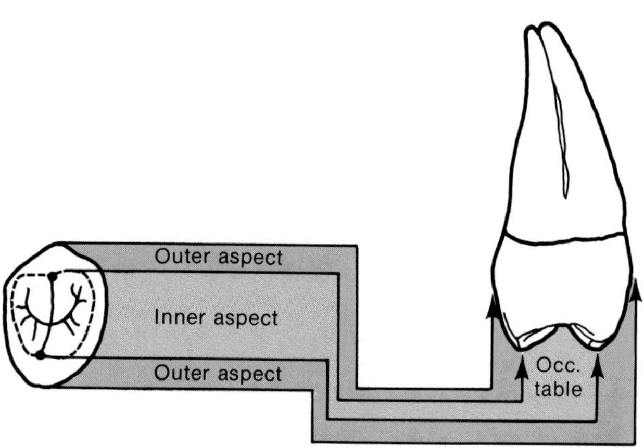

Figure 13.22

If one examines the crown of a well-formed posterior tooth one notes that a distinct line angle is present where the occlusal (*OCC*) surface meets the facial or lingual surfaces. These bucco-occlusal and linguo-occlusal line angles divide the cusps of the posterior tooth into *inner* and *outer aspects*.

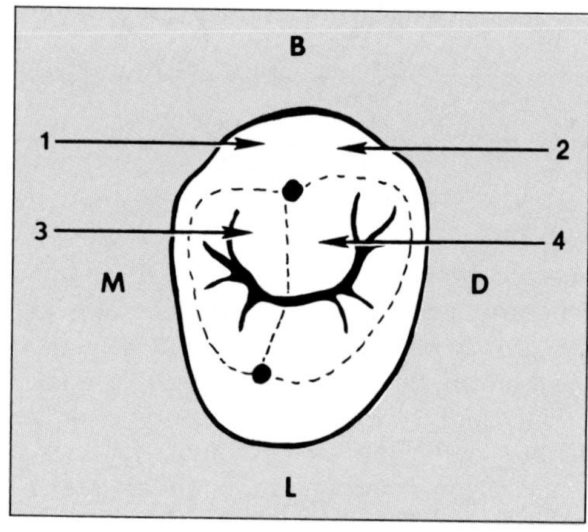

Figure 13.23

This idea simplifies the identification of occlusal inclined planes that are present.

1, the mesial (*M*) outer aspect of the buccal (*B*) cusp; *2*, the distal (*D*) outer aspect of the buccal cusp; *3*, the mesial inner aspect of the buccal cusp; *4*, the distal inner aspect of the buccal cusp; *L*, lingual.

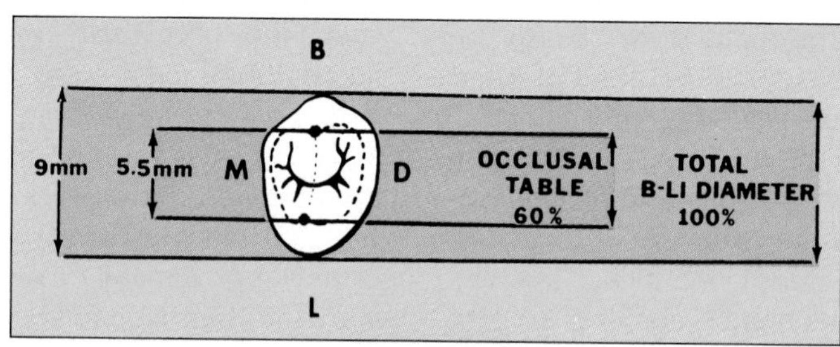

Figure 13.24

The inner inclines of the buccal and lingual cusps form the *occlusal table* of the tooth. The *occlusal table*, which is the recipient of the biting force, is generally only 50 to 60 percent of the overall buccolingual dimension (*B-LI diameter*) and is positioned over the center of root support. The occlusal table of each posterior tooth is composed of a supporting and guiding element. In the normal alignment of the human dentition the buccal (*B*) cusps of the lower arch and the lingual (*L*) cusps of the upper arch articulate within the opposing occlusal tables. *D*, distal; *M*, mesial.

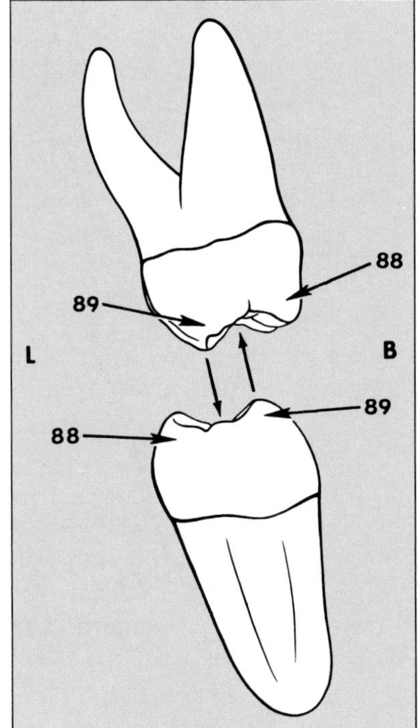

Figure 13.25

Since these cusps are responsible for supporting the occlusal vertical dimension in the intercuspal position they are referred to as the *supporting cusps* (*89*).

The buccal cusps of the upper arch and the lingual cusps of the lower arch have potential for occlusal contact only when the mandible is performing horizontal glide (contact) movements. Should these cusps contact during a given mandibular glide movement they provide guidance for such movement. The buccal cusps of the upper arch and the lingual cusps of the lower arch, therefore, are referred to as the *guiding cusps* (*88*).

Each of the two cusp groups, supporting and guiding, contain characteristics that link their members into what might be considered cuspal families.

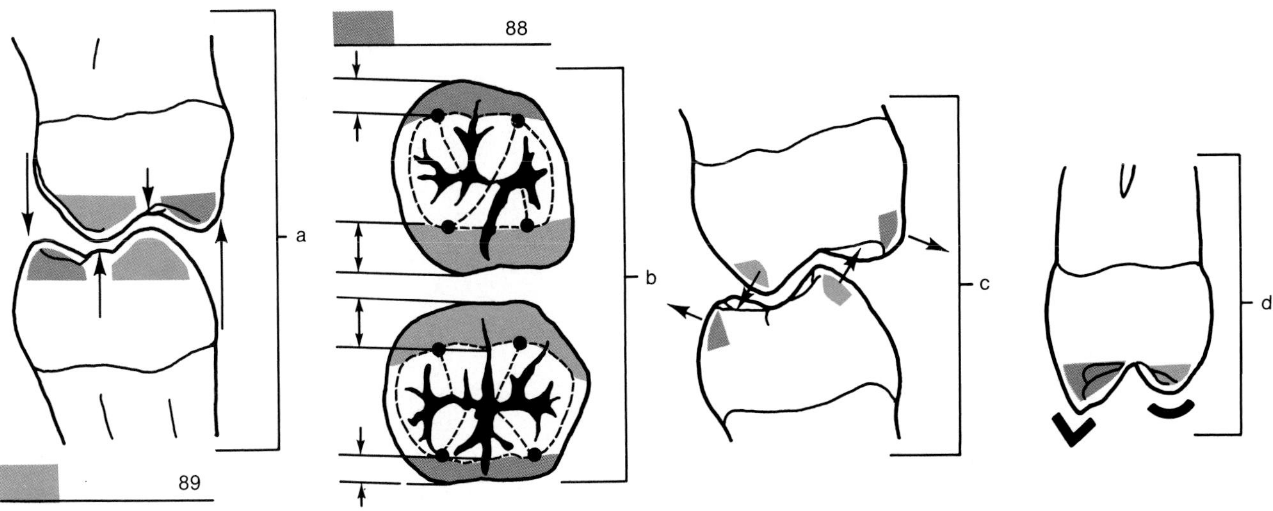

Figure 13.26

Similarities for All Supporting Cusps

a, The supporting cusps articulate within an opposing occlusal table and support the occlusal vertical dimension in the intercuspal position. *b,* The supporting cusps are positioned further from their outer aspects than are the guiding cusps so that there are usually greater amounts of supporting outer aspect visible from the occlusal view. *c,* The supporting cusps have outer aspects that have potential for occlusal contact. *d,* The supporting cusps are generally rounder than the guiding cusps.

Similarities for All Guiding Cusps

a, They have potentials for contact only when the mandible is in a horizontal glide movement and are articulated outside of the opposing occlusal tables. *b,* The guiding cusps are positioned closer to their outer aspect as seen from the occlusal. *c,* The outer aspects of the guiding cusps do not have potential for occlusal contact. *d,* The guiding cusps are generally sharper than the supporting cusps.

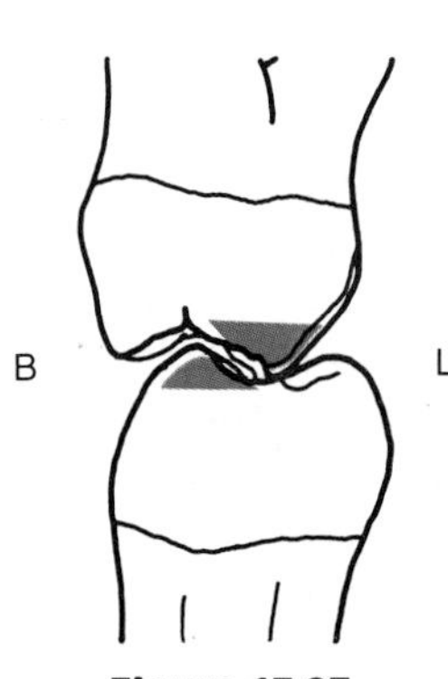

Figure 13.27

How much of the outer aspects of the supporting cusp may be considered functional? The outer aspect of the supporting cusp plays an important functional role since it enables the tip of the cusp to be cradled within the opposing occlusal table.

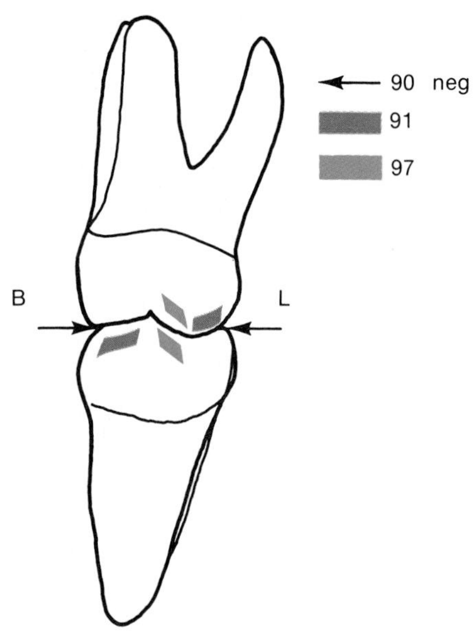

Figure 13.28

However, if the outer aspect of the supporting cusp were in complete contact, there would be a loss of the horizontal overlap which is necessary for the protection of the lip-cheek-tongue system. *90,* Mucosal protective overjet; *91,* functional outer aspect (FOA); *97,* inner aspect supporting cusp.

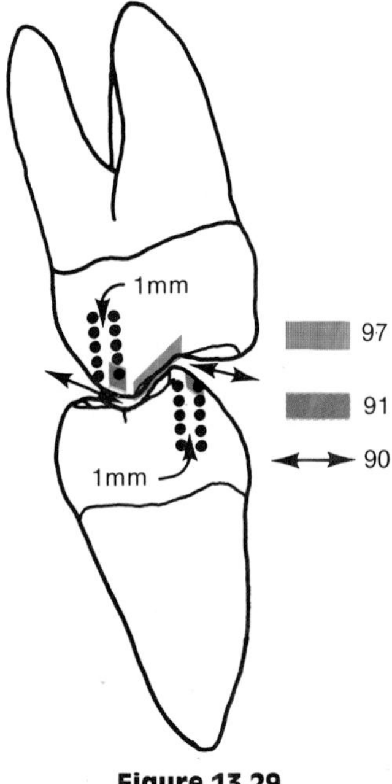

Figure 13.29

In the normal support of the intercuspal position, only a small area of the outer aspect of the supporting cusp is necessary to enable it to be properly cradled within the opposing occlusal table. The amount is only about 1 mm or less. *97,* Inner aspect supporting cusp; *91,* functional outer aspect (FOA); *90,* mucosal protective overjet.

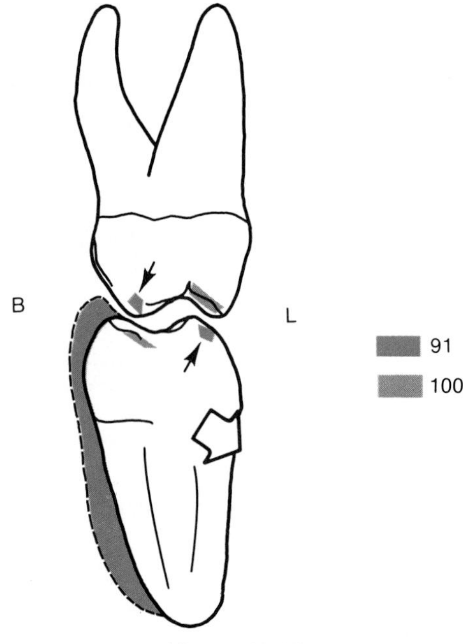

Figure 13.30

This zone on the outer aspect of the supporting cusp is referred to as the *functional outer aspect* or simply as the *FOA*. The functional outer aspect is also the portion of the supporting cusp that has the potential for making contact with the inner incline of the guiding cusps. *91,* FOA of supporting cusps; *100,* guiding incline of guiding cusps. *Large arrow* indicates mandibular glide movement.

The Relation of the Landmarks of the Occlusal Surfaces of Opposing Teeth in the Intercuspal Position

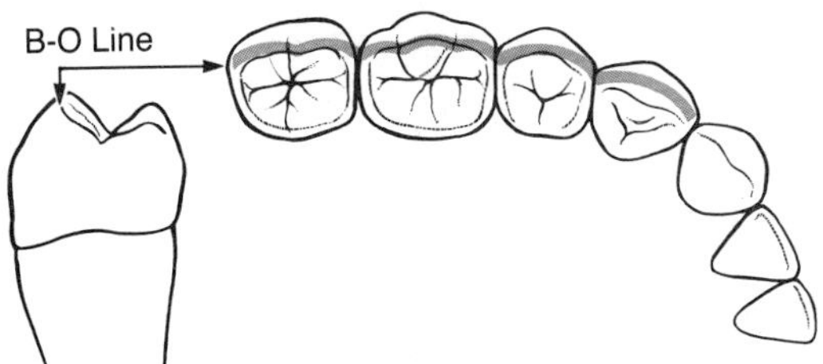

Figure 13.31

The Bucco-occlusal (B-O) Line

This is the line angle formed by the junction of the buccal and occlusal surfaces (junction of inner and outer aspects) of the buccal cusps. A well-aligned arch forms a continuous imaginary B-O line.

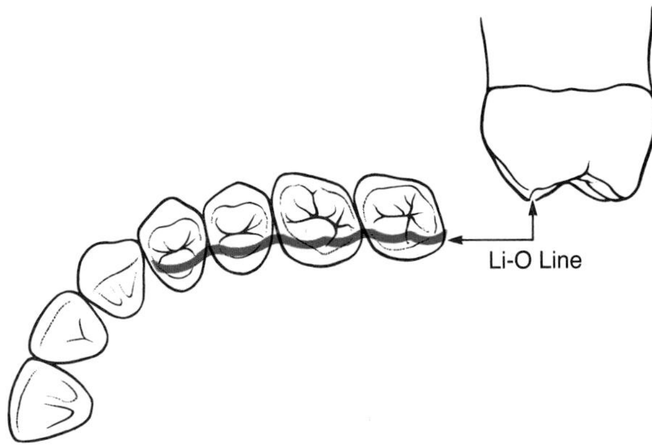

Figure 13.32

The Linguo-occlusal (Li-O) Line

This is the line angle formed by the junction of the lingual and occlusal surfaces (junction of the inner and outer aspects) of the lingual cusps. A well-aligned dentition forms a continuous imaginary Li-O line.

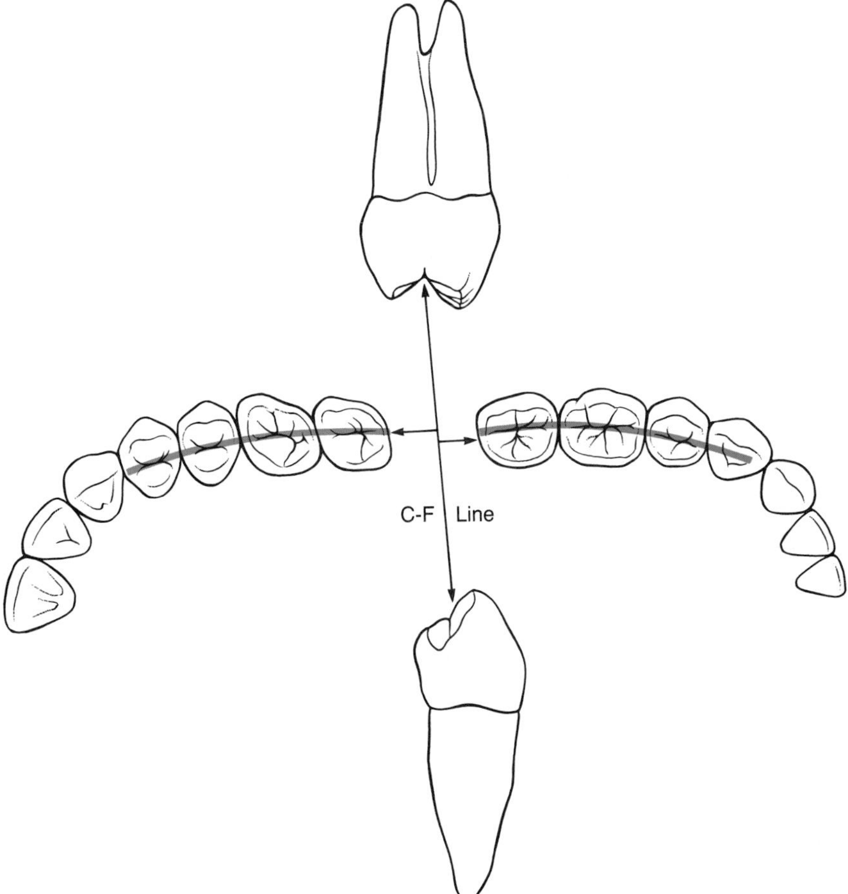

Figure 13.33

The Central Fossa (C-F) Line

This is an imaginary line that connects all the central developmental grooves of the posterior teeth. A well-aligned arch forms a continuous C-F line.

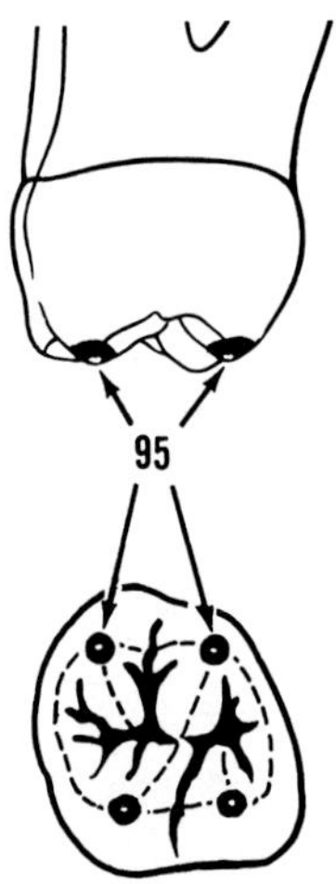

Figure 13.34

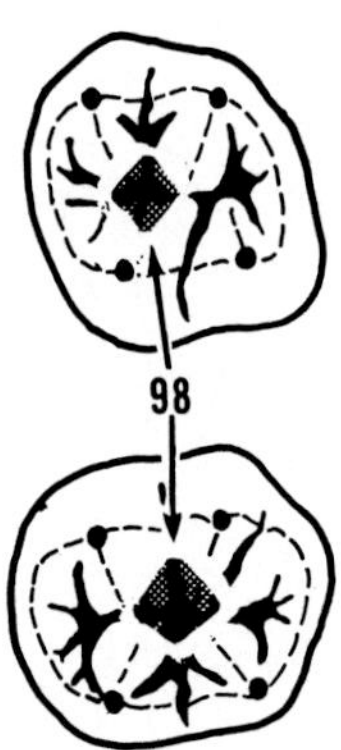

Figure 13.35

The Cusp Tip

The cusp tip, when used as a landmark, refers to a circular area with the true cusp apex as a center and with a radius about 0.05 mm in dimension. *95,* Articulating cusp tip.

The Central Fossa

The central fossa, when used as a landmark, refers to the true anatomic central valley of the molars. This is an area in the central portion of the occlusal table well designed to cradle a supporting cusp. *98,* Articulating central fossa.

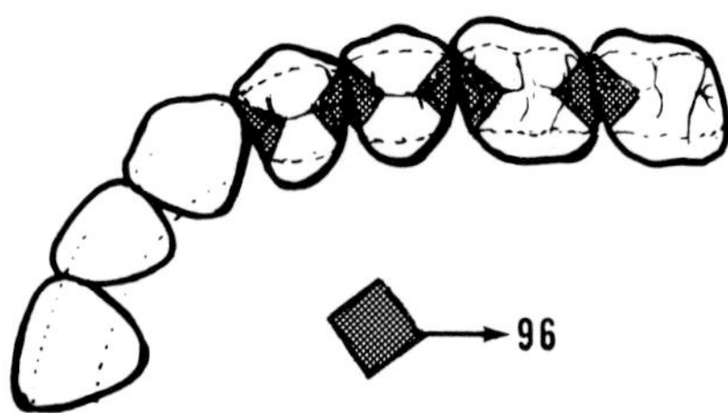

Figure 13.36

The Interproximal Marginal Ridge Areas

This refers to the platform area which is generally diamond shaped and very flat, and is created by adjacent marginal ridges. It is bounded by the supplemental grooves of the mesial and distal triangular fossae of adjacent teeth. This is an area well designed to cradle a supporting cusp. *96,* Articulating interproximal marginal ridge areas.

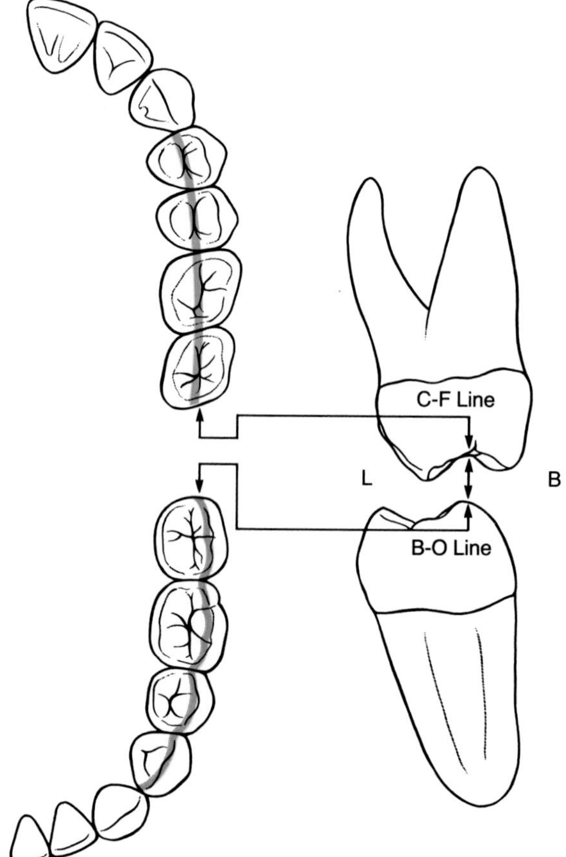

Figure 13.37

The Relation of the Occlusal Landmarks in the Intercuspal Position

Buccolingual Landmark Relations

The bucco-occlusal (*B-O*) line of the lower teeth is related to the central fossa (*C-F*) line of the upper teeth.

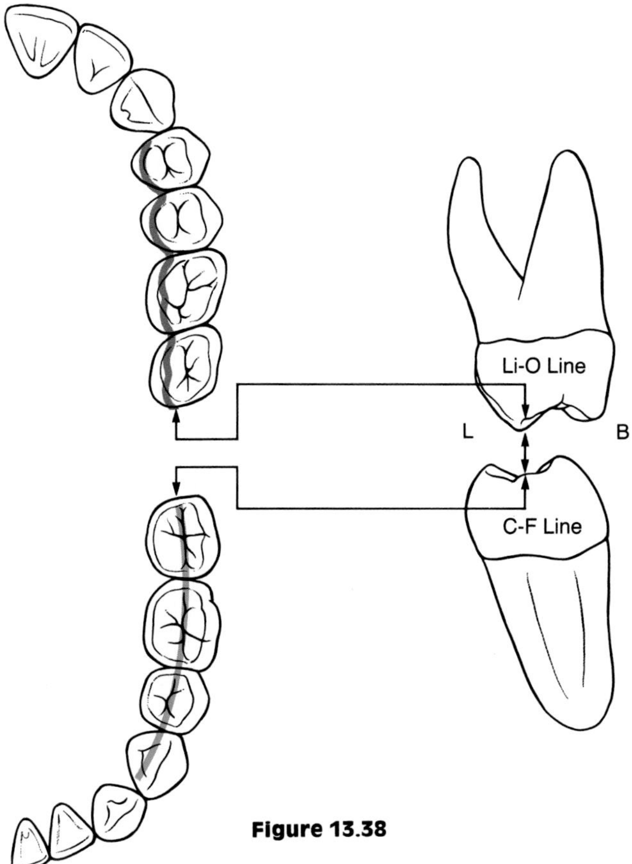

Figure 13.38

The linguo-occlusal (*Li-O*) line of the upper teeth is related to the central fossa (*C-F*) line of the lower teeth.

This means that if one examines the occlusal surface of the lower arch and looks at the bucco-occlusal line one must immediately think in terms of the opposing central fossa line or vice versa.

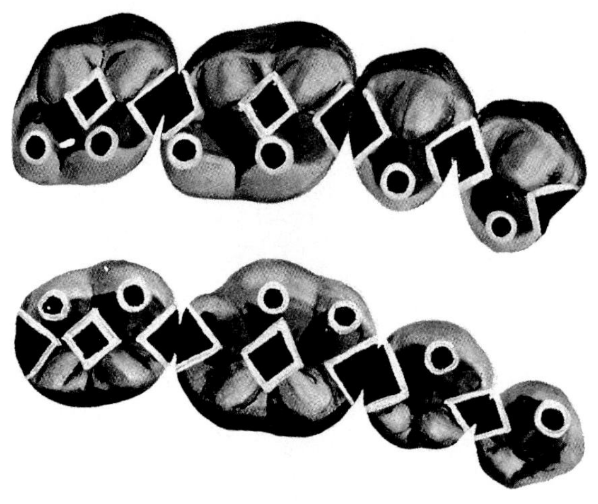

Figure 13.39

Mesiodistal View

In a quadrant, all but two supporting cusp tips are cradled in opposing adjacent marginal ridge areas. The two which are the exceptions are cradled in opposing central fossae. The exceptions are the mesiolingual cusps of upper molars and the distobuccal cusps of the lower molars.

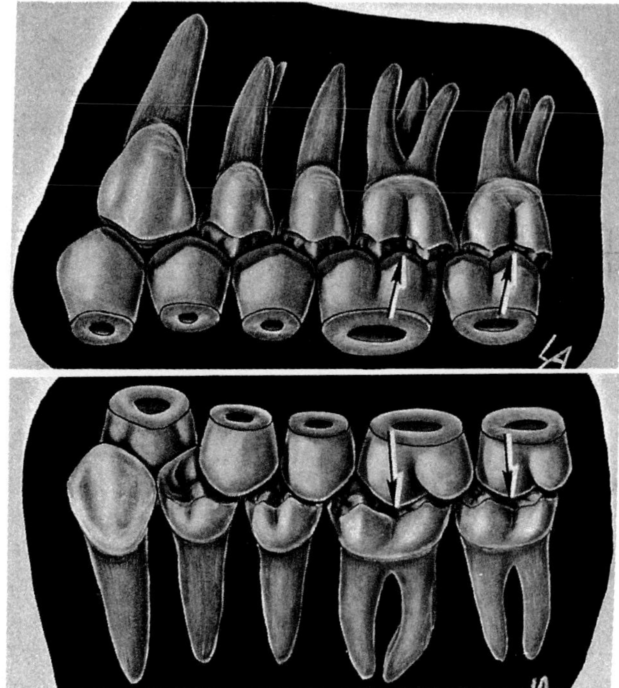

Figure 13.40

Buccal and Lingual View

Again, if one inspects the mandibular supporting cusps from the occlusal view one is able to envision the interproximal marginal ridge and central fossa areas responsible for cradling these cusps. Likewise, if one examines the mandibular interproximal marginal ridge and central fossa areas one is able to envision the cusp tips of the maxilla which articulate in these areas.

Arrows indicate cusp tips which articulate into central fossa.

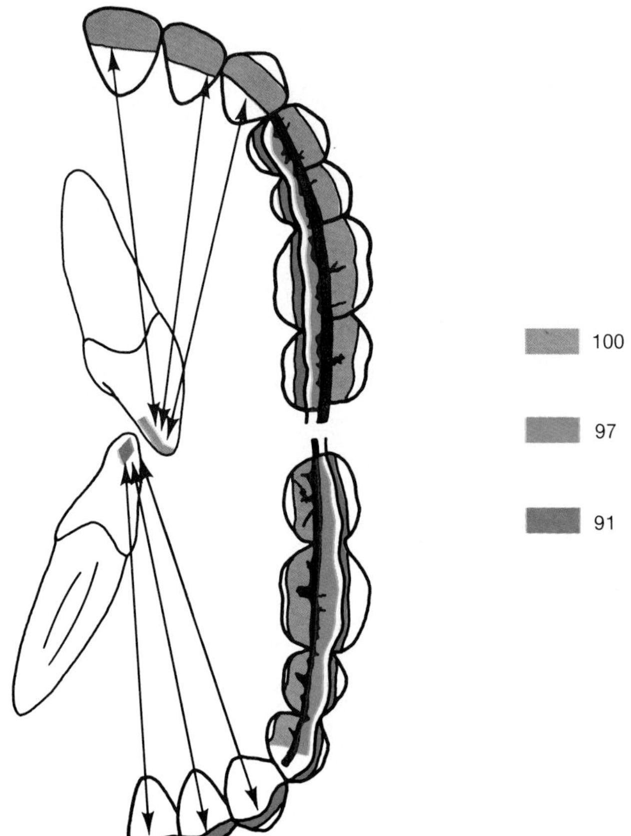

Figure 13.41

Articulating Properties of the Posterior Teeth Found in the Anterior Teeth

The lower incisors generally do not have incisal contact that will contribute to the support of the occlusal vertical dimension in the intercuspal position. However, when the mandible engages in horizontal glide movements the labioincisal edge has potential for contact with lingual inclines of the maxillary anterior teeth. The contacting portion of the lower incisal edge is considered to be a functional outer aspect.

The functional outer aspect of the lower arch, therefore, can be described as a continuous ribbon, less than 1 mm in width, that runs from the buccal of the right third molar to the buccal of the left third molar, and covers the incisal edges of the lower anterior teeth.

The lingual inclines of the upper anterior teeth are the chief guides for jaw movement. For this reason the lingual inclines of the maxillary incisors and canines are thought of as guiding inclines. *100,* Inner aspects of guiding cusps; *97,* inner aspect of supporting cusp; *91,* functional outer aspect (FOA).

It is evident that some elements of cuspal function are present in the anterior teeth.

Tooth Articulation in Mandibular Glide Movements (Contact Movements) (Figs. 13.42 and 13.43)

There is a great deal of conjecture as to the precise manner in which the natural human dentition should be articulated in the "ideal" state.

It is our belief that a very simple plan of articulation will account for the hypothetical ideal; namely, that the upper and lower posterior teeth represent negative counterparts of each other in the intercuspal position. It is further advocated that anterior teeth during contact movements will prevent contact of the posterior teeth. Mandibular contact movements occur in daily activity as a part of parafunctional states and not during normal physiological behavior of the masticatory system.

The concept of a bilaterally balanced occlusion with maximum intercuspation as "nature's intent" is extremely presumptuous and inexact when applied to the natural dentition of man. This concept, which has almost completely retreated from the professional scene, is a direct carryover from the ideas originally advocated by Bonwill in 1866. It must be remembered that Bonwill devised the theory of bilateral balance in order better to stabilize full denture bases. The concept of a bilaterally balanced occlusion is contrary to

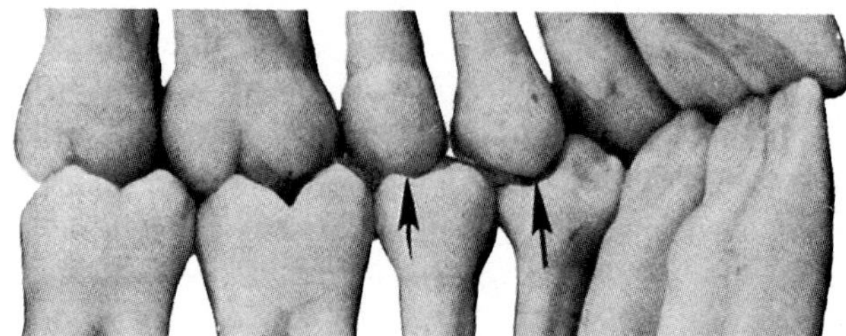

Figure 13.42

The maxillary premolars very often have the tips of their lingual cusps positioned in the distal fossa of the mandibular premolars (*arrows*). This idea was not discussed in the previous section in order to reduce intercuspation to its simplest terms.

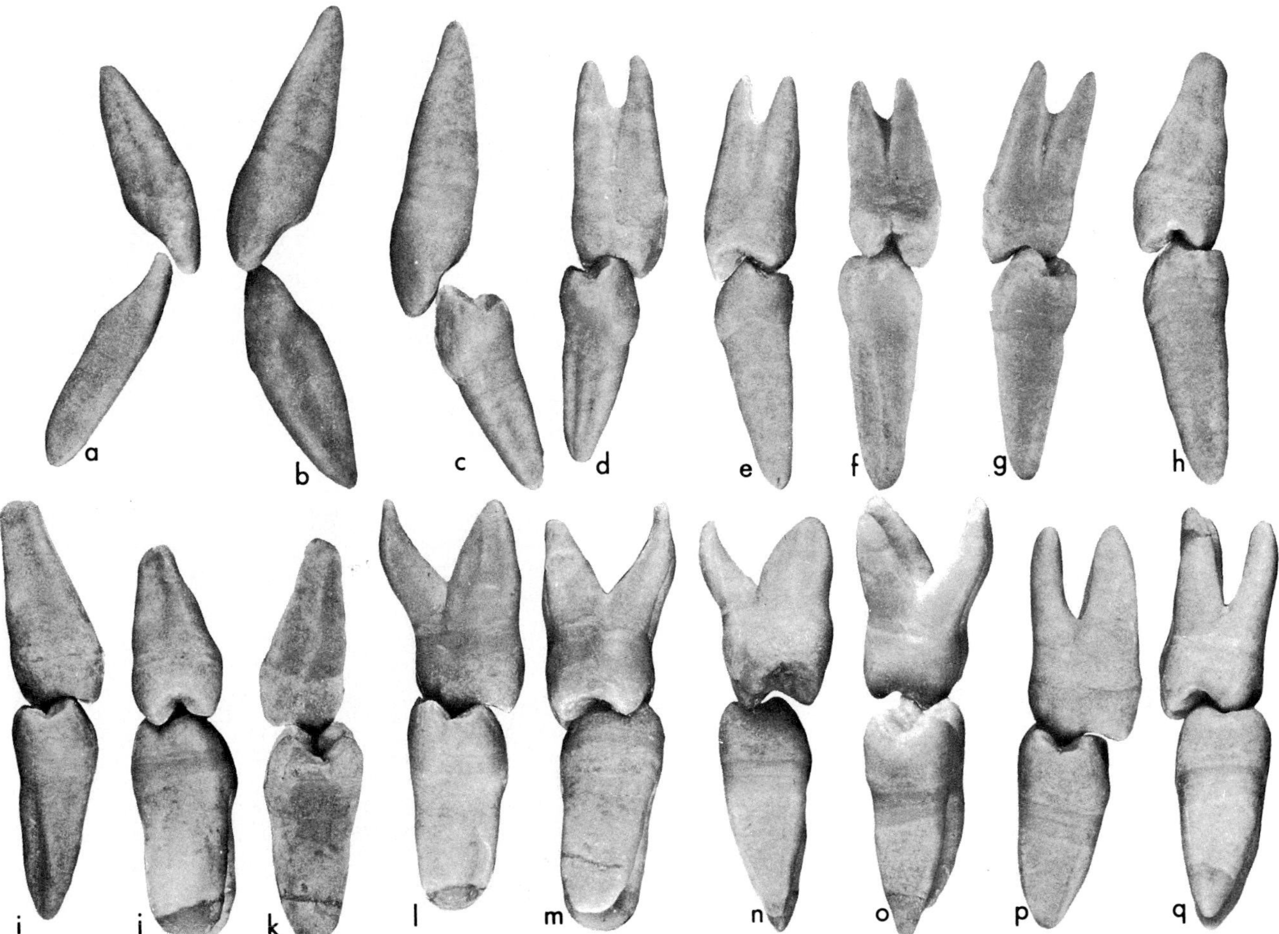

Figure 13.43

The proximal view of the articulation of teeth in the intercuspal position: *a*, central incisors, note absence of contact; *b*, canine relations; *c*, maxillary canine mandibular premolar relations; *d*, first premolars, mesial view; *e*, first premolars, distal view; *f*, maxillary first premolar, mandibular second premolar, mesial view; *g*, maxillary first premolar, mandibular second premolar, distal view; *h*, second premolars, mesial view; *i*, second premolars, distal view; *j*, maxillary second premolar, mandibular first molar, mesial view; *k*, maxillary second premolar, mandibular first molar, distal view; *l*, first molars, mesial view; *m*, first molars, distal view; *n*, maxillary first molar, mandibular second molar, mesial view; *o*, maxillary first molar, mandibular second molar, distal view; *p*, second molars, mesial view; *q*, second molars, distal view.

what is known about man's method of masticating food. Mastication takes place essentially as a unilateral activity on the preferred side and only slightly does tooth contact occur while food is in the mouth. Further, if a balanced occlusion is a phenomenon of the human dentition, it is observed only after some degree of occlusal attrition has taken place. This is evident when comparison has been made between "primitive" and "civilized" man. Even in primitive man with advanced occlusal attrition, however, the balanced contacts of teeth are confined to the working side only.

Bilaterally balanced occlusion, although not normally occurring, does offer excellent study opportunities, because it serves as a means of examining the mechanical possibilities for contact of opposing occlusal tables during all mandibular contact movements. Mandibular contact movements may be bilaterally symmetrical or asymmetrical, and may be further subdivided as follows.

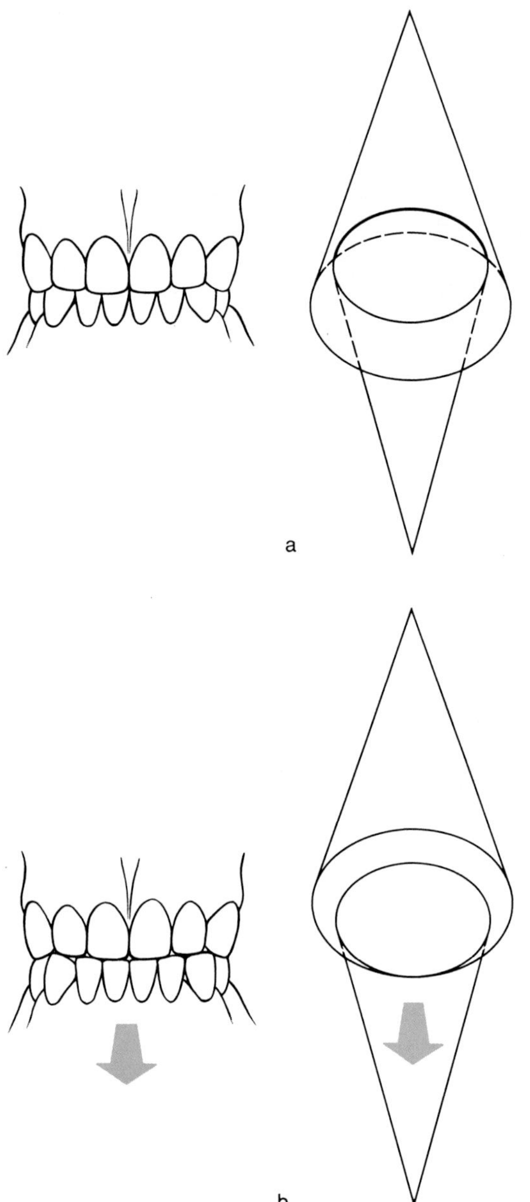

Figure 13.44
The incisal relations of the anterior teeth in protrusive glide: *a,* intercuspal position; *b,* protrusive edge-to-edge contacting position.

A. Symmetrical articulation
   1. Intercuspal position
   2. Protrusive glide and position
B. Asymmetrical articulation
   1. Lateral glide and position
      a. Working side
      b. Nonworking side
   2. Lateral protrusive glide and position
      a. Working side
      b. Nonworking side

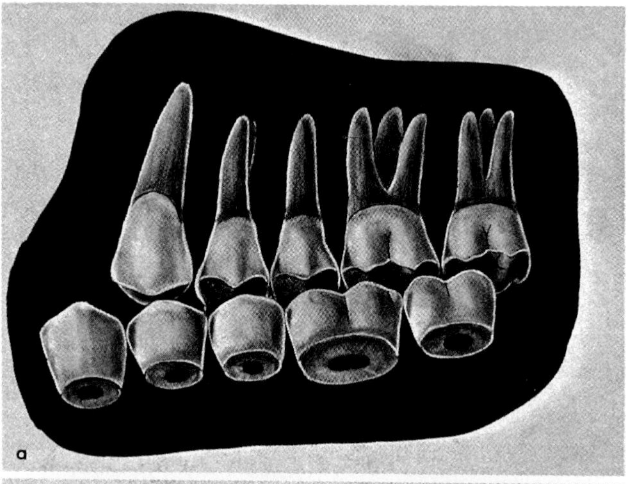

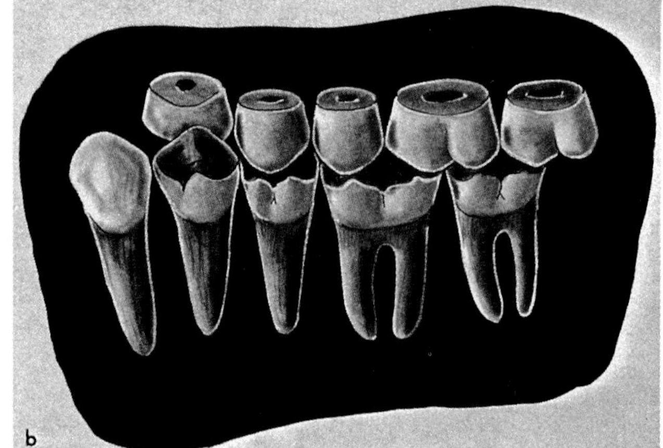

Figure 13.45
Protrusive tooth contacts: *a,* buccal; *b,* lingual.

All contact movements of the mandible, with the exception of the nonworking component of lateral glide, will occur between the FOA of one arch and the guiding inclines of the other. Further, glide tooth articulation, with the exception of the working side of lateral glide, takes place on mesial mandibular occlusal inclines and maxillary distal occlusal inclines.

Symmetrical Articulation

Intercuspal Position

Discussed earlier in this section.

Protrusive Glide and Position

Protrusive glide is accomplished when the mandible is propelled straight forward until the upper and lower incisors contact edge-to-edge. The movement is bilaterally symmetrical with both sides of the mandible moving in the same direction.

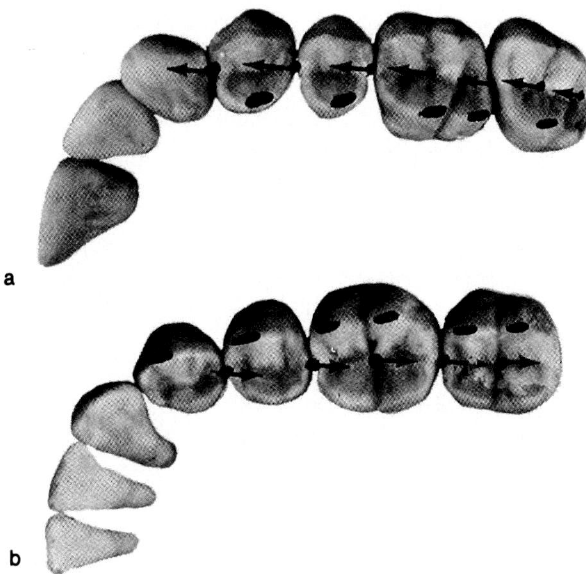

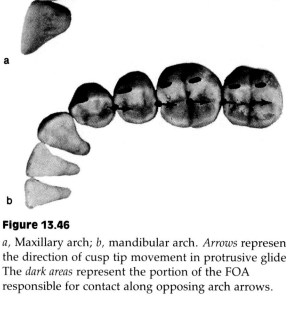

Figure 13.46

a, Maxillary arch; *b,* mandibular arch. *Arrows* represent the direction of cusp tip movement in protrusive glide. The *dark areas* represent the portion of the FOA responsible for contact along opposing arch arrows.

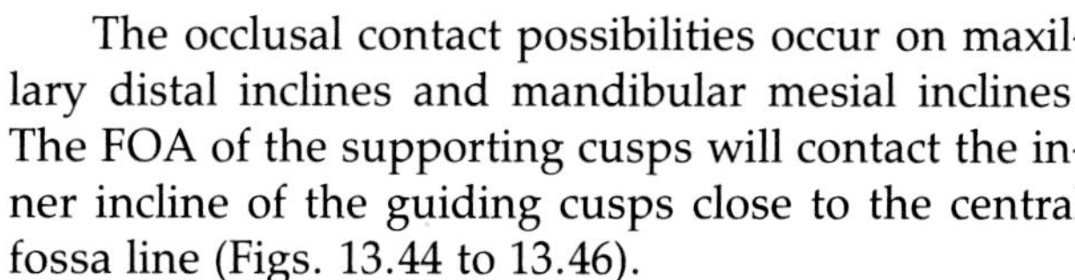

The occlusal contact possibilities occur on maxillary distal inclines and mandibular mesial inclines. The FOA of the supporting cusps will contact the inner incline of the guiding cusps close to the central fossa line (Figs. 13.44 to 13.46).

In the anterior teeth, at the same time, the FOA of the lower incisors will contact the guiding inclines of the upper incisor and canines.

It is to be remembered that the mesial half of the mandibular first premolar behaves identically to the canine.

Asymmetrical Articulation

Lateral Mandibular Glide (Lateral Excursion)

Here the mandible is moving toward the right or the left side. The side to which the mandible moves is referred to as the working side. The side *from* which the mandible is moving is referred to as the nonworking side (in full denture construction, the balancing side). Unlike in protrusive contact movement, each side behaves differently (Figs. 13.47 and 13.48).

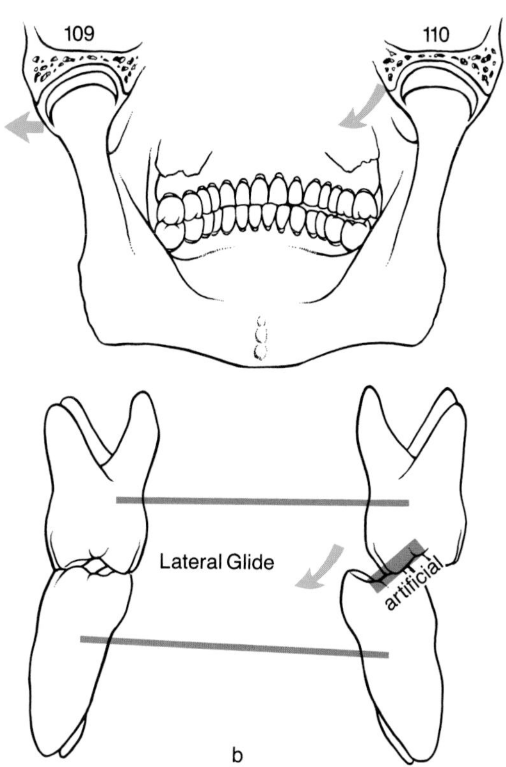

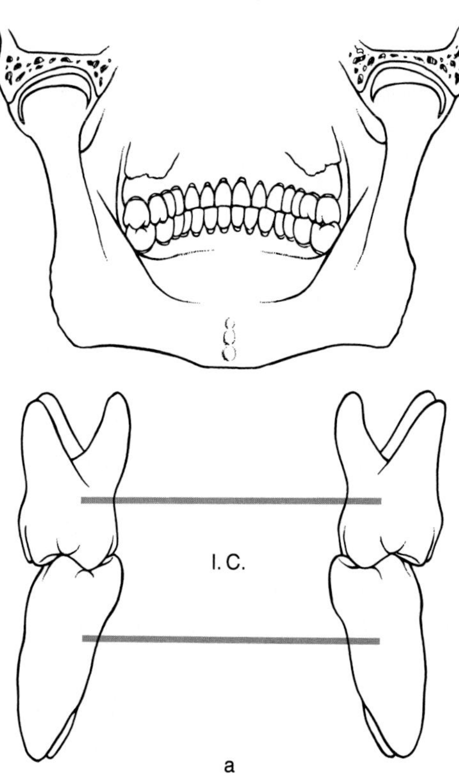

Figure 13.47

a, Intercuspal position; *b,* left lateral glide movement; *109,* working side; *110,* nonworking side. The nonworking tooth contracts are of the type seen in the artificial dentition. The movement space of these nonworking cusps will mimic the downward-forward movement of the nonworking condyle. For a given amount of incisal guidance the amount of interocclusal clearance (*IC.*) on the nonworking side will be a direct reflection of the amount of downward movement of the moving nonworking condyle.

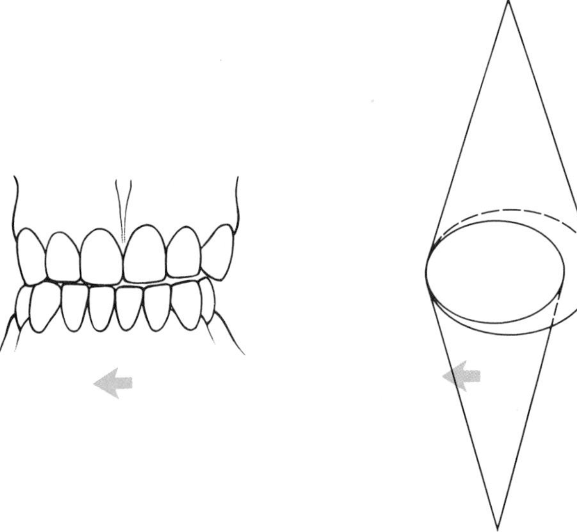

Figure 13.48

The anterior teeth relations in right lateral contact position. The mesial half of the mandibular first premolar behaves as if it were an anterior tooth.

Working-Side Contact On the working side the FOAs of the supporting cusps have the potentiality of sliding over the inner aspects of the guiding inclines with activity on both mesial and distal surfaces of both arches, so that the cusp tips pass between the opposing cusp tips.

Of special note is the behavior of the distobuccal cusp of the upper first molar, which will contact the groove between the fifth cusp and the distobuccal cusp of the lower first molar (Figs. 13.49 and 13.50).

Nonworking-Side Contact The contact on the nonworking side takes place on distal upper inclines and lower mesial inclines. The contact area possibilities here are unique because they involve the inner aspects of supporting cusps only. This is the only time that the inner inclines of the supporting cusps can contact outside the intercuspal position.

Of special interest is the behavior of the oblique ridge and the mesiolingual cusp of the upper first molars. This area will contact the developmental

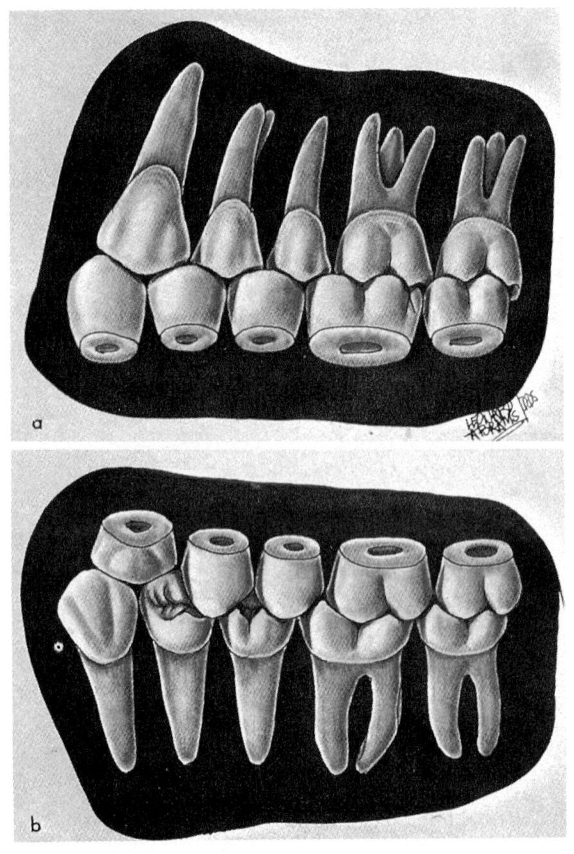

Figure 13.49

Working-side contacts: *a*, buccal; *b*, lingual.

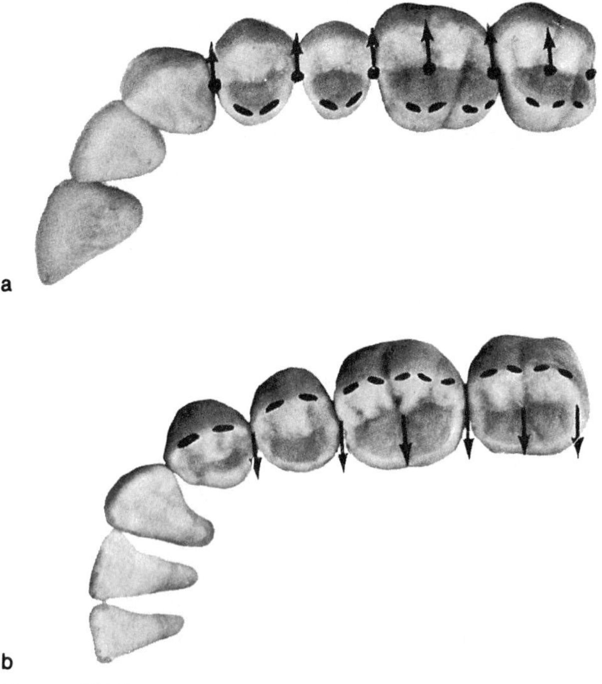

Figure 13.50

a, Maxillary arch; *b*, mandibular arch. Working-side cusp directions are indicated by *arrows*. *Shaded areas* indicate the FOA areas, which engage the guiding inclines.

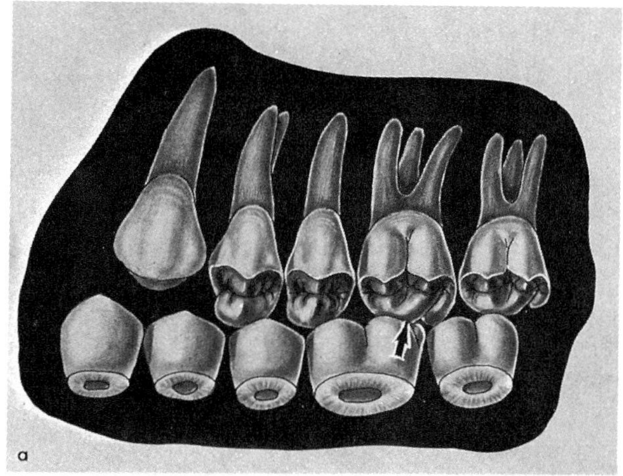

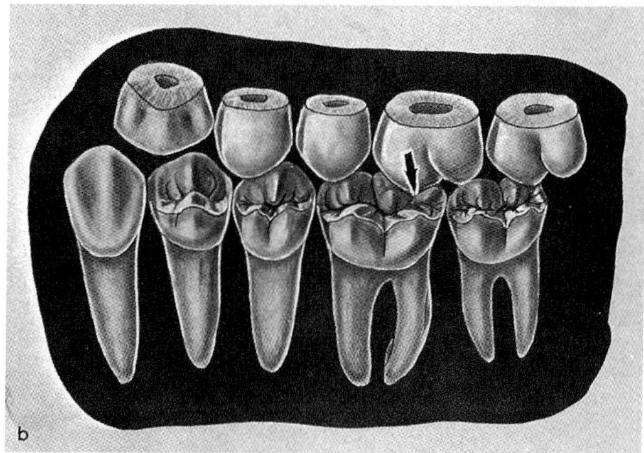

Figure 13.51

Nonworking contact: *a,* buccal; *b,* lingual. The *arrow* indicates the relation between the mesiolingual cusp and the groove between the fifth and distobuccal cups of the first molar.

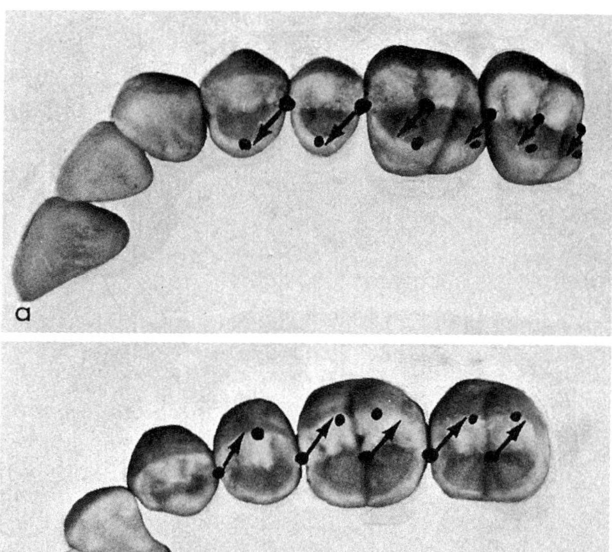

Figure 13.52

a, Maxillary arch; *b,* mandibular arch. *Arrows* indicate cusp directions. In this instance, *arrow markings* of the upper and lower arch are *superimposable.*

groove on the occlusal surface that separates the distobuccal and fifth cusps of the lower molars.

Contact on the nonworking side will take place on the surface of concentric curves that are parallel to the movement pattern of the nonworking condyle (Figs. 13.51 and 13.52).

Lateral Protrusive Mandibular Guide

This is a combination of a protruded and lateral glide. Although each side behaves differently, only contact on the working side is possible. Here contact takes place between distal upper inclines and mesial lower inclines. The FOAs of the supporting cusps follow a path diagonally across the inner aspect of the opposing guiding incline terminating cusp tip-to-cusp tip (Figs. 13.53 to 13.55).

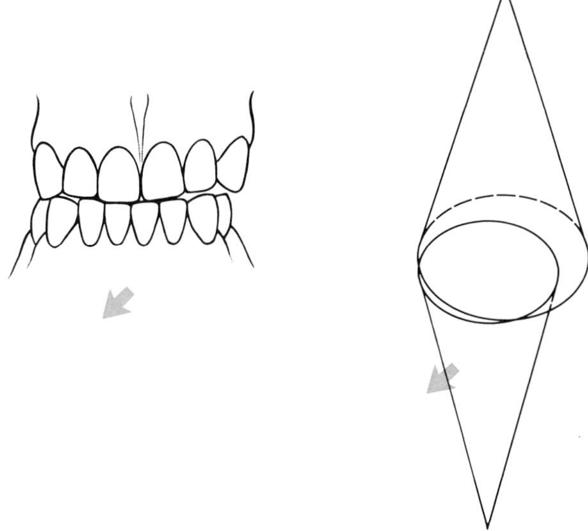

Figure 13.53

The anterior teeth in lateral protrusive contact movement (*arrows*).

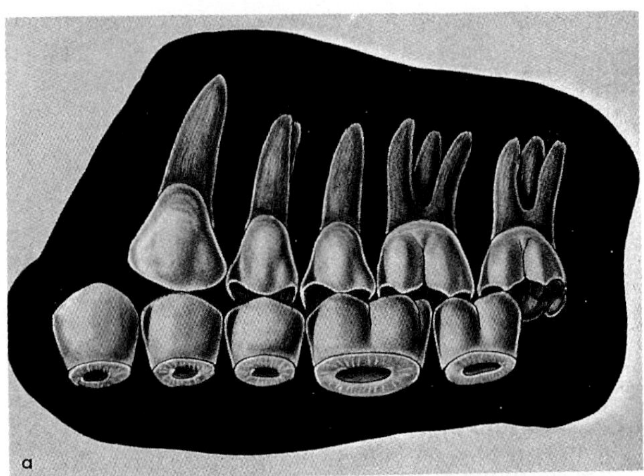

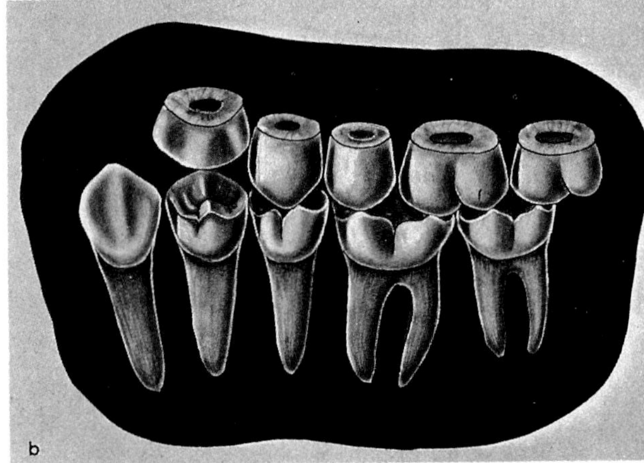

Figure 13.54

a, Buccal; *b,* lingual. The cusp tip-to-cusp tip relation of the working side in lateral protrusive contact position.

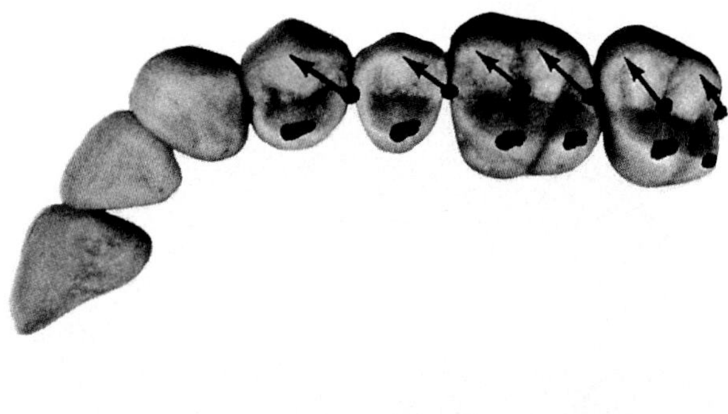

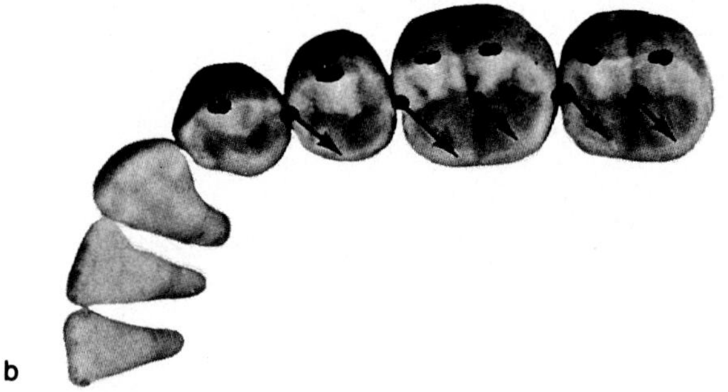

Figure 13.55

a, Maxillary arch; *b,* mandibular arch. The *arrows* indicate the direction of the supporting cusp tips across the guiding inclines to guiding cusp tips.

The Self-Protective Features of the Dentition

The dental profession subscribes to the hypothesis that teeth with proper form and alignment will tend to protect their supporting structures during normal functioning. Although there is no scientific evidence to support this belief, the observed correlation between destructive diseases and poor form and function tends to strengthen it. In the pages that follow we discuss the significance of tooth form in its physiologic setting as it is related to the so-called protective features.

The Effect of Axial Positioning on Tooth Form

When an extracted tooth is examined in the hand, the tooth is usually held in a completely upright position. There is an inherent error in this type of orientation that should be recognized. Teeth are almost never aligned in the dental arches with their center axes parallel to a vertical line. Generally there is a slight mesial and a buccal or lingual inclination of the crown to varying degrees, with resultant alterations in the vertical inclination of the center axis causing definite changes in the *effective* crown forms. In order to obviate misconceptions of tooth form and function, it is important that extracted teeth be examined with every effort made to approximate the correct axial (physiologic) position (Figs. 14.1 to 14.3).

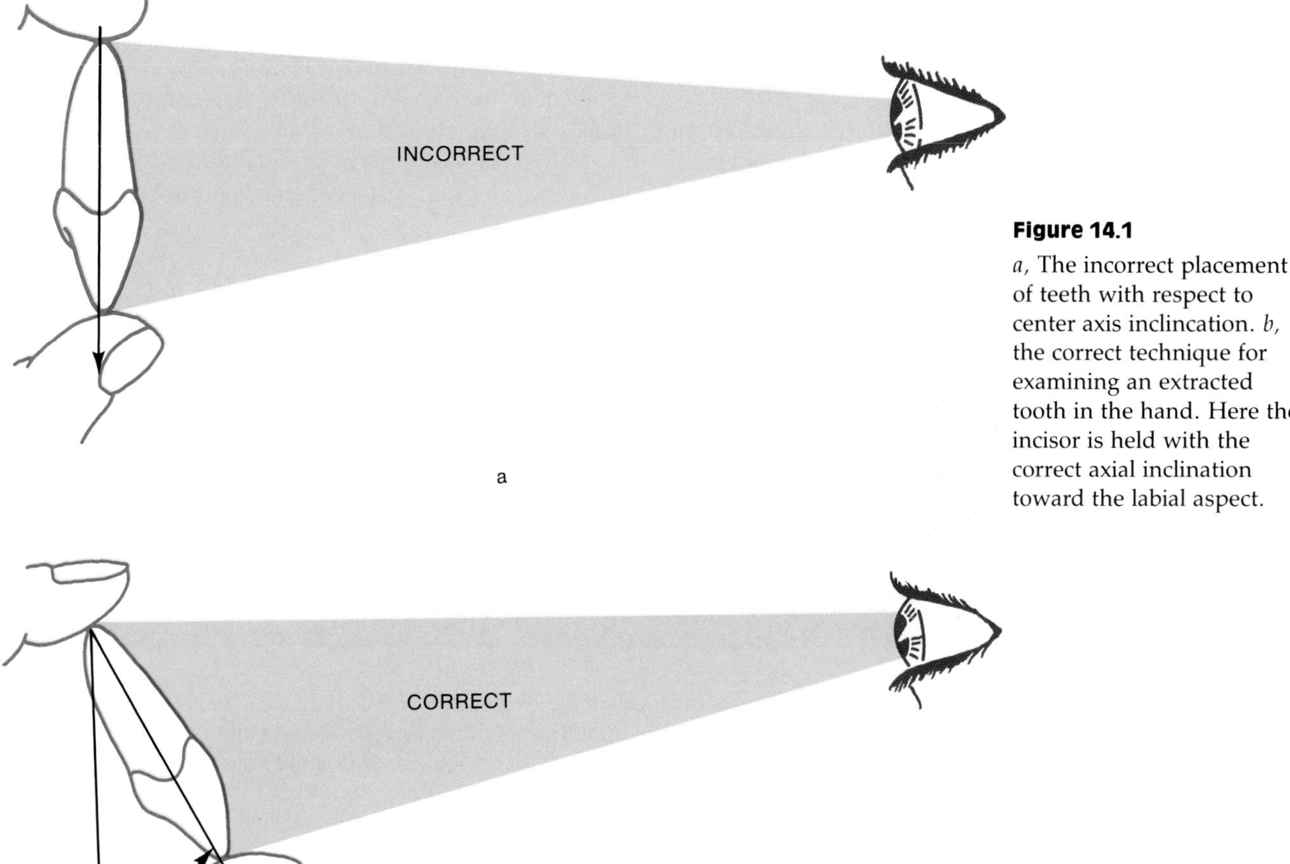

Figure 14.1

a, The incorrect placement of teeth with respect to center axis inclincation. *b,* the correct technique for examining an extracted tooth in the hand. Here the incisor is held with the correct axial inclination toward the labial aspect.

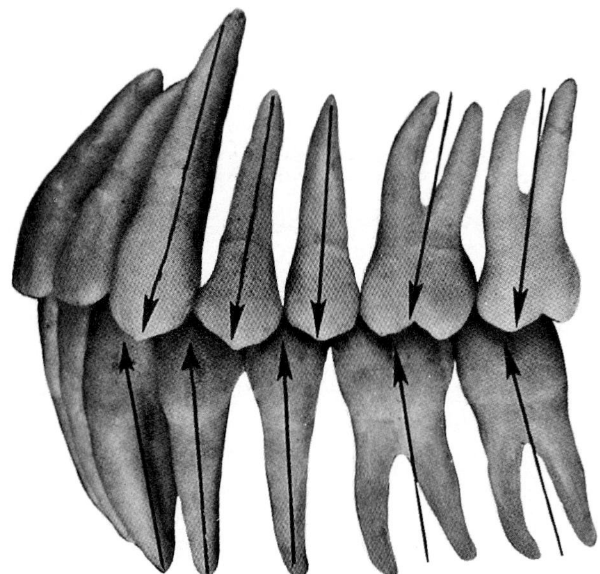

Figure 14.2
Most posterior teeth are inclined with their crowns toward the mesial. The *arrows* are placed so as to closely approximate the center axes of the teeth.

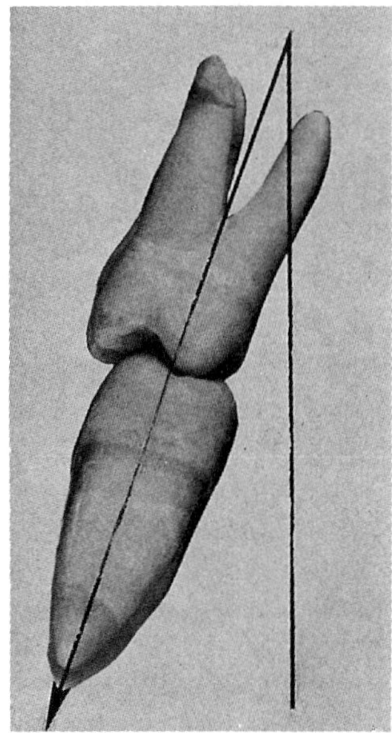

Figure 14.3
An example of the faciolingual inclination of teeth. Here the buccolingual inclination of the maxillary and mandibular molars is quite marked.

Protection to the Periodontium

In normal function, the teeth serve to protect the two basic areas of the periodontium, the gingival tissues and the attachment apparatus.

The gingival tissues appear to be dependent upon functional stimulation to retain their normal, healthy character. The ability for normal masticatory activity to serve as a stimulant rather than as an irritant is a product of the protective capacity that teeth possess by virtue of their individual coronal contours and collective alignment.

When one side of the arch is ignored in function, the clinician often observes that food debris and den-

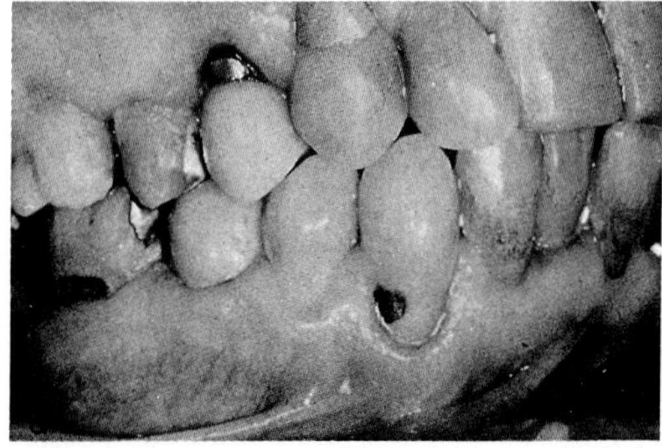

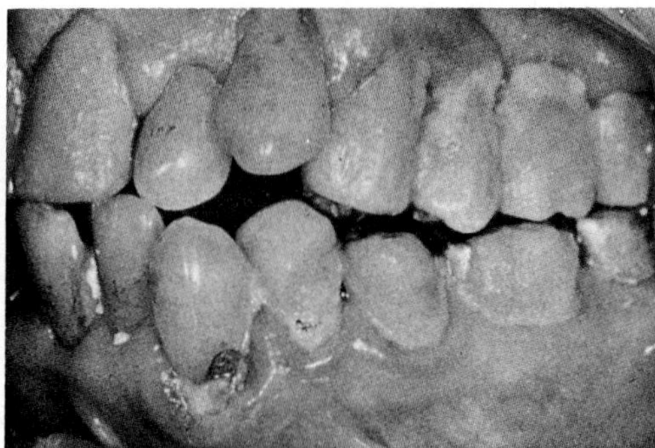

Figure 14.4
The effects of lack of occlusal function on gingival health in a patient who does not brush his teeth. *a*, the side of the mouth used in mastication. Note that there is an absence of debris and the gingival tissues appear firm, stippled, and free of inflammation. *b*, the unused side of the mouth. Here lack of function is manifested in the increased debris and plaque deposition. The gingiva appears swollen and reddened and lacks stippling.

tal plaque tend to stagnate with an accompanying increase in calculus formation, gingival inflammation, and cervical caries. Figure 14.4 presents typical examples of the effects of lack of function.

The Role of Crown Form in Gingival Health

In healthy individuals the necks of the teeth are surrounded by the attached gingiva. This seemingly well-adapted tissue does present, however, an area extremely vulnerable to periodontal disease, the gingival crevice. The gingival crevice (or sulcus) is bounded by tooth, free gingiva, and epithelial attachment to the enamel, as discussed in Chapter 10. It is lined by nonkeratinized epithelium that is only two to eight cells thick. A fluid exchange can and does occur in this area. The crevice is believed to be the primary site of marginal inflammatory periondontal disease due to accumulation of microbial plaque, so-called microcosm, in the area of the free gingival margin.

The form and alignment of the teeth tend to be such that the *vulnerable gingival crevice is sheltered from the adversities of increased microbial plaque formation by the proper location of coronal convexities and concavities.* The relation between the form and location of the gingiva and the tooth contour both individually and collectively creates a situation in which minimal free gingival margin is exposed for deposition of bacterial plaque debris.

The Facial and Lingual Crown Contours

Practically all facial and lingual surfaces of the tooth that are covered by enamel present a slight convex area located in the gingival third of the crown. The amount of convexity is about 0.5 mm per surface and thus permits a continuity of form from the crown to the attached gingiva with a minimum of ledge-like crevicular depository area. This relation enables the frictional activity of the lips, cheeks, tongue, resilient foods, and artificial cleansing devices to render the sulcular area free of dental plaque (Figs. 14.5 to 14.9).

On the lingual surface of the lower molars the amount and position of crown bulge are altered. As shown in Figure 14.9 the height of contour is located in the middle third of the crown and is about 1 mm

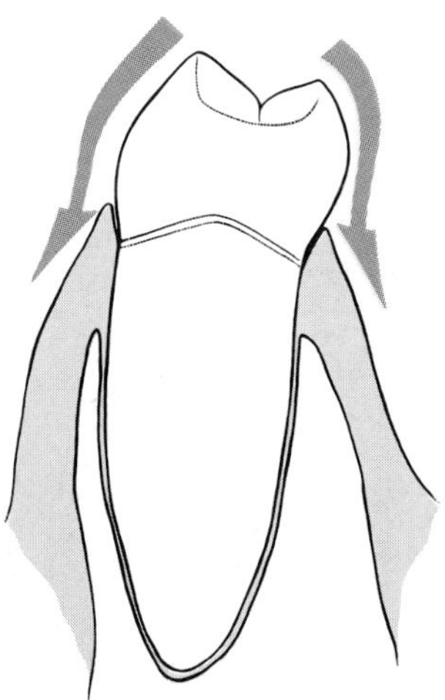

Figure 14.5

The hypothetical relation between correct crown contour and gingival health. The facial and lingual surfaces of the crowns contain just enough convexity so that the food is deflected away from the gingival sulcus. In this manner the gingival crevice is protected from becoming a depository for microbial plaque and food debris.

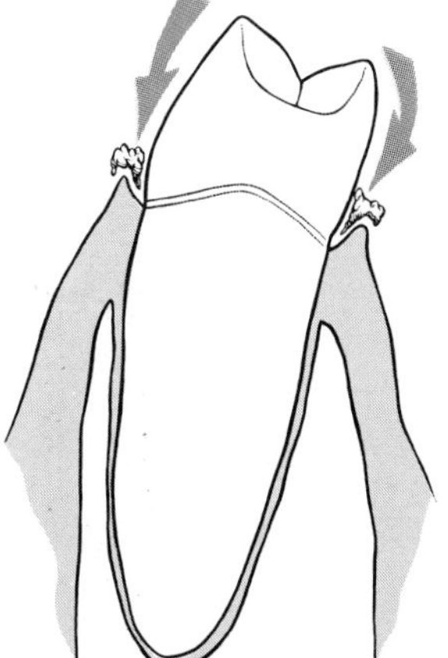

Figure 14.6

Incorrect crown contour in the form of facial and lingual surfaces that are too flat for the adjacent soft tissue. The result of this form is usually that microbial plaque and food debris become lodged in the gingival sulcus. Gingival inflammation often results.

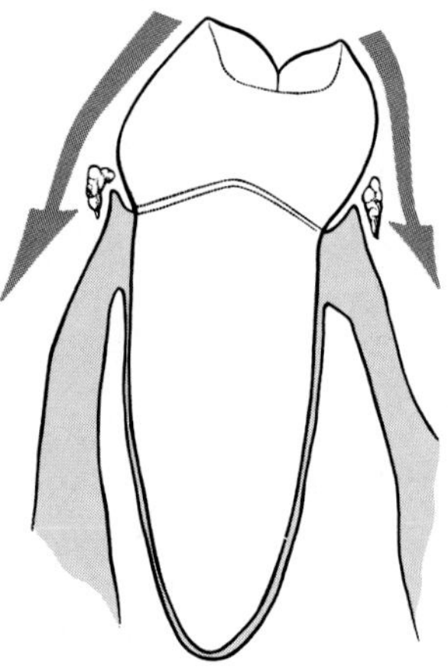

Figure 14.7

Incorrect crown contour in the form of facial and lingual surfaces that are too "bulbous" for the adjacent soft tissues. In this case microbial plaque and food debris tend to accumulate under the pronounced height of contour. Increased plaque in this area can lead to cervical caries in addition to gingival inflammation.

thick. The crown form differences here are apparently necessary because of the severe lingual inclinations which this tooth assumes in the arch. The lower molars have a decided lingual inclination (Fig. 14.10), and as a result cause the effective protective area of the crown to be lowered apically. The resultant position requires that the original crown convexity be positioned higher occlusally on the crown. Additional crown thickness is necessary, also, because of the thicker gingival tissues generally found covering the subjacent osseous ledge usually found in this area.

The thickness of the cervical crown bulge is not an exact measurement but is relative to the surrounding tissue dimensions. It appears, therefore, that teeth with heavier enamel bulges were designed as if to function in the mouth with heavier osseous and gingival forms (Fig. 14.11). This latter idea is apparently true in primary molars, which would be unable to function in fully erupted state within the size of the growing alveolus.

The Proximal Surfaces of the Crowns of the Teeth

The proximal surfaces of the crowns of all teeth are in many instances somewhat concave or at least are decidedly less convex than are the facial and lingual surfaces. This apparently permits approximating teeth to create an interproximal embrasure that will provide sufficient room to house and protect the interdental tissue and allow for a minimum of col formation. In teeth that possess greater cervical bulges of enamel on the facial and lingual surfaces, there generally is found a greater degree of proximal convexity. In all cases, however, the proximal surface is flatter than the facial or lingual surface.

The axial line angle that forms the transition between the flat or concave proximal surface and the convex facial or lingual surface deserves special attention. This area is referred to as the *transitional line angle*. This angle generally exhibits the same contour as the proximal surface and forms the opening for the residence of the interdental tissue. Inability to recognize the transitional line angle in clinical dentistry

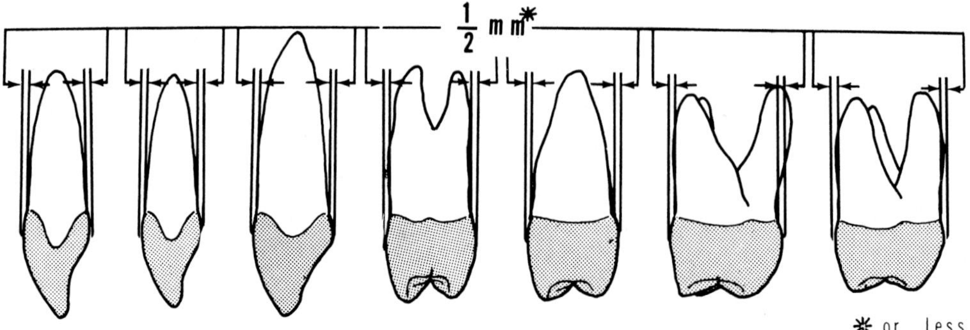

Figure 14.8

The amount of facial and lingual convexity of the crowns of the maxillary arch is shown. All facial and lingual surfaces have a convexity of 0.5 mm or less. The height of contour is located at the junction of the cervical and middle thirds of the crown. (Drawn with modification from Wheeler RC. A textbook of dental anatomy and physiology. 3rd ed. Philadelphia: WB Saunders, 1958.)

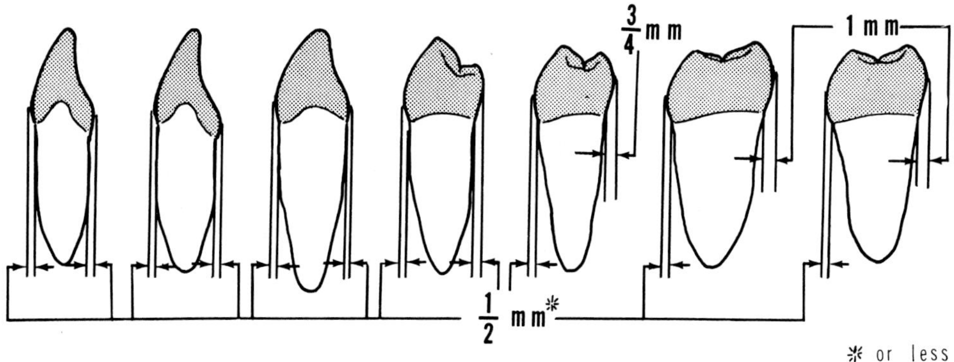

Figure 14.9

The amount of facial and lingual convexity of the crowns of the mandibular arch is shown. As in the maxillary arch, with the exception of the lingual surface of the second premolar and first and second molars, the facial and lingual surfaces have a convexity of about 0.5 mm or less. The mandibular second premolar will often have a lingual convexity of about 0.75 mm, and the mandibular molars will often demonstrate a lingual convexity of about 1 mm. The reason for the increases in convexity in the above areas is demonstrated in Figure 14.10. (Drawn with modification from Wheeler RC. A textbook of dental anatomy and physiology. 3rd ed. Philadelphia: WB Saunders, 1958.)

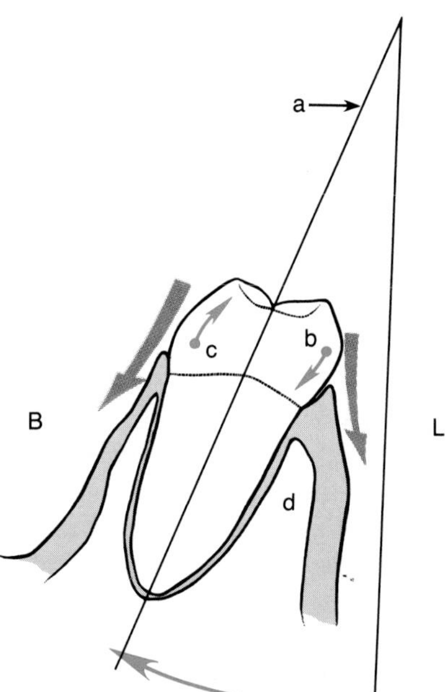

Figure 14.10

The positioning of the axial center (*a*) of the molar is such that the crown is inclined toward the lingual (*L*) and away from the buccal (*B*). This causes the height of crown contour (*b*) of the lingual to be depressed apically. At the same time the height of crown contour on the buccal surface (*c*) is elevated coronally. Also note that the increased contour on the lingual surface is apparently well designed to function with the increased thickness of the osseous and soft tissues (*d*) found on the lingual surface of the mandibular molar.

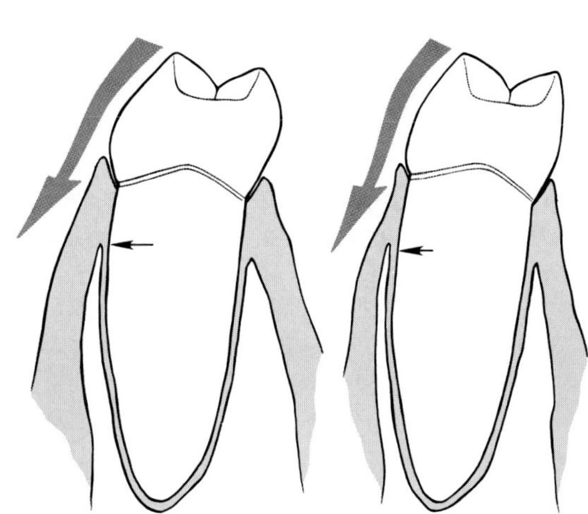

Figure 14.11

The proper relations between amount of crown contour and the thickness of the periodontal tissues. *a,* a severely convex crown form is properly related to the thick tissues. This results in a continuity of crown form and tissue form and creates a sulcular area less likely to accumulate microbial plaque and debris. *b,* the desirable objectives of crown form and gingival health are created by having a flatter crown contour properly related to thinner periodontal tissues.

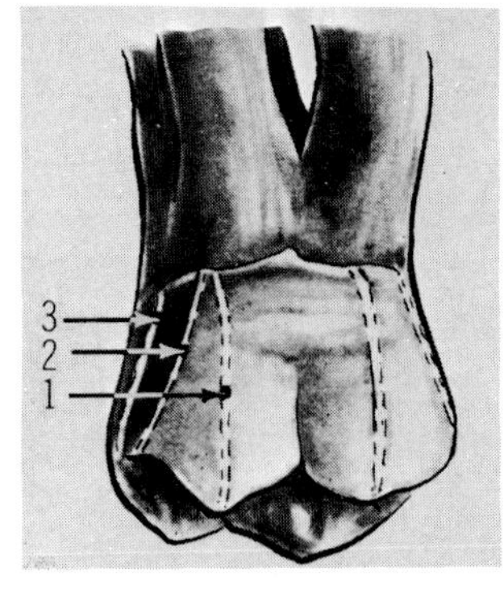

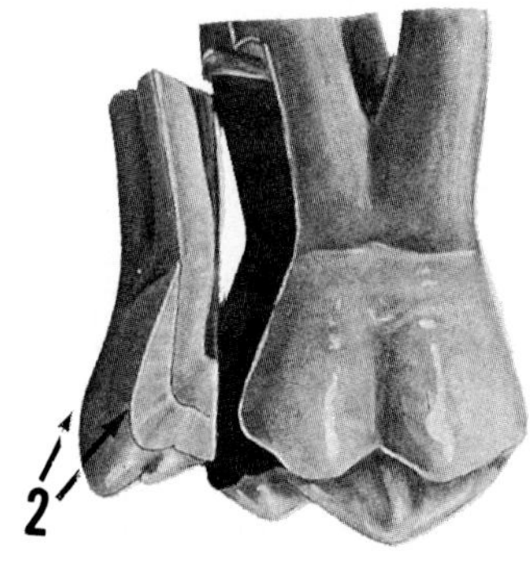

Figure 14.12

The "survey" lines of crown contour. The convexity of the facial and lingual surfaces (*1*); the flatness or slight concavity of the transitional line angle or the blending of the proximal with the facial or lingual surfaces (*2*); the flatness or concavity of the proximal surfaces (*3*).

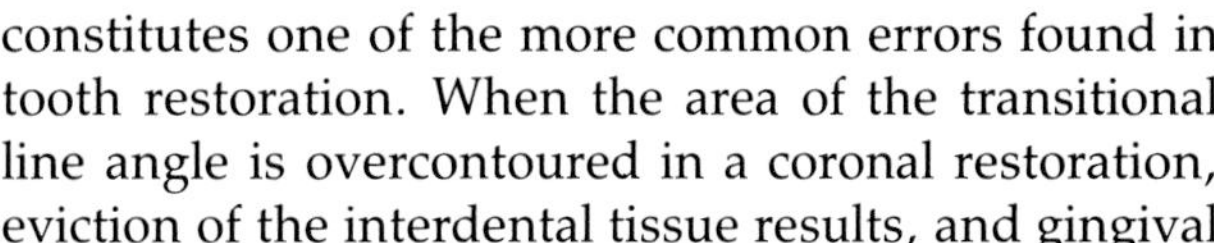

constitutes one of the more common errors found in tooth restoration. When the area of the transitional line angle is overcontoured in a coronal restoration, eviction of the interdental tissue results, and gingival deformation follows. Figure 14.12 demonstrates the proportionate differences in the contour "survey lines" of the three areas (Fig. 14.13).

Variations in Crown Contour Among Comparative Mammalian Forms

The degree of cervical convexity of the facial and lingual crown form in mammals varies from total absence to extreme cingulum formation. There appears to be a strong correlation between form and the special functions that the mammalian dentition may perform. Most grass-eating animals present totally flattened facial and lingual surfaces. There is apparently no need for food deflection in mastication. In carnivores, the development of pronounced facial and lingual cingula are compatible with the special needs of a diet that includes crushed bony spicules. In the hyena, a scavenger with a dentition specialized for bone crushing, one finds the most pronounced cervical cingulum formation among the carnivores. It has been postulated that if it were not for the deflecting nature of the exaggerated enamel cingulum, the gingival tissues would be heavily lacerated by the bony slivers of the diet (Fig. 14.14.).

The Collective Action of Tooth Alignment

When teeth approximate each other in the arch and the interproximal embrasure is formed, a canopy is thereby created, which houses the interdental tissue. Under normal circumstances, the interdental gingival tissue (interdental papilla) completely fills the interproximal space. The aforementioned flattened proximal surfaces should permit sufficient room for the interdental tissue to remain healthy and at the same time protect the area from becoming a depository of dental plaque and food debris by providing a profile continuous with the soft tissue.

The interproximal embrasure space created by the correct adjacent contacts of teeth should possess the following properties: (1) contact areas of the teeth should be located at the junction of occlusal and middle thirds of the proximal surface, closer to the facial aspect on posterior teeth and centrally located in the anterior teeth; (2) the proximal surfaces of adjacent teeth should tend to be mirror images of each other, so that a symmetrical canopy is created; (3) adjacent marginal ridges should be the same height; (4) adjacent cementoenamel junctions should be of equal height; (5) adjacent transitional line angles should be symmetrically positioned; (6) contact of teeth should be sufficiently tight so as to prevent food impaction and at the same time contribute to the stability of the arch (Fig. 14.15). It should be noted that the contact surface area increases with age as a result of proximal attrition.

Since the interdental embrasure is a primary site of dental disease, both gingival and carious, it bears close surveillance in clinical practice. The canopy that

(*text continues on page 273*)

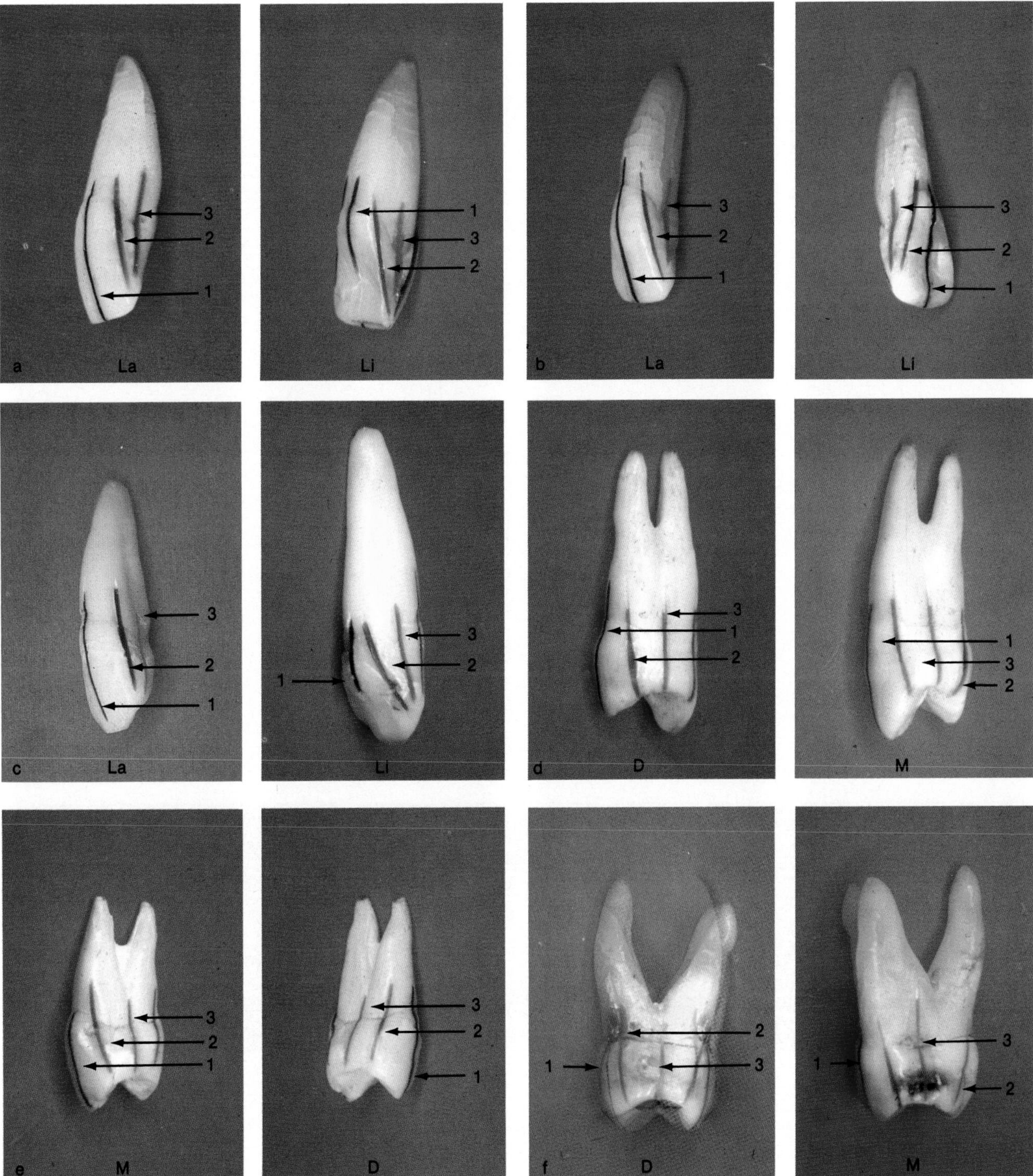

Figure 14.13

The "survey" lines of teeth that were determined by scoring extracted teeth. Note the contrast in form between the facial (*La.*) lingual (*Li.*) convexity (*1*), the transitional line angle (*2*), and the proximal surface (*3*). *M,* mesial; *D,* distal. *a,* maxillary central incisor; *b,* maxillary lateral incisor; *c,* maxillary canine; *d,* maxillary first premolar (flat contour); *e,* maxillary first premolar (thicker contour); *f,* maxillary first molar; (*continued*)

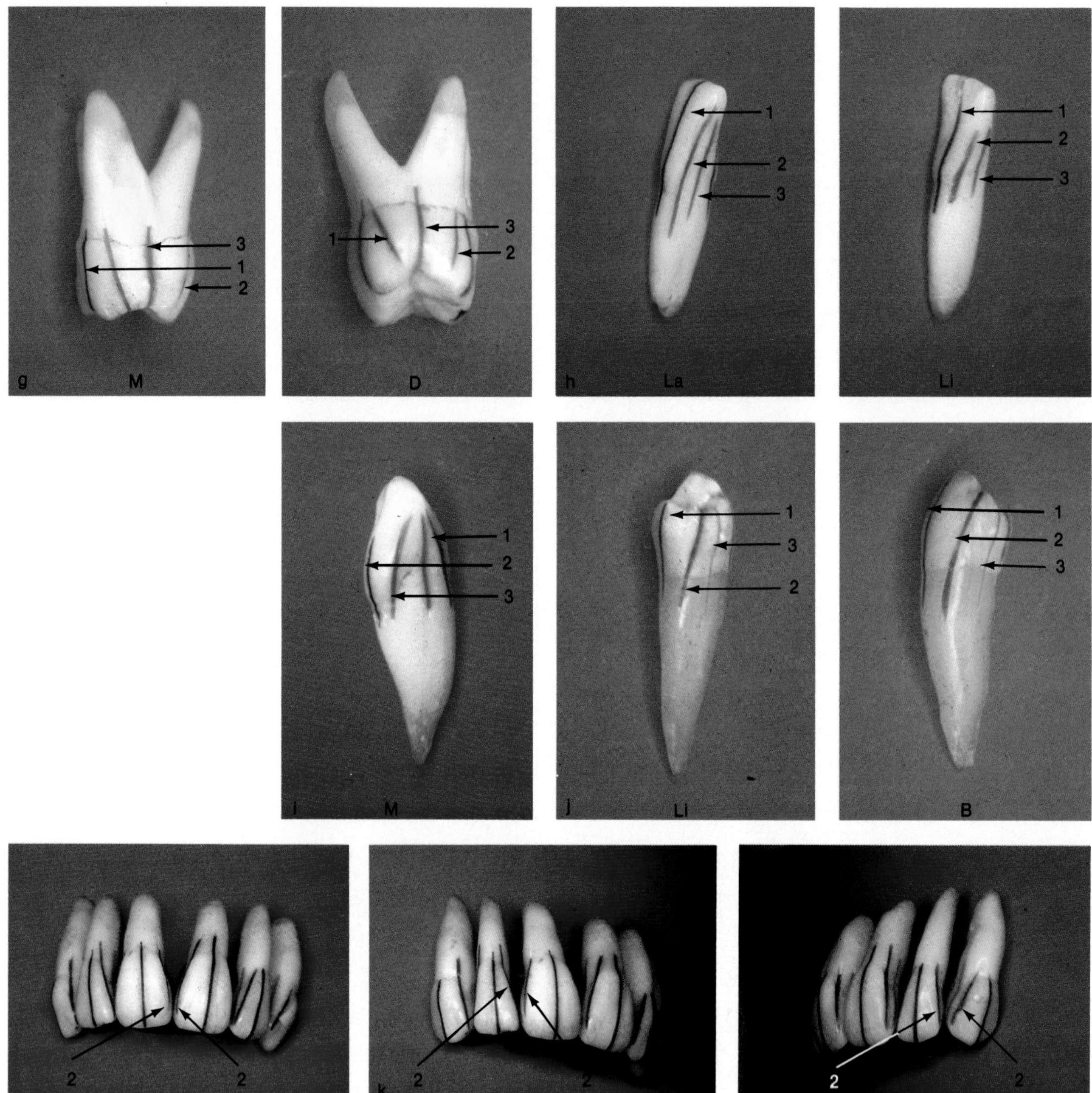

Figure 14.13, ***cont'd.***

g, maxillary second molar; *h*, mandibular central incisor; *i*, mandibular canine; *j*, mandibular first premolar; *k*, six maxillary anterior teeth from the same mouth. The adjacent transitional line angles (2) tend to be mirror images of each other.

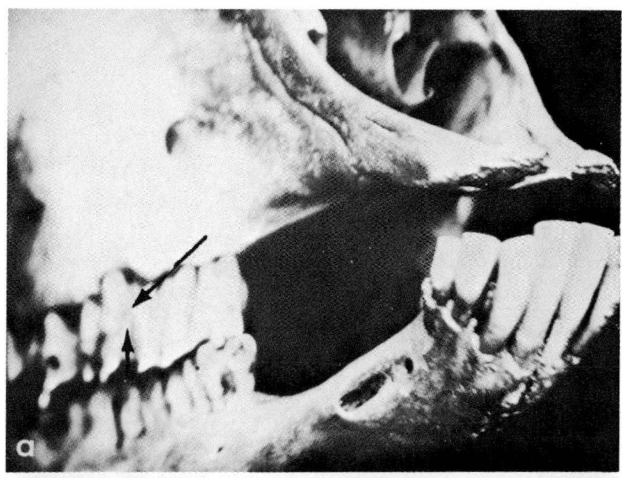

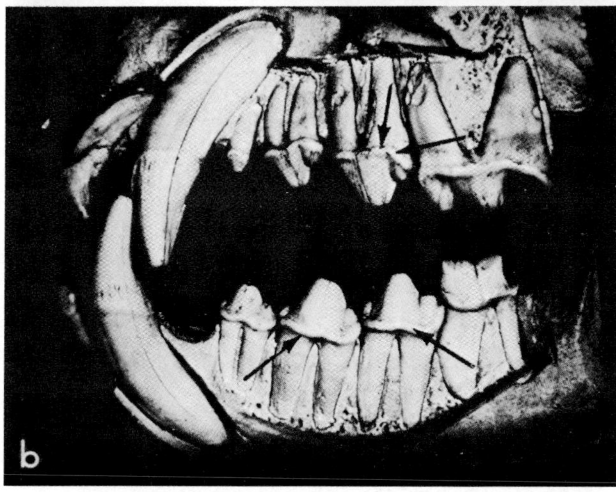

Figure 14.14

Crown contour in comparative mammalian forms. *a*, dentition of a cow. Note the extremely flat facial surfaces typical of grass-eating animals. *b*, dentition of an hyena. Note the enamel cingulae or bulges (*arrows*) that appear necessary to direct the bony spicules of the diet away from the gingiva.

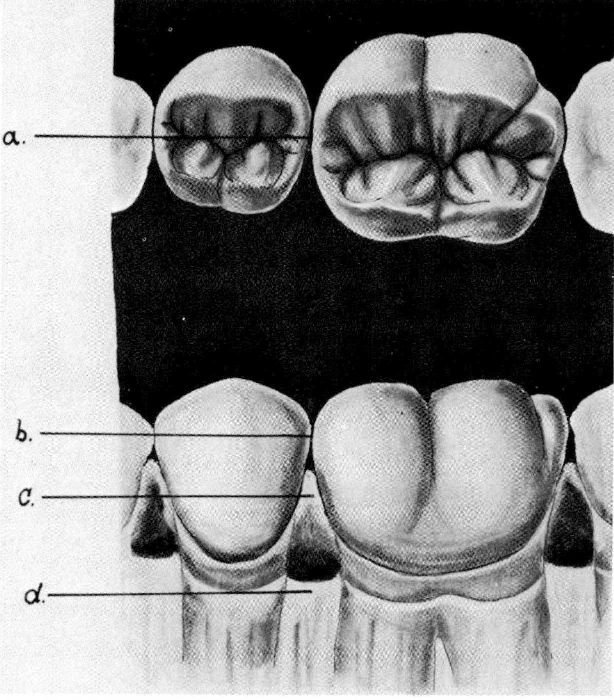

Figure 14.15

The normal interdental embrasure as exemplified by the mandibular second premolar and first molar. *a* and *b*, contact "point" which is in reality an area located slightly closer to the buccal surface and on the occlusal third of the crowns; *c*, the interdental papilla which completely fills the interproximal space and presents a contour which is continuous with the adjacent root surfaces; *d*, the position of the alveolar bone crest.

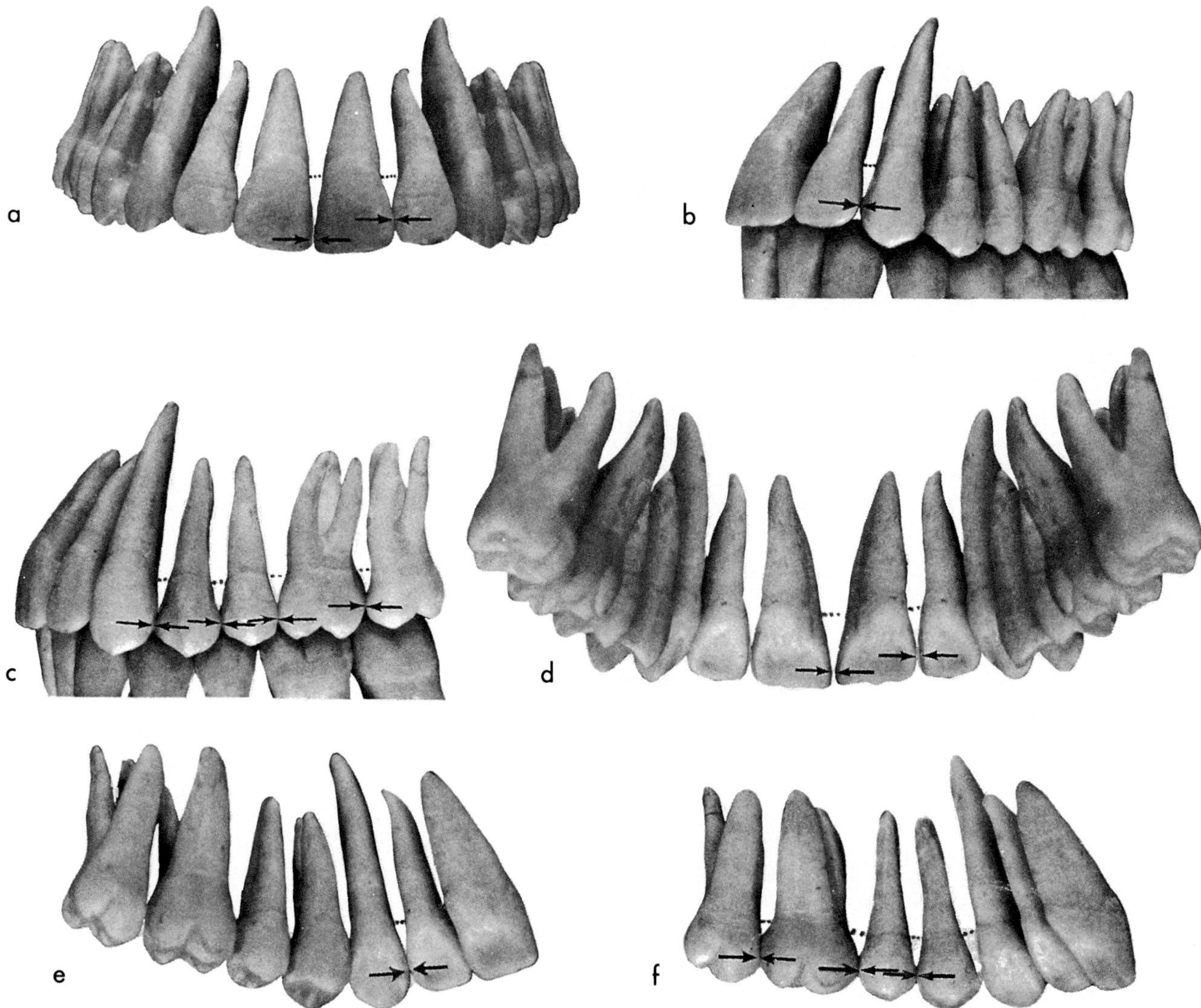

Figure 14.16

The continuity of the maxillary arch. Proximal contact indicated by *arrows*; adjacent cementoenamel junction indicated by *dotted line*. *a*, the gradual change apically in the position of the contact area of the central incisors from the mesial to the distal; *b*, the transition in form by means of the contact area of the lateral incisor and canine; *c*, the continued transition at the interproximal areas from the canine to the second molar; *d*, lingual view of the incisors showing that the adjacent marginal ridges have mirror forms and are at the same level; *e*, lingual view of the canine area demonstrating that adjacent marginal ridges are level and are mirror images; *f*, the continuity of tooth alignment in the molar area as viewed from the lingual aspect.

houses the interdental tissue has a roof that is created by the very tight positioning of the contact areas of the teeth. The walls are formed by the proximal surfaces of adjacent teeth. The base is formed by the cementoenamel junction (CEJ) of adjacent proximal surfaces. Correct interproximal embrasures result in a proper arch alignment, which possesses a definite continuity of tooth forms. This continuity is expressed as a gradual modification in form from anterior to posterior teeth and demonstrates a continuous alignment of occlusal tables, central fossae, and cusp tips.

Symmetry of the Embrasures

The basic hypothesis offered here is that adjacent proximal tooth surfaces tend to be almost mirror counterparts of each other, so that the continuity of tooth forms will then allow for the gradual distal transition from the central incisor to the second molar without abrupt departures from an harmonious alignment.

Continuity of Forms in the Maxillary Arch

The adjacent central incisors will have profiles that permit the proximal contact areas to be at the same level (Fig. 14.16). The adjacent mesial surfaces are somewhat flattened in their outline as viewed from the labial profile. The distal profile of the central incisor presents a more rounded form as if to prepare for its diminutive edition, the lateral incisor. The roundness of the distolabial profile raises the contact area of the central incisor apically to allow for level contact with the lateral incisor. The roundness of the distal profile of the lateral incisor, both from incisal and labial view, strongly suggests the mesial form of the canine that it contacts.

In the canine-first premolar area, there appear to be a number of changes necessary for a gradual transition from an anterior to a posterior tooth form (Fig. 14.17).

In the canine, the following is observed (Fig. 14.17): (1) the canine is wider labiolingually than the incisors, with the incisal edge placed closer to the buccal surface; (2) the lingual cingulum is exaggerated; (3) the distal marginal ridge is elevated incisally; (4) the contour of the labial surface in mesiodistal direction tends to mimic the two adjacent teeth. The mesial half of the canine's labial surface exhibits the flattened convexity found on the lateral incisor, while the distal half reflects the slight concavity typical of the mesial half of the buccal surface of the first premolar.

In the first premolars the following is observed: (1) the mesial marginal ridge is divided by a characteristic deep groove; (2) the buccal segment of the mesial occlusal surface is extremely canine-like in appearance.

The remainder of the posterior teeth align themselves in an orderly, even fashion with the possible exception of the interproximal embrasure between the first and second molar. Here the approximating surfaces are often aligned as negative counterparts rather than mirror images, with the contact areas located in the middle third of the proximal surfaces. The interproximal embrasure between the maxillary first and second molars has long been recognized as one of the more susceptible and early sites for both carious and periodontal interproximal disease.

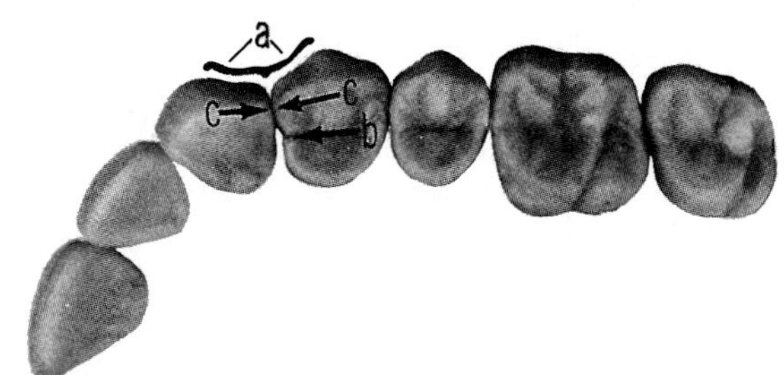

Figure 14.17

The occlusal view of the maxillary arch showing the continuous alignment of the teeth, their central fossa lines, and occlusal tables. The gradual transition from an anterior tooth form to a posterior tooth form is facilitated by the groove (*b*), which divides the mesial marginal ridge of the first premolar into a buccal and lingual segment. The buccal segment is an almost duplicate mirror image of the canine and forms an harmonious contact area (*c*) with the canine. The distal half of the labial surface of the canine contains the same pronounced depression (*a*) that runs vertically on the mesial half of the buccal surface of the first premolar.

The Continuity of Forms in the Mandibular Arch

The lower central incisors are characterized as being nearly symmetrical bilaterally, and one finds essentially the same form on both the mesial and distal aspects of the central incisor and on the mesial aspect of the lateral incisor. Because of the shape of the mandible, the incisor roots are positioned with their flattened proximal surfaces parallel to one another. The arch, however, rarely presents a straight line of incisal edges so that a twisting of the lateral incisor crown on its long axis takes place, as if to accommodate the gradual curvature of the arch (Figs. 14.18 to 14.20).

The distal profile of the labial surface of the lateral incisor is similar to the mesial profile of the adjacent canine. Both are strongly curved. This results in a more apical placement of the proximal contact area.

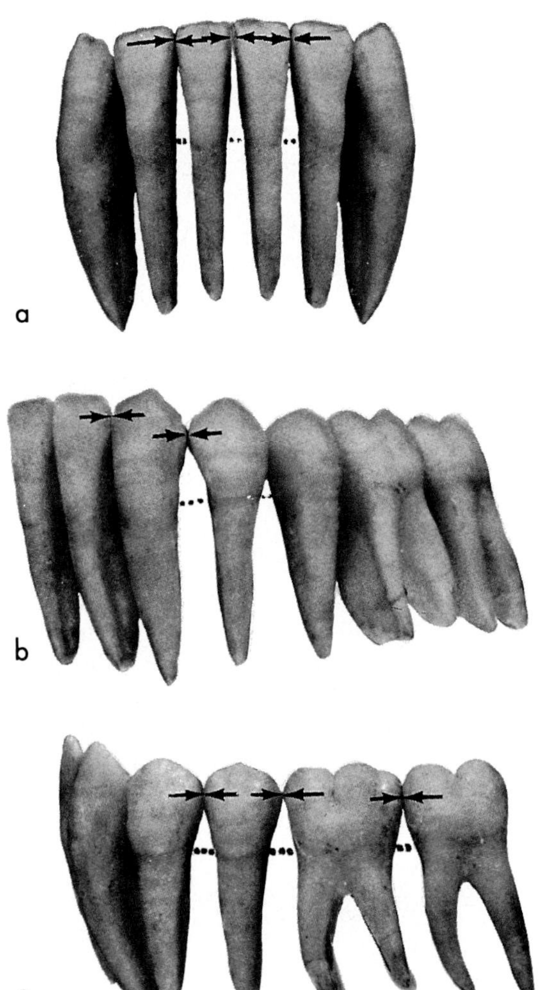

Figure 14.18

The continuity of the mandibular arch. Proximal contact indicated by *arrows*; adjacent cementoenamel junctions indicated by *dotted lines*. *a*, the labial view of the mandibular incisors. Note that the identical proximal forms are present from the mesial of the right lateral incisor to the mesial of the left lateral incisor. *b*, the canine area. Note that the contact area "steps down" from the height of the lateral incisor to the height of the first premolar by virtue of the "scoliosed" appearance of the canine. Obvious also is the mirror-like similarity between the mesial of the canine and the distal of the lateral incisor. *c*, the alignment of the posterior segment is seen as continuous with adjacent marginal ridges and cementoenamel junctions as the same level.

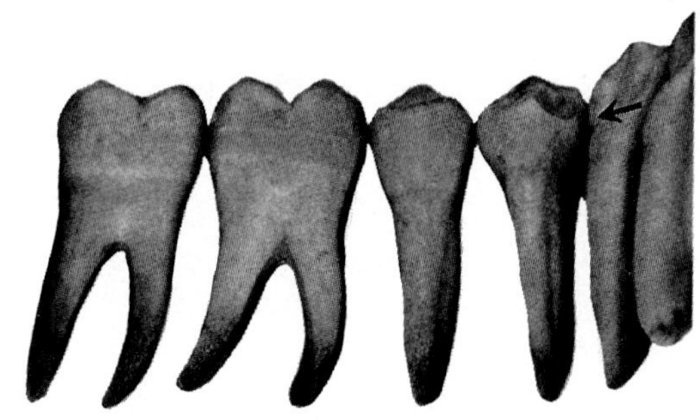

Figure 14.19

The alignment of the posterior segment as viewed from the lingual aspect. Note that the mesial marginal ridge of the mandibular first premolar is more apically positioned and resembles closely its canine neighbor. This enables a gradual transition from an anterior to a posterior tooth form.

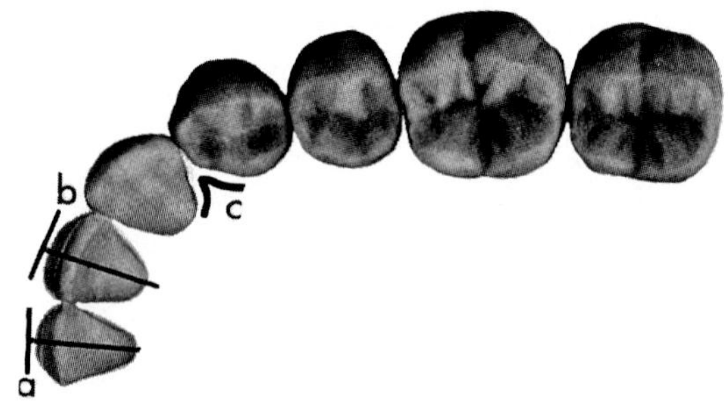

Figure 14.20

The occlusal view of the lower arch. Note that the occlusal tables and central fossa lines are aligned so that there is no abrupt departure from a continuous form. The continuity of the arch is enhanced by the change from the perpendicular incisal edge of the central incisor (*a*) that is "twisted" in the lateral incisor (*b*). The gradual transition from anterior to posterior segment occurs at the first premolar with its mesial half (*c*) closely resembling the distal half of the canine.

The canine, in turn, allows for a gradual transition from lateral incisor to first premolar by the increased curvature of the distal profile of its labial surface. The latter further moves the contact area apically and creates the so-called scoliosed appearance typical of the lower canine tooth (Fig. 14.18*b*).

In the lower arch, the transition from anterior to posterior tooth form occurs within the first premolar, which must be considered essentially part canine and part premolar. The mesial half functions as a canine. There is a canine antagonist. There is no mesial occlusal table. The transverse ridge, which connects the buccal cusp with a rudimentary lingual cusp, divides the posterior tooth form of the distal half of the crown from the anterior tooth form of the mesial half. In many instances, the mesial half of the lingual surface is further reduced in prominence by a mesiolingual groove (Figs. 14.20 and 14.21). On the other hand, the distal half of the mandibular first premolar does present an occlusal contact area for the lingual cusp of the maxillary first premolar, and functions as a true posterior tooth.

The remainder of the posterior teeth follow the fundamental alignment with respect to symmetry, leveling of the marginal ridges, and adequate embrasure space (Figs. 14.18*c* and 14.19).

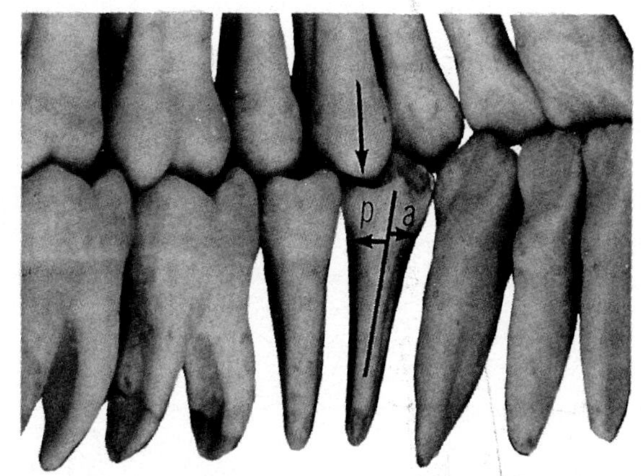

Figure 14.21

The mandibular first premolar is both an anterior and a posterior tooth. The mesial half (*a*) is the anterior tooth form since it does not possess a functional occlusal table, has no occlusal antagonistic cusp, and resembles the canine. The distal half (*p*) is the posterior tooth form and as such possesses a functional occlusal table with an antagonistic cusp.

The Evidence of Symmetry and Continuity of Tooth Forms Offered by the Adjacent Cementoenamel Junction

The epithelial attachment at the base of the gingival crevice follows the curvature of the CEJ. Also, the contour of the osseous alveolar crest follows the form of the CEJ of the tooth. Since the base of the interproximal embrasure is determined by the curvature of the CEJ, true mirror-image symmetry of adjacent teeth demands that the CEJs of the approximating tooth surfaces be located at the same level.

Studies in tooth form conducted by Wheeler (1958), and in periodontal form by Orban and Ritchie, have strongly substantiated the claim that adjacent CEJ of properly aligned teeth will be at the same level.

The curvature of the CEJ is measured in millimeters, using the position of the most apical level of the CEJ on the given proximal surface as the distance to be measured (Fig. 14.22*a* and *b*).

Definite behavioral tendencies seem to exist with respect to CEJ curvatures of teeth within a given arch: (1) the curvatures of CEJ gradually diminish from the incisors (3.5 mm) to the molars (0 mm); (2) all adjacent CEJs tend to be at the same level; (3) the mesial curvature of the CEJ of a given tooth is usually greater than its distal curvature; (4) the mesial CEJ curvature of the tooth immediately distal is usually greater than the distal curvature of the tooth immediately mesial (Fig. 14.23*a* and *b*).

The last observation, although appearing contradictory, seems to be necessary because compensation for the slight mesial axial inclination present in most roots is necessary (Fig. 14.23).

The end result of correct crown contour and embrasure form, therefore, is the establishment of a series of contours that will either prevent debris and plaque retention or allow the normal processes of detergent mastication and lip-cheek-tongue action to render the area clean.

This fine harmony of tooth form and resultant soft tissue protection is predicated not only upon the proper crown contour and alignment, but also upon the proper architecture and positioning of the gingival tissues.

Even though the dental arch may possess a desirable continuity of tooth forms, all of this may be

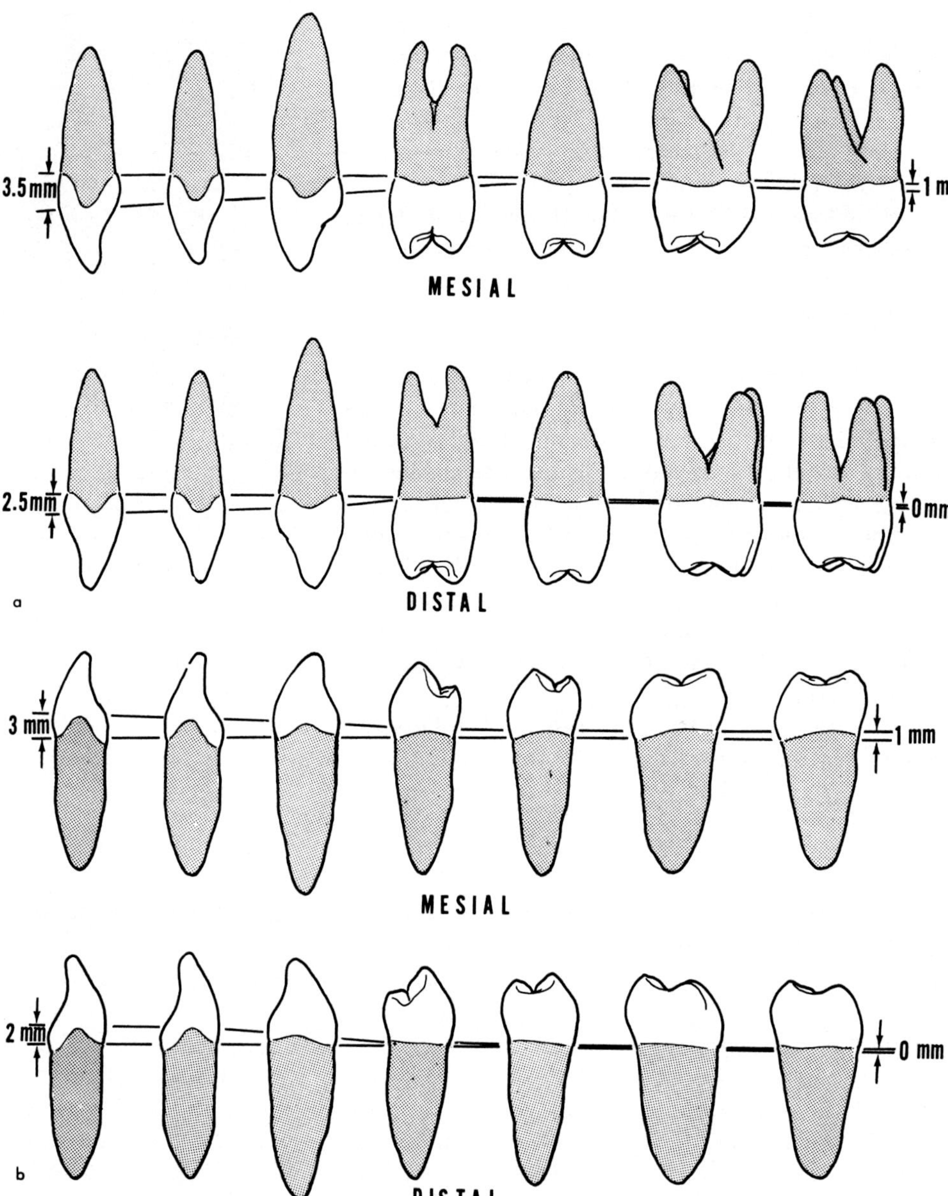

Figure 14.22

a, The curvatures of the cementoenamel junctions on the proximal surfaces of maxillary teeth. On the mesial surface, note the gradual reduction from 3.5 mm on the central incisor to 1 mm on the second molar. The distal surface shows a gradual reduction from 2.5 mm on the central incisor to 0 mm on the second molar. Note that the curvature on the posterior teeth is practically flat. *b,* the relative curvatures of the proximal cementoenamel junctions of the mandibular arch. This demonstrates the same properties as the maxillary arch. (Drawn with modification from Wheeler RC. A textbook of dental anatomy. 3rd ed. Philadelphia: WB Saunders, 1958.)

negated by any changes in gingival positioning in either a coronal or an apical direction.

In summation, therefore, one can say that the gingiva is protected by the correct relations of crown contour and arch continuity, while at the same time, the gingival tissues protect the teeth by covering that tooth substance (cementum) most vulnerable to caries.

Protection to the Attachment Apparatus

The attachment apparatus is responsible for anchoring the root of the tooth in the jaw. It is composed of the periodontal ligament and those structures to which the ligament is anchored—cementum and alveolar bone. Resistance to tooth displacement by the attachment apparatus is directly related to the amount of principal fibers available for stretch.

The importance of direction of force resulting from a given occlusal load and its tolerance by the attachment apparatus has been well established. Forces transmitted in an axial direction are best withstood because there is a minimum of compression of the periodontal fibers (Fig. 14.24).

The axial positions of the posterior teeth help accomplish this goal by being aligned so that the axial centers of the teeth are parallel to the direction of the force. Further, the location and design of the occlusal table of the posterior tooth tends to accomplish this end by the following means: (1) the buccolingual width of the occlusal table is generally no more than 50 to 60 percent of the overall buccolingual width of the tooth; (2) the occlusal table is located over the axial center of the root; (3) the occlusal table is perpendicular to the axial center of the root. All of this tends to place the area of the posterior tooth that receives the force directly over the axial center of the root. The above relationship, together with the root alignment which tends to parallel the direction of mandibular movement, serves to direct occlusal load vertically.

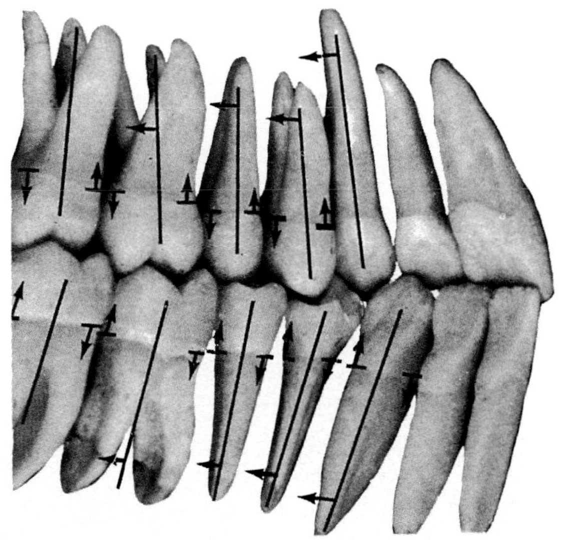

Figure 14.23

The axial inclinations of teeth cause the apex to be inclined distally. This causes the mesial cementoenamel junction level to be raised apically and the distal level to be raised coronally. If the cementoenamel junctions are to be at the same level, the mesial cementoenamel junction must be more coronal than the distal junction of the tooth immediately anterior to it when the tooth is in a pure vertical position. (Drawn with modification from Wheeler RC. A textbook of dental anatomy. 3rd ed. Philadelphia: WB Saunders, 1958.)

The occlusal tables of posterior teeth perform their protective function during maximum jaw closure in the bracing (intercuspal) position. It is at this time that the greatest occlusal load is normally applied. The forces of closure in the intercuspal position could prove damaging to the maxillary incisors because of the absence of occlusal tables and the inability of these teeth to transmit forces axially. The maxillary canines and incisors, therefore, require protection from the possibilities of horizontally directed forces during maximum jaw closure. This necessary protection is provided by the posterior teeth, which create the proper stability and support to the mandible during bracing.

The anterior teeth appear to be designed as guideposts to the functional movements of the jaw. It is suspected that in this role they play a sensory function as well. This affords a reciprocal protective action to the posterior teeth by causing them to be disarticulated when the mandible moves out of the intercuspal position.

In summation, it can be postulated that when the mandible is in the bracing position of maximum occlusion, apparently only posterior teeth are designed to sustain the load. This, in turn, protects the anterior teeth from horizontal overloading. When the mandible glides to and from the intercuspal position, the anterior teeth, with their guidances, both mechanical and sensory, reciprocate by disarticulating the posterior teeth and thus preventing horizontal overloading and excessive wear.

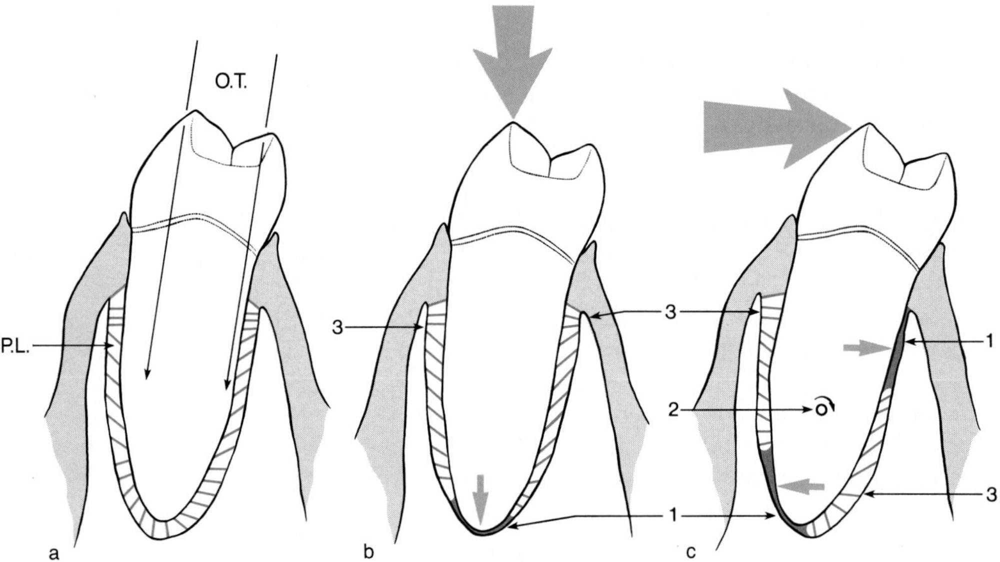

Figure 14.24

Protection of the attachment apparatus. *a,* diagrammatic representation of a tooth and its periodontium. The occlusal table (*O.T.*) is located over the root support and is about one-half of the overall buccolingual width of the tooth. This permits forces to be transmitted axially where they are best withstood. *b,* when vertical force (*large arrow*) is applied to the tooth the zone of crush (*1*) is minimized and the zone of stretch (*3*) or resistance is increased. Therefore, vertical forces are best withstood. *c,* when horizontal force (*large arrows*) is applied to the tooth, a fulcrum (*2*) is created about which the root rotates within the alveolus, causing an increased zone of crush (*1*) or destruction and a decreased zone of stretch (*3*) or resistance. Horizontal forces are not tolerated as well as vertical forces. *P.L.,* periodontal ligament.

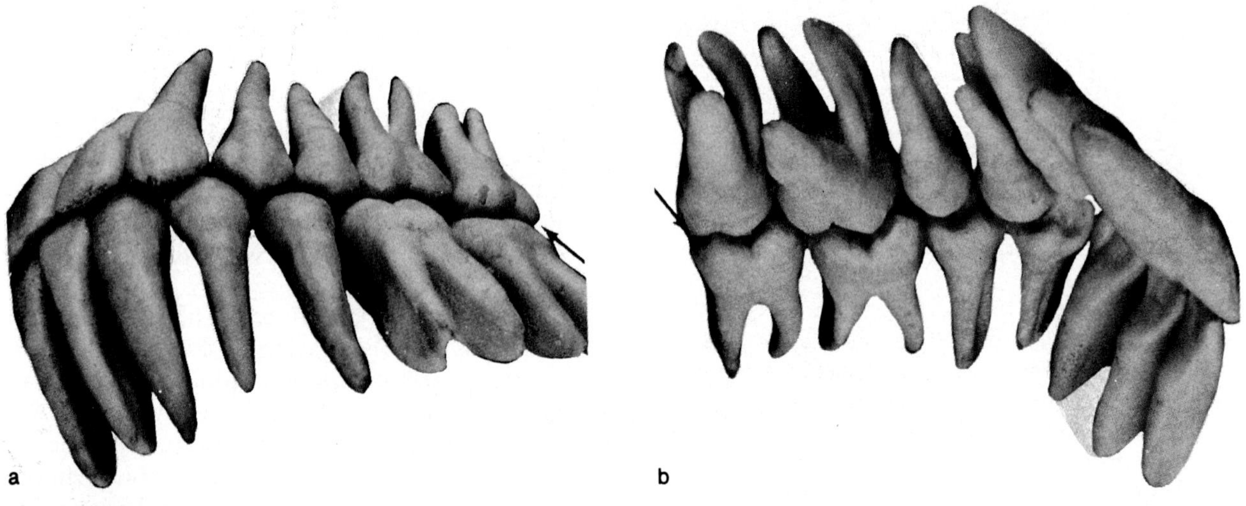

Figure 14.25

Protection to the lip-cheek-tongue system. *a,* the buccal overjet of teeth (horizontal overlap) keeps the cheek away from teeth during mastication and protects the mucosa from undue trauma. *b,* the lingual overjet protects by keeping the tongue away and acts in much the same way as the buccal overjet.

Protection to the Lip, Cheek, and Tongue System

The arrangement of the teeth in occlusion must be such as to prevent injury to the surrounding mucosal surfaces that are adjacent to the occlusal plane. In order to accomplish this end, a horizontal overlap facially, lingually, and distally to the arches appears mandatory.

In a well-aligned and articulated dentition the buccal horizontal overlap of the upper posterior teeth serves to keep the lip and cheek mucosa away from the cutting surfaces of the mandibular teeth. The lingual horizontal overlap of the lower posterior teeth in turn keeps the tongue away from the cutting surfaces of the upper teeth. The distal horizontal overlap of the upper second molar also protects the cheek musculature from injury in jaw closure (Fig. 14.25).

Frequently Occurring Variations of Tooth Form That Adversely Affect the Control of Advancing Periodontal Disease

Among the clinical problems created by normal variations in tooth form, two deserve special consideration because of the frequency of their occurrence. The two variations in tooth structure are the enamel projection and the bifurcational ridge.

The *enamel projection* is an apical extension of enamel at the cementoenamel junction onto the root surface in the area of the furcation of multirooted teeth. The degree of enamel projection may vary from slight, in the form of a small dip of enamel (Grade I), to severe, in which the projection may extend into the furcation proper (Grade III). An intermediate form (Grade II) may extend up to but not into the furcation itself.

The clinical problems caused by this phenomenon are related to the fact that the fibers of the gingival unit must be embedded in cementum in order to be anchored to tooth structure. When enamel covers the root surface of the tooth, the only type of gingival fixation that is possible is through the epithelial attachment. The epithelial attachment mirrors the form of the underlying enamel surface. It has been fairly well established that the gingival attachment over the enamel projection is more vulnerable to advancing periodontal disease than is the remainder of an intact periodontium. According to Masters and Hoskins (1964), 90 percent of all teeth with isolated bifurcational periodontal problems are teeth that possessed enamel projections at the disease site (Fig. 14.26). Of 304 mandibular molar teeth, 28.6 percent demonstrated enamel projections (Fig. 14.27). Projections occurred more frequently on buccal rather than on lingual surfaces.

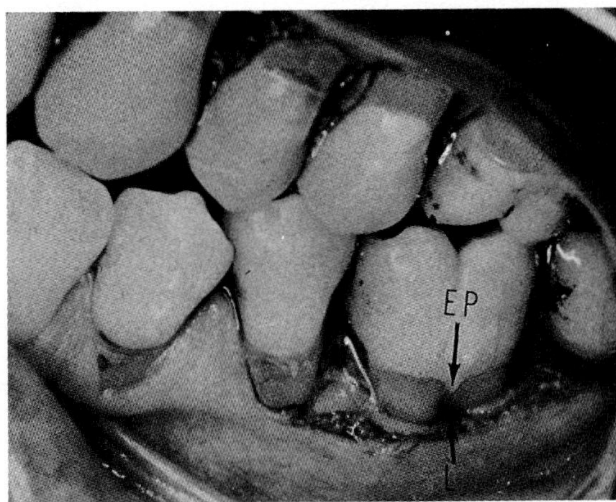

Figure 14.26

Surgical exposure for the treatment of an isolated intraradicular lesion (*L*) of a mandibular molar. The lesion takes the form of a deep pocket into the bifurcation. The enamel projection (*EP*) is seen extending between the roots. (Courtesy of Dr. Clifford Ochsenbein.)

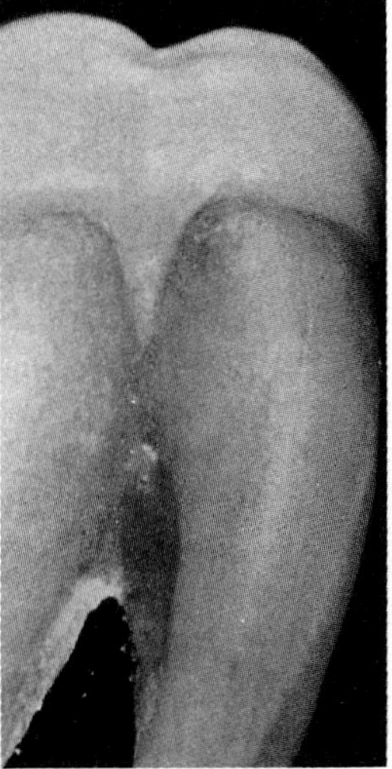

Figure 14.27

Enamel projection extending into buccal bifurcation of a lower molar

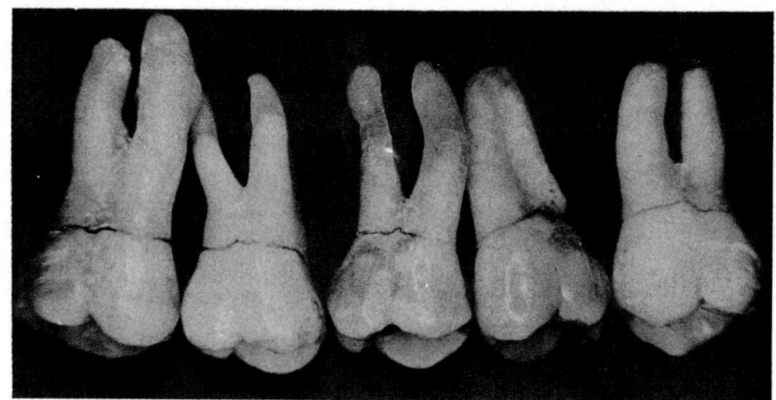

Figure 14.28

The buccal surface of maxillary molars showing variations in the enamel projection in the area of the buccal furcation.

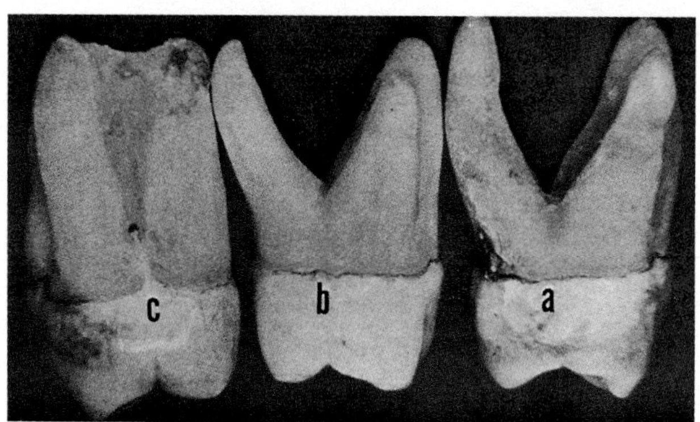

Figure 14.29

The distal surfaces of maxillary molars. *a*, flat, regular cementoenamel junction with no enamel projection; *b*, slight "bump" to cementoenamel junction; *c*, enamel projection (Grade III) extending into distal furcation.

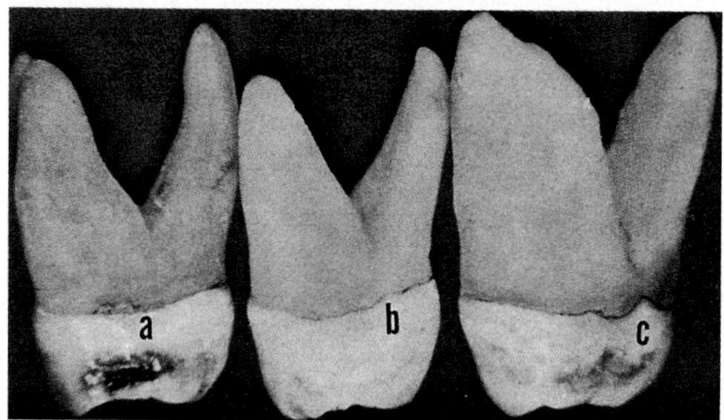

Figure 14.30

The mesial surfaces of maxillary molars. *a*, flat, regular cementoenamel junction with no enamel projection; *b*, slight "bump" to cementoenamel junction; *c*, enamel projection (Grade II) extending up to but not into the furcation. These are the same teeth that are shown in Fig. 14.29, and the degree of enamel projection on the mesial surfaces closely parallels that of the distal surfaces.

Table 14.1
Prevalence of Bifurcational Ridges

	Intermediate Bifurcational Ridge						Contour at Height of Bifurcation in a Buccolingual Direction						Relative Acuteness of Lingual Buccal Bifurcational Ridge					
	Pronounced		*Noticeable*		*Absent*		*Concavity*		*Convexity*		*Plane*		*Buccal More Acute*		*Lingual More Acute*		*No. Diff. Noticeable*	
	No. of Teeth	*% of Teeth*	*No. of Teeth*	*% of Teeth*	*No. of Teeth*	*% of Teeth*	*No. of Teeth*	*% of Teeth*	*No. of Teeth*	*% of Teeth*	*No. of Teeth*	*% of Teeth*	*No. of Teeth*	*% of Teeth*	*No. of Teeth*	*% of Teeth*	*No. of Teeth*	*% of Teeth*
Group 1, distal root (107 teeth)	54		24		29		14		38		55							
Group 2, mesial root (112 teeth)	47		38		27		21		44		47							
Group 3, amputation (109 teeth)	43		33		33		14		46		49		44		25		40	
Total (328)	144	44	95	29	89	27	49	15	128	39	151	46	44	40	25	23	40	37

Modified from Everett *et al.*, The intermediate bifurcation. J Dent Res 1958:37; by permission of the *Journal of Dental Research*.

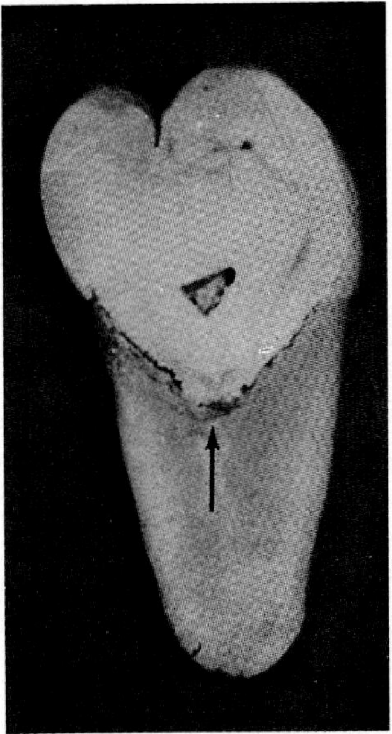

Figure 14.31

The intermediate bifurcational ridge as seen in a lower molar that has been sectioned buccolingually between the roots. Note that in this specimen the roof of the bifurcation is convex and contains neither buccal nor lingual bifurcational ridges.

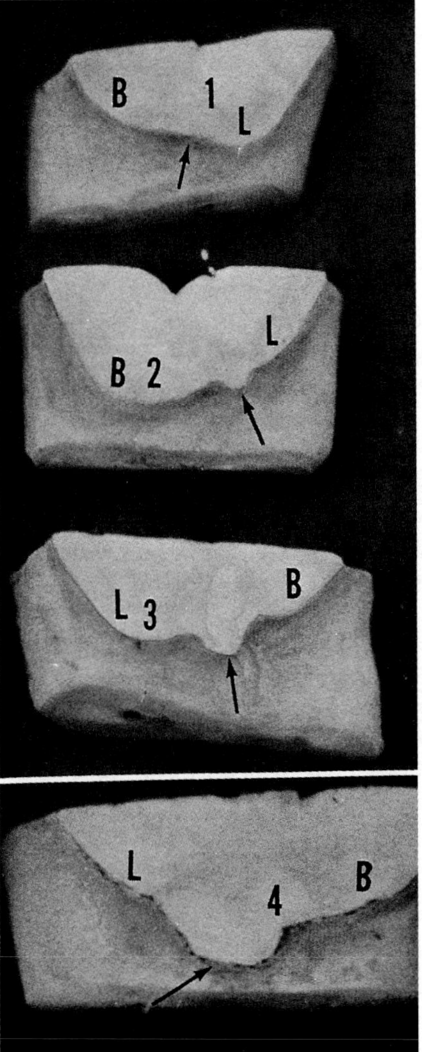

Figure 14.32

Comparison in size between buccal (*B*) and lingual (*L*) bifurcational ridges. *1,* the lingual bifurcational ridge is larger than the buccal. The *arrow* indicates absence of an intermediate bifurcational ridge with a concave bifurcational roof. *2,* the buccal bifurcational ridge is larger than the lingual. The *arrow* points to a rather small intermediate ridge. *3,* the lingual bifurcational ridge is larger than the buccal; the intermediate ridge (*arrow*) is of moderate size. *4,* the buccal bifurcational ridge is present, whereas the lingual ridge is completely absent. The intermediate ridge is quite pronounced.

Among maxillary molars, 17 percent demonstrated enamel projections in the buccal and distal surfaces, and like their lower counterparts, the buccal demonstrated the greater frequency (Figs. 14.28 and 14.29). Contrary to the published reports of Masters and Hoskins, we have been able to demonstrate occasional enamel projections on the mesial surface of maxillary molars (Fig. 14.30) and on the mesial surface of maxillary first premolars as well.

When isolated periodontal pockets are treated in the areas of the affected furcations, it is important that the enamel extension be removed and the root surface be polished so that healing may be facilitated.

The *bifurcational ridges* are prominences of tooth structure that traverse the "roof" of lower molar bifurcations in a mesiodistal direction (Everett *et al.,* 1958). The most prominent of these structures is the intermediate bifurcational ridge, which runs from the mesial surface of the more posterior root to the distal concave surface of the more anterior root and is nearly centered between the buccal and lingual surfaces (Fig. 14.31). The ridge is composed mainly of cementum with a slight dentin foundation for its form. In 328 lower molars examined, the intermediate bifurcational ridge was pronounced in 44 percent, noticeable in 29 percent, and absent in 27 percent (Table 14.1).

The roof of the bifurcational area was examined for degree of convexity or concavity in a buccolingual direction; 15 percent of the teeth presented concave surfaces, 39 percent of the teeth presented convex surfaces, and 46 percent of the teeth presented flat surfaces (Table 14.1). Whenever a concave surface was present there were sharp delineating line angles that extended mesiodistally on the buccal or lingual surfaces of the bifurcation and were referred to as *buccal* or *lingual bifurcational* ridges (Fig. 14.32). Buccal bifurcational ridges were more prominent in 40 percent of the teeth; the lingual bifurcational ridges were more pronounced in 23 percent of the specimens. No difference between prominence of the buccal and lingual bifurcational ridges occurred 37 percent of the time (Table 14.1). The buccal and lingual ridges, unlike the intermediate ridge, are covered by a thin layer of cementum and take their shape almost entirely from the underlying dentin.

The dentin which forms the floor of the pulp chamber appears to be morphologically different than the remaining dentin body and is cone shaped. The base of the cone forms the roof of the bifurcation and is coincident with the area of the intermediate bifurcational ridge. The apex of the cone touches the floor of the pulp chamber. The periphery of the cone often presents many nutrient canals.

The relationship between age and disease to the formation of the intermediate bifurcational ridge is not known. Prominent ridges have been described in young teeth with very expanded pulp chambers, and reduced ridges have been found in older teeth with constricted pulp chambers. Clinically, the bifurcational ridges are important because, at present, the dental profession is being called upon to treat and maintain teeth with periodontal involvement of the bifurcational area. In so doing, the clinician must be able not only to determine the presence of the bifurcational ridge but also be prepared to reshape the tooth in order to make the area more easily cleaned.

Conclusion

The masticatory system as a functional unit is a very complicated and highly coordinated mechanism. It is placed at the entrance to the digestive and respiratory systems and is provided with possibilities for discrimination between neutral and harmful substances and effects from the surroundings. This calls for a high degree of sensitivity and functional ability. It is in many ways a fine example of the intimate interdependency between form and function. A thorough knowledge of the functional anatomy and an understanding of the form-function relationships and their implements is essential in the evaluation not only of the normal and adequately functioning masticatory system (physiologic occlusion) but also of the changes found in functional disease (pathologic occlusion).

References

Aarstad T. The capsular ligaments of the temperomandibular joint and retrusion facets of the dentition in relationship to mandibular movements. Oslo: Akademisk Forlag, 1954.

Ash MM Jr. Wheeler's dental anatomy, physiology, and occlusion. 6th ed. Philadelphia: WB Saunders, 1984.

Brenman HS, Black A, Coslet J. Interrelationship between the electromyographic silent period and dental occlusion. J Dent Res 1968; 47:582.

Brenman HS, Weiss RC, Black M. Sound as a diagnostic aid in the detection of occlusal discrepancies. Penn Dental Journal, 1966; 69(2):33.

Beyron H. Occlusal relations and mastication in Australian aborigines. Acta Odont Scand 1964; 22:597.

Celenza FV. The centric position: replacement and character. J Pros Dent 1973 (Oct):591.

Dempster WI, Adams WJ, Duddles RA. Arrangement in the jaws of the roots of the teeth. J Am Dent Assoc 1963; 67:7.

Everett FG, Jump EB, Holder TD, Williams GC. The intermediate bifurcational ridge: A study of the morphology of the bifurcation of the lower first molar. J Dent Res 1958; 37:162.

Flanagan JB Jr. Twenty-four hour pattern of swallowing in man. J Am Dent Res 1963; 41:76.

Granit R. Receptors and sensory perception. New Haven: Yale University Press, 1955.

Hannam AG, Sessle BJ. Mastication and swallowing, biological and clinical correlates. Toronto: University of Toronto Press, 1976.

Homma S, ed. Understanding the stretch reflex. Progress In Brain Research. Vol 44. Amsterdam, Oxford, and New York: Elsevier, 1976.

Howell AH, Manley RS. Electronic strain gauge for measuring oral forces. J Dent Res 1948; 27:705.

Jankelson E, Hoffman GM, Hendron JA. The physiology of the masticatory system. J Am Dent Assoc 1953; 46:375.

Masters DH, Hoskins SW. Projection of cervical enamel into molar functions. J Periodont 1964; 35:49.

Matthews BC. Mammalian muscle receptors and their central actions. London: Edward Arnold, 1972.

Moller E. The chewing apparatus. Acta Phys Scand 1966; 69 Suppl 280:17.

Osborne JW. Investigation into the interdental forces occurring between the teeth of the same arch during the clenching of the jaws. Arch Oral Biol 1961; 5: 2002.

Posselt U. Movement areas of the mandible. J Pros Dent 1957; 7:375.

Rees LA. Structure and function of the mandibular joint. Br Dent J 1954; 96:125.

Silverman SI. Oral Physiology. 1st ed. St. Louis: CV Mosby, 1961.

Yurkstas A. Effects of missing teeth on masticatory performance and efficiency. J Pros Dent 1954; 4:120.

Part Four

The Human Dentition in Biological Perspective

15

Introduction

The crown of the human tooth even in its minute details represents but little that is fortuitous. It is the resultant of inherited ancestral conditions, modifying further by evolution and involution.

A. Hrdlicka, 1924

The dental system [thus] presents many and peculiar attractions to the anatomist and naturalist, for independently of the variety, beauty and even occasional singularity of the form and structure of the teeth themselves, they are so intimately related to the food and habits of the animal as to become important if not essential aids to the classification of existing species.

And while the value of dental characters is enhanced by the facility with which, from the position of the teeth, they may be ascertained in living or recent animals, the durability of the teeth renders them not less available to the Palaeontologist in the determination of the nature and affinities of extinct species, of whose organization the teeth are not unfrequently the sole remains.

Richard Owen, F.R.S.
Odontography
(London, 1845)

Thus far our attention has been directed entirely to the teeth of a single species, *Homo sapiens*, and we have concentrated upon their general configuration (gross anatomy), their microscopic arrangement (histology), and their mode of function within the oral environment (occlusion). It is easy to fall into the comforting assumption that in so focusing our energies we have reached the acme of understanding of the nature and function of the human dentition. It is true, perhaps, that as a clinician one might conduct a successful practice if one's knowledge of dental anatomy were confined to the first three parts of this book, but nothing could be more erroneous than to conclude that one truly understands the human dentition as a highly sophisticated professional student of the subject might be expected to understand it. Studies of teeth have been conducted by scholars of almost all fields of the sciences, both physical and natural. Their interests in the dentition have originated from many different points of view and from diverse backgrounds. Foremost among these students have been the anthropologists, paleontologists, anatomists, and geneticists. A survey of some of the results of their research and the problems that yet await solution will afford the dentist a much deeper appreciation of the clinical field, and broaden and excite interest in rapidly expanding areas of dental research.

The dentist is trained to observe the tooth as a structure that is prone to disease and susceptible to alteration because of wear, malalignment, diet, and other environmental agencies. The clinician also is concerned with the teeth as a whole (the dentition) which function within an integrated anatomic component of the body (the masticatory apparatus). He or she has the ability to diagnose malfunctioning and to plan treatment aimed at removing or intercepting the causes. The dental needs of patients occupy the major portion of his or her time and energies. However, dentists, like other professional people, have intellectual needs and curiosities that transcend the immediate problems of patients and office. These needs can find satisfaction in the very field in which they have devoted their lives, were they but aware of the academic challenges that are posed. With a background in the anatomy and physiology of the dentition, who is better able to appreciate the role of the teeth in reconstructing the evolution of the vertebrates, including mankind, or to muse upon the significance of individual and racial variability expressed in crown structure? Is there a practicing dentist who has not come upon oddly shaped, supernumerary, missing, or ectopic teeth, and then found similar conditions occurring in the siblings and parents of the patient? How often does he or she not treat the patient as any other patient, only momentarily piqued by this striking but not clinically important entity? Dentists are in a unique and potentially significant position. They are continuously looking at teeth. Nobody else is as apt to observe unusual dental conditions that occur in individuals or among members of a family. The dentist is, so to speak, "in the front line trenches." Unfortunately, most dentists are not trained to observe and record such conditions unless these are directly involved with the dental health of the patient. Thus, much valuable data, of firsthand significance for science, are perforce lost. It is, therefore, a matter of some scientific urgency that dentists be made aware of the importance of the dentition for fields other than the clinical one in which their major interest lies.

Clinicians and scientists must work together to

the greater enlightenment of both and to the greater advancement of dental research. There is, of course, some precedent for this type of collaboration. We think of the fruitful researches of William King Gregory, a paleontologist, of Milo Hellman, an orthodontist, and of Wilton Marion Krogman, the physical anthropologist, and his many dental colleagues. In recent years there appears to be a definite trend toward the buildup of basic science departments within the dental schools, and it is hoped that this will encourage the mutual stimulation and indoctrination of clinician and scientist, and even promote worthwhile collaboration in dental research.

In Chapters 15 to 22 our primary purpose is to open the door to the wider biological vistas afforded by the study of the dentition. It is our hope that in so doing we shall provide for the dental student the broad perspective from which to view the profession with increased respect, deeper appreciation, and more critical understanding. In this way the dentist's stature as a truly professional practitioner of the healing arts will be increased.

It may sound paradoxical but it is nevertheless true that if only human teeth are studied, knowledge of human teeth would be extremely limited and often questionable. It is impossible to describe a forest by examining a single tree; by confining examination to that single tree very little can be learned about it. In other words, knowledge based on a sample of one is self-limiting.

If we were to attempt to describe teeth *in general* from what we know of human dentition, we would make the following statements: (1) the dentition is composed of different kinds of teeth; (2) the function of teeth is to slice, crush, and grind food; (3) there are two sets of teeth, primary and permanent; (4) there are two incisors, one canine, two premolars, and three molars in the permanent dentition; (5) the crowns of teeth are completely covered with enamel; (6) the roots of teeth are embedded in bony sockets. All of these statements, if applied to teeth in general, are false. They do not apply exclusively to man, nor do they apply to all tooth-bearing animals. One can not learn about the anatomy, histology, function, eruption, development, and pathology of all dentitions by studying only the human dentition.

The comparative study of animal dentitions, plus the study of dental evolution, throws much greater light upon the human dentition and puts it in an entirely new perspective. Even a cursory glance at the teeth of various animals suggests that there is a great variety of different types and shapes of teeth, and that the different forms of teeth are related to the functions they perform. What is more, the locations of the dentitions in different animals relative to the eyes, brain, nostrils, and palate further indicate the type of activities carried on by the teeth. In terrestrial quadrupeds (four-footed land animals) the most anterior part of the body is the snout with its complement of teeth. These are the first organs to contact the environment, be it hostile or friendly. Not only are teeth used in offensive and defensive battle, but in catching and killing other animals for food, in digging for edible roots, in breaking or cracking hard-shelled fruit, in combing the fur, in gnawing wood, and in grasping and holding animate or inanimate objects. Of course, a primary function always remains the mastication of food. One could never deduce these many dental functions simply by observing the way man uses his teeth.

As we shall observe in the next few pages, the functions that a dentition performs are reflected in the shape and disposition of the individual teeth. This is certainly true for animals in the wild state. Two very important questions then arise: "Do the teeth of man likewise predict in their structure the uses to which they are put? And if not, why not?" The answer is to be found in the story of evolution.

The form and function of the human dentition is better appreciated against a background of understanding of variations that exist in animal dentitions by making comparisons—hence the science of comparative odontology. Such comparisons not only help explain the specific morphology and functions of modern human teeth, but also throw light on dental evolution and the changing shapes of teeth from the past to the present. Teeth in fact are extraordinarily important artifacts of evolutionary evidence, for they are the hardest structures of biological development and accordingly are the most durable survivors of decay after death. It is somewhat paradoxical that teeth are so susceptible to decay during life. Much of the evidence of the existence of many extinct species rests entirely upon their dentitions, which are the only remnants of their skeletons to have survived as fossil relics.

The intricate nature of many dentitions reflects a complex pattern of evolution and thereby of their genetic endowment. The phenotypic expression of a tooth—its morphological appearance—very accurately reflects its genotype—the inherited determinant of dental morphology. Accordingly, inherited dental traits are significant genetic markers, providing insights into lineages of familial inheritance. The various patterns of tooth morphology, both fossil and extant, are evidence of evolutionary trends over eons of time. Dental anomalies of genetic origin, such as congenitally absent or malformed teeth, are increasingly being used by geneticists to trace the geneology of malformation syndromes. The easy access to teeth in living individuals allows their direct comparison with the teeth of the long deceased, or even fossil teeth, which facilitates tracing genetic, and thereby, evolutionary affinities in a manner not possible with any other organs of the body. The main, and often only, link between genetics and the paleontologic record is that of the dentition. The differences in dental morphology between various forms of early mankind—prehominids and hominids—provide evidence of underlying genetic changes. Upon this evidence can the frequency and direction of microevolutionary changes be determined.

Teeth not only provide evidence of their own genetic endowment, but may also provide significant information about the nature of the diet and thereby, indirectly, about the evolutionary and cultural status of their original owners. The shapes of teeth correlate strongly with habitual diets. Carnivory, insectivory, and piscivory are associated with sharp-cusped pointed teeth for predatory ingestion, whereas herbivorous or omnivorous creatures possess flat-cusped grinding teeth for mastication. Scratch marks left on teeth by different diets, particularly of extinct creatures, provide insights into the consistency of habitually ingested foods that are significant in anthropological research for past populations, and of assistance in forensic odontology in present populations.

Racial variations in modern human dentitions reflect microevolutionary trends that are best understood against a background of paleoanthropology reflecting the evolution of mankind. An appreciation of the variety of human skull and jaw shapes and how they evolved is a useful aid in forensic identification of deceased individuals and facilitates current clinical practice in restorative dentistry and orthodontics.

Accordingly, comparative odontology and physical anthropology are significant components of a full understanding of the modern human dentition from biologic, morphologic, functional, and therapeutic perspectives.

Dental Anthropology

The significance of the dentition in studying variations of mankind is evident from the introductory observations, and, consequently, a specialized field of anthropology is devoted exclusively to teeth. Dental anthropology can include the study of tooth development and growth; theories on tooth cusp and fissure origins and their inheritance; primate dentitions and population variations of dental characteristics, both recent and archeological. These broad areas of inquiry incorporate in-depth studies of dental morphology, dental dimensions (odontometrics), evolution, genetics, forensic odontology, dental pathology and health, tooth usage and abuse, and ethnographic factors.

Populations

Affinities between different population groups can be based on odontometric descriptions. These include dimensions of not only whole teeth but also individual components, e.g., cusps, crown heights, root lengths, and pulp chambers, from which numerous indices can be derived and comparisons made between populations. Crown traits that form extra cusps, styles, tubercles, accessory ridges, or pits are generally inherited and are discrete (absent or present) in their expression. These can provide evolutionary markers and indicate associations of twins, families, and populations. These strongly genetic traits can also assist in delineating inherited versus environmental factors that influence dental development. This delineation is particularly significant in assessing whether anomalies of the dentition are idiopathic, iatrogenic, or inherited. Microdontia, macrodontia, anodontia (absent teeth), hypodontia (few teeth), and hyperdontia (supernumerary teeth) are all controlled by the same system of multifactorial polygenic modes of inheritance and allow for clinical determination of genetic distances. Agenesis of specific categories of teeth, e.g., third molars or maxillary lateral incisors, has a high familial and racial affinity, providing genetic identification.

Tooth size (mesiodistal and buccolingual crown diameters) has been used as a discriminant factor in differentiating population groups. Among extant human populations, Australian aborigines have the largest overall tooth size, some 30 to 35 percent larger than the smallest-toothed groups of Lapps and Bushmen. Among fossil hominids, the moderate-sized teeth of the most ancient hominids diverged into a dental aggrandizement, culminating in a megadontic *Australopithecus boisei* and a dental minification that characterizes the small cheek (posterior) teeth of *Homo sapiens*.

Certain morphological traits of tooth crowns are present or absent in various racial groups with sufficient frequency to become an identifying characteristic of a racial group. The between-group different frequencies of such traits as the Carabelli cusp or pit, shovel-shaped incisors, and an extra molar cusp 6 are so explicit that "typical" Caucasoid or Mongoloid dental complexes are recognized, and associations between populations are based solely upon this dental evidence. The Carabelli trait has a high incidence of expression in Caucasoid populations with a low level of frequency of shovel-shaped incisors. Conversely, the Carabelli trait is seldom fully expressed in Mongoloid populations, which possess a high frequency of shovel-shaped incisors. Numerous other dental traits, such as three-rooted lower first molars, cervical extensions of enamel onto roots, and extra or absent cusps, have been used to delineate population groups. These traits, correlated with serological genetics, have been used to estimate times of evolutionary divergence between local races, their ancestry, and migration patterns of populations. Dental traits are also used for forensic identification of unknown skeletons.

Genetics

The genetics underlying dental characteristics that are directly observable has enabled rates and degrees of gene flow to be calculated and genetic drift to be estimated in divergent populations. Mutations may be traced in this manner, and the selective advantages of particular dental conformations might account for dental microevolution. Simplification of complex crown structure would make teeth less susceptible to caries by providing fewer food traps, whereas conversely, accessory cusps or ridges would enhance the masticatory capability of teeth. Correlations of various tooth structures with the nature of different diets would appear self-evident.

Diets

Not only diet but also culture-specific behaviors might be observed in dental wear patterns. Distinctions between primitive hunter-gatherers subsisting on meat diets and agriculturists consuming abrasive grains might be inferred from abrasional wear of teeth. The study of scratch marks on the grinding surfaces of teeth has become a highly specialized science in interpreting dietary intake. The chipping of enamel may be related to bone crunching or implemental usage of teeth. The pathological grinding of teeth (bruxism) inflicts attritional wear that characterizes anxiety states. Habitual masticatory patterns create characteristic occlusal plane curves of Spee and Monson and helicoidal occlusal wear planes that are used in anthropological identification and determining the textural nature of the food normally triturated.

Cultures

Oral cultural practices can leave their imprint on the dentition. The use of anterior teeth as a vise in manipulating bow strings and ropes or in opening bobby pins and capped bottles characteristically grooves or even fractures teeth. The wearing of labrets (lip ornaments) in certain societies produces distinctive wear facets on the buccal and labial surfaces of teeth. The habitual use of toothpicks to remove food debris may leave distinctive interproximal grooves, and abrasional toothbrush wear is indicated in cervical erosion cavities that provide insights into oral hygiene practices.

Besides the deposits of tar on the teeth of heavy smokers, the habitual clamping on a pipestem abrades upper and lower teeth to create an interocclusal void that may be of anthropological, if not pathological, interest.

The intentional mutilation of teeth to conform to cultural practices is another aspect of dental anthropology with which dentists need to be acquainted. Such mutilations constitute some of the most primitive forms of dental practice as part of initiation ceremonies or following fashion dictates or status differentiation. The extraction of specific teeth—usually incisors—to provide oral access for fellatio, is considered an attractive sign of beauty in some populations. The chipping or filing usually of anterior teeth imparts a fang-like appearance to which some cultures aspire. The insertion of precious metal inlays or gemstones into upper anterior teeth constitutes a dental cultural modification demanding considerable dental practice skills. The wearing of orthodontic bands has achieved something of a status symbol in North American society.

Facial configurations, which vary among different racial groups, need to be considered in achieving "ideal" facial esthetics in orthodontic and orthopaedic therapy. The prognathic (projecting) profile of Black populations is to be contrasted with the orthognathic (flat-faced) profile of Mongoloid peoples, and prodontism (projecting front teeth), considered esthetically acceptable in some cultures, is a basis for orthodontic dental retrusion in other societies.

Dental Disease

The fact that teeth may permanently record metabolic disturbances occurring during their embryological development makes them a valuable source of information of stressed populations. Severe malnutrition or epidemic diseases in early childhood that interfere with normal amelogenesis or dentinogenesis causing dental hypoplasia or hypocalcification are identifiable in skeletal remains and account for extensive evidence in anthropology of not only dental health but also general health of archaic populations. Such investigations form a considerable component of paleoanthropology, and provide insights into the nutritional status and incidence of epidemics in earlier populations. The incidences of dental caries, periodontal disease, and dental anomalies are of course permanently imprinted on the dentition and jaws of both living and extinct populations and allow for their epidemiological evaluation.

In these numerous and diverse ways, the study of dental anthropology contributes to a greater understanding of mankind's past and present and may serve as a basis for predictions of its future. Teeth truly tell tales of the living and the deceased.

Suggested Reading

Davies DM. The influence of teeth, diet and habits on the human face. London: William Heinemann, 1972.

Hrdlicka A. New data on the teeth of early man and certain fossil European apes. Am J Phys Anthrop 1924; 7:109–132.

Iscan MY. The emergence of dental anthropology. Am J Phys Anthrop 1989; 78:1.

16

The Vertebrates

Animals possessing a vertebral column—a feature characteristic of the subphylum Vertebrata of the phylum Chordata—comprise the fishes, amphibians, reptiles, birds and mammals. The vertebrate skeleton consists of a cranium, a vertebral column and two pairs of limbs. Vertebrates distinctively possess paired branchial arches, the basis of the respiratory and masticatory systems. The earliest known vertebrates, living 500 million years ago, were jawless fish (Agnatha), rather similar to contemporary lampreys. Some groups evolved more rapidly than others, and many conservative groups remain in existence with little structural change. Such "living fossils" throw light on the past, but direct evidence of evolution requires the paleontologic record of fossils.

Preservation of body parts as fossils entails petrification—replacement of once living structures by stone. The hardest structures of the body are the most likely to become fossilized. Teeth, being the most densely mineralized biologic structures (with enamel being a "fossilized" tissue even in life) provide the most extensive fossil history of all the anatomic structures. Interpretation of the relationships of fossil remnants depends upon knowledge of living animals in which nonfossilized soft parts can be investigated. Paleontology, comparative anatomy, and more recently, molecular biology combine to provide a picture of the course of evolution.

Classification of the Vertebrates

The animal kingdom is divided into a number of major sections or phyla, of which only the phylum Chordata concerns us here. The Chordata consist of those animals which at least during their development possess a notochord beneath the nerve cord along the back, and gill-slits opening from the pharynx to the exterior. The Vertebrata are a subphylum of the Chordata, distinguished by the formation of vertebrae around the notochord and nerve cord, and also by numerous characters of the brain, heart, kidney, and other organs. Besides the vertebrates, the Chordata include Amphioxus and tunicates.

The Vertebrata are in turn divided into a number of classes:

1. Agnatha, lampreys and hagfishes. These have no jaws, and their teeth are horny, keratinized epidermal structures that do not resemble the teeth of other vertebrates.
2. Elasmobranchii, sharks and rays. These fish have no bone, but only a cartilaginous skeleton. Nevertheless, they have biting jaws provided with true teeth.
3. Teleosts, the bony fish, making up the majority of living fish. Most of them have teeth.
4. Amphibia, frogs and salamanders. These have true teeth.
5. Reptilia, turtles, lizards, snakes, and crocodiles. Many of these have teeth, but the turtles are toothless, their jaws being covered with a horny sheath.
6. Aves, the birds. These have no teeth today, but fossils show that birds had teeth in former times. Interestingly, they retain "dental" genes that are suppressed in their phenotypic expression.
7. Mammalia, the mammals, including man.

The evolutionary timetable of the vertebrates is presented in Figure 16.1.

Basic Features of the Teeth of Vertebrates

Vertebrate teeth always develop as a result of the interaction between two tissues. One of these is the epithelium of the mouth lining, which is of ectodermal origin; the other is the underlying mesenchyme, which is of neural crest origin. In reptiles and mammals these give rise respectively to the enamel and

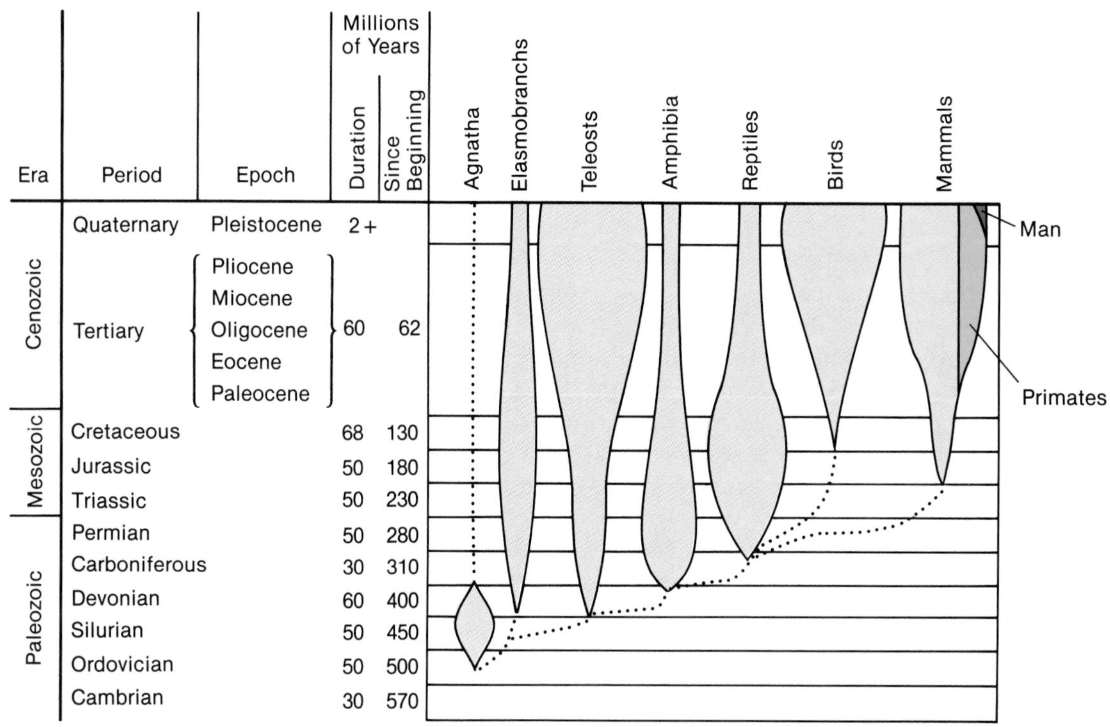

Figure 16.1
Chronology of the vertebrates.

the dentin. True enamel does not develop in most fish; instead, the surface of the tooth is composed of "enameloid," the highly calcified outer layer of dentin. However, even in fish the epithelium forms a cap-like structure around the developing tooth, corresponding to the enamel organ of mammals. Inside the cavity of the enamel organ is the mesenchymal papilla, which becomes converted into dentin, beginning at its outer surface. Dentin is one of the oldest of vertebrate tissues. It has been recognized in fossil remains as far back as the Ordovician period, more than 400 million years ago.

These early examples of dentin do not come from teeth but from skeletal plates (denticles) that formed a head shield in the Agnatha. The living lampreys and hagfishes do not have any calcified skeleton, but their fossil relatives had a well-developed system of plates of armor in the skin. These ossicles of dentin were initially not dental tissues, but rather sensory and protective organs, which later in evolution migrated to the mouth region to become attached to newly developed bone from the branchial arches (the jaws), as found in the placoderms. The modern elasmobranchs also have toothlike structures in their skin, known as placoid scales. These fishes have the capacity to form teeth not only in the mouth but over the surface of the body. Placoid scales are also found in some teleosts.

Within the mouth, teeth are frequently found not only along the edges of the jaws but also on the palate (Fig. 16.2). Palatal teeth are usually present in bony fishes, in salamanders, in lizards, and in snakes, being borne on such bones as the vomers, palatines, and pterygoids. Moreover, many bony fish have pharyngeal teeth on the gill arches. In the mammals, teeth have become restricted to the premaxillary, maxillary, and dentary bones.

Teeth, then, are primarily structures that develop in the skin or the mouth lining, and only secondarily do they become attached to underlying bones. The dentitions of the elasmobranchs and teleosts differ in character. In the cartilaginous group (e.g., sharks, rays), the teeth are all alike (homodont), simple-cusped in shape (haplodont) and are constantly replaced with successive generations (polyphyodont) (Fig. 16.3). In some bony fishes these primitive dental characteristics evolve into more complex variably shaped teeth (heterodont) with fewer replacement generations and more rigid attachment to the jaws. In the cartilaginous fish, which have no bones, the placoid scales and teeth are merely embedded at their base in the fibrous layer of the dermis overlying the jaw cartilage. In the dermis the placoid scale develops the basal plate, consisting of a tissue known as osteodentin, ramified by pulp canals containing blood vessels and lined with odontoblasts. In other vertebrates, teeth generally form some attachment to bone, but the attachment can take a number of differ-

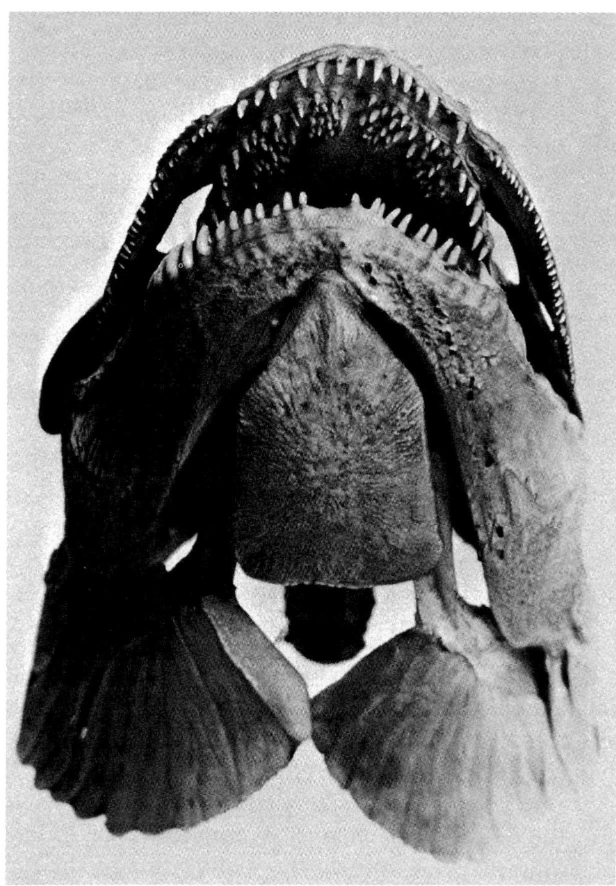

Figure 16.2
Skull of Amia (Bowfin) in ventral view to show palatal teeth.

ent forms. In many teleosts the tooth becomes fused to the surface of the bone (ankylosis); this occurs also in lizards and snakes. In some lizards the side of the tooth fuses to the lingual side of the vertical edge of the maxilla or dentary. In some fish the teeth do not fuse to the underlying bone, but are connected by elastic fibers, so arranged that the tooth can be bent over as by a hinge, allowing prey to pass into the mouth, and then flipping up to prevent escape. Among living reptiles, only the crocodiles and alligators bear their teeth in sockets (Fig. 16.4). In these, as in mammals, the tooth is not fused to the bone but connected to it by a layer of periodontal fibers. The crocodilians also resemble mammals in that the base of the tooth is covered with a thin layer of cementum, a tissue resembling bone but lacking in blood vessels, and thus it is possible in these forms to speak of the root of the tooth as distinct from the crown. Only in the mammals do we find teeth provided with more than one root.

The way in which new teeth originate is by differentiation of the enamel organ directly from the oral

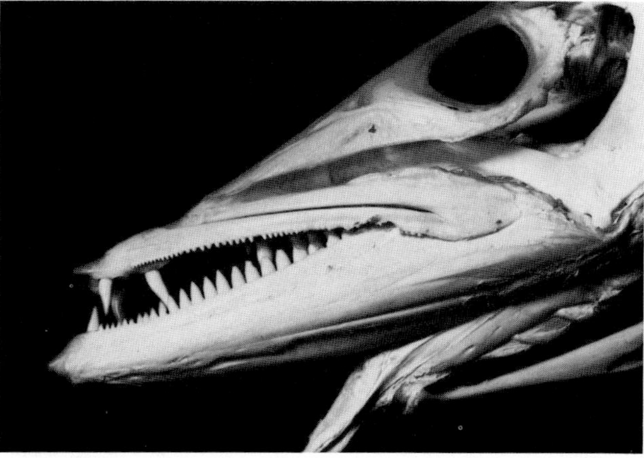

Figure 16.3
Barracuda jaws: the haplodont homodont conical teeth of this fish are arrayed in two rows in the upper jaw, an outer row of tiny teeth and an irregular inner row of larger teeth for capture of prey. (University of Alberta Dental Museum)

epithelium, part of its germinative layer becoming converted into the ameloblast layer of the tooth germ. This is the usual way in which the teeth of teleosts arise; the placoid scales of elasmobranchs develop in a similar manner (Fig. 16.5). The first-formed teeth of salamanders and crocodiles are also formed directly from the oral epithelium, but later on the tooth-forming area of epithelium grows down into the underlying tissues and becomes a dental lamina. In elasmobranchs the teeth of the mouth are also formed from a dental lamina. The palatal teeth of lizards, snakes, and amphibians develop from a dental lamina separate from that which forms the marginal teeth of the maxilla. Mammals of course have a dental lam-

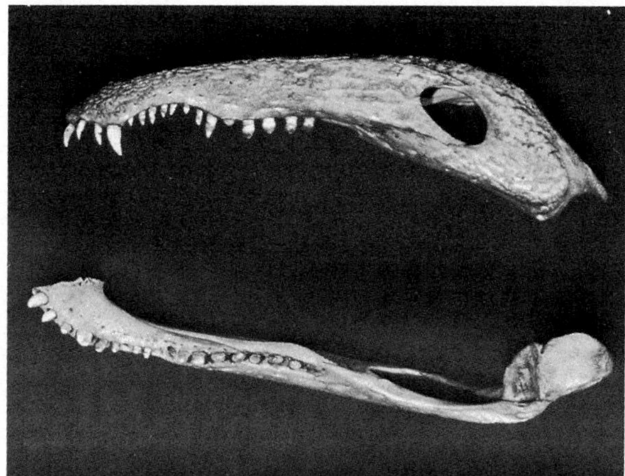

Figure 16.4
Mandibles of an alligator. The right mandible is seen from the lateral side, the left mandible is seen from above. Note that teeth are in sockets.

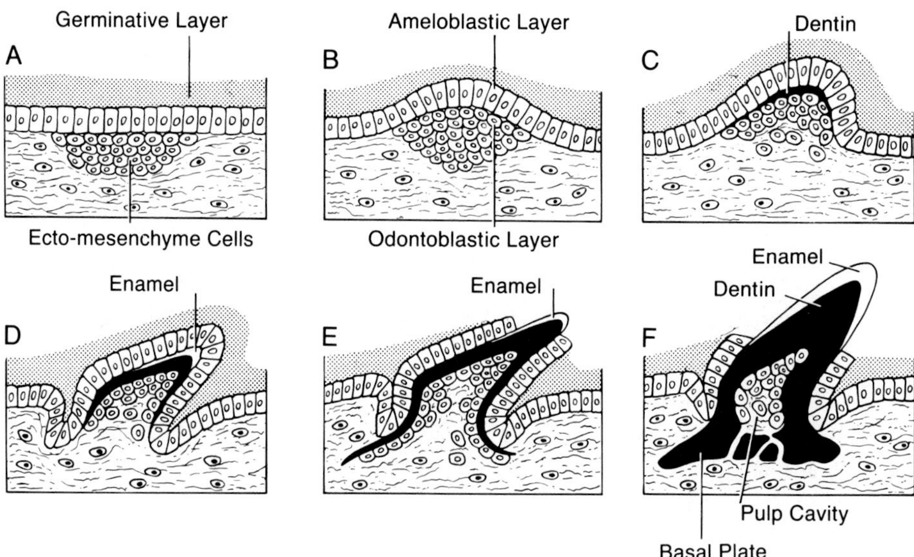

Figure 16.5
Development of placoid scale.

ina, but in some cases the teeth begin to develop at a time when the lamina has just begun to sink in. Whether or not teeth form from a lamina, they can always be regarded as developing from the oral epithelium; the lamina is simply a specialized part of this epithelium.

In most vertebrates the process of forming new teeth continues throughout life (polyphyodont dentitions) so that the animal is constantly provided with replacements as the old teeth become worn or broken. When teeth form a row along the edges of the jaw, the new teeth develop from the oral epithelium or the lamina on the lingual side of the old ones, and when the old teeth are shed the new teeth move buccally to take their places in the functional row. In sharks there are several rows of functional teeth, and lingually several more rows are at various stages of development (Fig. 16.6). New teeth appear at the deep edge of the lamina and move buccally as they develop.

Tooth shedding and replacement are not random, but are sequenced in alternate rows. Sharks' teeth form a battery of sharp narrow blades for predatory attack. Constant shedding of shark's teeth has

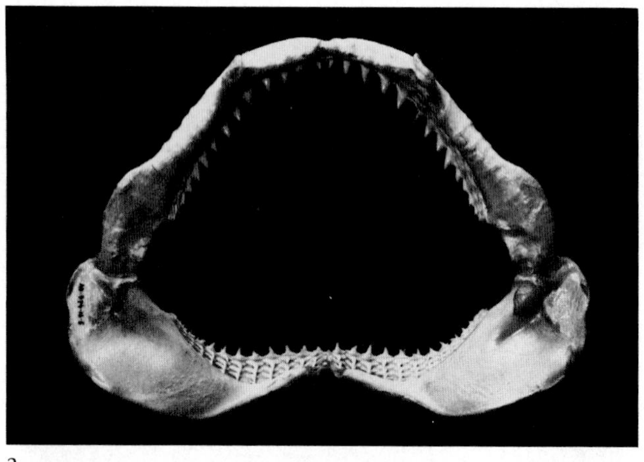
a

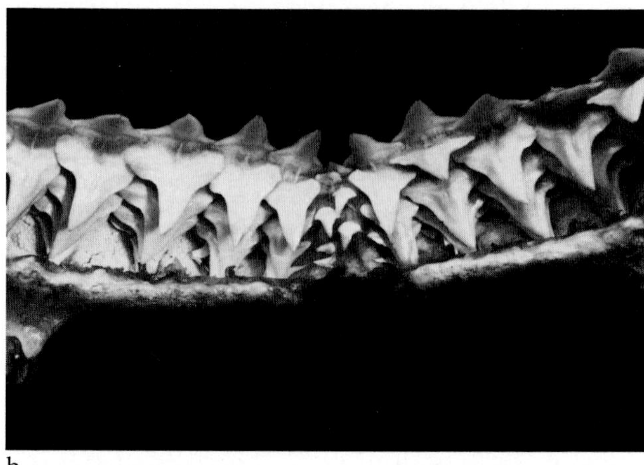
b

Figure 16.6
Shark's jaw: the imbricated layers of successive generations (polyphyodont) of haplodont, homodont teeth. The layers move into function as escalator stairs.

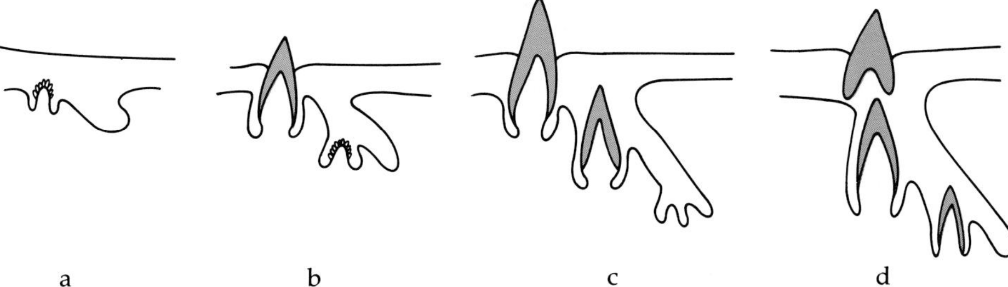

Figure 16.7
Method of tooth replacement in reptiles.

occurred over millions of years, resulting in the floors of the ocean being covered with their discarded teeth. In crocodiles and lizards the new tooth moves into a cavity that is resorbed out of the base of the old tooth, so that eventually the new tooth lies directly below the old one; when the old tooth is shed the new tooth is already in place and has only to erupt (Fig. 16.7). The situation in mammals is rather similar to this. The fangs of snakes are highly specialized teeth fused to the maxilla. Poisonous snakes have a groove or canal in the fang through which poison is injected into the prey. New fangs lie horizontally in the roof of the mouth, and when the old fang is lost a new fang rotates into position and fuses to the maxilla to become functional. In some vertebrates, in which the teeth are large and durable, replacement takes place rarely or even not at all; this is true of the mammals, which typically replace their deciduous teeth only once with a permanent set constituting a diphyodont dentition. The permanent molars are never replaced at all.

The simplest form of vertebrate tooth is a gently curved conical structure, a haplodont tooth. Such teeth are found in the majority of elasmobranchs and in many reptiles. They function mainly in holding prey. Sometimes the tip is blunt or rounded, and then the teeth are used for crushing food, as in fish that live on mollusks or crustaceans. In other cases the mesial and distal surfaces of the cone are sharpened to form cutting ridges as in some sharks and reptiles. In sharks the ridges are usually serrated to increase the cutting power, and some species possess accessory cusps developed on the ridges (Fig. 16.8). Some lizards, too, possess mesial and distal accessory cusps, so that the tooth has three cusps in a mesiodistal row. Frogs and salamanders frequently possess an accessory cusp on the buccal side of the main cusp. However, none of the other classes of vertebrates has such complex crown patterns as the mammals.

In many vertebrates all the teeth in the jaw are alike (homodontism), differing from each other only in size. In the alligator some teeth are much larger than others, although they all have a similar shape. Some fish, however, have more than one sort of tooth, a condition described as heterodontism. For example, the mesial teeth may be adapted for rasping food off the surface of rocks, and the distal teeth for crushing the food that has been taken into the mouth. Only in the mammals, however, is the dentition fully heterodont, consisting of a number of different sorts of teeth that perform different functions, so that we can distinguish incisors, canines, premolars, and molars.

Fishes and most reptiles have hinged jaws that can open wide and shut down on prey, which is processed little if at all before it is swallowed. The capability for anteroposterior jaw movement with the development of a sliding jaw joint with heterodont teeth marks a few advanced crocodilian reptiles and characterizes mammals. This chewing capability, associated with secondary palate development, has enabled exploitation of diets very different from those species with limited hinge movement.

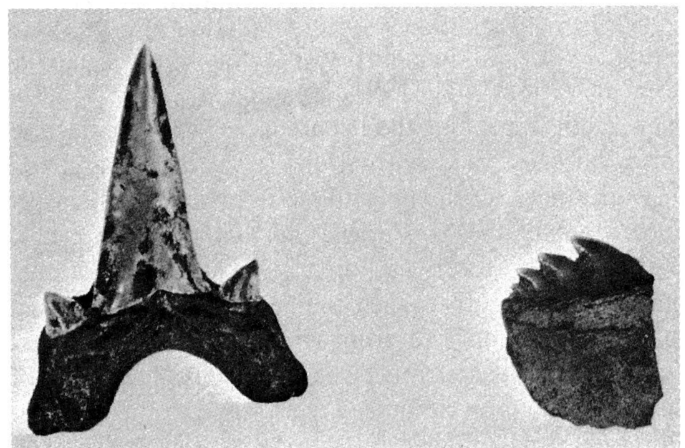

Figure 16.8
Teeth of two fossil sharks, showing multiple cusps.

Characteristics of the Mammalian Masticatory Apparatus

Against the background of vertebrate jaws and teeth in general we can now point out some of the main characteristics of the mammalian masticatory apparatus: (1) teeth are confined to the edges of the mouth and associated with the premaxillary, maxillary, and dentary bones; (2) they are provided with roots, usually more than one root to each tooth except on the simple teeth at the anterior end of the jaw. The roots are covered with cementum, and are connected by periodontal fibers to sockets in the alveolar bones (gomphosis); (3) teeth develop from a dental lamina and are replaced at most only once (diphyodont), or, in the case of the permanent molars, or in rodents not at all (monophyodont); (4) they are heterodont, so that it is possible in each jaw to distinguish incisors, canines, premolars, and molars; (5) the molars, and often also the premolars, have a complex crown pattern, with more than one cusp; (6) there is a process of mastication, in which the cusps of opposing teeth relate together in a regular way.

One of the main reasons for the complexity of the dentition of mammals is that this class of vertebrates has developed to a high degree the function of chewing food. Mammals have a high rate of metabolism. Unlike reptiles, which obtain heat by basking in the sun and become torpid when the external temperature falls (poikilothermic), mammals keep warm by heat produced in their own bodies (homothermic). Their hairy covering and subcutaneous fat enable them to retain heat, but the source of this heat is ultimately the energy taken in as food. A small mammal has a much larger area of skin (through which heat is lost), in proportion to the volume of muscle (in which heat is produced), than has a large mammal; and so we find that small mammals take in relatively larger quantities of food. We know from fossil evidence that all of the early mammals were small creatures, most of them not much bigger than mice or rats, and they must have been very efficient at obtaining and digesting large quantities of food. This efficiency has been inherited by all the living members of the class.

Bearing this in mind, we can understand some of the characteristic features of the mammalian (hence human) mouth and jaws. The flexible lips and cheeks are provided with muscles, innervated by the facial nerve, which help in picking up food and manipulating it in the mouth. These muscles are absent in other vertebrates. The development of a secondary palate by the union of palatal folds resulted in separation of the respiratory passage from the mouth, enabling the mammal to go on breathing while its mouth is full of food, thus enabling respiration and mastication to take place concurrently. In reptiles the two passages are incompletely separated, and the food has to be swallowed quickly. Mammals retain this primitive inability to swallow and inspire at the same time. Any attempt to do so sets off coughing spells. Being able to retain food in its mouth, the mammal masticates, using its tongue and cheeks but especially its molar teeth, which grind and break up the food thus allowing it to be mixed with saliva. The saliva differs from that of other vertebrates in containing a digestive enzyme, so that digestion begins even before the food is swallowed. The process of mastication involves a strong development of lip, cheek, tongue, and jaw musculature to control the food bolus over the molar teeth. The jaw muscles are differentiated into tem-

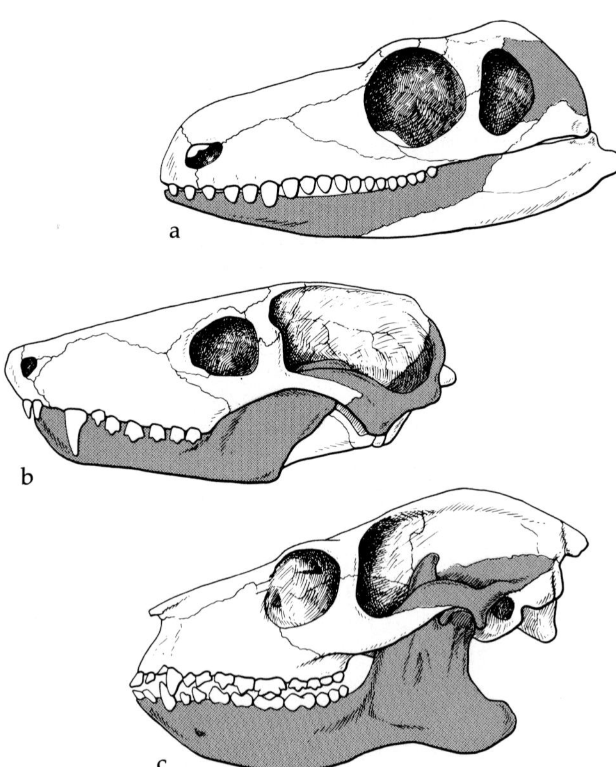

Figure 16.9

Transformation of reptile into mammal: *a*, an early mammal-like reptile from the Lower Permian period (Permian Pelycosaur); *b*, a more advanced mammal-like reptile from the Lower Permian period (Triassic Cynodont); *c*, a primitive mammal (Eocene Lemuroid). Note the approach of the dentary and spuamosal bones (shaded) and the eventual formation of a joint between them, replacing the reptilian jaw joint between quadrate and articular.

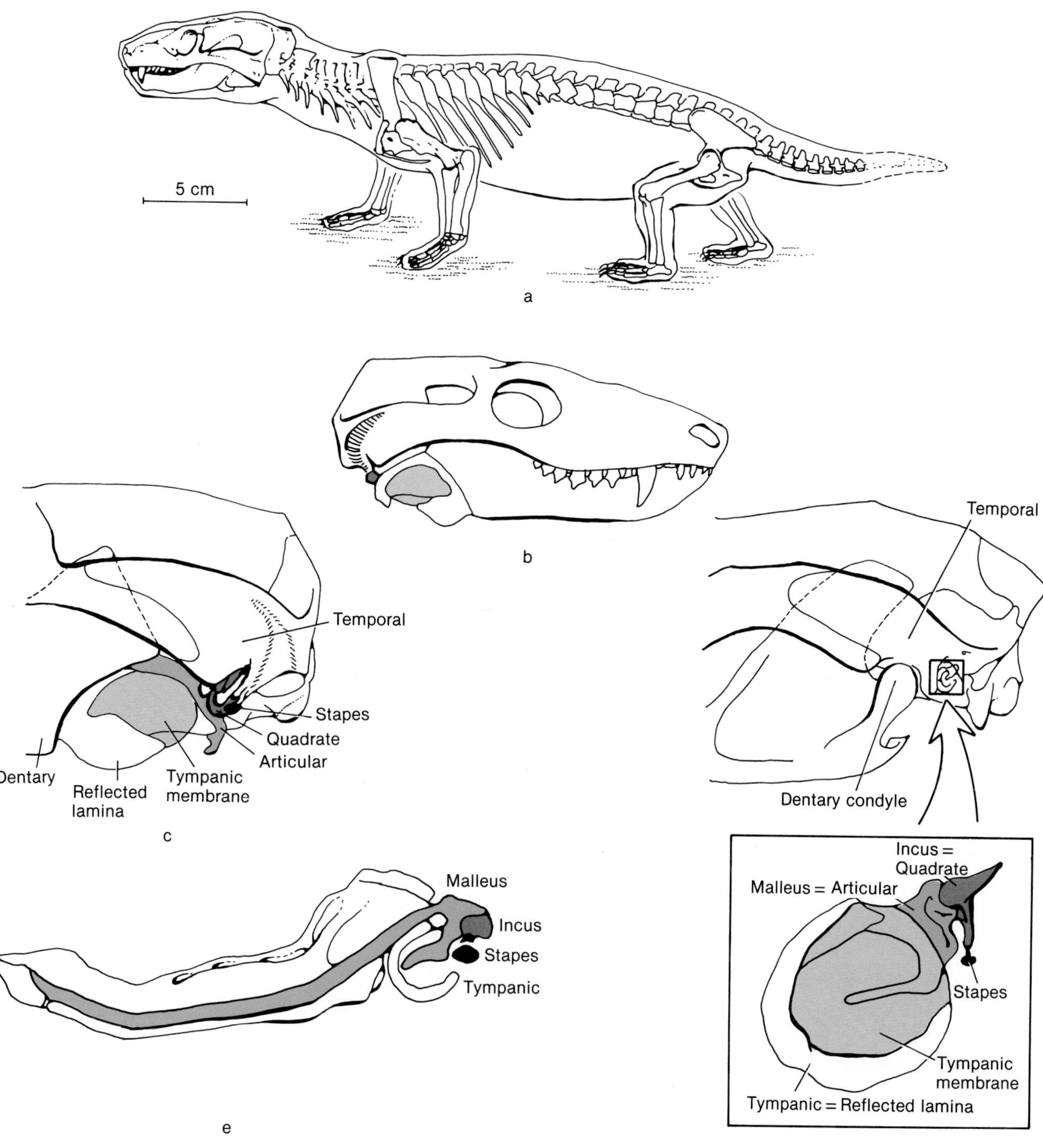

Figure 16.10

a, Reconstruction of an Early Triassic (230 million years old) mammal-like reptile, *Thrinaxodon; b,* its skull—note the heterodont dentition, with triconodont cheek teeth; *c* and *d,* comparison of the jaw joint and middle ear of *Thrinaxodon* (*c*) and a mammal (opossum, *d*); *e,* the jaw of a fetal mammal in which the primitive joint is still present. (From Crompton AW. Developmental aspects of temporomandibular joint disorders. Carlson DS, McNamara JA, Ribbens KA, eds. Monograph 16, Craniofacial Growth Series. Ann Arbor: University of Michigan, Center for Human Growth and Development, 1988; with permission.)

poralis, masseter, medial, and lateral pterygoids and digastric muscles. These enable not only opening and closing, but also transverse and protrusive-retrusive movements of the mandible. Mastication is also associated with development of a peculiar type of jaw joint; in other vertebrates the lower jaw consists of several bones, and the joint is formed by two of them, the articular and the quadrate, whereas in mammals the mandible consists of the dentary alone, articulating with the squamosal (which equals part of the temporal bone in man). Some of the bones that originally formed part of the reptilian jaw are preserved in the mammalian ear: the angular supports the ear drum and becomes the tympanic; the articular and quadrate become ear ossicles, respectively malleus and incus. The stapes is retained as the original reptilian ear ossicle. Fetal mammals still develop the primitive jaw joint, and the earliest fetal jaw movements occur through the articular-quadrate or malleo-incudal joint. It is retained after birth by marsupials, being replaced by the dentary-squamosal or temporomandibular joint in eutherian mammals.

The newly established temporomandibular joint differs from other synovial joints that are cartilage-derived. Both components of this joint are membrane-bone derived, accounting for the lack of hyaline cartilage (present in other synovial joints) at the site of articulation. The temporomandibular joint, in company with the only other membranous bone-derived joints, the sternoclavicular and acromiocla-

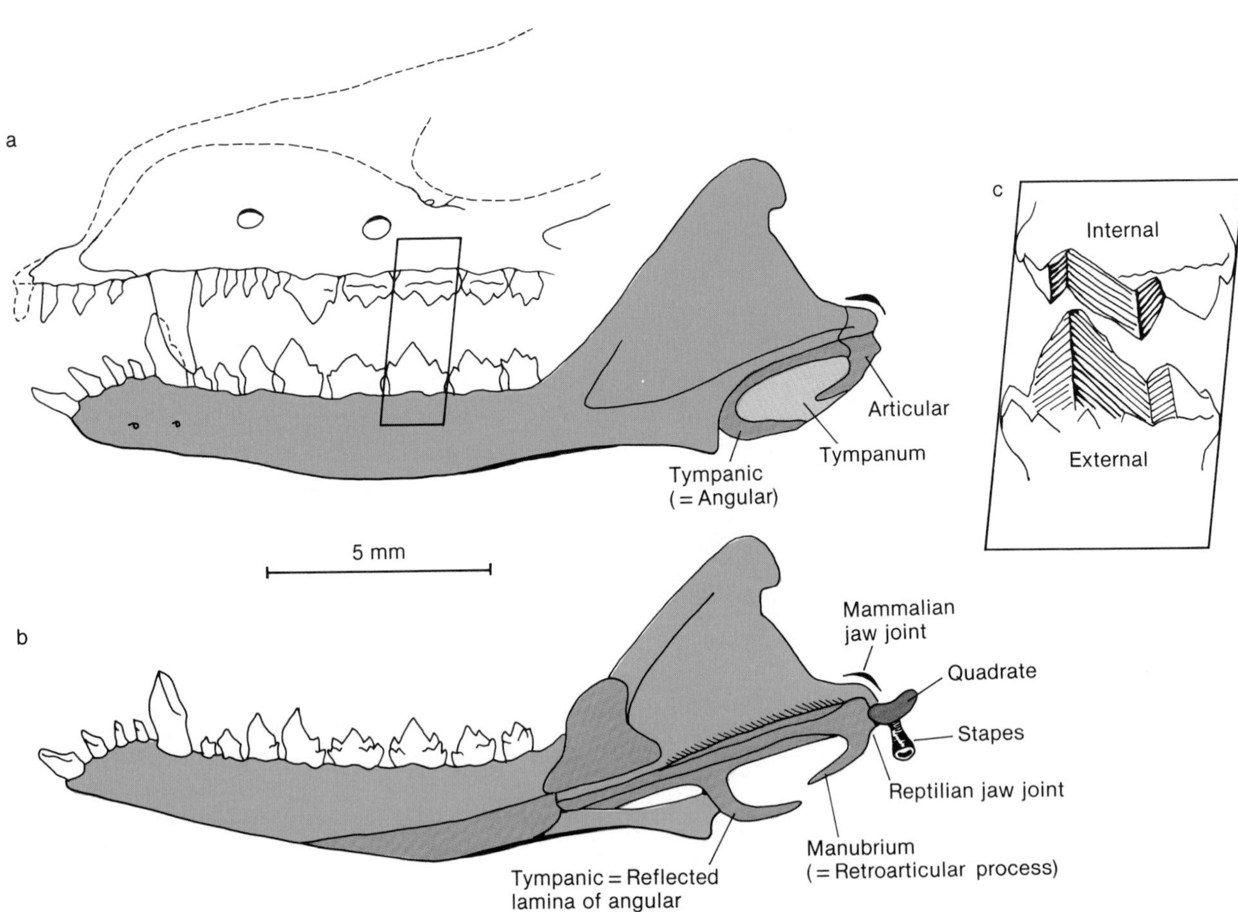

Figure 16.11

a, Jaws of *Morganucodon,* an Early Jurassic (180 million years old) mammal; note the fully heterodont dentition; *b,* the internal view of the lower jaw—both the reptilian and the mammalian jaw joints are present; *c,* the molar occlusion—the upper molar is depicted in lingual view, as if transparent, to show the wear facets. (From Crompton AW. In: Lillegraven JA, Kielan-Jaworoska Z, Clemens WA, eds. Mesozoic mammals: The first two-thirds of mammalian history. Berkeley, CA: University of California Press, 1979:63; © 1979 The Regents of the University of California; with permission.)

vicular joints, have fibrous tissue rather than hyaline cartilage covered ends of bones.

It is clear that the teeth cannot be understood by themselves; they are part of a complex comprising jaws, muscles, cheeks, tongue, palate, and ear.

All these characteristics of mammals did not arise in one step. There was a long process of evolution resulting in the attainment of the mammalian organization. Many of the stages in the process can be traced in the fossil record, among the so-called mammal-like reptiles, or Synapsida. These show, for example, stages in the formation of a secondary palate, the gradual development of heterodontism, and the enlargement of the dentary bone, until finally it met the squamosal and took part in the jaw joint (Figs. 16.9, 16.10, and 16.11).

Classification of Mammals

Mammals first appeared at the end of the Triassic period, but little is known of them during the first 100 million years of their history, which coincided with the age of dinosaurs (Jurassic and Cretaceous). The early mammals were small animals, about the size of mice or shrews. From their teeth the majority appear to have been insectivorous, but some probably fed on larger prey and others were more likely to have been herbivorous. At the end of the Cretaceous period we come across the first representatives of orders that still live today, forerunners of the great variety of mammals that characterized the Tertiary period, sometimes called the Age of Mammals.

The most important of the orders into which living mammals are divided are as follows.

1. **Monotremeta**, the egg-laying mammals of Australia. These very archaic forms, the duck-billed platypus and the echidna, stand far apart from all other mammals. They throw little light on dental evolution: the echidna is a toothless anteater, and the platypus is an aquatic animal that loses its teeth early in life and develops horny epidermal plates for crushing crustacea and mollusks.

2. **Marsupialia**, in which the young are born in a very undeveloped stage and are carried about attached to the mother's nipples, usually in a pouch. These include the opossum, and also many Australian mammals such as the kangaroo and koala bear. The group dates back to the Cretaceous period.

The dental formula of marsupials differs from that of the remaining orders of mammals which are collectively referred to as the Eutheria. On each side of the mouth, there may be as many as five incisors in the premaxilla and four in the mandible; in addition each jaw has one canine, three premolars, and four molars. Only one tooth, the last premolar, has a deciduous predecessor, although there are rudimentary teeth in the incisor region, which probably represent a deciduous dentition that has almost disappeared.

Eutheria: The subclass Eutheria includes several orders, of which the most important are listed below. They commonly have a "typical" dental formula of three incisors, a canine, four premolars and three molars in each quadrant, although in modern forms the number of teeth is usually less than this. All the teeth except the permanent molars have deciduous predecessors, except in some specialized forms.

3. **Insectivora**, small insect-eating mammals such as moles and shrews.

4. **Scandentia**, the tree-shrews such as *Tupaia*, of Southeast Asia; small squirrel-like animals thought to link the Insectivora with the Primates.

5. **Primates**, the order that includes man as well as apes, monkeys, and prosimians.

6. **Chiroptera**, the bats.

7. **Edentata**, a mainly South American group, which lacks enamel on the teeth (armadillo, sloth) or has no teeth at all (anteater).

8. **Rodentia**, the largest order of mammals, including squirrels, porcupines, beavers, rats, and mice.

9. **Lagomorpha**, rabbits and hares.

10. **Carnivora**, a large order, which includes not only cats, dogs, weasels, raccoons, and bears, but also the seals and sea lions.

11. **Cetacea**, whales, porpoises, dolphins.

12. **Perissodactyla** (odd-toed ungulates), an order including horses, rhinoceroses, and tapirs.

13. **Artiodactyla** (even-toed ungulates), those mammals which "divide the hoof," including pig, hippopotamus, deer, camel, cattle, sheep, and antelope.

14. **Proboscidea**, the elephants.

15. **Sirenia**, the dugong and the manatee.

Of the Eutherian orders in existence, the Insectivora are probably the most ancient, with the probability that the Primates are derived from them. Little detail is known of the phylogenetic relationships between the various orders.

Evolution of the Mammalian Molar Tooth

The Tritubercular Theory and Nomenclature of Molar Cusps

The evolution of the homodont, haplodont reptilian dentition to the heterodont mammalian form involved reduction in the number of teeth in the jaws and reduction in the number of replacements. Thus, polyphyodontism evolved into di- or monophyodontism. The cheek teeth evolved to form molars consisting of a series of cusps, comprised of a single cone (*protocone* in the upper jaw, *protoconid* in the lower jaw) with mesial (*paracone,* upper, or *paraconid,* lower) and distal (*metacone,* upper, or *metaconid,* lower) small cusps. Among the earliest mammals the order Triconodonta, named after their dentition, had three-cusped cheek teeth. As in reptiles, the upper and lower teeth alternated in the jaws, allowing the teeth to interdigitate on jaw closing. This arrangement was modified in later orders by increasing the size of the accessory cusps, and rotating the cusps relative to the principal cusp to form triangular teeth, with the addition of sharp crests (lophs) between the cusps creating *lophodont* teeth. The relations of the upper and lower triangles to each other were reversed by the upper protocone becoming lingually displaced, while the lower protoconid was buccally displaced, allowing interdigitation of the triangles. Teeth of this type characterize the order Symmetrodonta of the Jurassic period.

These tritubercular or trigon(id) teeth function not only by puncturing food between the cusps, but also by slicing food through a shearing action of the crests acting against each other. The next evolutionary stage involved development of a distal "heel" or *talonid* in the lower molars, which formed a platform for crushing food against the protocone of the upper molar. These cuspal patterns form *tribosphenic* molars (Greek *tribein*: to rub; *sphen*: a wedge) that are ancestral to the cuspal patterns of primate molars.

Later, an additional cusp developed on the distal aspect of the upper molar (the *hypocone*) to form a rectangular four-cusped tooth. Small additional cusps that form on the mesial and distal margins of the trigon are the *protoconule* and *metaconule.* Cusps developing along the buccal margins of the upper molar are *styles*: a *parastyle* at the mesial margin, a *mesostyle* in the middle, and a *metastyle* at the distal margin.

The lower molar talonid gave rise to three cusps—the *hypoconid* (buccal), the *entoconid* (lingual), and the *hypoconulid* (distal)—producing a six-cusped lower molar. Such four-cusped upper molars and six-cusped lower molars are found in lower primates and occur in the living Tarsius. It is important to realize

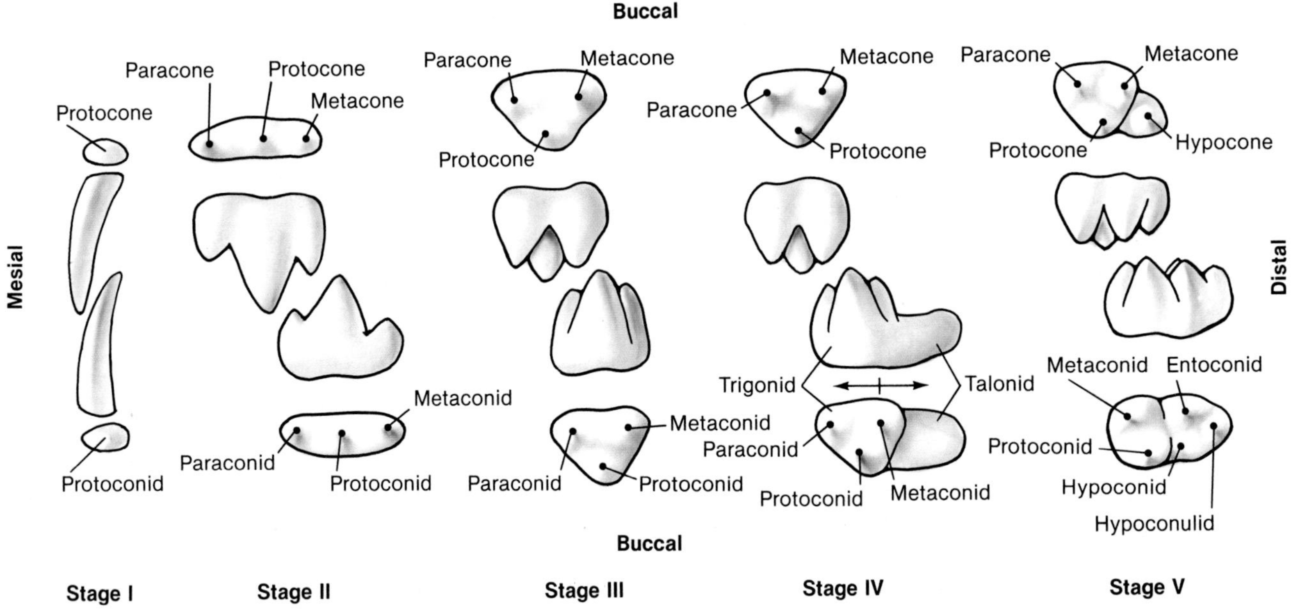

Figure 16.12

The main stages in molar evolution according to the tritubercular theory (modified).

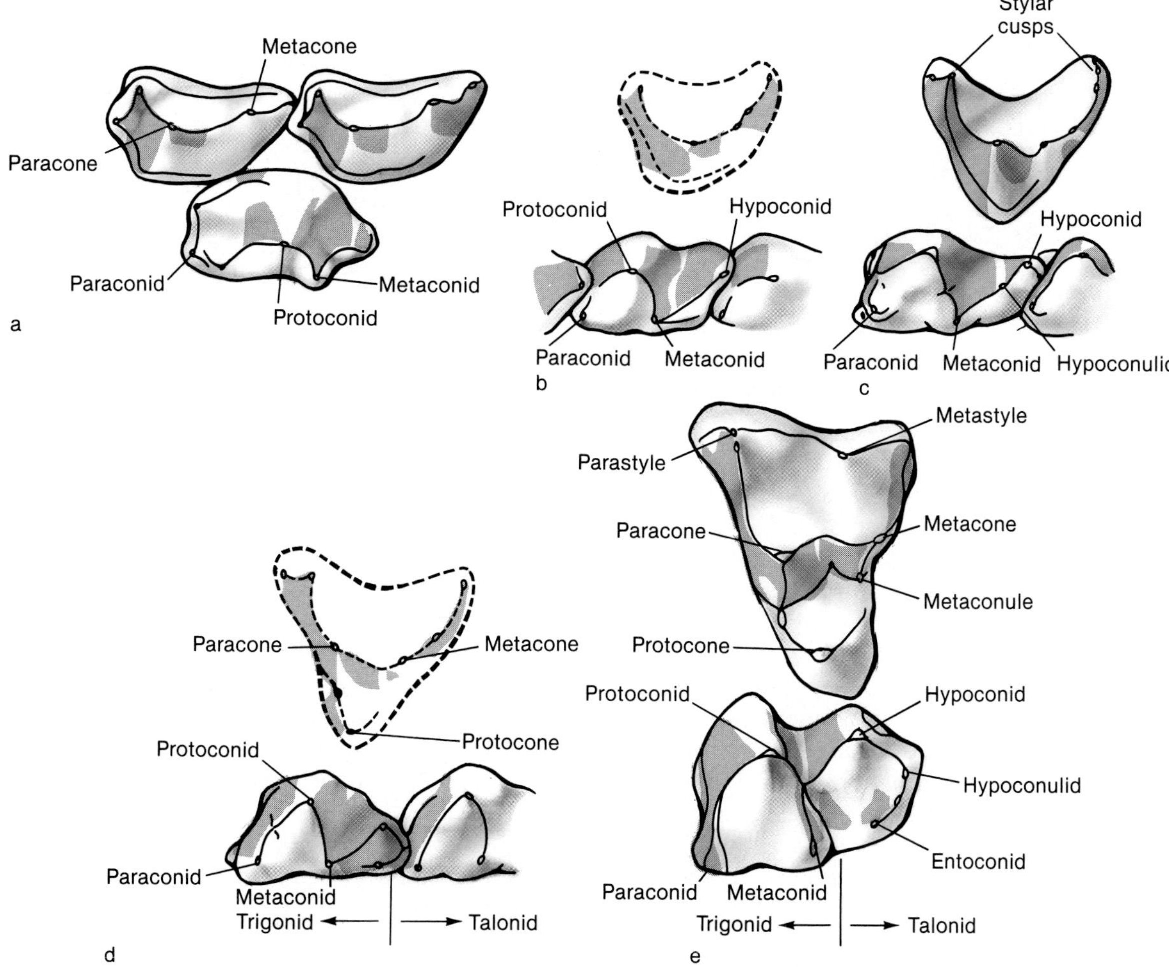

Figure 16.13

Fossil teeth of primitive mammals illustrating stages in the evolution of tribosphenic molars. The wear-facets are shaded: *a, Kueneotherium,* a primitive Symmetrodont from the Late Triassic and early Jurassic period; the lower molars lacked a talonid, and the upper molars lacked a protocone; *b, Amphitherium,* a Pantothere of the Middle Jurassic period; the lower molars developed a talonid, represented by the hypoconid; *c, Peramus,* an advanced Pantothere of the Late Jurassic period, with a more complex molar pattern; *d, Aegialodon,* a primitive tribosphenic mammal of the Early Cretaceous period; the protocone developed at this stage; *e, Didelphodus,* an insectivore of the Eocene epoch; a complex molar cusp pattern had developed to crush insects. The upper molars of *Amphitherium* (*b*) and *Aegialodon* (*d*) have not been recovered, and their structure was reconstructed from the wear-facets on the lower molars. (Adapted from Bown TM, Kraus MJ. In: Lillegraven JA, Kielan-Jaworoska Z, Clemens WA, eds. Mesozoic mammals: The first two-thirds of mammalian history. Berkeley, CA: University of California Press, 1979:176; © 1979 The Regents of the University of California; with permission.)

that upper and lower molars evolved together as complementary parts of a single functional complex. Each cusp has definite occlusal relationships to cusps of the opposing dentition, revealed by the wear-facets. Like the cusps, corresponding wear-facets can be identified on teeth at different stages of evolution. Differences in the size, shape, and position of the cusps result in differences in the size and orientation of the wear-facets and reflect evolutionary changes in molar function (Fig. 16.12).

These stages in the evolution of tribosphenic molars were developed in various primitive mammals

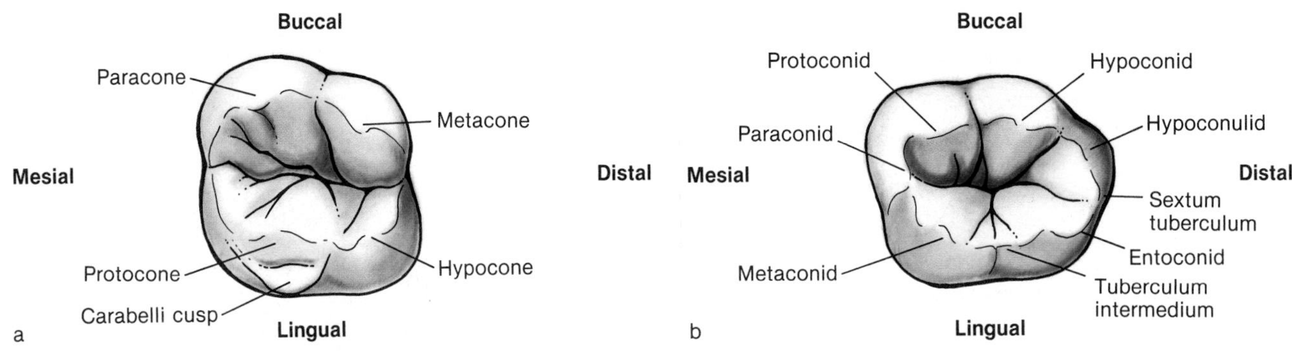

Figure 16.14

The odontological cusp terminology for human molar teeth. (*a*) Upper molar teeth; (*b*) lower molar teeth.

and are represented in the fossilized teeth of early mammalian orders. The triconodonts had molars with three prominent cusps aligned mesiodistally. The fossil symmetrodonts had symmetrical triangular trigonid molars lacking a posterior talonid basin. The fossil pantotheres had developed in stages a talonid attached to the trigonid molars. Further modifications in tribosphenic molars evolved to adapt to ecological opportunities offered, producing carnivores, herbivores, insectivores, and omnivores, reflected in their varying dental morphologies (Fig. 16.13).

In humans, the paraconid in first lower molars is lost, producing a five-cusped tooth; additionally, the hypoconulid (distal cusp) is also lost in second lower molars, producing a four-cusped tooth. The five-cusped molar occurs in anthropoid apes and man (Fig. 16.14). The Y-5 molar pattern, named after the Y-shaped pattern of fissures separating the five cusps, first appeared in a fossil pongid, *Dryopithecus*, that existed 24 million years ago and represents a very conservative genetically determined pattern still present in 90 percent of lower first permanent molars of modern man. The second and third molars are less conservative and more variable in their cusp and fissure patterns, departing from the archetypal Dryopithecus molar pattern.

These observations are limited to the molars of later mammalian orders and do not apply to variations of incisors, canines, and premolars. A full explanation of the evolution of tooth form awaits more fossil evidence from mammal-like reptiles and the early mammalian orders. Much remains to be elucidated regarding the relationships of tooth form, jaw movements, facial development, and diet.

Attachments of Teeth

The attachment of teeth to the underlying jaws may be categorized into four types: (1) fibrous, (2) hinged, (3) ankylosis, and (4) gomphosis. The first three types are confined to non-mammalian dentitions, and the complex gomphotic attachment characterizes mammalian dentitions. Fibrous attachments are generally associated with polyphyodont dentitions, which allow for rapid replacement of successive generations of teeth. Examples are found in sharks and rays. Hinged attachments allow for the inward bending of teeth to facilitate swallowing of prey that are prevented from escaping by the uprighting of hinged teeth. Examples occur in fishes such as cod, hake, angler, and pike. Ankylosis forms the firmest attachment of teeth to bone, because there is no intervening soft tissue. Dentin and bone are so intimately fused that an intermediate osteodentin blends imperceptibly into the dentin of the tooth and the bone of the jaw. Examples are found in barracuda, haddock, frogs, eels, and pythons. Loss of their teeth incurs fracture of the osteodentin.

Gomphosis attachments require a socketed root in alveolar bone, characteristic of mammalian dentitions. The development of specialized tissues of attachment, cementum and a fibrous periodontal ligament, signifies most gomphoses, as seen in mammals. However, gomphotic dental attachments exist in some reptiles (crocodiles) and in some fish (pristis or sawfish) in which succeeding teeth erupt into the same sockets as the preceding ones ("thecodont" dentitions). The sawfish (pristis) has gomphosed teeth of persistent growth.

Some Mammalian Dentitions

Insectivores

It is probable that all mammals originally fed on insects, and this diet has been retained today mainly in two orders, Insectivora and Chiroptera. They include some forms that have taken to other diets, such as the flying fox, which eats fruit, and the vampire bat, which lives on blood. The insectivorous bats, though primitive in their food, are not primitive in their method of feeding. Whereas other insectivorous mammals search for their prey on the ground or among vegetation, the bats have perfected the power of flight and catch insects on the wing. They are also remarkable in the use of a form of echolocation to find their prey. When young, they have sharp hooked deciduous teeth by which they cling to the mother, who carries them about in her flights. The permanent premolars and molars of bats have high sharp cusps, connected by ridges. The upper and lower molars fit into each other as the jaw closes. This enables the bat to cut up its food, the crests of the opposing teeth acting like the blades of scissors. As the jaw closes it moves medially because of a sliding action of the condyles, so that the lower molar glides across the upper molar to some extent, increasing the effectiveness of the cutting action. The premolars, though simpler in pattern, also have a deeply interlocking articulation. The canines are high-cusped teeth and assist in holding the prey. The incisors are reduced; in the upper jaw the premaxillae are small and fail to meet in the midline, leaving a free path for the emission of high-frequency sound waves. A similarly interlocking type of cheek dentition is found in other insectivorous mammals such as the shrews, although these are very different from bats in their anterior teeth; their incisors form a pair of forceps for picking up insects.

Carnivores

Meat eating generally demands hunting and killing prey, requiring a highly specialized dentition. Most prominent are enlarged canine teeth, for killing, combined with relatively small incisor teeth for prehension. The cheek teeth are reduced in number and greatly modified into sectorial blades for slicing. The scissor blades are formed (in cats) by a sharp crest on the last upper premolar (P^4) and another on the mesial part of the first lower molar. Both blades extend mesiodistally, and the lower blade passes to the lingual side of the upper blade as the jaw closes. The teeth so modified are known as carnassials (Fig. 16.15), and they function to cut through sinews and other tough parts of meat. The remaining premolars are simple, peg-like teeth that are used merely for holding food, e.g., when the animal is carrying its prey. At the distal end of the dentition there is a crushing region consisting of the molars. In the case of the first lower molar, however, only the distal portion (talonid) of the tooth takes part in the crushing function, as the mesial portion (trigonid) forms the carnassial blade. The first lower molar occludes with two upper teeth: distally against the first upper molar and mesially against the last upper premolar. In the cat the crushing region has degenerated: in the upper jaw only a rudimentary first upper molar remains, and the first lower molar consists almost entirely of the carnassial blade.

The jaw action of carnivores is a simple hinge movement: the cylindrical condyle rotates in a transversely extended glenoid cavity. Lateral movement of the mandible is reduced to a minimum, but it is not completely eliminated, since the animal needs to vary the closeness of contact between the upper and lower carnassial blades. The condyle is strongly supported by bony ridges, preventing dislocation when the animal is holding struggling prey with its canines. In the skull, the well-developed sagittal crest and the widely flared zygomatic arches are evidence of the presence of powerful jaw muscles. Young carnivores have carnassials in the deciduous dentition, but because of the shorter jaws the deciduous carnassials occupy a more mesial position in the dentition than

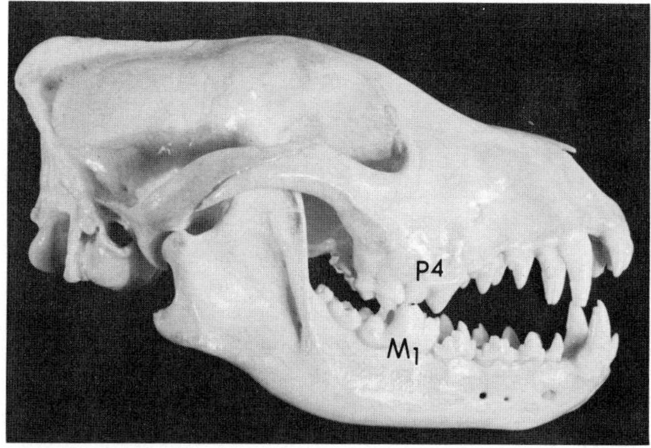

Figure 16.15
Skull of a wild dog (*Lycaon pictus*) showing the carnassial teeth, P^4 above and M_1 below, that occlude in a scissor-like fashion to slice meat. (Courtesy of University of Alberta Dental Museum)

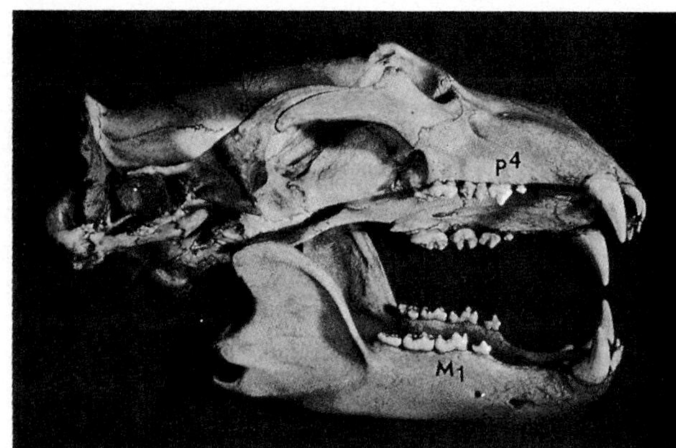

Figure 16.16
Skull and mandible of a bear. Note that P^4 and M_1 are poorly differentiated.

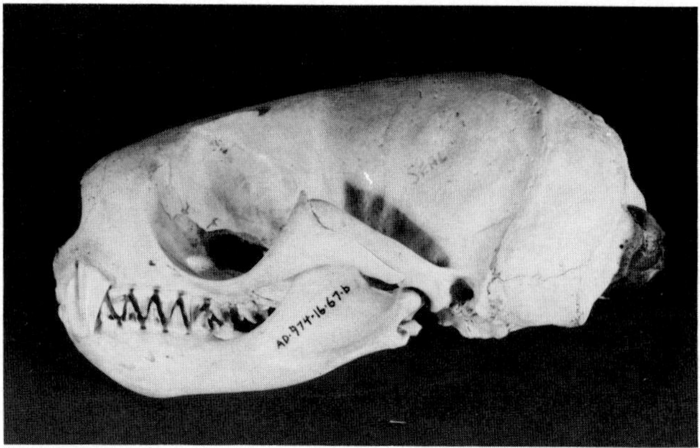

Figure 16.17
Skull of a seal (*Phoca vitulina*) showing simplified (haplodont) postcanine dentition adapted for its piscivorous diet.

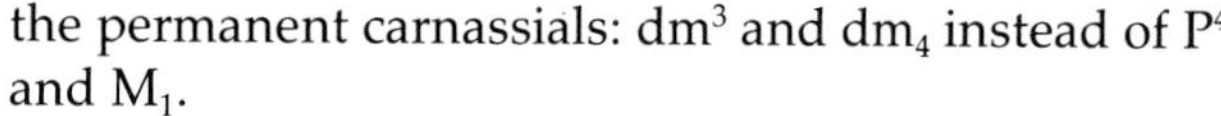

the permanent carnassials: dm^3 and dm_4 instead of P^4 and M_1.

Some members of the order Carnivora, such as bears (Fig. 16.16), have lost the carnassial blades and have enlarged the distal cheek teeth to form flattened crushing structures. This is an adaptation to a more omnivorous diet.

The seals and sea lions also belong to the Carnivora, but their diet of fish requires a dentition for holding the slippery food, which is swallowed whole. This is achieved by the anterior teeth; the maxillary incisors have a labial and lingual cusp each separated by a valley into which a mandibular incisor fits (see Fig. 16.17). The cheek teeth have become simplified pegs, sometimes with accessory mesial and distal cusps. The deciduous teeth are very reduced, and in some species they erupt and are shed even before birth. Even greater simplification of the teeth has taken place in porpoises, dolphins, and other members of the order Cetacea. Here all the teeth are alike; they have only one cusp and one root, a secondary regression to a reptile-like haplodont, homodont condition. Some whales obtain their food by straining water through plates of "whale-bone," keratinous structures developed from the palate, and in these the teeth do not develop beyond an embryonic condition.

Simplification of the dentition has also taken place in some mammals that feed on ants and termites. Thus the anteater obtains its food by means of a very long tongue, made sticky with saliva and extruded through a very small mouth (Fig. 16.18). The food, consisting of numerous small insects, does not

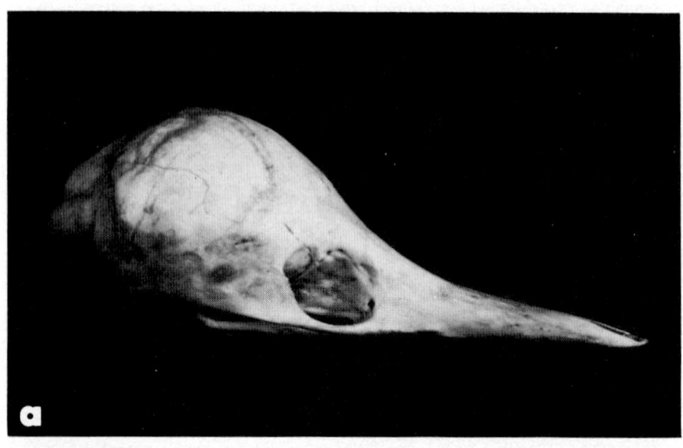

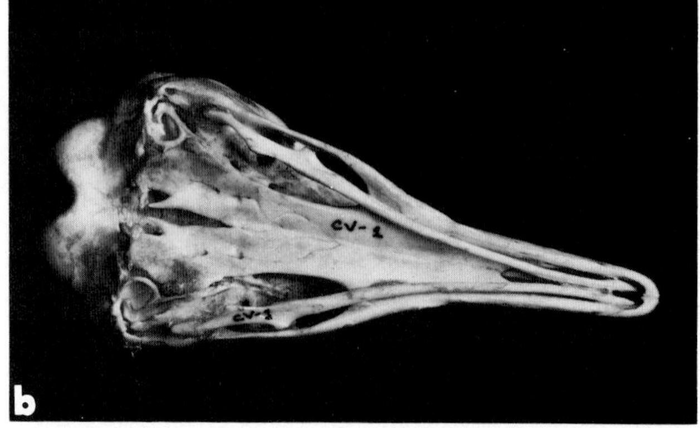

Figure 16.18
Skull of echidna or spiny anteater (*Tachyglossus aculeatus*), whose sticky tongue captures its insect diet: *a,* lateral view: the mandible is largely hidden from view; *b,* undersurface: there are no teeth, but horny serrations on the back of the tongue grind insects against palatal ridges. (Photos courtesy of the A. W. Ward/Atkinson Museum, San Francisco.)

need chewing, and teeth are absent. Jaw muscles are very weakly developed and the mandible is reduced to a rodlike structure.

Herbivores

Most species of mammals are herbivorous. Their plant food requires a great deal of mastication to break up the cellulose cell walls and allow the digestive juices access to the nutritive contents. In ruminants such as the cow and sheep the herbage is at first swallowed quickly; it remains in a special portion of the stomach for a time, during which bacteria and other microorganisms assist in softening the cell walls; then it is returned to the mouth and chewed as cud. The rabbit and other mammals have a process called refection that subserves a similar function: the animal passes night feces which are taken from the anus back to the mouth. The anterior teeth of herbivores differ between perissodactyls (odd-toed ungulates, e.g., horses) that have edge-to-edge incisors and artiodactyls (even-toed ungulates, e.g., sheep) that have lost their upper incisors, which have been replaced by a fibrous gum pad. Herbivores tend to retain most of the mammalian cheek tooth number.

The cheek teeth of herbivores function like millstones: they have flattened occlusal surfaces that rub across each other during horizontal excursions of the mandible, grinding the food. Grinding power is increased by roughening of the occlusal surface: folds of enamel project as ridges above the softer dentin on the worn surface of the tooth. In the sheep, cow, and horse the grinding movement is transverse to the jaw, the mandible moving buccolingually while the teeth are in contact; in the elephant and in many rodents, on the other hand, the mandible moves mesiodistally. Just as in a millstone, the ridges are perpendicular to the direction of movement: mesiodistal in the sheep and buccolingual in the elephant and beaver. Not all herbivores have grinding teeth working on this principle, however; in the rabbit, for example, in which grinding is transverse (buccolingual), ridges work in grooves on the opposing teeth. The kangaroo and the tapir provide other examples of ridges working in grooves, but in these there is a shearing action between the distal surfaces of lower ridges and the mesial surfaces of upper ridges; such teeth are more useful for cutting up leaves and other soft vegetation than for grinding grass.

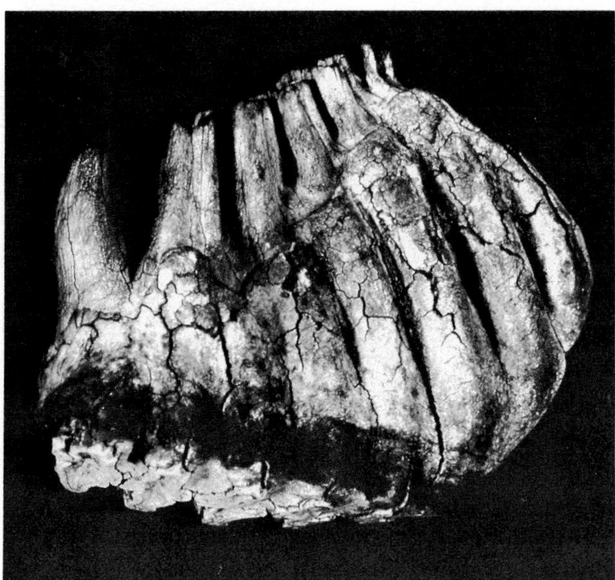

Figure 16.19
The hypsodont upper molar of an African elephant.

Grinding teeth suffer a great deal of abrasion, especially when the diet consists of grass, which contains silica in its cell walls. To compensate for abrasion, the height of the crown of the tooth is increased, at the expense of the roots, which form late in the development of the tooth or not at all. In the latter case the tooth can continue to grow at the apex while being worn away on the crown. High-crowned teeth are described as *hypsodont,* as opposed to *brachyodont.* Examples of hypsodont teeth are those of the horse, elephant (Fig. 16.19), and sheep, which have short roots, and those of the rabbit and guinea pig, which are permanently growing. Hypsodont incisors are characteristic of the rodents, in which enamel is present only on the labial surface, so that the end of the tooth retains a chisel shape as it wears down (Fig. 16.20). As the crown of a hypsodont tooth increases in height, the valleys between the cusps and ridges deepen to form vertical grooves or tubes passing down the length of the tooth. These grooves become filled with cementum, which forms not only over the root but all over the crown. Thus, in the elephant the tooth has a series of transverse ridges which when worn appear as islands of dentin bordered by enamel, the whole series set in a mass of cementum (Figs. 16.21, 16.22). Each incisor of the horse has a deep pit, filled with cementum, and known as the "mark"; as the tooth wears down the mark changes in size and it may be used in determining the age of the horse.

The premolars of herbivores assist the molars in forming the grinding surface, and in many cases they are molarized, having become like the molars in structure. The horse is a good example of this. The canines of herbivores are usually small, so as not to impede the movements of the mandible. In the lower jaw of cow and sheep the canines resemble the incisors in pattern; the corresponding teeth of the upper

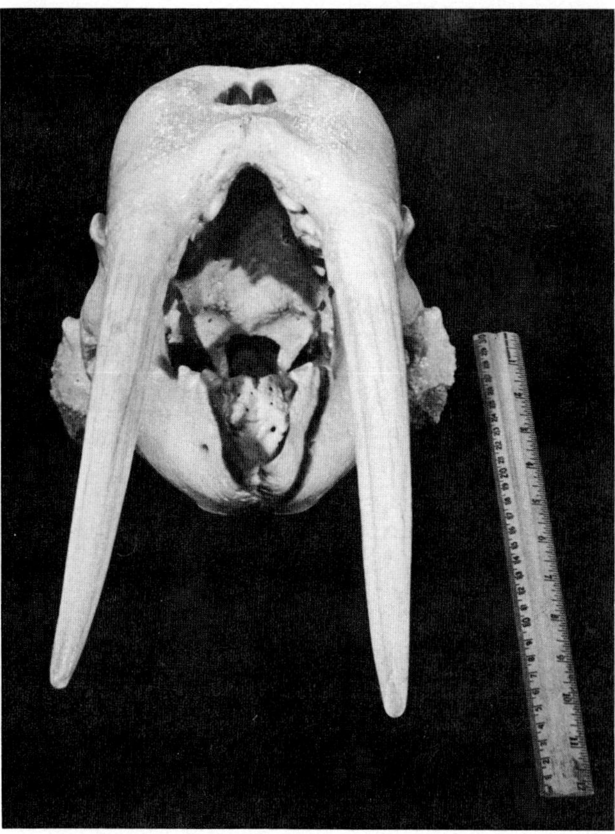

Figure 16.20

The upper canine tusks of a male walrus skull (*Odobenus rosmarus*). (Scale rule is 45 cm long.) (University of Alberta Dental Museum)

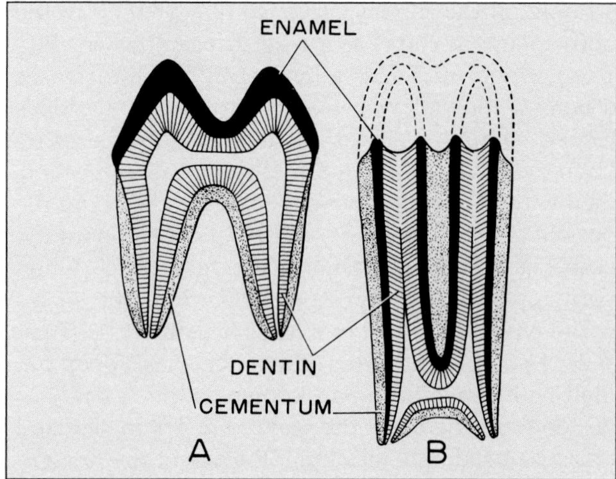

Figure 16.21

Sections through a brachyodont and hypsodont molar. Enamel is *black*, dentin is *line-shaded*, cementum is *stippled*. In the hypsodont tooth crown formation continues for a long time and root formation is retarded. Cementum, confined to the roots in brachyodont teeth, is laid down over the crown in hypsodont teeth. At the worn surface, the enamel, being harder, stands up above the dentin and cementum.

jaw are absent. Canines are lacking in rodents and in the rabbit. There is usually a gap, or diastema, mesial to the grinding teeth of herbivores: it enables the jaws to become elongated so that the animal can reach the ground when grazing; it provides a space in which food can be manipulated by the tongue and cheeks into the right position for passing back between the grinding teeth; in rodents it allows a fold of skin to close off the mouth behind the incisors when these are used in gnawing.

Tusks

Persistent growth of anterior teeth that are not abraded results in tusks that protrude out of the mouth. Tusks may be either incisors (e.g., elephants) or canines (e.g., walruses) and are employed as instruments of aggression and for tree-felling, porterage, and digging. The commercial significance of tusks is their dentin content, known as ivory, which is sought as a medium of art expression and once was used to make billiard balls and piano keys.

Because of their persistent growth, there is no sharp definition between the crowns and roots of tusks, and their enamel cover is sparse. The apex of the tusk root remains open throughout life to maintain a central pulp that continually produces dentin or ivory, resulting in the largest tusks in the oldest animals. Tusks generally follow a spiral growth pattern, and the quality of ivory varies among species and their habitats.

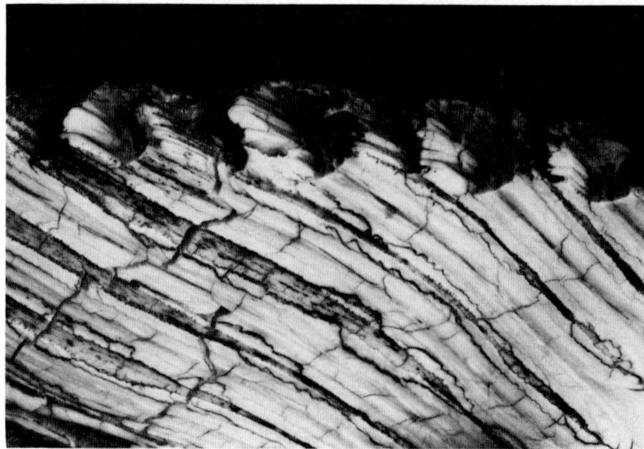

Figure 16.22

Sectioned elephant molar tooth: the elephant's molars are composed of angled plates of dentin cores covered by enamel with cementum between successive plates. The uneven surface wear, due to different hardnesses of the three dental tissues, creates a rough masticatory surface.

Examples of Dental Variation

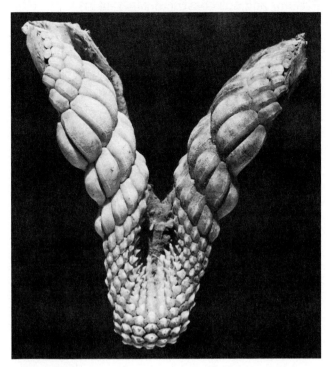

Figure 16.23
Port Jackson shark (Heterodontus) jaw: the teeth differ from those of typical sharks in being lamelliform. The front teeth are small, recurved, serrated, and are used for prehension. The posterior teeth, which are large and rounded, are used for crushing shells. (Photo courtesy of A. W. Ward/Atkinson Museum, San Francisco.)

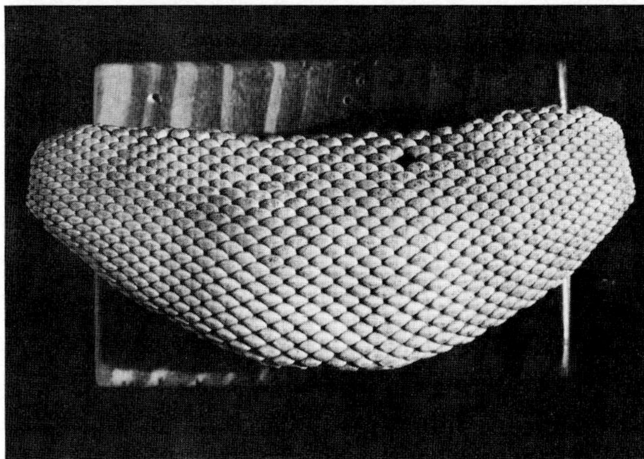

Figure 16.24
Ray jaw: the blunt homodont teeth form a tesselated pavement used for crushing the coverings of molluscs, crustaceans, and clams. (Photo courtesy of A. W. Ward/ Atkinson Museum, San Francisco.)

It is impossible within the scope of this text to present all the variations of dental morphology that exist in the animal world. Only a limited sample of the great diversity of tooth forms are presented here to illustrate the wide range of comparative odontology.

Fishes

Sharks

The several rows of teeth in shark jaws represent *polyphyodontism* with successive generations of homodont teeth rising like escalator stairs into functional rows that are discarded with use. The shapes of the teeth vary with different species and provide a means of identification of the species.

Heterodontus (*Cestracion phillipi*) (Fig. 16.23)

Variations in the size and shapes of the teeth (*heterodontism*) distinguish the Port Jackson shark from other shark species characterized by homodontism. The sharply pointed anterior teeth differ from the large flat posterior teeth that crush the shellfish on which the shark subsists.

Rays and Skates (Fig. 16.24)

The mosaic pavement arrangement of the homodont teeth provides for crushing the shells of molluscs and crustaceans that form the diet of rays and skates.

Sawfish (*Pristis antiquorum*) (Fig. 16.25)

This fish is a ray in which the intraoral teeth are pavement-like as in other rays. The rostral snout projects haplodont, homodont teeth of persistent growth, attached, unusually, in sockets. The rostrum is a weapon of attack, the sharp teeth ripping open the bodies of large prey.

Barracuda Pike

The lower jaw protrudes beyond the upper jaw, and the numerous homodont, haplodont teeth are fused by ankylosis to the jaws.

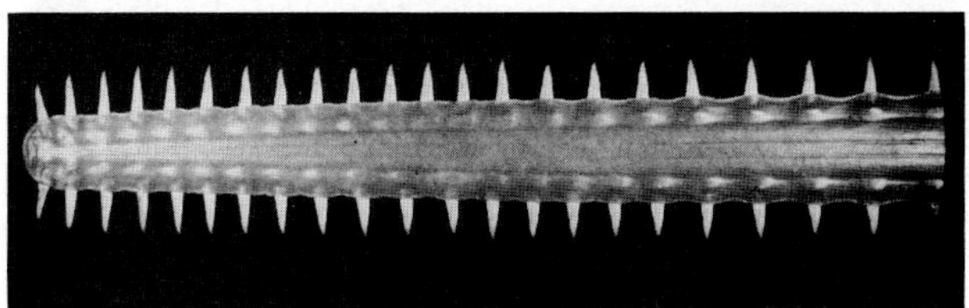

Figure 16.25
The cartilage rostrum of a saw-fish (pristis) containing laterally protruding socketed teeth of persistent growth.

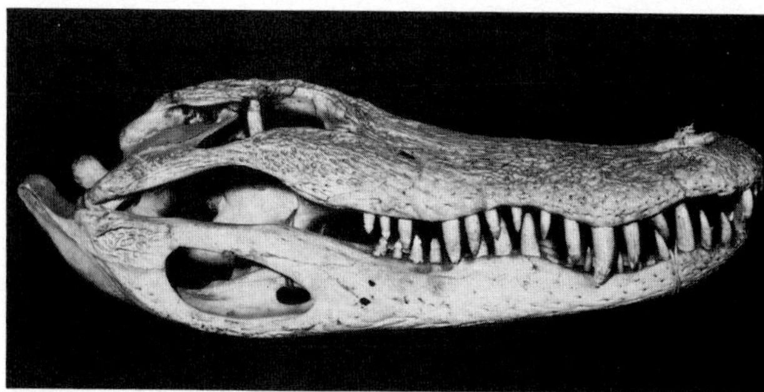

Figure 16.26

Alligator skull: the haplodont teeth vary in size and interdigitate haphazardly for a purely prehensile function. (Photo courtesy of A. W. Ward/Atkinson Museum, San Francisco.)

Reptiles

Alligators and Crocodiles (Fig. 16.26)

The polyphyodont teeth are slightly heterodont in that specialized lower teeth consistently bite into pits in the upper jaw. The teeth are attached by a thecodont gomphosis, in which successional teeth erupt into the same sockets as their predecessors.

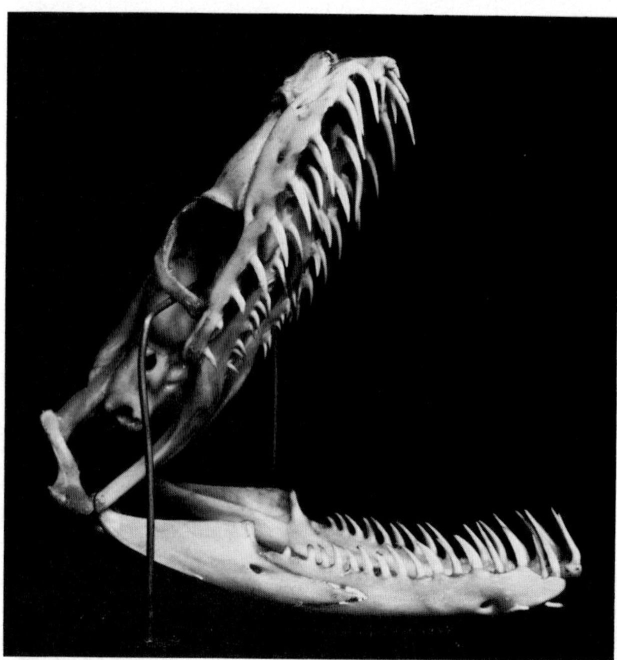

Figure 16.27

Python skull: the haplodont, homodont teeth, which form a double row in the upper jaw and a single row in the lower jaw, are used solely for prehension of prey. (Photo courtesy of A. W. Ward/Atkinson Museum, San Francisco.)

Ophidia (Snakes)

Pythons and Boa Constrictors (Fig. 16.27)

These nonpoisonous snakes kill their prey by crushing. They have two rows of teeth in the upper jaw and a single row of teeth in the lower jaw. The polyphyodont, haplodont, homodont recurved teeth are ankylosed to the jaws and are used simply for prehension. The double jaw articulation, through the intervening quadrate bone, allows exceedingly wide opening, facilitated by separate lower jaws, which retract alternatively when swallowing large prey.

Rattlesnakes (*Crotalus scutulatus*) (Fig. 16.28)

The specialized upper anterior fang teeth are canaliculated for the injection of poison. These fangs provided the basis for the concept of syringe needles. The fangs lie flattened in the closed mouth, becoming erect upon opening. Polyphyodontism prevails, meaning that lost fangs are replaced. The posterior upper and all lower teeth are noncanaliculated and are used solely for prehension.

Mammals

The enormous variety of mammalian dentitions means that only a small number of selected examples can be described here, and represent the more interesting variations on the "typical" mammalian dental for-

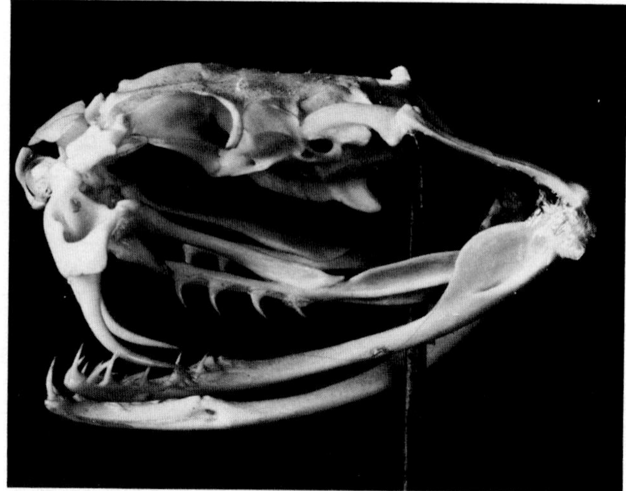

Figure 16.28

Rattlesnake skull: the upper poison fangs are set separately in the movable maxillae, allowing for their erection when striking. The remaining smaller teeth are used for prehension of prey. (Photo courtesy of A. W. Ward/Atkinson Museum, San Francisco.)

mula of heterodont teeth: i.e., incisors 3/3, canines 1/1, premolars 4/4, molars 3/3.

Cetacea

Aquatic mammals possess monophyodont homodont dentitions, which facilitates the capture of their piscivorous diets. The odontoceti are the toothed whales; the mystacoceti are edentulous, although their fetuses possess rudimentary heterodont teeth that are resorbed before birth. The mystacoceti possess whalebone or baleen plates, suspended from the palate as epithelial downgrowths, that act as filters for the krill and plankton upon which they feed.

Narwhal (*Monodon monoceras*) (Fig. 16.29)

This rare animal is remarkable for its single (left) incisor tusk occurring in males only. All other teeth are suppressed. The spiral grooving of the tusk, which rotates as it erupts, led to the early belief that isolated tusks were the "horns" of unicorns.

Spermwhale (*Physeter macrocephalus*) (Fig. 16.30)

Edentulous in the maxilla, with suppressed tooth germs, the mandible contains a constant 54 large, conical, recurved homodont teeth that fit into pits in the maxilla.

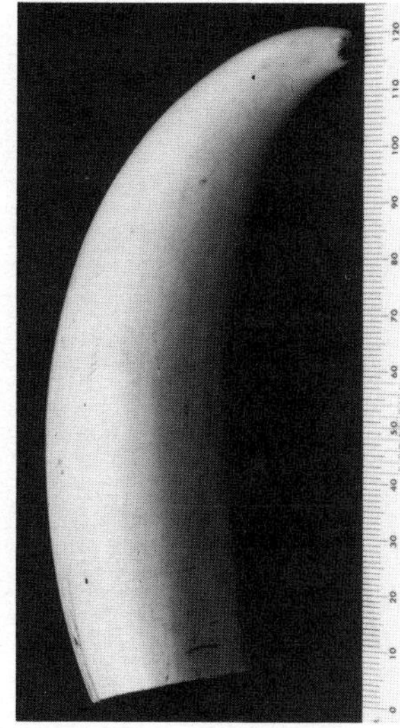

Figure 16.30

Sperm whale (*Physeter macrocephalus*) tooth. A haplodont tooth recurved distally for predatory capture of a piscivorous diet. Only the tip of the tooth is covered with enamel, the root having been cut off. (Scale in mm.)

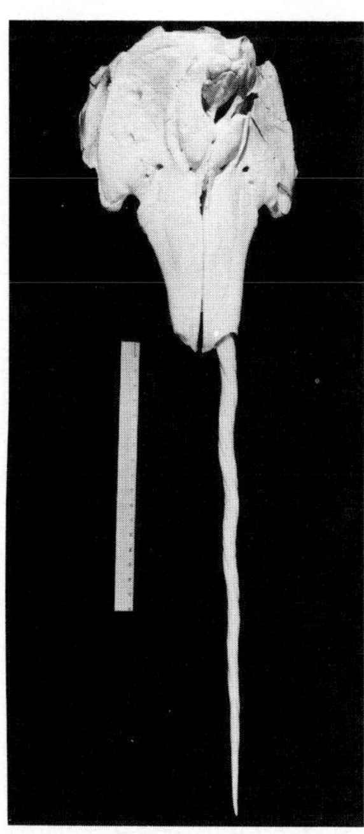

Figure 16.29

The left-side incisor protruding from a skull of a male narwhal (*Monodon monocerus*). The incisor grows into a single spirally twisted straight tusk. The tusk is confined to the male of the species, the incisors being repressed in the females, representing the most extreme example of sexual dimorphism in dentitions. (Scale rule is 45 cm long.) (Photo courtesy of the University of Alberta Dental Museum.)

Ungulates

Most members of the order are herbivorous, which is reflected in their dentitions, although the suidae (boars and pigs) are omnivorous. Ungulates usually have a reduced number of incisors, a gap (diastema) between the anterior and posterior (cheek) teeth, and

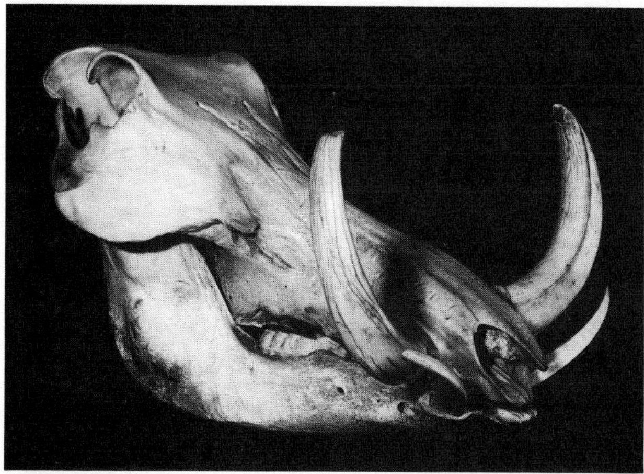

Figure 16.31

Wart-hog skull: the continuously growing and greatly enlarged canine teeth form projecting tusks, used for digging roots. The procumbent anterior lower teeth aid the digging process. (Photo courtesy of A. W. Ward/ Atkinson Museum, San Francisco.)

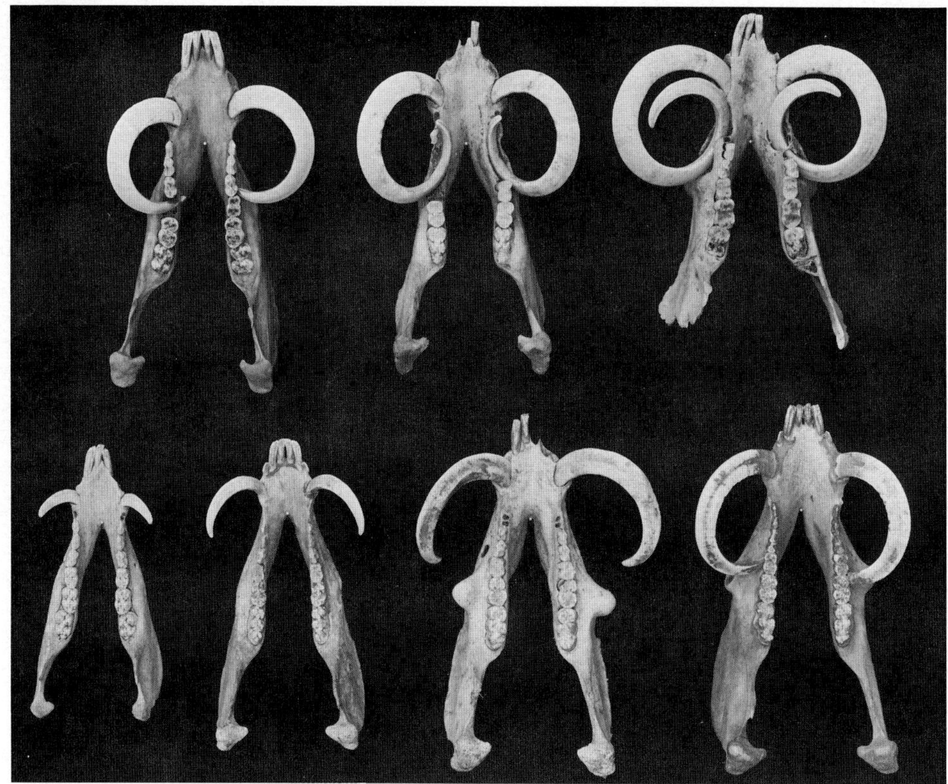

Figure 16.32

A series of wild boar mandibles portraying the continuous growth of the canine tusks consequent to the opposite maxillary canines having been removed during life, thereby eliminating normal attritional wear. The spiral tusks are used for ornamentation by the natives of New Hebrides, South Pacific. (Photo courtesy of Field Museum of Natural History, Chicago.)

cementum covers the crowns of the cheek teeth. The wearing of the cementum to the underlying enamel provides roughened surfaces for herbivorous mastication.

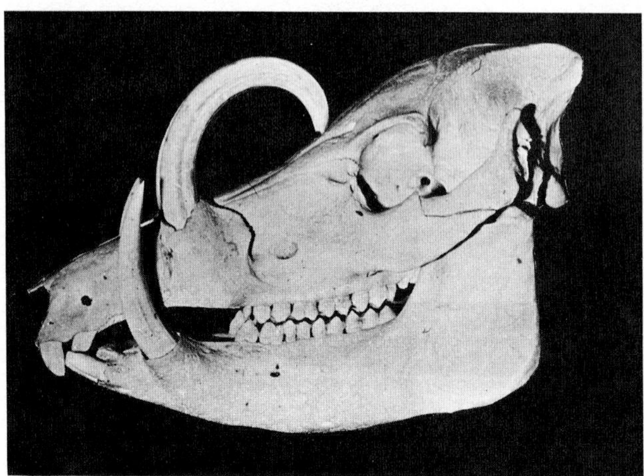

Figure 16.33

The extraoral canine tusks of the wild Malayan pig (*Sus babirussa.*)

Suidae (Pigs and Boars)

The full mammalian dental formula of 44 teeth of this suborder is characteristically bunodont (blunt rounded molar crowns). The canines are sexually dimorphic, being larger in males, and of continuous growth, enlarging into tusks in wild boars (Figs. 16.31 and 16.32). The rare *Sus babirussa* (Fig. 16.33) has upper canine tusks growing upward, of unknown function.

Ruminants

This class of animals chews the cud and possesses molars with crescentic ridges (selenodonts) to aid in cutting grasses. They include cattle, sheep, antelopes,

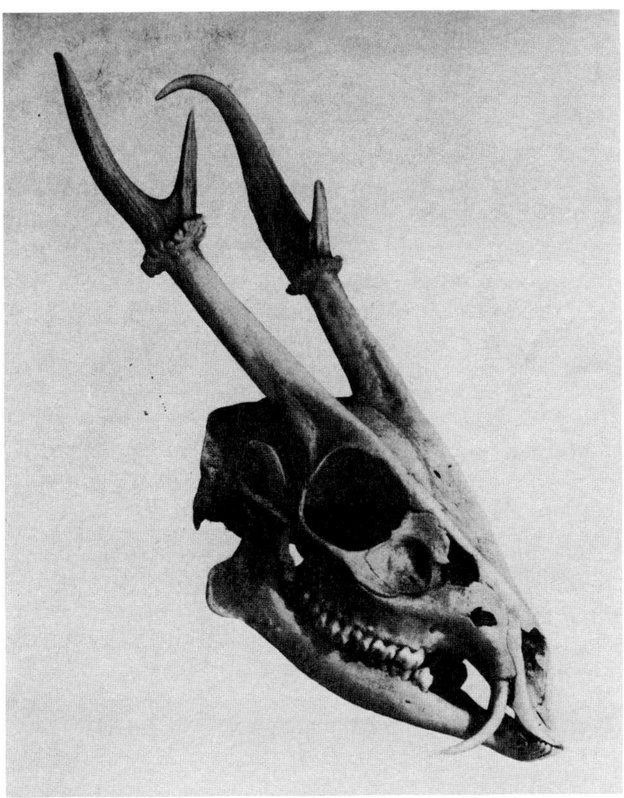

Figure 16.34

Muntjac deer skull: lacking upper incisors, this male deer possesses tusk-like upper canines that can be used in conjunction with its horns for defensive slashing. (Photo courtesy of A. W. Ward/Atkinson Museum, San Francisco.)

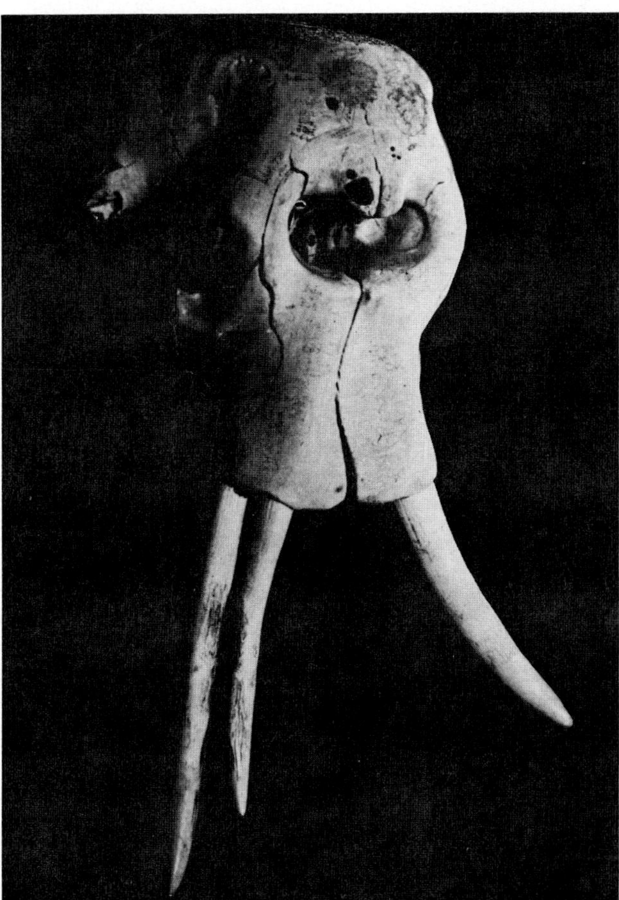

Figure 16.35

A triple-tusked African elephant (*Loxodonta africana*) skull. The tusks are usually the lateral incisors, with suppression of the central incisors. This rare example has one central as well as two lateral incisor tusks. (Photo courtesy of G. H. Sperber)

giraffe and deer, generally possessing horns, mostly in males. Characteristically, the upper incisors are absent, being replaced by a gum pad against which the procumbent lower incisors and canines occlude.

Muntjac Deer (Fig. 16.34)

Most deer possess upper canines, which grow into tusks in males but are of limited growth in females. The male muntjac has hinged canine tusks that move back and forth in wide sockets.

Proboscidea (Figs. 16.35 and 16.36)

The dental formula of the two species of this genus (African and Indian elephants) is incisors 1/0, canines 0/0, premolars 0/0, molars 3/3 in which the upper incisor forms a tusk of continuous growth. The three permanent molars erupt successively in a rotary fashion, resembling a polyphyodont condition, with each molar extruding after approximately 20 years' function (Fig. 16.36). The large molars are composed of vertical plates of dentin, covered by enamel, and the whole tooth is enclosed in a mass of cementum. Masticatory abrasion of these dental tissues, that differ in hardness, creates a very rough occlusal surface for trituration of grasses.

Rodentia

The Rodentia include beavers, squirrels, rabbits, hares, rats, and mice. The dental formula varies among the species, but characteristically the canines are absent, creating a diastema into which the cheek folds, allowing division of the mouth into an anterior gnawing compartment and a posterior masticating compartment. The upper and lower incisors are of continuous growth, which by their attritional wear

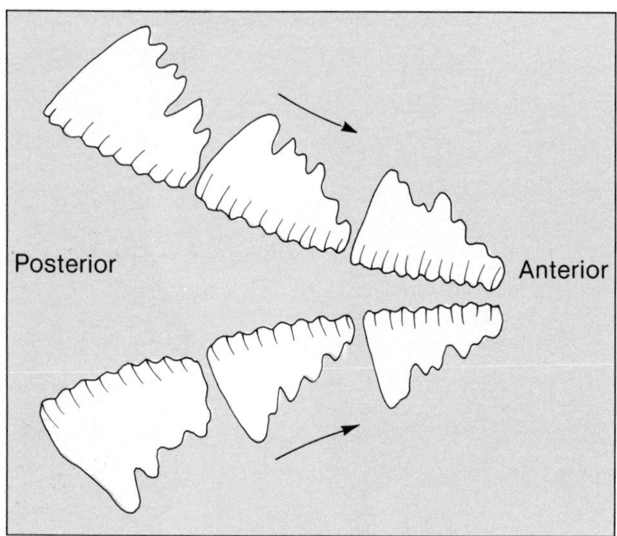

Figure 16.36

Schematic depiction of molar tooth eruption in elephants. The teeth migrate forward in escalator-like fashion. Each molar is exfoliated after an average of 20 years.

against each other (gnawing) sharpen these teeth into chisel-shaped edges. This characteristic is due to enamel, the hardest tissue, being located only on the labial surface. The softer dentin and cementum wear more rapidly, creating the angled chisel edge. Bright yellow and red pigmentation characterizes rat and beaver incisor enamel (Fig. 16.37). Rodent incisors are widely used for experimentation; owing to their continuous growth, all stages of odontogenesis and eruption are found in a single tooth.

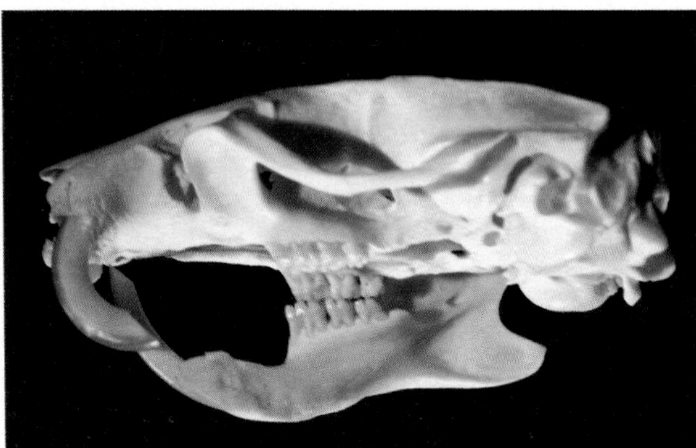

Figure 16.37

Beaver skull: the continuously growing upper and lower incisors form gnawing chisels that are separated by a diastema, owing to canine absence, from the masticatory molars.

Insectivora

The diet of insects and worms of this order determines their specialized teeth that are adapted to crushing chitinous coverings. A full mammalian dental formula is found in many insectivora, with modifications of tooth types such as incisiform canines and caniniform mandibular premolars, which makes precise determination of dental formulae difficult. The occlusal surface of the molar crowns has a W or V pattern composed of numerous sharp cusps.

Flying Lemur (*Galeopithecus*) (Fig. 16.38)

The lower incisors project forward to create a comblike effect that may facilitate a fructivorous diet in piercing fruits. It has been suggested that they use their projecting incisors to comb their fur.

Tree Shrew (*Tupaia chrysoptera*) (Fig. 16.39)

Representative of the order Scandentia, intermediate between Insectivora and Primates, this creature, with a dental formula of incisors 3/2, canines 1/0, premo-

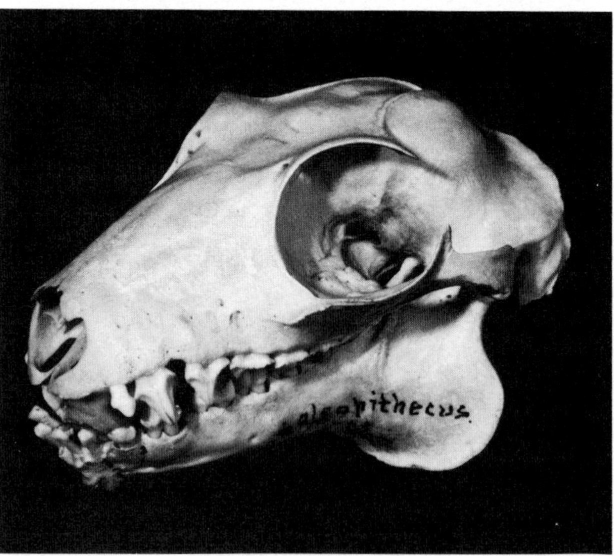

Figure 16.38

Flying lemur (*Galeopithecus*) skull: the pointed maxillary incisors are separated by a wide median diastema into which the procumbent mandibular incisors and canines bite. This peculiar arrangement is adapted to a fructivorous diet. Note the large pointed sharp maxillary canines and caniniform first premolars. (Photo courtesy of A. W. Ward/Atkinson Museum, San Francisco.)

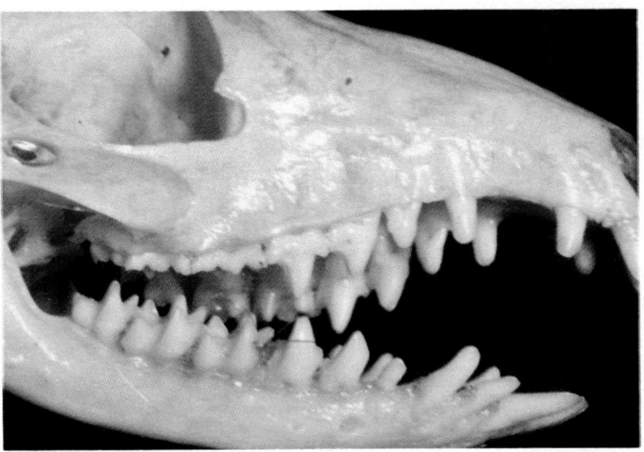

Figure 16.39

Tree shrew skull: the procumbent lower anterior teeth include incisors, canines, and caniniform first premolars, all forming a fruit-piercing and possibly hair-combing apparatus. The upper molars are tritubercular.

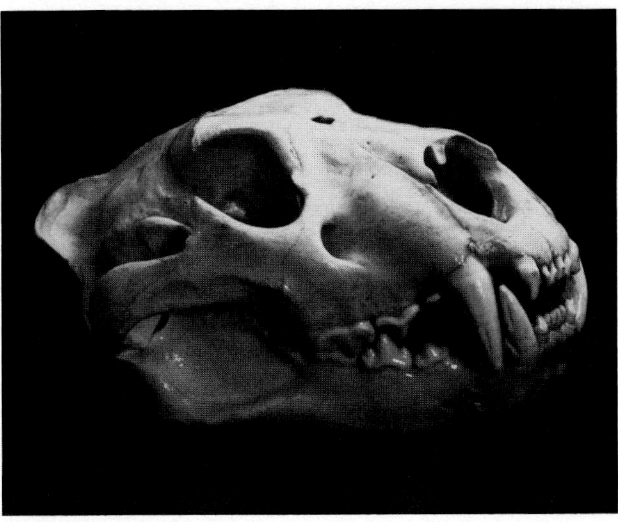

Figure 16.40

Lion (*Panthera leo*) skull: this typical carnivore has diminutive incisors, massive canines for killing prey, and blade-like cheek teeth for slicing meat.

lars 3/1, molars 3/3 has peculiar first incisors. The large, maxillary first incisor is notched, into which the bent tips of the horizontal elongated first mandibular incisor fits. The cheek teeth are typical of an insectivore, i.e., W-shaped with numerous sharp cusps.

Carnivora

The flesh diet of carnivores determines a highly specialized dentition for predation and scissor-like sectioning of meat. The incisor series is complete, although generally diminutive, but the canines are greatly enlarged, requiring a diastema to allow complete closure of the jaws. The premolars and molars are sectorial (blade-like) and generally reduced in number. The cheek teeth are broader in less carnivorous species, e.g., bears.

Lion (*Panthera leo*) (Fig. 16.40)

Dental formula: incisors 3/3, canines 1/1, molars 3/3. The massive canine teeth, used for predation, project into diastemata in the closed jaws. The cheek teeth are elongated into sectorial blades for slicing.

Bear (*Ursus americanus*) (Fig 16.41)

Dental formula: incisors 3/3, canines 1/1, premolars 4/4, molars 2/3. The dentition is adapted to a mixed diet, with reduced canines and broad-topped cheek teeth, resembling those of humans. The predilection of bears for honey makes them the only wild animals susceptible to natural dental caries.

Primates

All primates are heterodont and diphyodont. Their generally omnivorous diets makes their dentitions relatively unspecialized. This complex order of mammals, to which mankind belongs, may be divided as follows.

Prosimii

The suborder Prosimii consists of primitive forms that have survived in the tropical parts of the Old World comprising the following superfamilies:

1. Lemuroidea, the lemurs of Madagascar
2. Lorisoidea, the galago (bush baby) and the potto of Africa, together with the loris of Southeast Asia
3. Tarsioidea, the tarsier of Southeast Asia, which resembles the higher primates in a number of characters such as the placenta, and is probably more closely related to them than to lemurs and lorises

Anthropoidea

The suborder Anthropoidea, the higher primates, consists of three superfamilies:

1. Ceboidea, South American monkeys and marmosets. They frequently have prehensile tails.
2. Cercopithecoidea, Old World monkeys, mainly in Africa and southern Asia, but one species extends to Gibraltar, and another to Japan. The tail is retained but it is not prehensile.

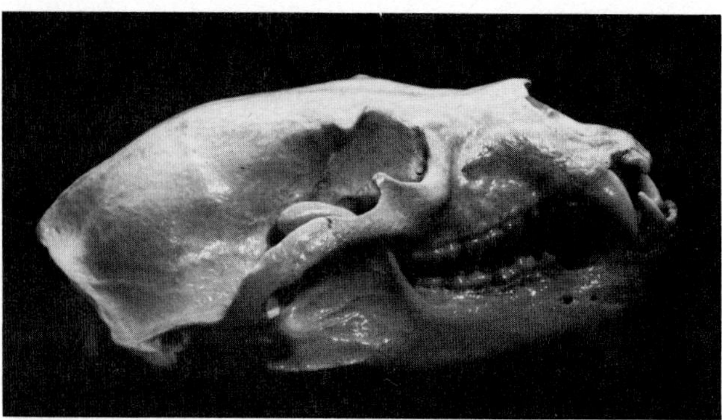

Figure 16.41
Bear (*Ursus americanus*) skull: the omnivorous diet of this carnivore is reflected in modifications of its cheek teeth for crushing, rather than the slicing action characteristic of carnivores.

3. Hominoidea, tailless forms with comparatively large brains. They include (a) the Hylobatidae, or gibbons, of Southeast Asia; (b) the Pongidae, or great apes, orangutan of Southeast Asia, and gorilla and chimpanzee of Africa; and (c) the Hominidae, or mankind, who most probably originated in Africa. The hominoids and cercopithecoids are closely related and are grouped together in the infraorder Catarrhini, as opposed to the ceboids which are Platyrhini.

The primates are essentially a tropical group, mainly associated with forests, but some forms, such as the baboons, have adopted a ground-living life in open country, and this stage must have occurred at some time in the antecedents of man. Typical primates are acrobatic tree climbers, with hands and feet—and sometimes also tails—that can cling to branches of trees. The hand, which was originally a climbing organ, is also used to pick up food and convey it to the mouth, and so the jaws and anterior teeth are no longer needed for this purpose; as a result, the jaws tend to be reduced in length, and the neck is short. Typical primates feed mainly on fruit and other soft vegetable matter, but they also eat insects and bird eggs. Their diet does not require a high degree of specialization of the teeth either for cutting or grinding, and the cheek teeth usually have comparatively low, blunt cusps. Such teeth are described as bunodont. Man is the most carnivorous of the primates, but he depends upon cutting implements and cooking to reduce his food to a form suitable for ingestion. Only in the tropics is fruit available all the year round, and no doubt man's ability to subsist on a meat diet, made possible by his use of flint tools and fire, permitted his spread to the temperate regions of the world and his eventual entry into America from Asia about 15,000 years ago.

Fossil primates are common in Early Tertiary rocks of North America and Europe, an indication that the climate of those continents was warmer than at present. The oldest known primate, *Purgatorius*, dates from the end of the Cretaceous, about 65 million years ago and a wide variety of fossil primates are found in the Paleocene and Eocene, some of which are probably fairly closely related to the lemurs and tarsiers of today. The oldest catarrhines are from the Oligocene of Africa, about 30 million years old. Presumably because of deterioration of the climate, primates disappeared from North America and Europe in the Oligocene.

The insectivorous ancestors of the primates had a "typical" mammalian dental formula of three incisors, a canine, four premolars, and three molars in each quadrant $\left(\frac{3143}{3143}\right)$, but with shortening of the jaws the number of teeth has been reduced by loss of the third incisor and usually the first two premolars. American monkeys (Ceboidea) and most prosimians still have three premolars (Fig. 16.42). The number of molars remained at three except in the marmoset, which has lost the last molar. Absence of the last molar occurs in a number of species, including man, as an individual variation.

The anterior teeth show much variety of size and form, especially in prosimians. For example, in the lemur the lower incisors and canines are narrow, horizontally placed teeth which are used for combing the fur; the mesial lower premolar (P_2) is enlarged and functions as a canine (see Fig. 16.38). The ayeaye (*Daubentonia*), a peculiar lemuroid from Madagascar, has greatly enlarged, chisel-shaped incisors that are used for gnawing into rotten wood in order to obtain the insect larvae on which it feeds. In the Anthropoidea the incisors are flattened teeth used for biting into food held in the hand. The canines are usually pointed teeth, so arranged that the lower canine glides in front of the upper canine in transverse movements of the jaw, thus guiding the jaw and ensuring a correct alignment of the molar cusps when the animal chews. In some primates the canines are enlarged and are used as fighting weapons. In such instances, sexual dimorphism prevails, i.e., males possess larger canines than their female counterparts. The formidable canines of male baboons and macaque monkeys form part of a display pattern in aggressive behavior (Fig. 16.43). The canines of man are exceptionally small and meet edge-to-edge like the incisors. This permits a wider variety of horizontal

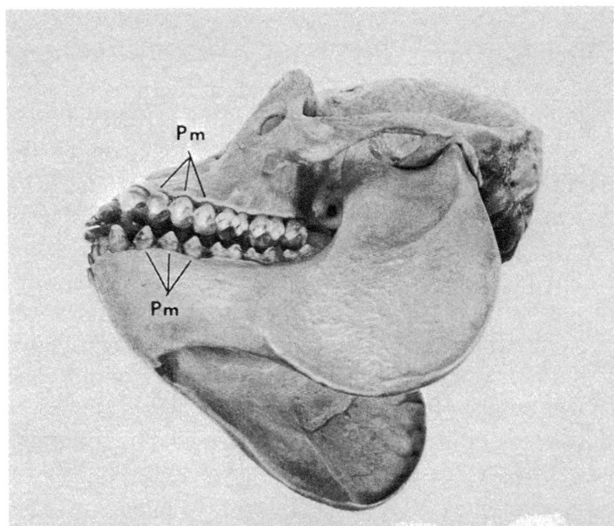

Figure 16.42
Skull and mandible of a howler monkey, a Ceboid. There are three premolars (P_m) in each jaw.

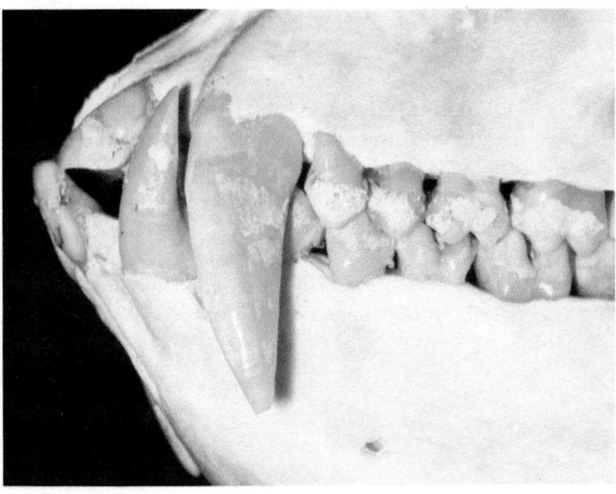

Figure 16.43
Macaque monkey dentition. The projecting dagger-line canine teeth have razor-sharp edges honed by mutual attrition. They form attack weapons. Note the calculus deposits on the tooth crowns.

jaw movements. In apes, but not in man, there is a gap, or diastema, mesial to the upper canine, to allow for lateral movements of the lower canine. The upper canine passes laterally to the lower first premolar (P_3) when the jaw closes, and enlargement of the canine is associated with specialization of this premolar. The premolar becomes drawn out at its mesial end to shear against the canine, perhaps functioning to keep the canine sharp (Fig. 16.44). In man, perhaps because of the small size of the upper canine, the two lower premolars are more alike in size and shape than in the apes.

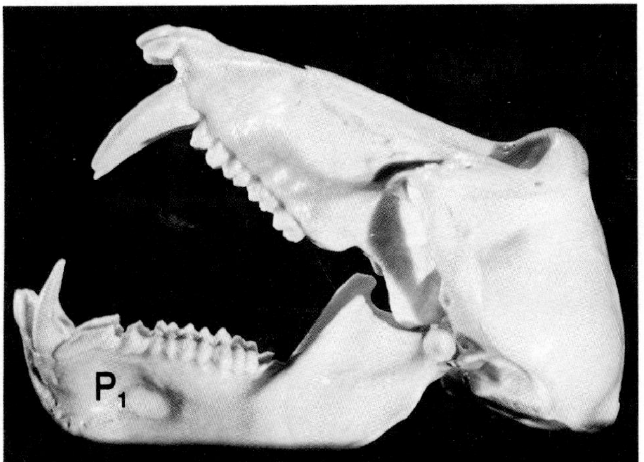

Figure 16.44
Skull and mandible of a baboon. Note the enlarged upper canine and the specialized mesial lower premolar (P_1) which shears against it.

The molars of the early primates were still of the primitive tribosphenic type, but they became transformed into more effective grinding teeth. Specialization of diet results in the leafeaters (folivores) having sharper cusped teeth with thin enamel, whereas fruit eaters (frugivores) have more rounded cusps with thicker enamel (bunodont teeth). In the lower molar the talonid approached more closely the trigonid in height, and the latter was reduced to two cusps by loss of the paraconid. The talonid increased in area so that it occupied more than half of the occlusal surface. On the third molar of most primates the talonid was still further enlarged by an increase in size of the distal cusp (hypoconulid), and in Hominoidea the hypoconulid is enlarged on all three molars. On the upper molars, especially M^1 and M^2, a fourth cusp (hypocone) developed on the distolingual part of the crown. The molar cusps, originally high and sharp, became lower and more rounded. This change seems to be due to an increase in the thickness of enamel, for if the enamel of human molars is removed by acid, the dentin cusps are seen to be sharp like those of primitive primates. When the enamel is thick it tends to close up the valleys between the cusps, reducing them to narrow grooves or fissures. Man lives longer than other primates, and the exceptional thickness of the enamel of his teeth would enable them to remain in use for a longer time.

References

Chivers D, Wood B, Bilsborough A (eds.). Food acquisition and processing in primates. New York: Plenum, 1984.

Clemens WA. *Purgatorius,* an early paromyomid primate. Science 1974; 184:903–905.

deBonis L, Bouvrain G, Geraads D, Koufos G. New hominid skull material from the late Miocene of Macedonia in Northern Greece. Nature 1990; 345:712–714.

Martin L. Significance of enamel thickness in hominoid evolution. Nature 1985; 314:260–263.

Molnar S, Molnar IM. Dental arch shape and tooth wear viability. Am J Phys Anthrop 1190; 82:385–395.

Sperber GH. Comparative primate dental enamel thickness: a radiodontological study. In Tobias PV (ed.), Hominid evolution: past, present and future. New York: Alan R. Liss, 1985, pp. 443–454.

17

The Evolutionary Pathway to Mankind

The Achievement of Upright Posture

In order to assess the biological significance of the dentition in man it is important to review the mechanical and functional changes that took place in the terrestrial, quadrupedal, mammalian skeleton to achieve its human qualities. It is generally agreed that the Primate order originated among those small arboreal four-footed animals classified as insectivores or insect eaters. The descendants of these Early Paleocene animals still live today with relatively little modification. If we examine the skeleton of one of these survivors (Fig. 17.1), some obvious characteristics are observed at once: (1) the head is long and is connected to the vertebral column at its most dorsal end; (2) the brain is located well in the back of the snout and skull. The orbits are likewise placed far behind the snout; (3) the fore- and hindlimbs bear the weight of the body, each approximately to an equal degree; (4) the weight of the body is transmitted to the limbs via the pectoral and pelvic girdles; (5) the vertebral column is like a suspension bridge, supporting the pendant weight of the thoracic and abdominal viscera. The individual vertebrae are so constructed that the entire column resembles a keystone arch; (6) the rib cage and the abdominal musculature support the weight only of the viscera immediately above. It is from this type of skeletal structure and organization that the primate (and peculiarly human) skeleton has developed over a period of about 70 million years. If the tree shrew skeleton is compared with the human skeleton, with the former oriented in an upright position (Fig. 17.2), it is easy to see what changes had to occur if evolution was to lead from the terrestrial quadrupedal to the terrestrial bipedal type of organization. Although we can theorize from Figure 17.2 the changes that must have taken place and postulate the step-by-step modifications that led to each, it is not necessary to rely on theory alone. There is sufficient documentation in the form of primate fossils recovered from the various Tertiary and Quaternary deposits to substantiate in considerable detail these theories and postulations. Indeed, it is possible to determine in many instances the sequence of events in skeletal modification and to assign them approximate dates.

From the vast number of hominoid fossils, collectively referred to as Australopithecinae, that were

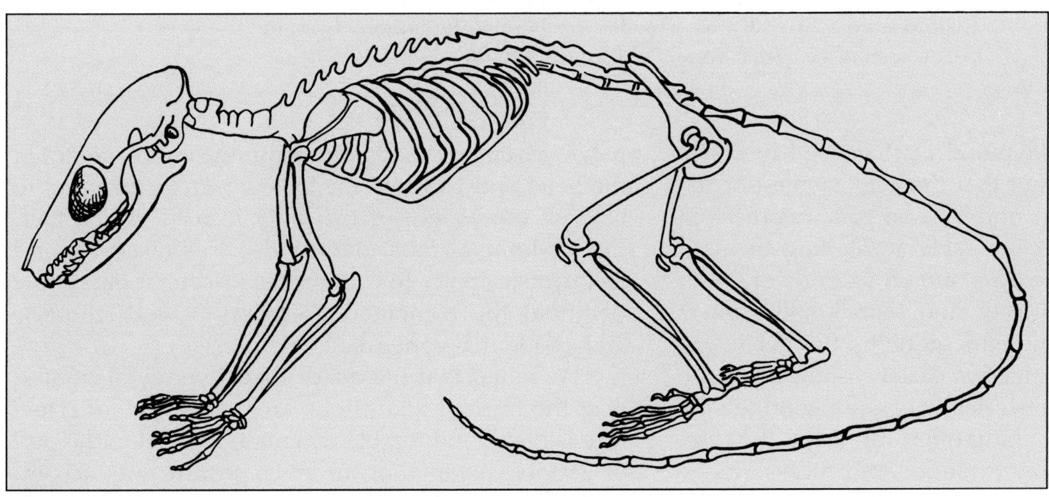

Figure 17.1

Skeleton of a modern insectivore (From Kraus, The Basis of Human Evolution, 1964, by permission of Harper & Row, Publishers, New York.)

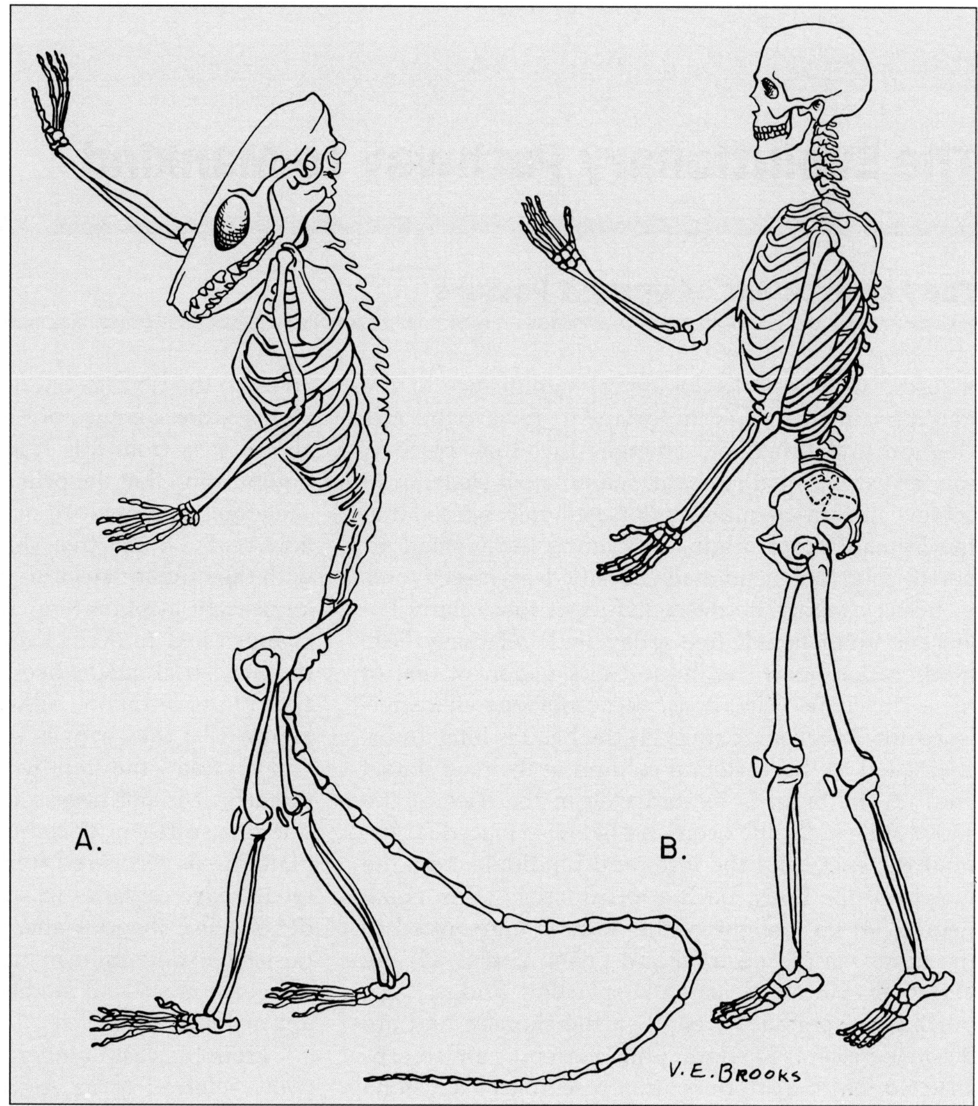

Figure 17.2
Skeletons of an insectivore (*A*) and man (*B*) compared in an upright position. (Not to scale.) (From Kraus, The Basis of Human Evolution, 1964, by permission of Harper & Row, Publishers, New York.)

first discovered by Raymond Dart in 1924 in South Africa, it is now certain that the achievement of habitual upright posture and bipedal gait was the first and major change in the skeleton leading to man. This is reflected in the now numerous finds of pelvic bones of these hominids of more than 3 million years ago. The modifications undergone by the pelvic girdle had to be accompanied or closely followed by significant changes in the vertebral column and the lower extremities. The assumption of erect posture, whether a slow or rapid evolutionary process, necessitated profound changes in structure and function in almost all parts of the body. The heart now had to pump blood uphill to the head, neck, and arms. The pelvic girdle now had to transmit the entire weight of the head and trunk to the legs, which in turn had to bear all the weight of the body instead of just half. The abdominal musculature also was taxed beyond its intrinsic ability to contain the viscera; it must now withhold the combined pressures of both thoracic and abdominal contents.

We noted that the quadrupedal vertebral column is in the form of a keystone arch. This type of structure is highly vulnerable when it is parallel to the pull of gravity. Adaptation to erect posture was accomplished, after a fashion, by modifications in the vertical dimensions of each vertebral corpus, resulting in a series of curves. The S-shaped vertebral column of man is by no means a perfect solution to the problems imposed by the vertical orientation of the body, as those of us with slipped disks, bony exostoses, and chronic backaches can so eloquently testify.

The pelvic girdle was given an added function, that of helping the abdominal musculature to support the weight of the viscera. If we look at the characteristic os coxae of a quadrupedal mammal, or even of a semi-erect chimpanzee, and compare it with that of fully erect man, we can see some important differences in structure, particularly in the blades of the ilia. They no longer lie in the same plane but curve around in a sort of cup-shaped depression toward the ventral part of the abdomen. Moreover, in four-footed animals as well as in all primates but man, the bony birth canal is smooth, rounded, and without bony impediment to the passage of the newborn. In the human pelvis the canal shows several bony processes projecting into the passageway. What is more, the sacrum, which is relatively straight in apes, is strongly curved in man and its caudal tip protrudes into the canal. These may well reflect the "attempt on the part of nature" to provide bony and ligamental support for the pendant viscera.

These, and many other changes in the skeleton of the trunk and lower extremities, may be regarded as direct consequences of the attainment of erect posture, indicating the course of evolutionary selection. There were, in addition, profound alterations in the head itself, and in its relationship to the neck and trunk. It is to these evolutionary modifications that we now turn our attention.

In reviewing the vertically oriented skeleton of the tree shrew (Fig. 17.2), we notice that the position of the occipital condyles at the rear of the skull would place the entire weight of the skull anterior to the joint with the vertebral column, resulting in the head hanging down upon the chest. To counteract this weight it would be necessary to have powerful back muscles inserting into the occiput. The play of these muscles upon the site of insertion on the occipital bone would produce large protuberances, tubercles, spines, or crests. This is actually the case in those primates like the chimpanzee and gorilla that have semi-erect posture and have both foramen magnum and occipital condyles posteriorly placed relative to the skull base. The massive trapezius muscle and the splenius, rectus, and oblique muscles of the head insert into very prominent superior and inferior nuchal crests on the occipital bone and indicate the great power needed to lift the head and hold it in a horizontal plane. It might be postulated that if the head were to become more centered upon the top of the vertebral column by gradual forward movement of the foramen magnum, the need for this heavy musculature would then be lessened and the rugged markings of their insertions would be correspondingly reduced. This is precisely the case, as has been attested by the various hominoid fossil finds. We do not know why this effect (the centering of the head upon the vertebral column in man) had adaptive significance. We can only say that it seems to have been a logical solution, in that the head became balanced upon the top of the body and could now rotate approximately 180 degrees, permitting a much wider field of vision. In primates, it must be remembered, the orbits became directed forward and moved closer together than in other mammals. Although this reduced the total simultaneous field of vision, it did permit a greater overlap of vision and hence allowed better development of stereoscopic vision (depth perception). In man, the restriction of the simultaneous field of vision could be compensated for by rotation of the head. This evolutionary development is reflected in the relatively massive muscles of head rotation, the sternocleidomastoids, and the consequent increase in the size of the mastoid processes into which they insert. The steady increase in size of these processes during the evolutionary process leading to man is likewise documented in the hominoid fossils (Fig. 17.3).

In all four-footed mammals the snout is more or less elongated, bearing long parallel rows of cheek teeth. The eyes are located to the side and behind the teeth, and the brain case is situated in the very back of the head. Since in these animals the head is generally the first part of the body to come into contact with the environment, the fighting and food-acquiring equipment (the teeth, particularly the incisors and canines) are strategically located in front, with the vital eyes and brain removed from the scene of action and possible damage. The adaptive value of such an arrangement was nullified when the head was lifted far from the ground by the acquisition of semi- and then fully erect posture and locomotion. With the head placed *hors de combat*, changes in its structures and internal proportions could proceed without endangering the essential functions of fighting and feeding. In erect bipedal creatures these functions were no longer performed by the teeth but rather by the forelimbs as directed by the eyes and brain.

The major phases of hominization were marked by the evolution of a small-brained *Australopithecus* stage, a medium-brained *Homo habilis* phase, a large-brained *Homo erectus* phase, and a gigantocephalic *Homo sapiens* phase. Concurrent with enlargement of the brain (and cranium) has been a diminution of the dentition and a concomitant reduction of the jaws. The combined influences of the enlarging brain and diminishing dentition upon the shape of the skull ac-

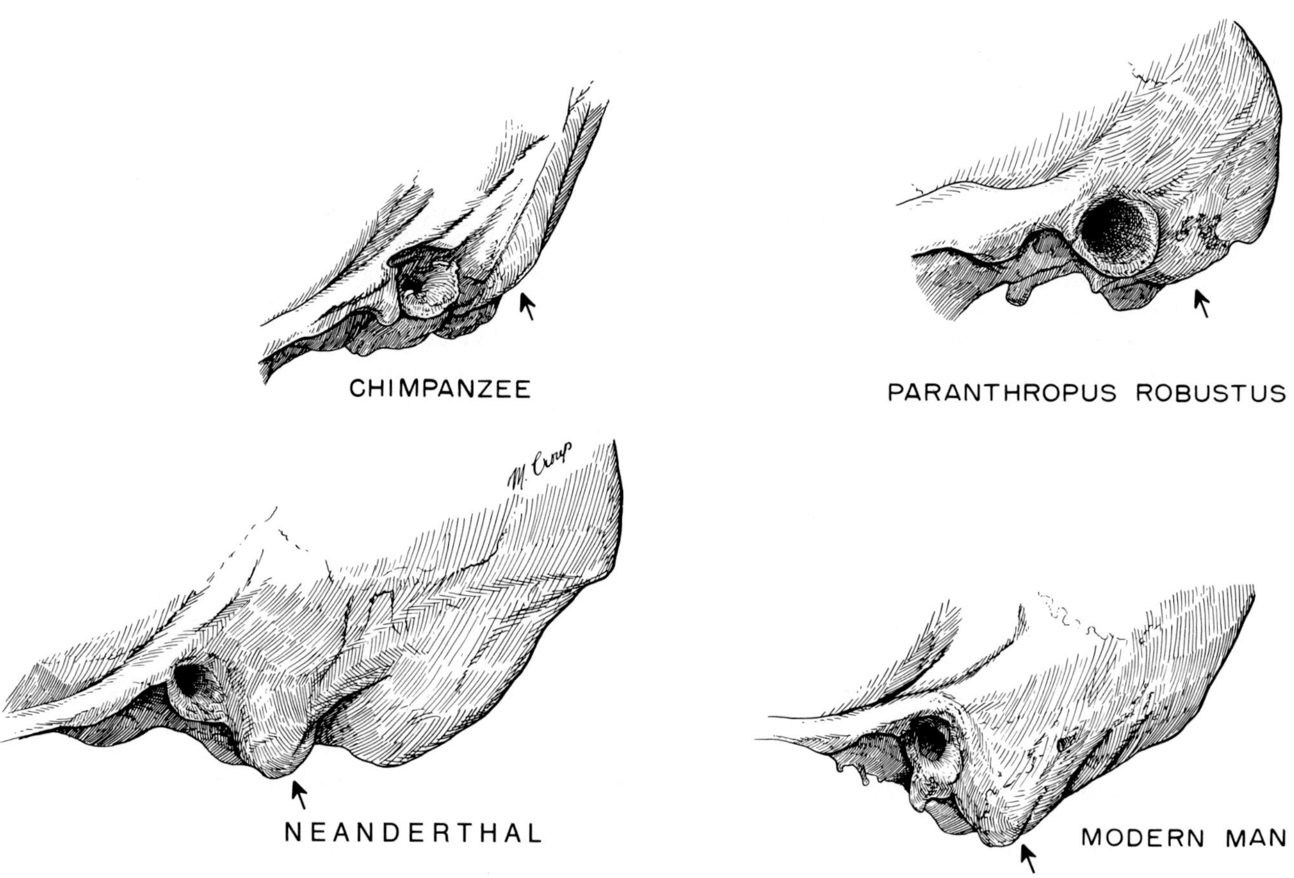

Figure 17.3
Increase of the size of the mastoid process in hominoid evolution.

counts for the increasing neurocranial predominance and the reducing facial features of the different stages of hominization (Figs. 17.4 and 17.5).

The prehensile primate hand, adapted for climbing trees, was used also to pick fruit and nuts and to convey food to the mouth. Chimpanzees use their long arms to swing in trees (brachiate), and when they come to the ground they walk on all fours, supporting themselves on their knuckles. However, they can also, when throwing sticks or carrying objects such as bunches of bananas, walk in an awkward bipedal manner. Early hominids must gradually have spent more time on the ground, perhaps because, owing to drying of the climate, trees were becoming more sparse. Characteristics making for more efficient bipedal walking would be an advantage and would be selected for in evolution. Footprints found at Laetoli, Tanzania, dating between 3.5 and 3.8 million years ago, provide striking proof that by that time fully bipedal walking had developed. They were made by *Australopithecus afarensis,* numerous remains of which have been found also at Hadar, Ethiopia. Though fully bipedal on the ground, *A. afarensis* was probably still partly arboreal, for the arms are longer in comparison with the legs than in modern man, the elbow-joint is stronger, and the longer toes seem to have been better able to grasp. Perhaps trees were used for sleeping and to escape predators.

Freed from the requirements of locomotion, the arms and hands of man became highly specialized for picking up, holding, and manipulating objects, including tools and weapons. The canines were no longer used for defense, and they were reduced in size. The teeth retained only the function of biting and chewing food already obtained and placed in the mouth by the hands. Even this role was reduced in importance when stone tools were used to cut up the food, and fire was used to soften it by cooking. It is an interesting evolutionary fact that the assumption of erect posture freed both forelimbs and teeth from important duties: the forelimbs from weight bearing and locomotion, the teeth from fighting, catching, and killing prey. A most important difference to remember is that *the forelimbs found other functions to fulfill; the teeth did not.* In the case of the forelimbs there was *positive* selection on the part of the evolutionary

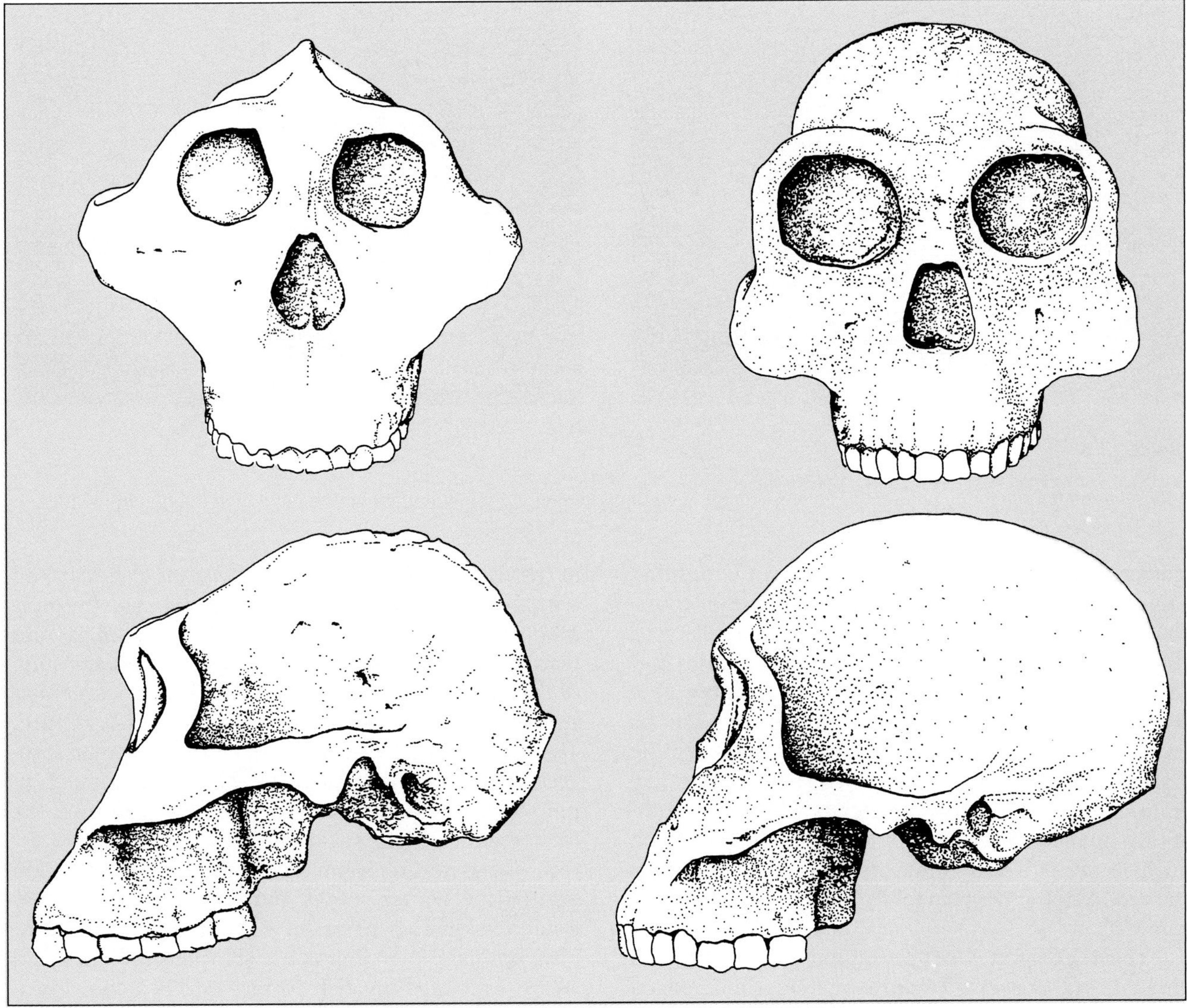

Figure 17.4

Skulls (restored) of two Early Pleistocene hominids from East Africa: *Australopithecus boisei* (*left*) and *Homo habilis* (*right*). (Reprinted by permission of the publishers from Evolution of African Mammals edited by Vincent J. Maglio and H.B.S. Cooke, Cambridge, MA: Harvard University Press. Copyright © 1978 by the President and Fellows of Harvard College.)

process to improve the adaptation of form to function. In the case of the dentition, there being a loss of former functions, changes could and did occur in a more or less haphazard way without affecting the survival of the animal. The differences that we now see in the dentition of man as compared with his next of kin, the anthropoid apes, or with his hominoid antecedents, are *undirected* differences. They are *without adaptive significance* and undoubtedly are the concomitances of other changes elsewhere throughout the body that had true adaptive value and were positively selected throughout hominoid evolution. This is tantamount to saying that the dentition does not have the same taxonomic worth in evaluating the phylogenetic status of a fossil hominoid as is the case with nonhominoid fossils. Much of the debate over the evolutionary significance for man of this or that primate fossil is the result of a failure to understand the nonadaptive role of the teeth in the last 1 or 2 million years of human evolution.

Although the relegation, after erect posture, of the dentition to a more or less purely masticatory function took place perhaps 2 million years ago, even this role was soon lost. The assumption of an habitual upright stance and gait left man's ancestors with no weapons and less speed. Perhaps the need for an im-

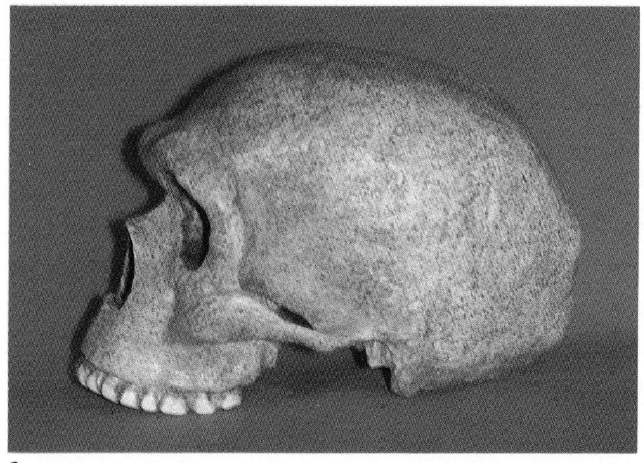

a

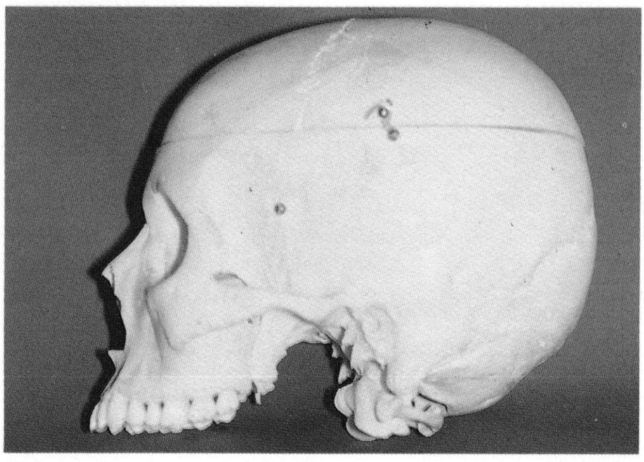

b

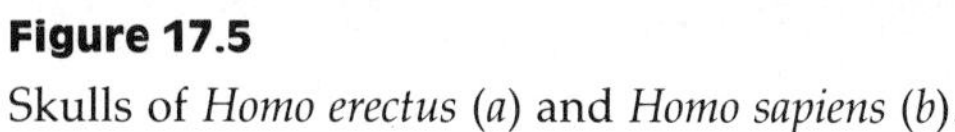

Figure 17.5

Skulls of *Homo erectus* (*a*) and *Homo sapiens* (*b*).

mediate substitute for this reduction in his fighting equipment led to a rapid selection of superior qualities and increased size of the brain, which in turn was able to make maximum use of the freed forelimbs and hands and the greater visual depth perception. One thing we feel is certain: there could have been no great lag of time between the achievement of fully erect posture and the development of a human-like brain capable of memory, speech, and thought; otherwise man's ancestors would have quickly fallen prey to other carnivorous animals or have been starved out by their inability to catch or destroy game.

The four species of australopithecines were all bipedal and possessed approximately similar-sized small brains, averaging about 500 cc, little more than one-third the size of modern human brains, which average 1300 cc. Their cranial characteristics account mainly for their division into separate species, *A. afarensis* being the most gracile, *A. africanus* having larger dimensions, the intermediate *A. robustus* being of more sturdy structure, and the hyperrobust *A. boisei* possessing a megadontic set of cheek teeth that greatly influenced the morphology of the surrounding skull. The varying size of the dentition, from the smallest *A. afarensis/africanus* teeth through the large-toothed *A. robustus* to the enormous-toothed *A. boisei,* distinctively differentiates one species from another. *Australopithecus afarensis* was about the same size as a chimpanzee and had a similar-sized brain (Fig. 17.6). Only with the appearance of *Homo habilis* in East Africa about 2 million years ago did the brain size exceed that of apes. *Homo habilis* is associated with the first stone tools, made by breaking small rocks and pebbles to give sharp edges, and known by archeologists as the Oldowan culture. There is also evidence of the construction of crude shelters out of stones and branches. *Homo habilis* completely changed the normal processes of evolution for both animals and plants—the creation of culture. From the beginning of the Pleistocene there is a wonderfully documented story of the step-by-step unfolding of human culture. The pace at first was incredibly slow as man progressed from a crude fracturing of stone to finer chipping by pressure flaking. Weapons changed from the ineffective clubs to spears and then to bow and arrow. Caves and rock shelters were used as protection against the winter snows and winds. Clothing consisted of skin and fur garments. Implements for skinning animals, piercing skins, sharpening bones and sticks, and catching fish were made of bone, horn, and shell. Life was a constant search for food and left no time for establishing any sort of permanent abode since the animals had to be followed in their wanderings and new sources of fish and vegetable foods had to be found. Animals were undoubtedly butchered with sharp stone knives rather than with teeth, and pieces were held over an open fire and roasted. Fruits and nuts with hard shells were opened by cracking or crushing with large hand-stones. What was formerly the function of the dentition was now transferred to a suitable cultural inventory. The role of teeth was thus further reduced. For the first time in evolutionary history the species could survive even with its teeth removed, broken, or unerupted. Certain edentulous Neanderthal skulls show evidence of healing (see Fig. 17.7).

Not many people could live in one group since the food resources of the immediate territory could not support more than a handful of families. Nor was there room in such society for the physically handicapped or aged. These could not keep up with the

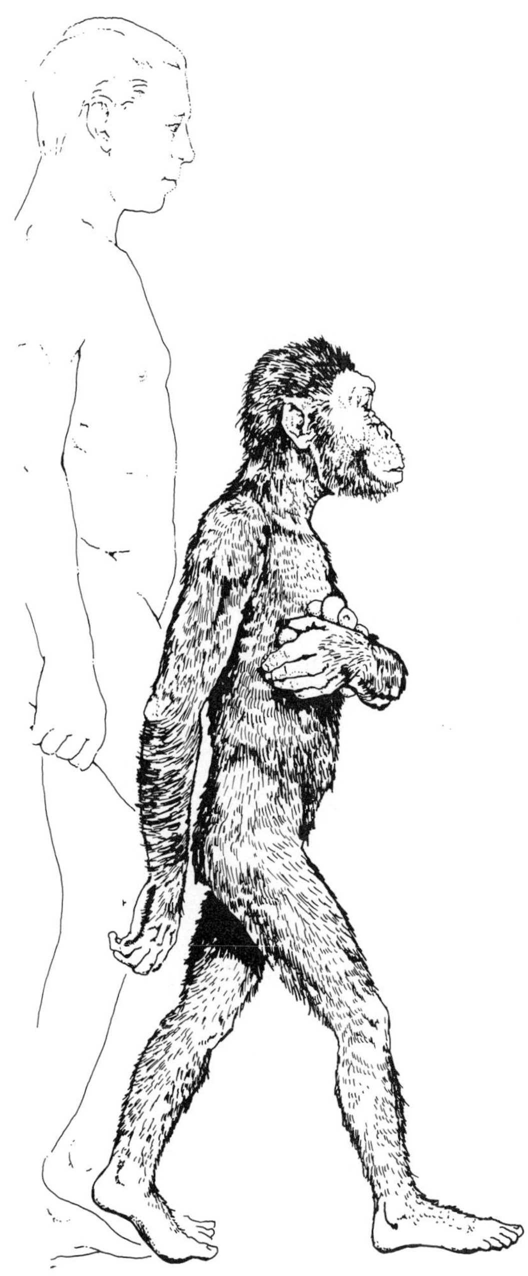

Figure 17.6

A reconstruction of *Australopithecus afarensis,* compared with modern man. (From Lambert D. The Cambridge Guide to Prehistoric Man. New York: Cambridge University Press, 1987; with permission.)

band or contribute to the general larder, so they were abandoned. Until very recently this practice was not uncommon among many primitive hunting and gathering groups.

Until about 10,000 years ago this way of life, with various modifications depending upon climate, locality, and available types of food, was universal throughout the continents of Europe, Asia, and Africa. North and South America, as we have noted, were relatively late in human occupation. Then, along the valleys of the Indus, Tigris, Nile, and Euphrates rivers certain wild grasses began to be cultivated by man, and the science of agriculture began. This great discovery had, and still has, far reaching consequences for mankind. It permitted the accumulation of surplus food, the concentration of many people in a small area, the rise of villages and cities, the development of specialized occupations and skills, the beginning of trade, the use of trade goods and then money, the leisure time to explore the secrets of nature and to practice the arts, and above all—from our present point of view—the invention of pottery. The latter was probably concomitant with the origins of agriculture and permitted the storage of the harvested grains as well as a new method of preparing food—by boiling. This type of cooking still further softened meat and grains to the consistency of pulp and gradually took away the last remaining vestigial functions of man's dentition—that of mastication. It would no longer matter if a molar bore three instead of five cusps, if a canine was peg shaped, or an incisor congenitally missing. The fact is that in terms of biological adaptiveness, species survival, and evolutionary significance, the human dentition ceased to perform any survival function after the invention of pottery permitted the boiling of food. Perhaps this trend was first established with the discovery and use of fire by man.

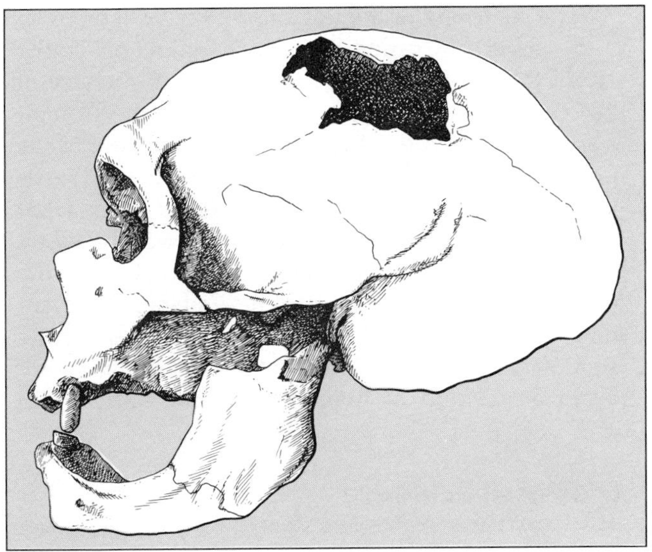

Figure 17.7

La Chapelle aux Saints. Neanderthal skull. The nearly endentulous jaws have healed after tooth extraction.

The centering of the head upon the vertebral column was accompanied by a great reduction in the size of the jaws and teeth, an increase in the size of the brain with a pronounced bulging of the frontal, parietal, and occipital portions, and a decrease in the nostrils and olfactory senses. The brain and eyes were now directly over the teeth, resulting in what anthropologists and orthodontists call *orthognathism*. The canines became smaller in size so that all the teeth were now in the same occlusal plane. The mandible, now quite gracile as compared with the huge jaws of early hominoids, developed a chin—a very recent acquisition of hominids (about 75,000 years ago). The lips became more or less everted, exposing the mucous portion that formerly formed part of the anterior wall of the oral cavity. The nasal bones, once arranged in the same flat plane as in the other primates, came to meet at an oblique angle to form the bridge of the nose—a peculiarly human trait. The heavy muscle markings on the external surface of the skull that characterized man's hominoid ancestors and are to be observed on male anthropoid apes became greatly reduced. The heavy brow ridges, sagittal crests, temporal lines, and occipital protuberances have almost disappeared, although a sex difference can still be noted.

The Fossil Evidence

The story of human evolution presented above may give the impression that it is one of steady progress from primitive primates to modern humans. The fossil evidence shows that this is far from being the case. The evolutionary tree has many branches, some of which survived to the present as the numerous species of monkeys and apes, and others have become extinct (Fig. 17.8). The 4 million years that separate

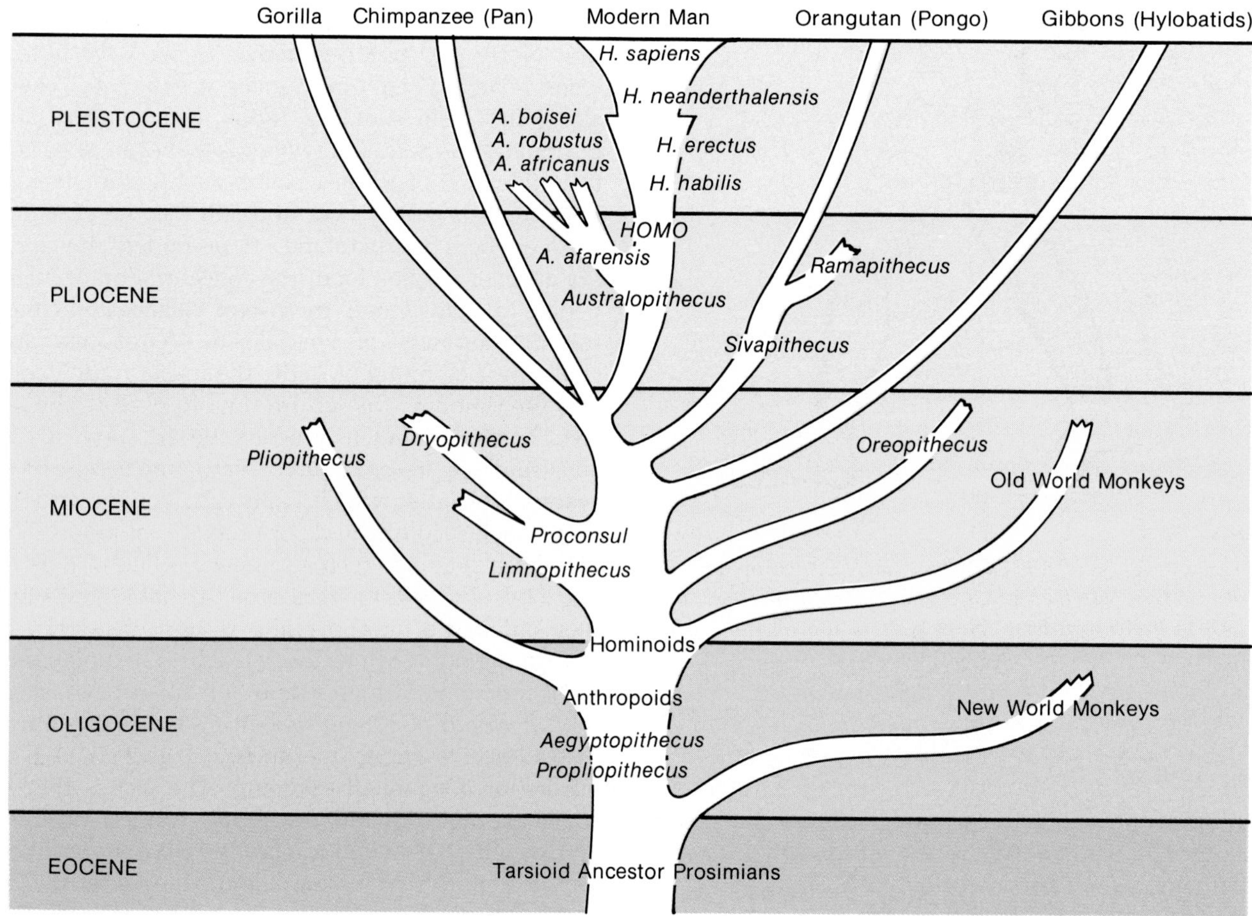

Figure 17.8
Postulated phylogenetic tree of the Anthropoidea.

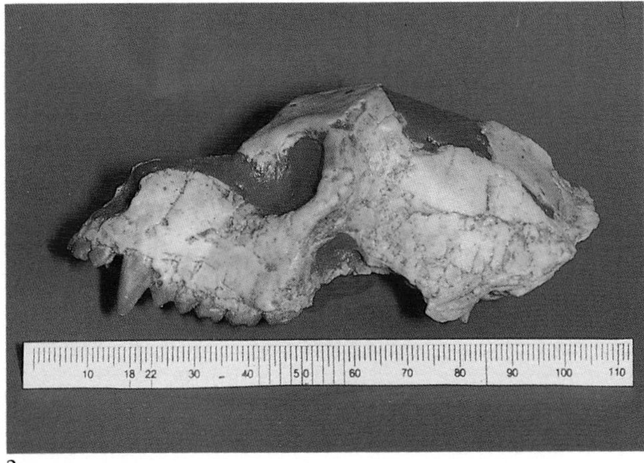

a

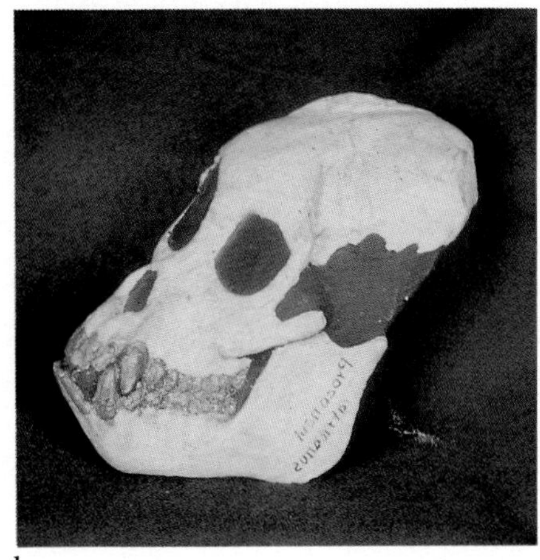
b

Figure 17.9
Aegyptopithecus (*a*) and *Dryopithecus* (*b*). Note the prominent canines.

us from *Australopithecus afarensis* may seem a long time, but it is short in comparison with the 65 million years of known primate history, going back to *Purgatorius.*

The earliest catarrhine fossils come from the Oligocene deposits in the Fayum lake beds of Egypt, about 30 million years old. Of these, *Aegyptopithecus* was an arboreal animal, the size of a gibbon, with teeth adapted for fruit-eating (Figs. 17.9 and 17.10). It is believed to be near the common ancestry of the cercopithecoid monkeys and the hominoid apes. These two groups had separated by the Miocene, but the monkeys were rare until toward the end of that period, when they spread out of Africa into Asia and Europe. They developed a distinctive type of molar tooth, known as bilophodont, in which buccal and lingual cusps were joined in pairs by transverse ridges. These teeth appear to have been adapted for slicing leaves.

Hominoids were common in the Early Miocene of East Africa, around 20 to 18 million years ago. A number of genera have been distinguished, ranging in size from *Proconsul,* one species of which, *P. major,* was as large as a gorilla, down to *Limnopithecus* and *Micropithecus,* of the size of gibbons. Formerly, they were believed to be related to these modern apes, but current opinion is that they are offshoots from a more primitive stage of hominoid evolution. They had large canines and molars with crenulated enamel and bluntly pointed cusps that resemble those of *Aegyptopithecus.* Their skeletons show that they were acrobatic tree-living animals.

About 14 million years ago a number of hominoids migrated from Africa, which previously had been cut off by sea, into Europe and Asia. In Europe appeared *Pliopithecus,* a primitive form that still had a tail, *Dryopithecus,* perhaps a relative of Proconsul, and *Oreopithecus,* a long-armed form with small canines that was thought by some to be related to man (Fig. 17.10). In Asia there were the *Sivapithecinae,* with thick enamel on the teeth. One member of the group, called *Ramapithecus,* was thought to be close to the ancestry of man, but the discovery of skulls showed that the sivapithecines are more nearly related to the orang, which also has thick enamel. They ranged from Hungary to China, and there are several species. Presumably the ancestors of the gibbons reached Southeast Asia from Africa at the same time, but there are no fossils to prove this.

The hominoids (anthropoid apes, gorilla, chimpanzee) and hominids (australopithecines and humans) are believed to have had a common ancestry in Africa. The difference in the structure of their proteins is so small that they must be genetically very similar; protein structure is determined by the structure of DNA. Taking into account the average rate of evolutionary change of DNA (the "molecular clock"), it is calculated that the pongids and hominids had a common ancestor between 9 and 5 million years ago—i.e., in the Late Miocene. Whether man is more closely related to the gorilla or to the chimpanzee, or whether he separated from the common ancestry of the two apes before they separated from one another, is disputed. As hominids were already walking upright nearly 4 million years ago, we have between 2 and 6 million years in which bipedal adaptations evolved, if the above calculations are correct.

The australopithecines were widely distributed in East and South Africa, and at least four species have been distinguished, from the chimpanzee-sized *A. afarensis* to *A.* (or *Paranthropus*) *boisei,* who was as tall as a modern man and survived until 1 million years

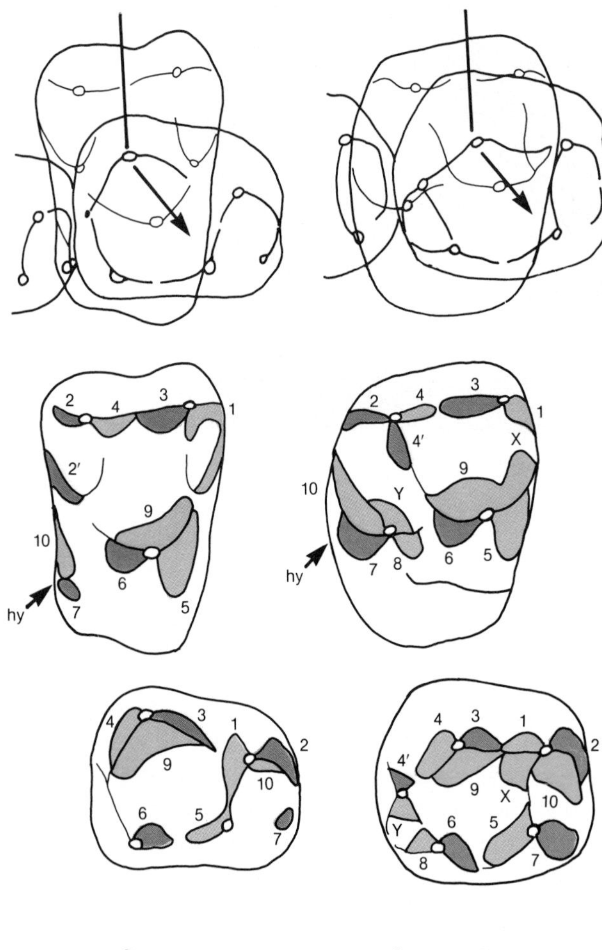

Figure 17.10

Molar occlusion in an Eocene tarsioid (*Omomys*) and an Oligocene catarrhine (*Aegyptopithecus*). The wear facets are shaded, and corresponding upper and lower facets are numbered. The arrows indicate the path of the lower molar across the upper molar when chewing. Note the enlargement of the hypocone. (From Butler. In: Wood B, Martin L, Andrews P, eds. Major Topics in Primate and Human Evolution. New York: Cambridge University Press, 1986; with permission.)

ago. *A. boisei* developed very large molars and premolars, contrasting with the small incisors and canines; the jaws were massive, and the powerful temporalis muscles spread over the small braincase, resulting in the formation of a median sagittal crest, especially in the males. The brain remained small, about one-third the size of a modern brain. The genus *Homo*, starting with *H. habilis*, probably derived, about 2 million years ago, from one of the early gracile forms of *Australopithecus;* opinion is divided on whether this was *A. afarensis* or the somewhat later *A. africanus*. For a million years *Homo habilis* and *Australopithecus* lived side by side in Africa. *H. habilis* was small, standing 4 or 5 feet high and estimated to have weighed about 110 lb. But his cranial capacity averaged 680 cc, compared with an average of 440 cc in *Australopithecus*. He did not have excessively large molars, but his teeth were proportionately like those of modern man, though larger (Figs. 17.12 to 17.14).

By about 1 million years ago the brain had increased to about 1000 cc, and the stage of *Homo erectus* was reached. It was at this stage that man spread from Africa into Asia and Europe. A skull cap of the species was first discovered in 1891 by Eugene Dubois, at Trinil, Java. The original find was known as *Pithecanthropus erectus* and was first regarded as the "missing link." Subsequently several other Middle Pleistocene pithecanthropines were found in Java, in addition to a whole group of fossils collectively called *Sinanthropus pekinesis,* found in an ancient cave near Beijing (Peking) China (see Fig. 17.16). These and other finds from the Middle Pleistocene of Africa and Europe are now regarded as all belonging to one variable species, *Homo erectus*. Compared with modern man, the brain was smaller, the forehead low and retreating, the eyebrow ridges prominent, the teeth larger (Fig. 17.16), and there was no chin.

The earliest finds that are morphologically indistinguishable from modern humans date in Europe and Asia only to 30,000 to 40,000 years ago. They were preceded by more primitive types that are collectively known as archaic *Homo sapiens* (Fig. 17.16). In Europe these date back more than 100,000 years. Among them are the Neanderthals, which evolved in Europe and Southwest Asia. The type site was at Neanderthal near Dusseldorf, Germany, where in 1856 a skull cap was found. Its then strange structure was duplicated in many other skulls found subsequently throughout Europe (see Figs. 17.7 and 17.17). The cultural remains of the Neanderthals, called Mousterian, show a high skill in the manufacture of flint tools, and they were the first people to regularly bury their dead. They were able to survive in the cold of the last glaciation. However, toward the end of that glaciation, modern man appeared in Europe, and the Neanderthal people and culture apparently were absorbed by them or were annihilated in an abrupt ending around 32,000 years ago.

All living humans form a single world-wide species, *Homo sapiens*. Man entered America from Asia across the Bering Strait, which was dry land during the Ice Age, and by 11,000 years ago he had reached the southern tip of South America. In the course of his extensive migrations he has undergone much morphological differentiation, and we now recognize four major varieties or "races" of mankind: Negroids,

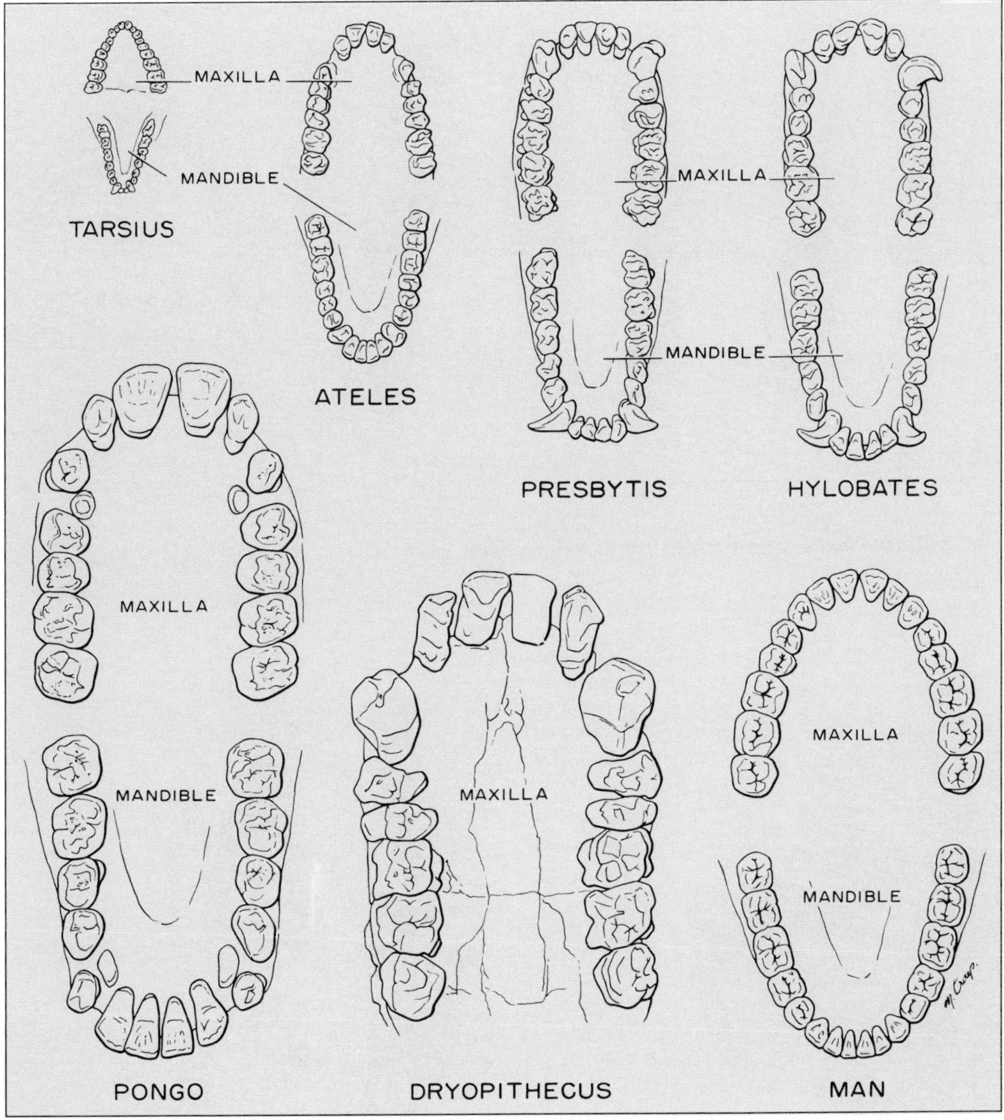

Figure 17.11
Dental arch forms in man, *Dryopithecus,* and other primates.

who originated in Africa; Caucasoids, in Europe and the Middle East; Mongoloids, in eastern Asia, and including the American Indians; and Australoids, the Australian aborigines. Besides differences of skin pigmentation and hair, there are racial differences in the teeth; for example, teeth are largest in Australoids and smallest in Caucasoids and Mongoloids, Carabelli's cusp is most frequent in Caucasoids, and shovel-shaped incisors are most frequent in Mongoloids. These broad divisions are not sharply distinct; they intergrade through populations of intermediate character, and moreover, within each race there is much regional variation. Some anthropologists maintain that the races of modern man descended from different regional populations of *Homo erectus:* Mongoloids from *Sinanthropus,* Australoids from *Pithecanthropus,* and so on. Others, however, believe that *Homo sapiens* represents a new dispersal from Africa, and replaced *H. erectus* in Asia and Europe.

We have seen in rough outline the evolutionary pathway leading from the earliest vertebrates to man, and we have looked at some of the fossil evidence strewn along the way. This gives us some appreciation of the antiquity of the human dentition and an understanding of its evolutionary and biological significance. But just what is evolution? How does one animal species evolve from another? What are the biological principles that guide the evolutionary process? And finally, what is the role of genes in evolution?

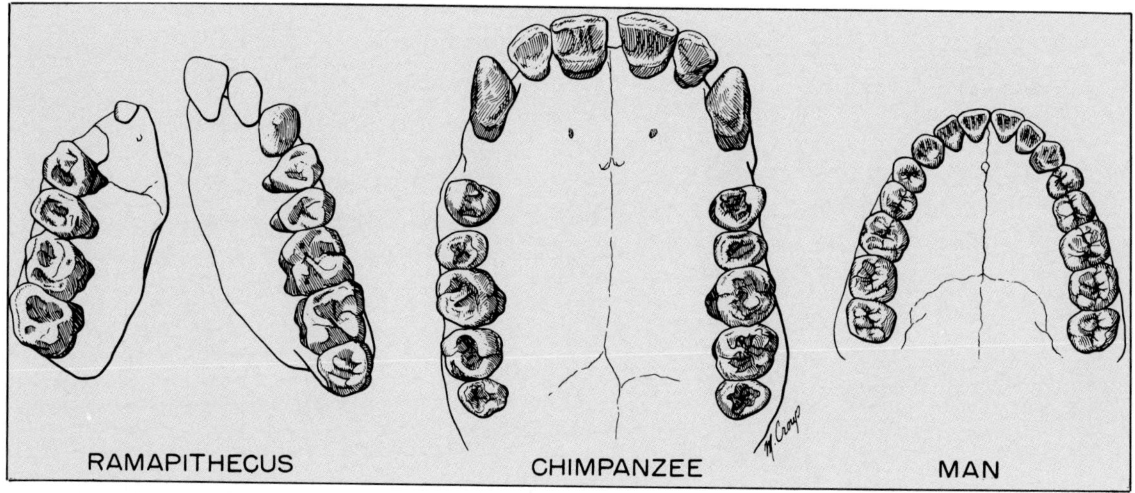

Figure 17.12
The dentitions of *Ramapithecus,* chimpanzee, and modern man.

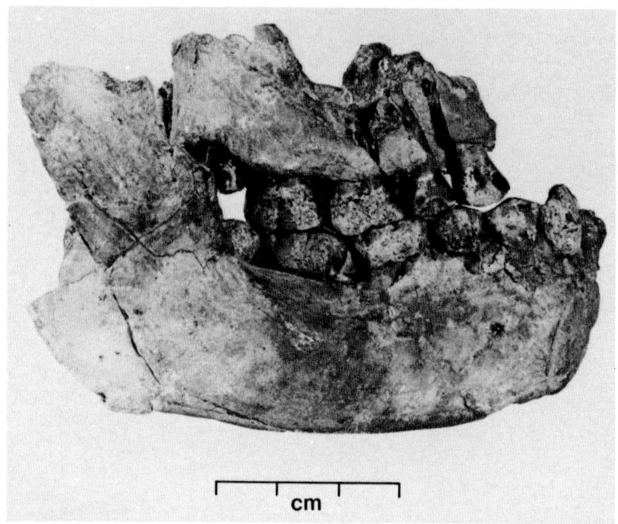

Figure 17.13
Maxilla and mandible of *Homo habilis* (OH13) from Olduvai Gorge, Tanzania. (Courtesy of P. V. Tobias. Olduvai Gorge, Vol. 4: The Skulls, Endocasts and Teeth of *Homo Habilis*. New York: Cambridge University Press; reprinted with permission of Cambridge University Press.)

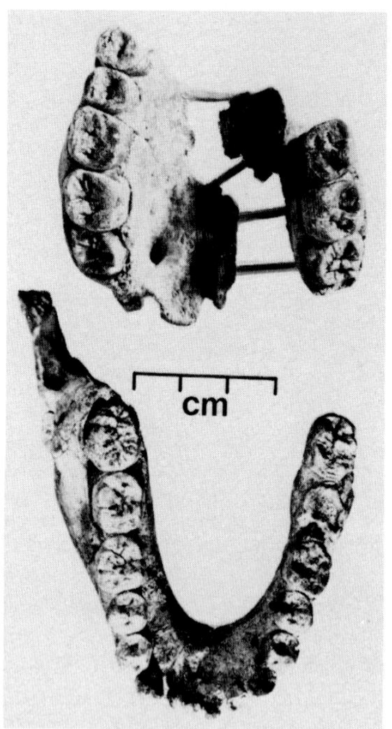

Figure 17.14
Homo habilis (OH13). Occlusal views of maxilla and mandible. Note that the third molars are just erupting, while the first and second molars have suffered considerable abrasional wear, indicative of a hard diet. (Courtesy of P. V. Tobias. Olduvai Gorge, Vol. 4: The Skulls, Endocasts and Teeth of *Homo Habilis*. New York: Cambridge University Press; reprinted with permission of Cambridge University Press.)

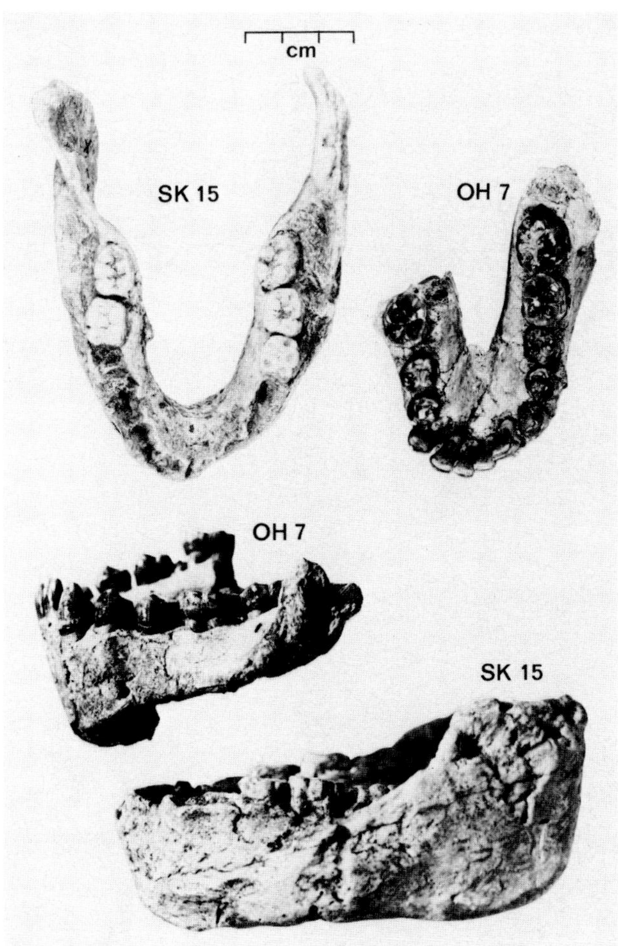

Figure 17.15

Occlusal and lateral views of fossil hominid mandibles: SK 15, *Homo erectus* from Swartkrans, South Africa; OH 7, *Homo habilis* from Olduvai Gorge, Tanzania. (Courtesy of P. V. Tobias. Olduvai Gorge, Vol. 4: The Skulls, Endocasts and Teeth of *Homo Habilis*. New York: Cambridge University Press; reprinted with permission of Cambridge University Press.)

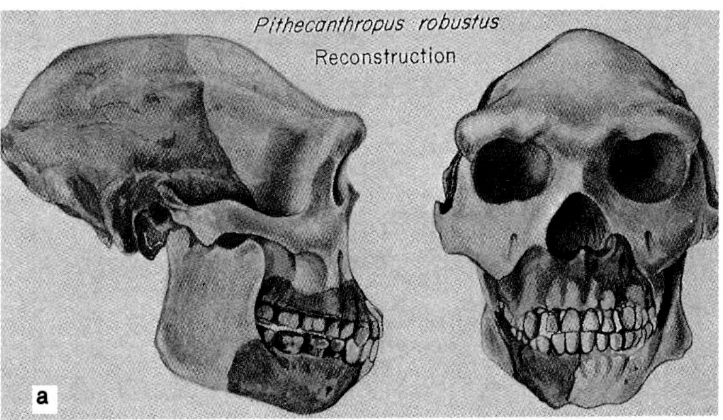

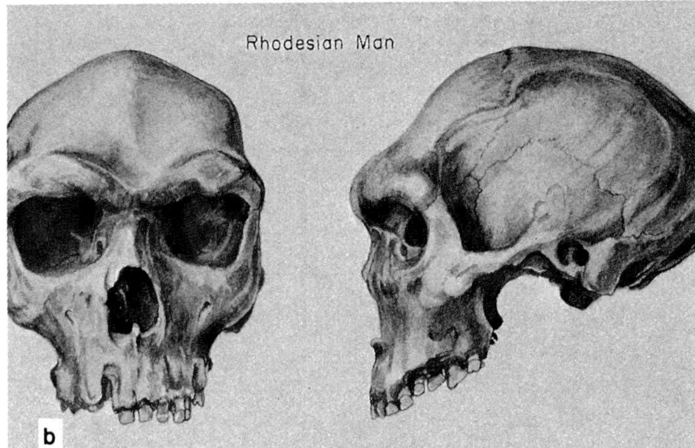

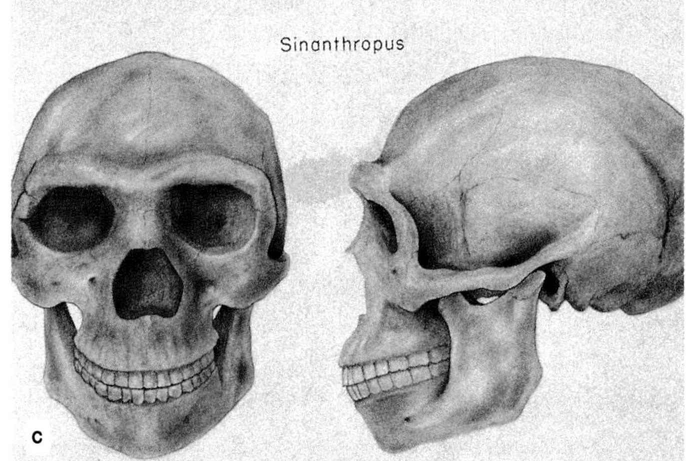

Figure 17.16

Middle Pleistocene hominids. *a, Pithecanthropus robustus* (*Homo erectus*); *b,* Rhodesian Man (Archaic *Homo sapiens*); *c,* Sinanthropus (*Homo erectus*).

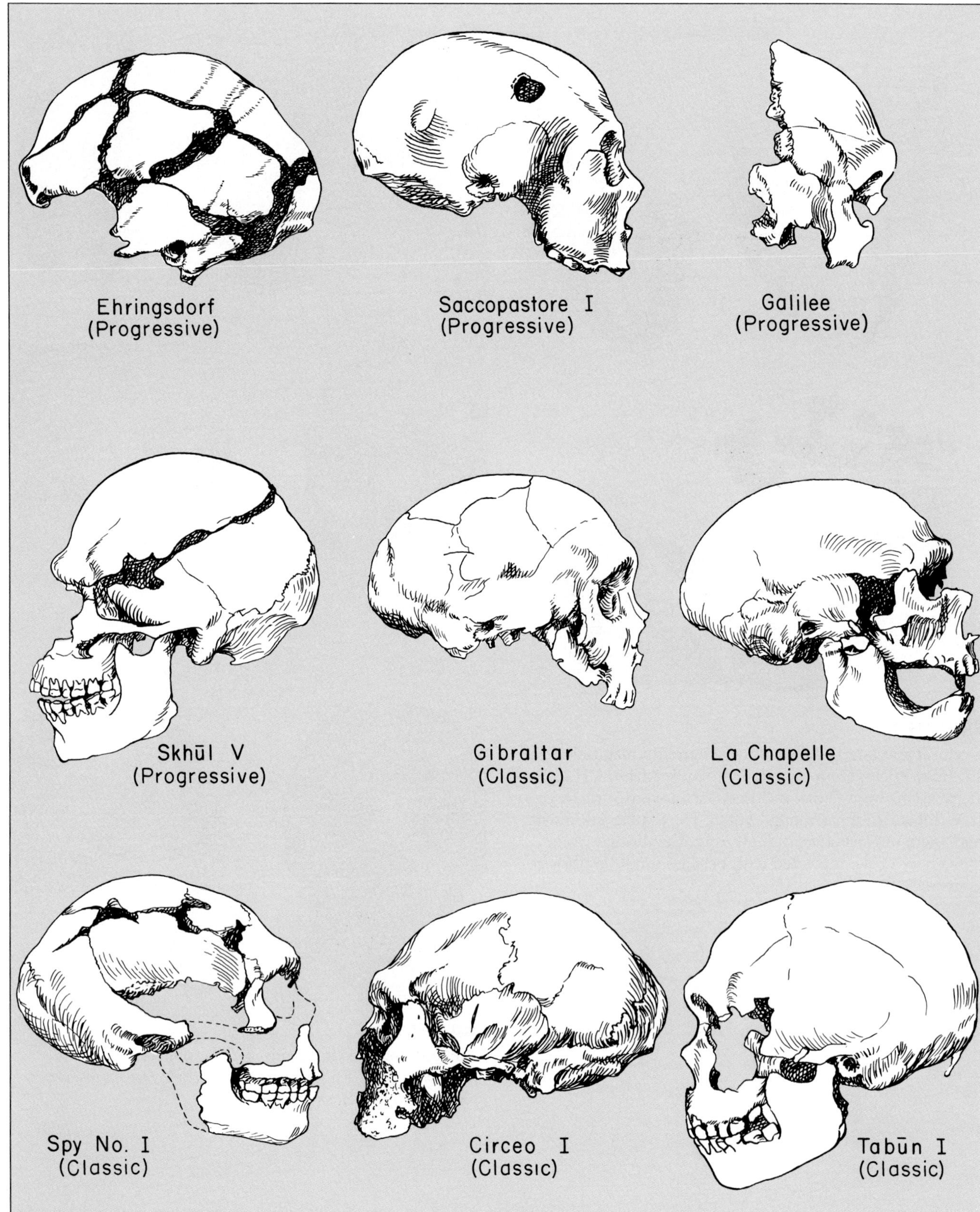

Figure 17.17

Late Pleistocene hominids, Classic and Progressive Neanderthaloids. (From Kraus, The Basis of Human Evolution, 1964, Harper & Row, Publishers, New York; with permission.)

References

Brown T, Rose K. Patterns of dental evolution in the Early Eocene anaptomorphine primates (Omomyidae) from the Bighorn basin, Wyoming. J Paleo Soc Mem 1987; 23:1–162.

Conroy G, Vannier M. Dental development in South African australopithecines. Am J Phys Anthrop 1990; 77.

Mann A. Some paleodemographic aspects of the South African australopithecines. University of Pennsylvania Publications in Anthropology. No. 1. Philadelphia: University of Pennsylvania, 1975.

McHenry H. Relative cheek tooth size in Australopithecus. Am J Phys Anthrop 1984; 64:297–306.

McHenry H. Implications of postcanine magadontia for the origin of *Homo.* In Delson E., ed. Ancestors: the hard evidence. New York: Alan R. Liss, 1985, pp. 178–183.

Richard AF. Primates in nature. New York: WH Freeman, 1985.

Tobias PV. Olduvai Gorge, Vol. 4. The skulls, endocasts and teeth of *Homo habilis.* New York: Cambridge University Press, 1990.

18

Some Principles of Evolution as Applied to Mankind

For detailed answers to the questions posed at the end of the previous chapter the student is advised to consult textbooks devoted to the subjects of evolution, genetics, and general biology. Here we can paint only a very broad general picture of the evolutionary process and merely point out the roles played by heredity and environment.

Evolution is an ongoing process that is the product of the continual interplay of many forces and conditions at any "moment" in time. One might look upon evolution as a battle between intrinsic (or endogenous) forces and extrinsic (or exogenous) forces for control over the destiny of life forms. The intrinsic forces are the genes, the sum total of which in any particular population constitute the *gene pool* of that population. The extrinsic forces are the multitudinous aspects of the environment: climate, vegetation, water, topography, soil composition, forms of life. But it must be remembered that environment is a relative term. When we are discussing the chromosomes of a single cell, the environment includes the other components of the cell: the nucleolus, mitochondria, Golgi substance, centrioles, lysosomes, vacuoles, membrane, and so on. In terms of a young embryo, the environment includes the fetal membranes, the uterus of the mother, and the various constituents of the mother's blood.

The interaction between these forces is responsible for the ways in which life on earth has unfolded into the many species, both extinct and living, that have occupied every conceivable "niche" on land, in the sea, and in the atmosphere. The species is "tossed between" these forces, so to speak, and is "molded" into forms that are constantly undergoing change. Now we examine the mechanism of this process as it applies to mammals.

Every population of mammals is made up of male and female individuals in about equal proportions. The members of one population are more like each other than they are like the members of any other population. Moreover they are more interested in each other sexually than they are in any other population. They interbreed within the population and produce viable offspring that tend to resemble the members of the parental generation. Such a population describes in a general way the term *species*. In a genetic sense, the species is a population that has a distinct gene pool as a result of breeding in isolation over an indeterminate period of time; the individual member simply is a "temporary vessel holding a small portion of the contents of the gene pool for a short period of time" (Mayr, 1963).

There are two built-in processes that occur in all bisexual species with importance for evolution, which must be firmly grasped if any real understanding of biology is to be realized. One is the phenomenon of *mutation*. Mutations are alterations of the deoxyribonucleic acid (DNA) chain molecules in the chromosomes, sections of which constitute the genes. They therefore result in changes in the structure or arrangement of genes. They can be brought about by certain types of environmental circumstances: some chemical substances such as mustard gas, and radiations such as ultraviolet light, cosmic rays, and those produced by radioactive materials. In addition, mutations can occur spontaneously, owing to variations in duplication of the DNA chains during cell division. It would be unreasonable to suppose that the great majority of mutations could be of any direct benefit to the individual organism. In fact, most of them are probably lethal and destroy the organism in the early embryonic period. But certainly a minority of them are without apparent harmful effect and can be carried throughout life by the individual, particularly when "masked" by a normal homologous mate (*allele*). Those individuals in a population who are carrying one or more of these nonharmful mutants in their genetic constitution comprise the "safety reserve" of the species. When environmental change demands certain modifications in the characteristics of a species if it is to continue to survive, these stored mutations may just happen to confer upon the individual those features that give it a better chance for survival under the changing conditions of the environment. How does this happen, if, as is generally the case, the mutant allele is recessive to its normal mate? Usually any mutant allele reaches a certain frequency (equilibrium) in the population, and this is maintained until the particular feature it produces in the individual acquires adaptive value as a result of a change in the environment. When this happens, all those individuals who happen to have two such mutant alleles (*homozygotes*) as a result of breeding between individuals with only one such mutant allele (*heterozygotes*) tend to have a *selective advantage* over the other members of the species. Their progeny gradually increase in number as a result of this selection and consequently the mutant allele increases in frequency relative to the former "normal" allele. The result is a change in *gene frequency*. When we consider that this process is going on all the time, and not merely with a single gene but with several, perhaps many, then it becomes apparent that evolution is really *change in gene frequency*, brought about by the *selection* of specific gene-mediated individual characteristics (*phenotypic traits*) which happen to have *adaptive value* in a new set of environmental circumstances.

We spoke of two processes, one of which was mutation. The other is the process of *meiosis*, a mechanism that occurs in the sex cells during the reproductive life of the individual and ensures that each gamete (sperm or ovum) will contain only half the number of chromosomes characteristic of the somatic cells of the individual. What is more, meiosis, which is found only in bisexual species, is nature's way of guaranteeing that *each sperm and each ovum will be genetically unique*. This means that the possibility of any two individuals of a species of mammals, past or present, being genetically identical is so slight as to be not worthy of mention. The exception, of course, is the occurrence of monozygotic individuals; this is discussed in detail in Chapter 19.

As a result of nature's assurance of biological individuality within each species through meiosis, the various alleles of each gene are "tried out" or "tested" in a vast number of combinations. Thus, each mutant allele is found in many different associations, some of which may produce phenotypic traits that prove of immediate or ultimate adaptive value. By the same token, unfavorable combinations of genes produce individuals that fail to survive or to have offspring. In a species of carnivorous mammal in which long canines have a very high adaptive value, mutant alleles that tend to produce a short canine or even agenesis of the canine will be eliminated or reduced to a very low frequency in the population, since the individual possessing such an allele in a homozygous state would not be able to survive.

It is of great importance to understand the significant role of teeth in any wild species, the genetic basis of tooth structure, and the very restricted range of variation that can be tolerated if the individual member of the species is to survive. Hence, mutant alleles that affect the dentition would tend to be kept at a low frequency in the population through the elimination of individuals possessing them. Although variation is inevitable because of mutations and meiosis, it must be kept within the bounds dictated by adaptation. If the form or arrangement of a bodily feature need not be precise or exact in order for the individual to adapt suitably, then the range of variation of the trait within the species will gradually become extended; this simply means that a certain number of mutant alleles that influence it can increase and be tolerated in numerous combinations. In other words, mutations affecting a trait that has little survival value can occur with impunity, so to speak. As a result, the trait itself will show considerable variation within the population.

In the case of man we have seen that the functional importance of the dentition was reduced when hominids assumed upright posture, and was still further reduced when his cultural inventory permitted him to roast and then boil his food. Finally, with the cultivation of cereal foods and methods of preserving cooked food, the survival value of the dentition was eliminated. This meant that the range of variation in tooth structure, chemistry, eruption, and so on could be extended without affecting the survival of the individual. It also meant, concomitantly, an increase in the number and frequency of mutant alleles involved in tooth development (increased *polymorphism*).

It must not be thought that an increase in the frequency of mutant alleles is without consequence in man simply because tooth variability can be tolerated. Genes have multiple functions, and although it is likely that each gene may have but one primary action, this in turn may influence numerous subsequent events in development. There are many *hereditary syndromes* in which widely separated structures and systems of the body, *including the dentition*, are abnormally formed because of a single mutant allele. These include: osteogenesis imperfecta, epidermolysis bullosa dystrophia, Fanconi syndrome, cleidocranial dysplasia, hypertrichosis universalis, rachitic diathesis, and Rothmund-Thomson syndrome.

By now it must be obvious that there is a fundamental difference in the evolutionary process between man and the rest of the animal kingdom. This difference concerns the nature of the environment in which the species operates. For all the rest of the animal species the environment to which they must adapt and which exercises a rigid system of selection on the members of the species is the *natural* environment. For mankind it has become his *culture* and his *society*. Because of clothing, houses, preserved foodstuffs, agriculture, animal husbandry, irrigation, transportation, medicine, surgery, vitamins, and many other inventions, the direct impact of the natural environment upon man has been diverted. Man adapts to his world through his culture and social organization, not by changing his structure or chemistry. It follows, then, that although evolution (change in gene frequency) continues in man, it is in directions and in ways that we do not yet understand and certainly cannot predict. We know only that his "load of mutations," is steadily increasing, since our culture has interfered with the negative selective forces of nature. Eventually, perhaps, no one will die immaturely and each individual's genes, mutant and otherwise, will be preserved in his offspring.

The oft-heard predictions concerning the eventual loss of man's fifth toe and "wisdom" teeth, the increasing size of his brain, the diminishing size of his face and legs, and other equally sensational changes, are *utterly without foundation.* What appears to be happening is the inevitable increase in the range of variation of almost all human traits as a consequence of the intercession of culture between man and his natural environment.

It is to consideration of variation as it pertains to the dentition that we now turn our attention.

References

Ciochon R, Corruccini R (eds.). New interpretations of ape and human ancestry. New York: Plenum, 1983.

Dutrillaux B. Chromosome evolution in primates. Folia Primatol 1988; 50:134–135.

Fleagle JG. Primate adaptation and evolution. San Diego: Academic Press, 1988.

Groves CP. A theory of human and primate evolution. New York: Oxford University Press, 1989.

Jully C (ed.). Early hominids of Africa. London: Duckworth, 1975.

Lewin R. Human evolution: an illustrated introduction. 2nd ed. Cambridge, MA: Blackwell Scientific, 1989.

Lovejoy O. The origin of man. Science 1981; 211:341–350.

Mayr E. Animal species and evolution. Cambridge, MA: Harvard University Press, 1963.

Miller WA. Evolution and comparative anatomy of vertebrate masticatory systems. In Mohl ND et al., eds. A textbook of occlusion. Chicago: Quintessence, 1988.

Stringer C (ed.). Aspects of human evolution. London: Taylor and Francis, 1981.

Szalay FS, Delson E. Evolutionary history of the primates. New York: Academic Press, 1979.

Genetic Control of Morphological Variability

We shall begin by a reconsideration of morphological variation. In Chapters 1 to 6 the basic diagnostic traits of each tooth were described, but in addition a few of the deviations within each basic pattern were depicted. In particular it was stated that the mandibular first premolar was one of the most variable teeth in the human dentition. It has been noted (Kraus and Furr, 1953) that there are at least 17 discrete traits that can be described for this tooth, each with two or more aspects. What is more, each aspect of each trait is randomly present with regard to the other 16 traits. Consider just three of these traits with their respective aspects.

Trait 1; the transverse ridge of the occlusal surface of the buccal cusp may consist of a single straight ridge or may bifurcate. Thus, there are two aspects for this trait: (a) nonbifurcated transverse ridge; (b) bifurcated transverse ridge.

Trait 2; the number of lingual cusps may vary from one to five, resulting in five different aspects: (a) one lingual cusp; (b) two lingual cusps; (c) three lingual cusps; (d) four lingual cusps; (e) five lingual cusps.

Trait 3; the number of transverse ridges may vary from one (the central one) to five (including the bifurcation of the central ridge as two ridges): (a) one transverse ridge; (b) two transverse ridges; (c) three transverse ridges; (d) four transverse ridges; (e) five transverse ridges.

Variations in crown structure of this tooth may take many forms (Figs. 19.1 to 19.4). If each trait (with its various aspects) may be present irrespective of what is present for the other traits, then there are 50 possible kinds of mandibular first premolars if just these three traits are considered. However, if all 17 traits with their aspects are included, 4,147,200 different kinds of mandibular first premolars are theoretically possible!

Naturally the aspects of any single trait do not appear in any one population or race with equal frequency. What is more, these aspect frequencies differ among the various populations. For example, among Caucasoid populations *two* transverse ridges are the most frequent aspect (46 percent) while the frequency of the *single* transverse ridge is 30 percent. Among Chinese, 50 percent of the first premolars show *three* transverse ridges. The Papago Indians of Arizona are notable in the relatively high frequency (32 percent) of premolars with *four* transverse ridges. Thus, the various aspects are distributed at different frequencies among the races, strongly suggesting a hereditary control over their presence or absence.

If there are, theoretically, over 4 million types of mandibular first premolars, then the chance of any two unrelated persons having identical types would be in the nature of 1 in 16 trillion, assuming that each aspect within a given trait had an equal probability of occurring. If we now assume that the other teeth—incisors, canines, premolars, and molars (both maxillary and mandibular)—present numerous traits with varying numbers of aspects, then the probability of any two unrelated persons having identical dentitions (in the morphological sense) becomes almost infinitesimally small, perhaps in the order of 10^{-50}! It is apparent, then, that variability is an important component of human dental structure. There must be some mechanism that ensures that no two individuals will be exactly alike in their total tooth complement. We can get a little closer to understanding this mechanism by examining the one exception to the above statement: the case of so-called "identical" twins.

In the United States Caucasoid population 1 of every 88 births is a twin birth. One out of three twin births consists of "identical" twins. Thus "identical" twins occur about once in 264 births. The other twin births are "fraternal" twins. The former are more appropriately designated *monozygotic* or *monovular* twins, since they result from the union of a single sperm and a single ovum and hence *must have identical genotypes.* The latter are termed *dizygotic* or *diovular* twins, each member of the pair the product of a different zygote, and each as different genetically from the other as any two siblings of different ages. Monozygotic twins are always the same sex, whereas dizygotic twins may be both males, both females, or one male and one female. Since monozygotic twins are genetically identical, any differences between them must be the result solely of environmental factors. Conversely, any trait in which monozygotic twins are different can not be strictly controlled by genes alone but must be subject to environmental in-

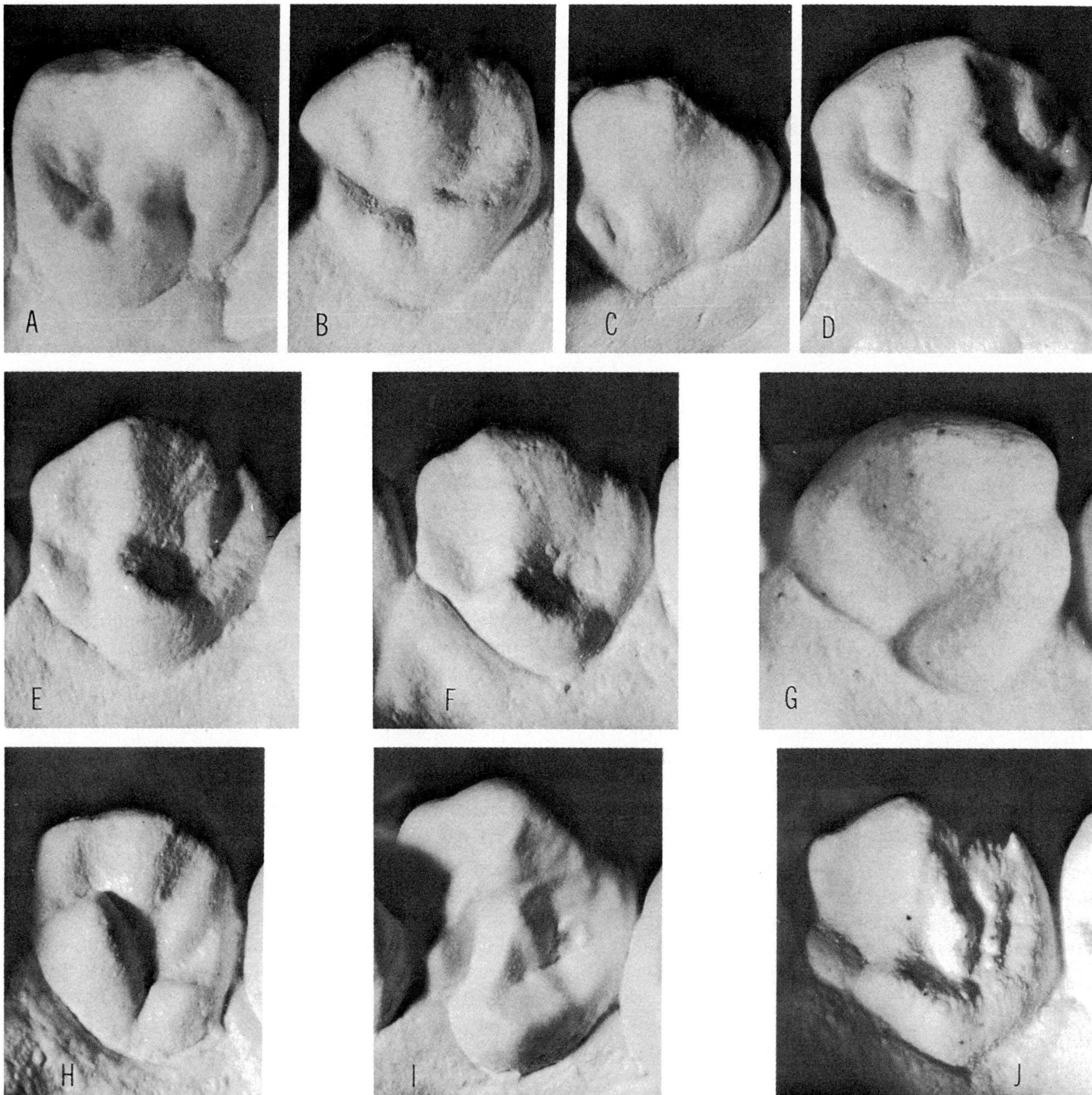

Figure 19.1

Morphological traits of the mandibular first premolar. *A, left,* complete distal marginal ridge; *B, left,* three small lingual cusps; *C, left,* absence of lingual cusp with presence of mesial marginal ridge; *D, left,* four occlusal ridges, two lingual grooves; *E, right,* blending of lingual with buccal cusp; *F, right,* single small lingual cusp; *G, right,* absence of lingual cusp and marginal ridges; *H, right,* two lingual cusps and mesial location of main lingual cusp; *I, right,* bifurcation of central occlusal ridge; *J, right,* three pronounced occlusal ridges.

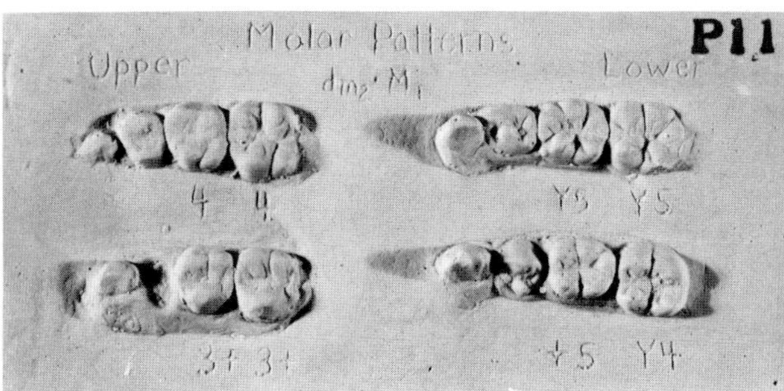

Figure 19.2

Relationship of occlusal surface patterns between deciduous and permanent molars. The models in this figure show where specific genetic morphological changes on the first permanent molars are also registered on the second deciduous molars. The model on the upper left shows four well-developed cusps on both of these teeth. The model on the lower left shows a markedly reduced hypocone on both. The upper right-hand model shows the same pattern of grooves and cusps on both teeth. However, the deciduous second molar is even more stable morphologically than the permanent first molar. Ancestral traits may be and frequently are retained in the former when they are lost in the latter. The model on the lower right shows the distal cusp (hypoconulid) portrayed on the deciduous tooth and lacking on the first permanent molar. This conforms to the established concepts of variability in the dentition. Another example of this is seen in the upper right model, in which the Carabelli's cusp (also a primary character) is present in the upper deciduous second molar and lacking in the upper permanent first molar. (Courtesy of A. A. Dahlberg and the Zoller Laboratory of Anthropology, University of Chicago.)

fluences. For example, with reference to the ABO blood groups, monozygotic twins are always identical since environment has apparently no influence on, nor plays any role in the determination of, the blood groups.

It is obvious, then, that the study of twins can be most useful in assessing the respective roles of heredity and environment in producing a specific phenotypic trait. By the use of statistics in analyzing the average intrapair differences for a series of monozygotic and dyzygotic twins, the heritability of a trait can be determined. Thus, it has been shown that there is a strong component of genetic variability for the mesiodistal tooth dimensions of the permanent anterior teeth, and hence a good argument for genetic control of general tooth size (Osborne et al, 1958).

A study of crown structure in the two kinds of twins shows that tooth by tooth there is identity between members of monozygotic pairs but in dizygotic twins the differences are as frequent as between un-

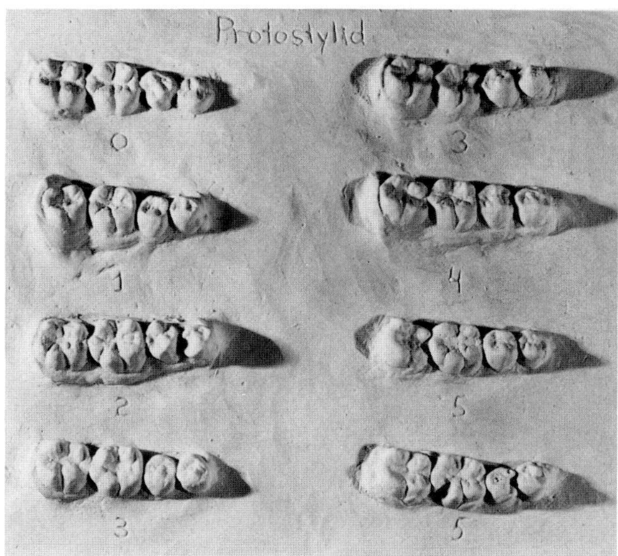

Figure 19.3

A sequence of casts illustrating the various degrees of expression of the protostylid and related structures. The protostylid is a primary character found on the buccal surface of the mesiobuccal cusp (protoconid) of lower molars. It, like Carabelli's cusp, is derived and specialized from the cingulum. It resembles the Carabelli's cusp in most ways except that rather than being a recently evolved structure it is currently a much modified one, having been extremely prominent in some of the fossil forms. It occurs with lesser frequency in man, but reports show a tendency for greater display of this cusp in Mongoloid peoples.

Model 0 shows no structure on the buccal surface other than the normal developmental grooves. Model 1 shows a large pit which has been considered to be a specialized area resulting from influences associated with the protostylid even when it is not present. Model 2 shows a distal deviation of the mesiobuccal groove. Both models marked 3 show a greater deviation of the groove plus a definite but small rise in the surface following the pattern of the typical large protostylid shown on the bottom and next to the models marked 5. Model 4 shows an intermediate stage. (Courtesy of A. A. Dahlberg and the Zoller Laboratory of Anthropology, University of Chicago.)

related pairs or siblings (Kraus et al, 1959). In Figure 19.5 the teeth of the lower left and upper right quadrants of two sets of triplets are shown. In Triplet Set I the *top two quadrants* illustrated (*A* and *B*) are those of identical twin boys, whereas the *bottom quadrant* (*C*) is that of their fraternal twin sister. *Arrows* point to some morphological features in the sister which are different from those in her identical twin brothers. The same situation holds for Triplet Set II, except that in this case the upper two photographs (*A* and *B*) are those of identical twin sisters, whereas the

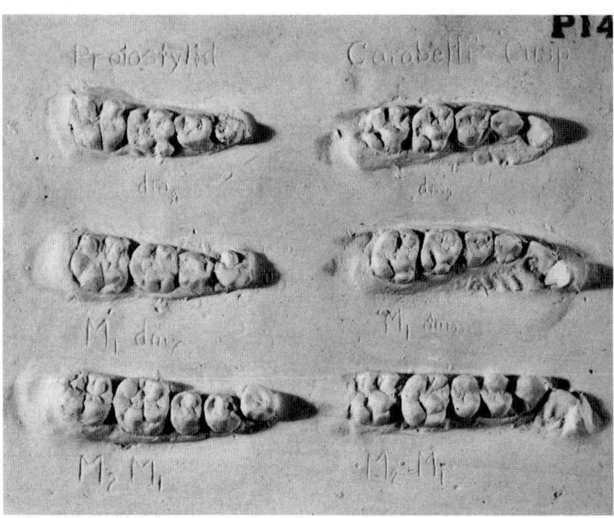

Figure 19.4

Illustration of varying penetrance of the protostylid and Carabelli's cusp in the deciduous-permanent series of molar teeth. It was pointed out in the legend for Fig. 19.2 that there is a definite morphological relationship between the deciduous molars and the permanent molars. This plaque demonstrates some of the principles involved. The upper two models show the extreme prominence of the protostylid and Carabelli's cusp (primary characters), respectively, on the deciduous second molars, but not on the permanent molars. This illustrates the even greater conservativeness or stability of the deciduous second molar in the composite molar groups in both the upper and lower molar series. The middle two models show the structures on both the deciduous and permanent teeth. The lower models show them on both the permanent molars. Such primary characters are sometimes shown on the third molars in addition to the others. The combination of character penetrance of primary characters is therefore (dm^2), (dm^2 M1), (dm^2 M1 M2), or (dm^2 M1 M2 M3). (Courtesy of A. A. Dahlberg and the Zoller Laboratory of Anthropology, University of Chicago.)

third and dizygotic member of the set (C) is a boy, whose mandibular left quadrant is shown in the lower photograph. Again, *arrows* point out some of the discordant traits. Note that in Sets I and II the teeth are practically identical in crown structure for the two monozygotic members of the sets.

Zygosity is generally studied by means of the various blood groups, dermatoglyphics (finger prints), taste sensitivity to PTC, and other phenotypic traits. Serology is particularly useful in providing dizygosity, but *cannot positively prove monozygosity*. Present indications are that dental concordance is one of the methods by which monozygosity can be positively determined, DNA fingerprinting being the other. Dental study models of twins allow a careful comparison of the crowns, tooth by tooth. The case for the use of the dentition in zygosity determination was first put forth in 1959 (Kraus et al, 1959) and later substantiated by Lundström (1963).

When we now contemplate the fact that the potentialities for morphological variation in the human dentition are enormous, yet that persons with the same genetic constitution show no discordance in dental crown features, we must come to the conclusion that (1) these traits are under very rigid genetic control, and (2) the genes that determine their expression are more or less independent of each other. This conclusion is further reinforced when it is recalled that the frequencies of certain crown characters differ among the various populations and races of mankind. For instance, the Carabelli trait shows definite racial variations. In so-called "pure" Mongoloids (Japanese, Chinese, Eskimo, and pre-Columbian American Indians) the maximum expression, a large tubercle or cusp, is absent. Instead there are found one or two grooves or pits, very slight tubercles or bulges, or complete absence of any expression. In Negroid and Caucasoid populations the entire range of expressions occur, including the pronounced tubercle. Among Melanesians the Carabelli cusp attains the size of the other cusps in many cases. In the case of hybrids (Mongoloid-Caucasoid or Mongoloid-Negroid) the Carabelli cusp is expressed, suggesting that the genes governing this aspect of the Carabelli trait were introduced by the Caucasoid or Negroid parent.

References

Kieser JA. An analysis of the Carabelli trait in the mixed deciduous and permanent human dentition. Arch Oral Biol 1984; 29:403–406.

Kieser JA, van der Merwe CA. Classifying reliability of the Carabelli trait in man. Arch Oral Biol 1984; 29:795–801.

Kraus B, Furr M. Lower first premolars. J Dent Res 1953; 32:554–564.

Kraus B, Wise W, Frei R. Heredity and the cranio-facial complex. Am J Orthodont 1959; 45:172–217.

Lundström A. Tooth morphology as a basis for distinguishing monozygotic and dizygotic twins. Am J Hum Genet 1963; 15:34–43.

Osborne R, Horowitz S, DeGeorge F. Genetic variation in tooth dimensions: a twin study of permanent anterior teeth. Am J Hum Genet 1958; 10:350–356.

Scott GR, Potter RHY. An analysis of tooth morphology in American twins. Anthropologie 1984; 22:223–231.

Townsend GC, Corruccini RS, Richards LC, Brown T. Genetic and environmental determinants of dental occlusal variation in South Australian twins. Austral Orthod J 1988; 10:231–235.

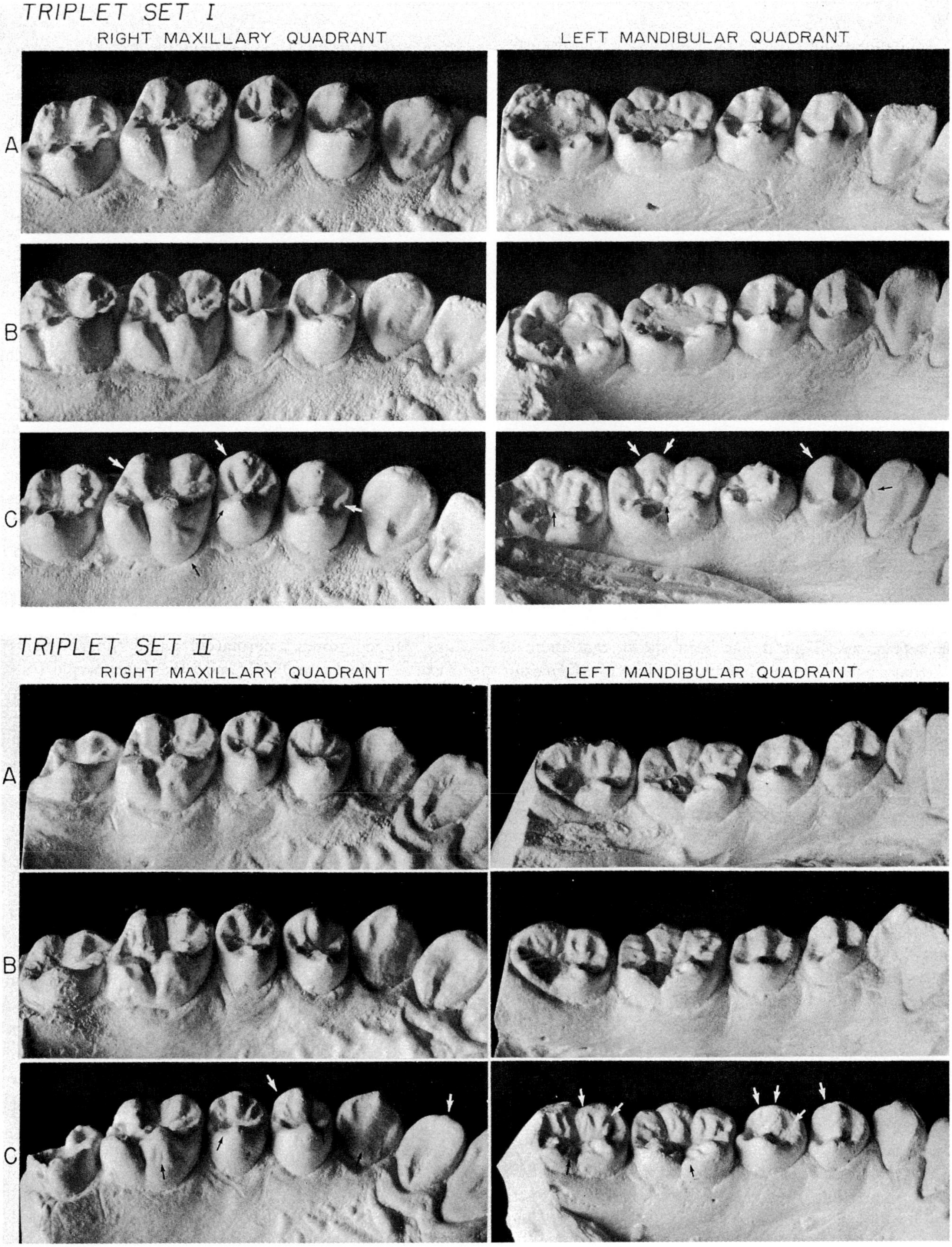

TRIPLET SET I

RIGHT MAXILLARY QUADRANT

LEFT MANDIBULAR QUADRANT

A

B

C

TRIPLET SET II

RIGHT MAXILLARY QUADRANT

LEFT MANDIBULAR QUADRANT

A

B

C

Figure 19.5

Mandibular left and maxillary right quadrants of two sets of triplets. *A* and *B* are monozygotic members of the triplet set; *C* is the dizygotic member. Arrows point to crown features of *C* that differ from corresponding features in *A* and *B*.

20

Embryology: The Attainment of Final Crown Structures

Although the evidence for the genetic regulation of tooth structure is overwhelming, the exact mode of inheritance has not been determined for a single normal dental trait. This potentially rich and promising area of human genetics has begun to yield to precise genetic analysis. While it is impossible to perform controlled breeding experiments with humans, it can be done with mice, in which a number of genes that influence the teeth have been identified. A more serious difficulty arises from the fact that the relationship between gene and character trait is by no means a simple one. Genes act by determining the proteins that are synthesized in cells, including the enzymes that control biochemical actions. The dentition is the end result of a complex process of development, starting long before birth and involving the activities of cells in the lamina, enamel organs, papillae, follicles, and surrounding tissues of the jaws, all of which are influenced by their genes. All the cells of an individual contain the same genes, but only some of the genes are active at any one time. Different genes are active in different sorts of cells and in the same cell at different phases of its development. The final structure is therefore the product of many genes, a mutation of any one of which will produce a changed end result, i.e., a variation. It is not surprising therefore to find that nearly all variant traits are polygenic, varying in expression as a result of the modifying action of several genes.

As an example we may consider the so-called "Y-5" or "Dryopithecus" pattern, formed by the grooves separating the cusps, the mesiobuccal from the distobuccal, the distobuccal from the distal, and the mesiolingual from the distolingual, is considered diagnostic of hominoid forms. In fact, however, the occurrence of the Y fissural pattern is independent of the number of cusps, whether four or five. At any rate, there is a continuous gradient of variations of the pattern, going from "+4" to a "Y-5" and +5" (Fig. 20.1). It is assumed that this trait, fissural pattern, is polygenic; that is, its expression is determined by combinations of alleles at two or more loci. The fissural pattern appears only in one of the last stages in molar development and is obviously, as we shall see, a product of final enamel deposition.

The Carabelli trait, on the other hand, is the expression of alleles at a single locus. It, too, has figured prominently in evaluations of taxonomical position. Neither the Carabelli nor the fissural pattern trait were known embryologically until 1965. Subsequently it was quite clear that the determinants for the Carabelli expression act early in tooth embryology, compared with those for the fissural pattern. There is some justification for speculating that the genes determining the Carabelli trait are phylogenetically older than those which produce the fissural pattern. Weidenreich pointed out that the Carabelli pit is a remnant of the lingual cingulum that is characteristic of all primates, but that the Carabelli cusp (tubercle) is merely an accidental variation "without phylogenetic significance" (1937). Both fossil and embryologic evidence argue against this point. The two are different forms of expression of the same genotype. What is more, the Carabelli cusp is the maximum expression of the lingual cingulum in man, whereas the pit (or groove) occurs when the cingulum is absent. The embryology of both pit and cusp is shown in Figure 20.2. The cusp is always preceded by the growth of a cingulum (*zona cingularis*), just as is the case with any cusp (see below). When a lingual cingulum fails to develop, a pit may (or may not) be present. There is no evidence to indicate that the pit is a "remnant" of the cingulum. It should also be pointed out that on no other site on a tooth does a tubercle or cusp alternate with a pit or groove.

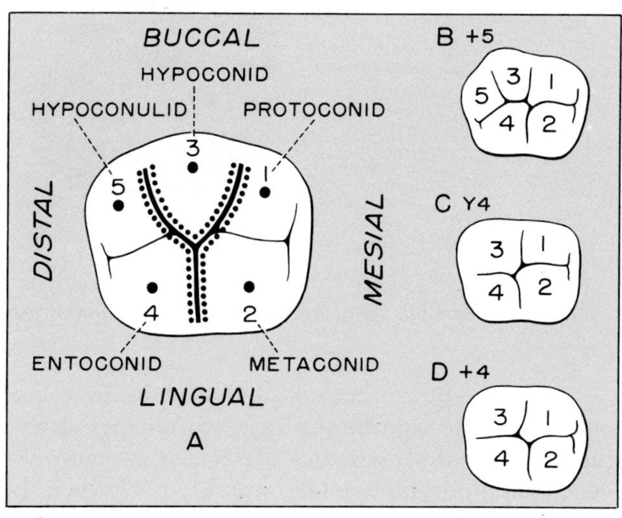

Figure 20.1

Fissural patterns of hominoid mandibular molars.

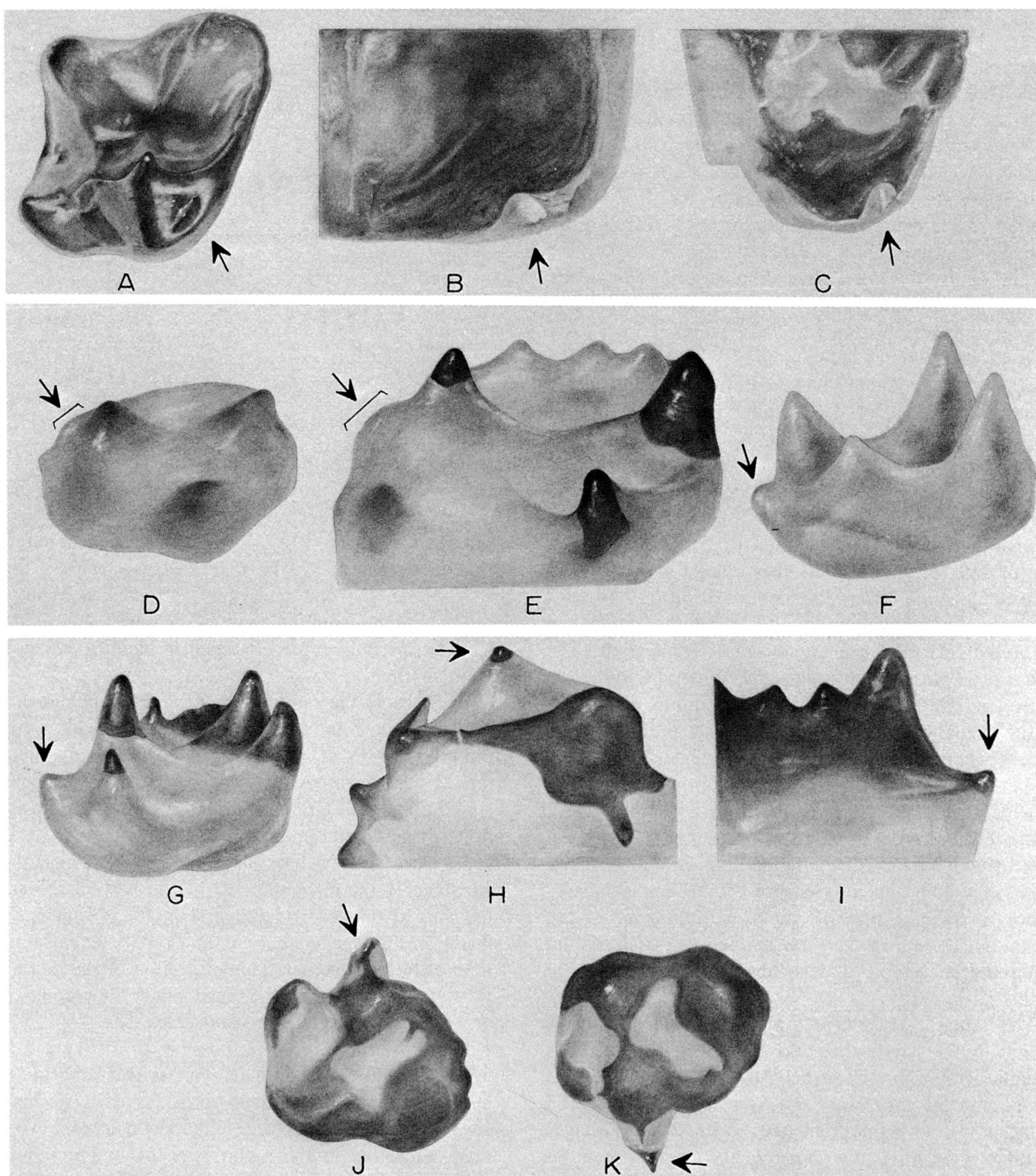

Figure 20.2
Incipient Carabelli cusps and pits (*arrows*) in human maxillary molar buds.

The attempt to interpret phylogenetically or taxonomically the significance of a morphological feature is fraught with many dangers if its morphogenesis and developmental course are not known. In order to interpret a morphological feature correctly, it is desirable to know how it develops. For this reason alone it is advisable that the embryologic stages leading to the final crown form of the primary mandibular first and second molars be briefly described and illustrated.

A young tooth germ consists of an enamel organ, derived from the oral ectoderm, and partly enclosing a mass of ectomesenchyme known as the dental papilla. The inner epithelial layer of the enamel organ, which will later become the ameloblast layer, is separated from the surface of the ectomesenchyme (later to develop into odontoblasts) by a basement membrane, the bilaminar amelodentinal membrane. The cusps, crests, and valleys of the crown of the tooth are formed as folds in this membrane, owing to unequal growth within the epithelium and ectomesenchyme. Eventually, when ameloblasts and odontoblasts differentiate externally and internally to the membrane and begin to deposit enamel and dentin, the shape of the membrane is preserved as the amelodentinal junction of the tooth. Formation of calcified tissues begins at the tips of the cusps and spreads downward, so that the deepest valleys and basins (fissures) are the last areas to calcify. While this is happening the tooth germ is growing, but growth can take place only in uncalcified areas. Once two cusps become joined by the spread of calcification along a connecting ridge their distance apart is fixed, but other cusps can still move apart, and small additional cusps can form in the still-growing uncalcified areas. Thus, formation of the crown pattern is highly organized, but there are differences from tooth to tooth, accounting for the final differences of their morphology.

Radiographs of the fetal jaws are not adequate for depicting the development of the tooth germs, either before or after calcification commences. In order to observe the tooth germ in detail and "in the round" it is necessary to dissect out the surrounding follicle (Fig. 20.3), carefully remove the follicle, and examine and photograph the tooth germ under a dissecting microscope. This procedure was followed for the complete dentitions of several hundred human fetuses from 10 to 40 weeks of age. The primary molars, as well as the first permanent molars, are first seen macroscopically as tiny hemispherical mounds (Fig. 20.4) measuring about 0.1 mm in diameter. We have termed this earliest form Stage I. In the first molar it is attained at about 12 weeks; in the second at about 12½ weeks. It is impossible at this stage of development to identify one molar from another.

In Stage II the mound-like elevation becomes more sharply defined and higher in both the first and second molars (Fig. 20.5). This is to be the future mesiobuccal cusp (protoconid). At this point it should be stated that in all human molars, as well as in those of other primates, the mesiobuccal cusp is the first to become elevated as well as the first to begin calcification. In Stage II the distal portion of the base of the cusp has spread outward; in the first molar it is mostly a distalward extension, but in the first the expansion is both distal and lingual. This projection of the bud outward from the base of a cusp might be termed the *developmental cingulum* or *zona cingularis.*

From Stage III on it is possible to differentiate the first from the second molar. This is true also for the maxillary molars. In other words, as early as about 13 weeks *type traits,* in a developmental sense, have already appeared in the molars. In the first molar the mesiolingual cusp (metaconid) has appeared, reach-

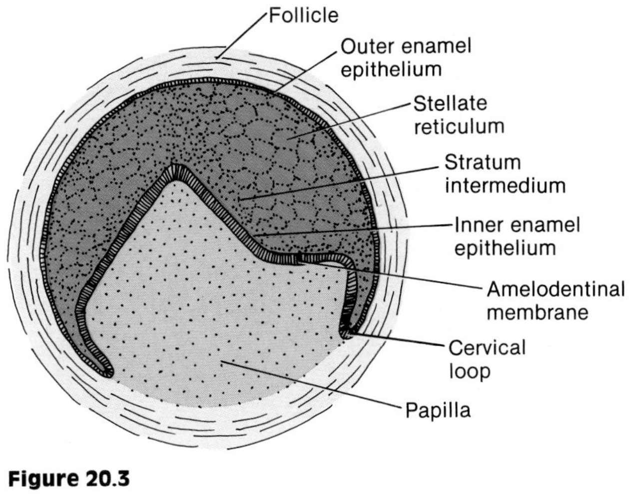

Figure 20.3

Diagrammatic vertical section through a tooth germ. (From Butler PM. The ontogeny of molar pattern. Biol Rev 1956;31:33; with permission.)

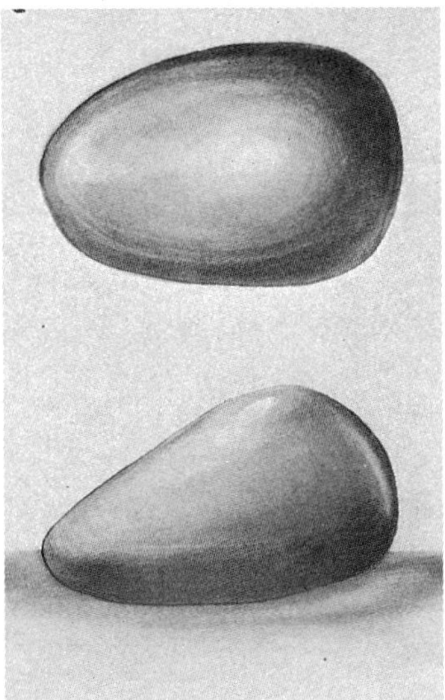

Figure 20.4

Stage I, mandibular first and second primary molars. (Reproduced from Kraus and Jordan, 1965, *The Human Dentition Before Birth;* by permission of Lea & Febiger, Philadelphia.)

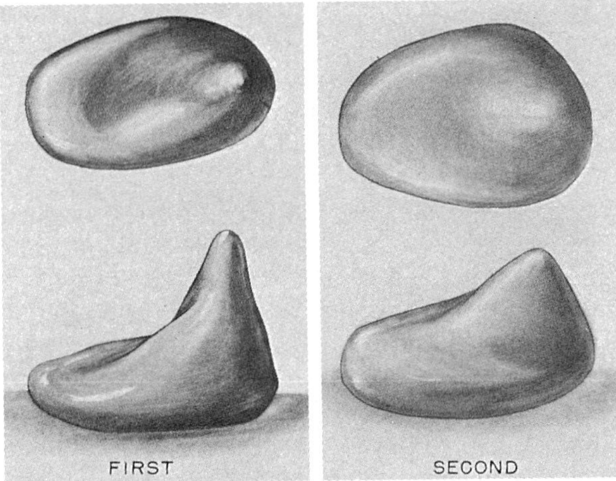

Figure 20.5

Stage II, mandibular first and second primary molars. (Reproduced from Kraus and Jordan, 1965, *The Human Dentition Before Birth;* by permission of Lea & Febiger, Philadelphia.)

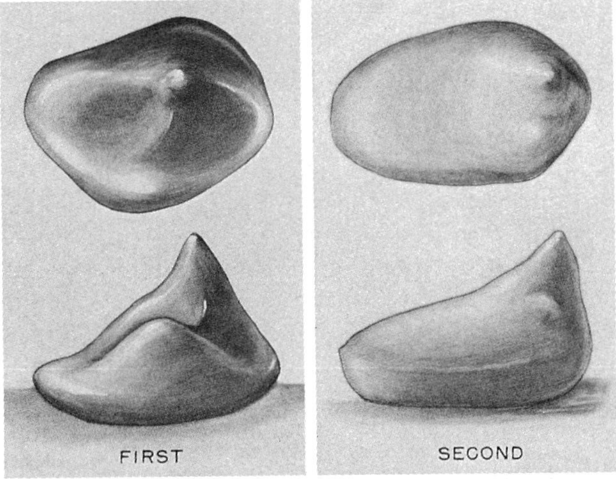

Figure 20.6

Stage III, mandibular first and second primary molars. (Reproduced from Kraus and Jordan, 1965, *The Human Dentition Before Birth;* by permission of Lea & Febiger, Philadelphia.)

ing about half the height of the protoconid. The two cusps occupy almost the entire mesiodistal extent of the bud. In the second molar, on the other hand, the metaconid is barely seen, whereas the protoconid is confined to the mesial half of the bud. The result is that the distal portion of the developmental cingulum in the second molar is more prominent than in the first molar, whereas the opposite is true with respect to the two cusps (Fig. 20.6). Stated another way, the talonid (distal moiety of the molar) has made its appearance in Stage III of the development of the second molar. The talonid, it will be recalled, is *phylogenetically* the newer or more recent portion of the molar. As can now be seen, it is *embryologically* the newer, as well.

In Stage IV the differences between the first and second molars become more marked. The talonid is but a small distal projection of the cingulum in the first, but has become a long shallow basin in the second. The metaconid is very slow in its development in the second molar but continues to rise sharply in the first (Fig. 20.7).

When the first molar has reached the two-cusp stage and the transverse ridge between the MB and

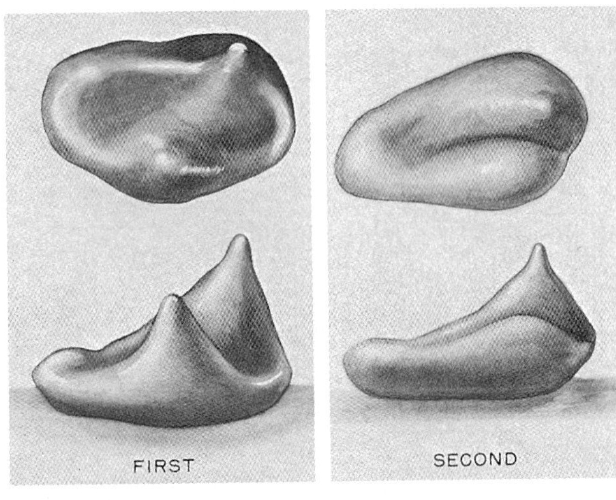

Figure 20.7

Stage IV, mandibular first and second primary molars. (Reproduced from Kraus and Jordan, 1965, *The Human Dentition Before Birth;* by permission of Lea & Febiger, Philadelphia.)

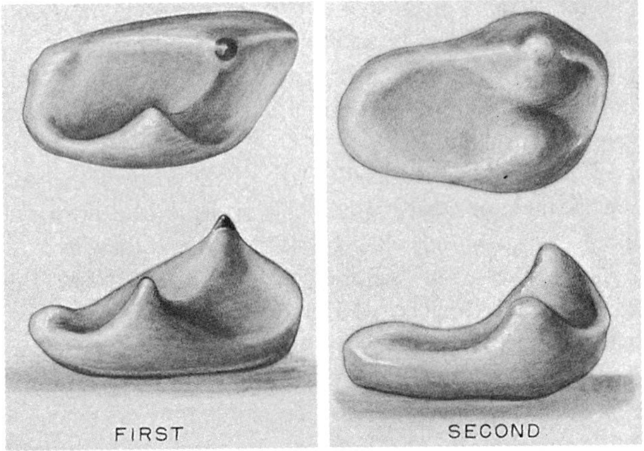

Figure 20.8

Stage V, mandibular first and second primary molars. *Shaded sections,* calcified. (Reproduced from Kraus and Jordan, 1965, *The Human Dentition Before Birth;* by permission of Lea & Febiger, Philadelphia.)

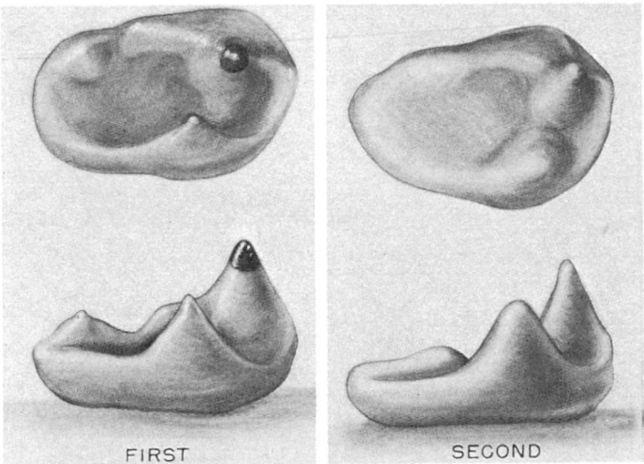

Figure 20.9
Stage VI, mandibular first and second primary molars. *Shaded sections,* calcified. (Reproduced from Kraus and Jordan, 1965, *The Human Dentition Before Birth;* by permission of Lea & Febiger, Philadelphia.)

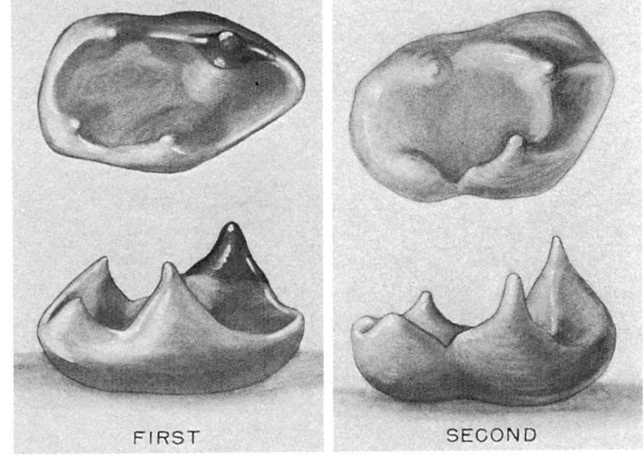

Figure 20.10
Stage VIII, mandibular first and second primary molars. *Shaded sections,* calcified. (Reproduced from Kraus and Jordan, 1965, *The Human Dentition Before Birth;* by permission of Lea & Febiger, Philadelphia.)

ML cusps is clearly defined, calcification on the tip of the mesiobuccal cusp commences (Fig. 20.8). In addition, both a mesial and a distal marginal ridge can now be seen. In this stage (Stage V) the second molar is in a similar state of development except that calcification will be delayed until all five cusps have appeared. Also, the transverse ridge has not yet developed.

Stage VI in both molars is marked by the appearance of the third cusp, the distobuccal (hypoconid). In the first molar it occurs near the distobuccal corner of the diminutive talonid; in the second it springs up near the middle of the distal margin of the tooth bud (Fig. 20.9). This, plus the fact that the MB cusp in the first molar is calcifying, makes it easy to distinguish between the two tooth buds.

In Stage VIII (Fig. 20.10) the two molars reach the four-cusp stage of development. The MB cusp of the first molar becomes more calcified down its slopes. The characteristic "prow-shape" of the mesial marginal ridge in this molar is accentuated. In both molars the two cusps of the ancient trigonid are much higher and more sharply pointed than are the two more recent cusps of the talonid.

In Stage IX (Fig. 20.11) the MB cusp of the second molar commences to calcify and the fifth cusp, the

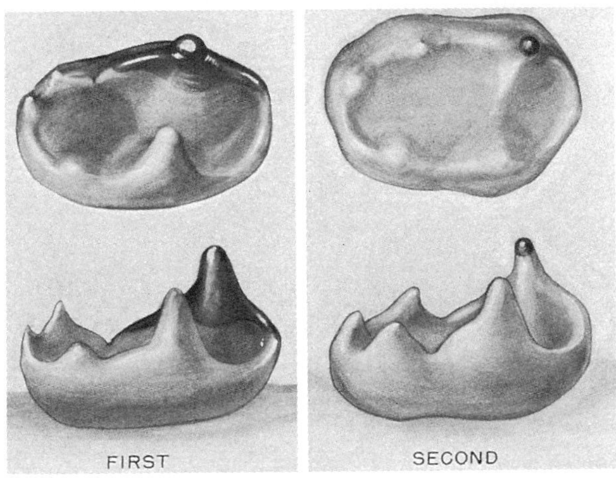

Figure 20.11
Stage IX, mandibular first and second primary molars. *Shaded sections,* calcified. (Reproduced from Kraus and Jordan, 1965, *The Human Dentition Before Birth;* by permission of Lea & Febiger, Philadelphia.)

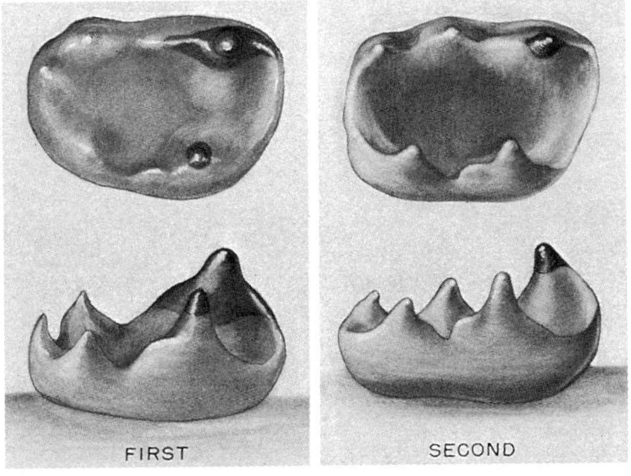

Figure 20.12
Stage X, mandibular first and second primary molars. *Shaded sections,* calcified. (Reproduced from Kraus and Jordan, 1965, *The Human Dentition Before Birth;* by permission of Lea & Febiger, Philadelphia.)

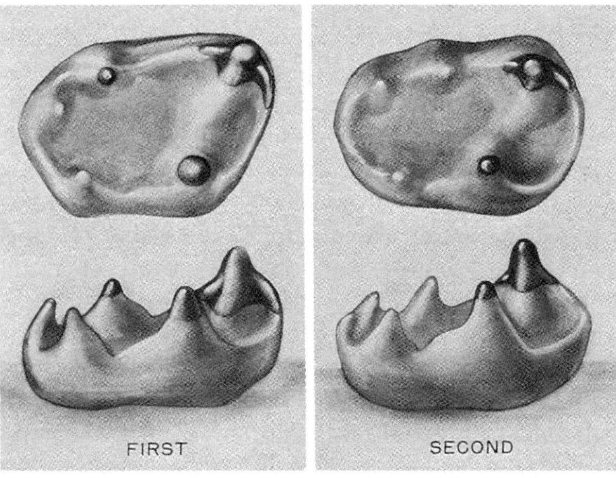

Figure 20.13

Stage XI, mandibular first and second primary molars. *Shaded sections,* calcified. (Reproduced from Kraus and Jordan, 1965, *The Human Dentition Before Birth;* by permission of Lea & Febiger, Philadelphia.)

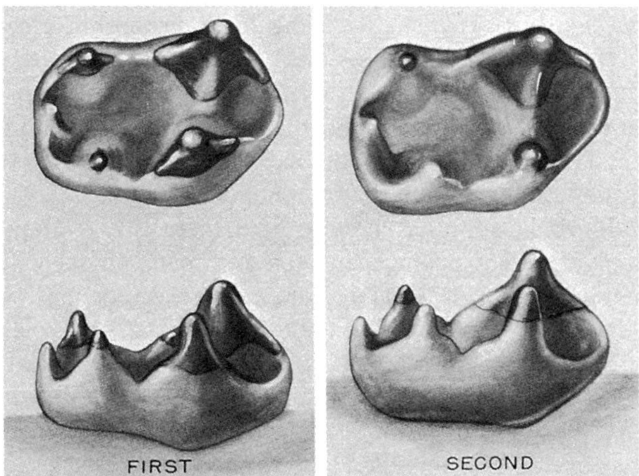

Figure 20.14

Stage XII, mandibular first and second primary molars. *Shaded sections,* calcified. (Reproduced from Kraus and Jordan, 1965, *The Human Dentition Before Birth;* by permission of Lea & Febiger, Philadelphia.)

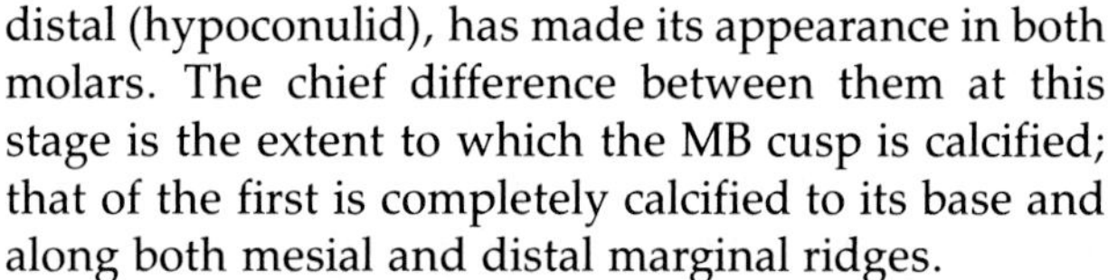

distal (hypoconulid), has made its appearance in both molars. The chief difference between them at this stage is the extent to which the MB cusp is calcified; that of the first is completely calcified to its base and along both mesial and distal marginal ridges.

The next few stages are defined mainly in terms of the sequence of calcification both on and between cusps. In Stage X (Fig. 20.12) the ML cusp of the first molar begins to calcify but in the second this event does not occur until Stage XI (Fig. 20.13), by which time the hypoconid has commenced to calcify on the first molar. In Stage XII the distolingual cusp (entoconid) of the first molar begins calcification as does the hypoconid on the second (Fig. 20.14). All five cusps of the first molar are undergoing calcification in Stage XIII, but only four cusps in the second molar (Fig. 20.15). By Stage XIV all five cusps of the second molar are in various degrees of calcification, but in the first molar calcified coalescence between the two buccal cusps has now taken place (Fig. 20.16). In the

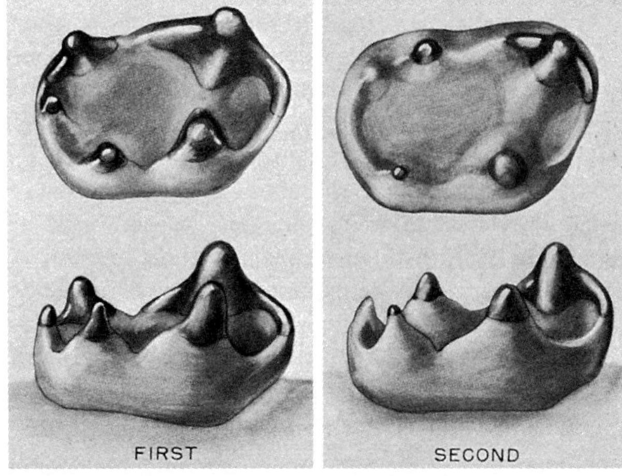

Figure 20.15

Stage XIII, mandibular first and second primary molars. *Shaded sections,* calcified. (Reproduced from Kraus and Jordan, 1965, *The Human Dentition Before Birth;* by permission of Lea & Febiger, Philadelphia.)

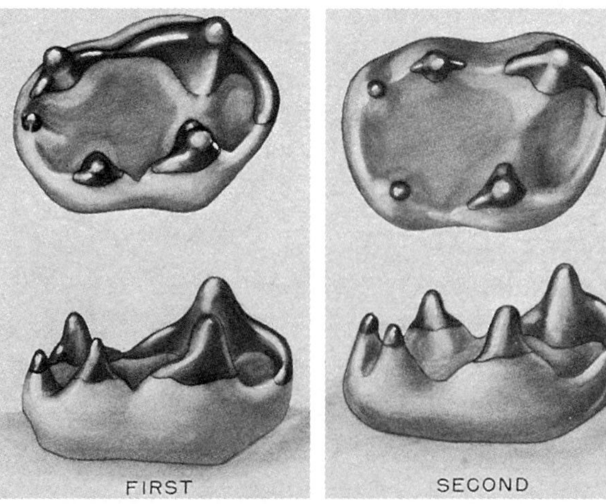

Figure 20.16

Stage XIV, mandibular first and second primary molars. *Shaded sections,* calcified. (Reproduced from Kraus and Jordan, 1965, *The Human Dentition Before Birth;* by permission of Lea & Febiger, Philadelphia.)

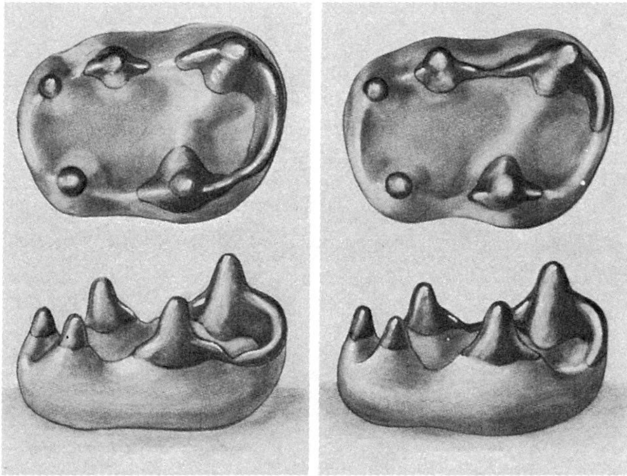

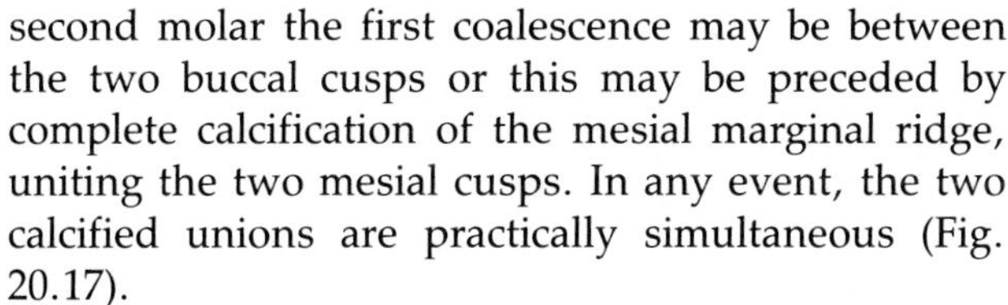

Figure 20.17

Stage XV, two orders of calcified coalescence in the mandibular second primary molar. *Shaded sections,* calcified. (Reproduced from Kraus and Jordan, 1965, *The Human Dentition Before Birth;* by permission of Lea & Febiger, Philadelphia.)

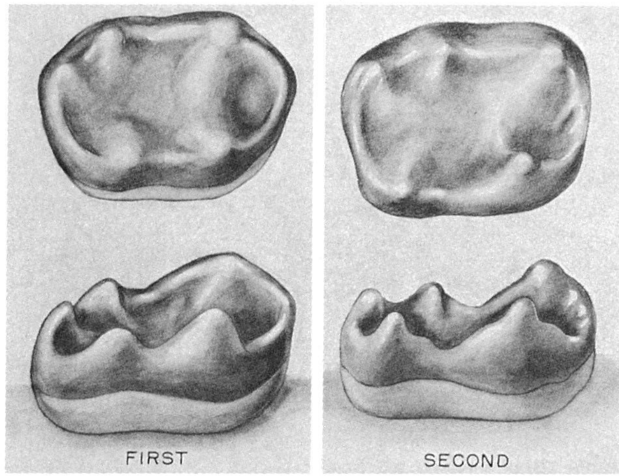

Figure 20.18

Stage XIX and XX in the mandibular first and second primary molars, respectively, at birth. *Shaded sections,* calcified. (Reproduced from Kraus and Jordan, 1965, *The Human Dentition Before Birth;* by permission of Lea & Febiger, Philadelphia.)

second molar the first coalescence may be between the two buccal cusps or this may be preceded by complete calcification of the mesial marginal ridge, uniting the two mesial cusps. In any event, the two calcified unions are practically simultaneous (Fig. 20.17).

An important difference between the two molars lies in the sequence of calcified coalescence. In the first molar the order is: (1) protoconid to hypoconid; (2) hypoconid to hypoconulid; (3) protoconid to metaconid (*over the transverse ridge*); (4) hypoconulid to entoconid; (5) entoconid to metaconid and protoconid to metaconid (*over the mesial marginal ridge*). In the second molar the order is: (1) protoconid to hypoconid and protoconid to metaconid (*over the mesial marginal ridge*); (2) hypoconid to hypoconulid and protoconid to metaconid (*over the transverse ridge*); (3) hypoconulid to entoconid and entoconid to metaconid. In both molars the central basin is the last portion of the occlusal surface to become calcified. By birth the two molar crowns are almost equally calcified in terms of area covered. The entire occlusal surface is under active calcification as is approximately the upper half of the sides of the crown (Fig. 20.18). It is of both interest and importance to note that the appearance of the molars at birth is most unlike that of the same molars when they erupt into the oral cavity as fully calcified crowns. Missing are the fully formed cusps each of equal height, the intercuspal grooves, and the many minor ridges and wrinkles. In fact, even the pedodontists would be hard put to identify them as human molars. The "finishing touches" are not applied to the human primary molar crowns until after birth and before eruption. These consist of additional activity of the ameloblasts as they continue to deposit enamel. If one compares the illustrations of the two molars at birth (Fig. 20.18) with those of the same molars at time of eruption (see Figs. 6.12*a* to *e* and 6.13*a* to *e*) one realizes that *the process that gives each molar its peculiarly human and highly individualized character is the postnatal deposition of enamel.* A complete chronology of morphogenetic stages for the four primary molars is presented in Tables 6.5 to 6.8.

The effect of enamel on the crown morphology of human teeth was demonstrated in another way by Korenhof (1963). He studied teeth from a medieval cemetery in Java, where, owing to unusual soil conditions, the dentin had decayed but the enamel remained intact. He was able to make casts of the internal surface of the enamel (i.e., the dentinoenamel junction) and compare them with the outer surface of the same teeth. Whereas on the outer surface the cusps were rounded and separated by fissures, the inner surface had pointed cusps, sharp ridges and rounded valleys, like those of developing tooth germs. Korenhof noted the resemblance of the dentinoenamel junction of man to the outer surface of primitive hominoids such as Pliopithecus and Proconsul. In these the enamel is thin, and the outer surface of the tooth is not so different from the surface of the dentin. A human, a chimp, and a gorilla man-

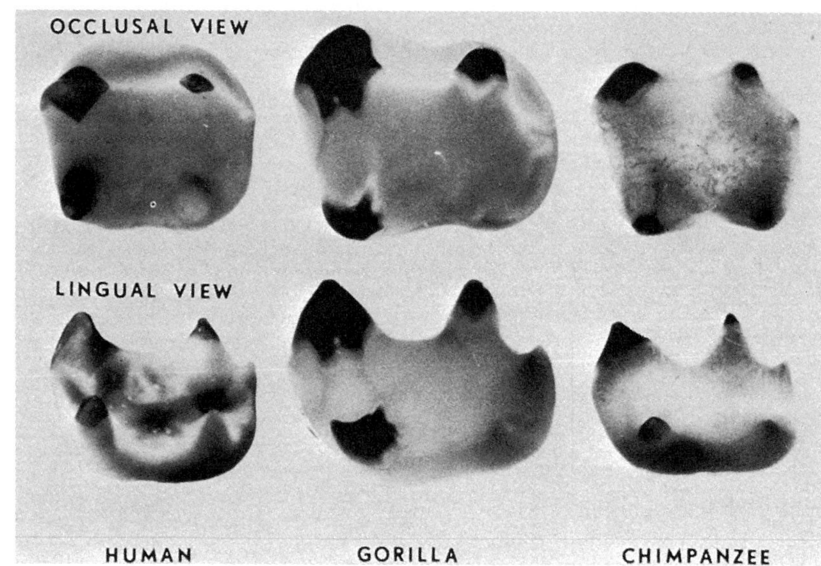

Figure 20.19

The mandibular first permanent molars of human, gorilla, and chimpanzee, full-term fetuses. *Dark sections,* calcified.

dibular first permanent molar are shown in Figure 20.19. They were extracted from full-term fetuses. Only an expert, upon careful examination, might be able to distinguish between them. There is no difficulty, however, in identifying these teeth once they have been completely calcified (Fig. 20.20). If, on the other hand, one were to examine the same molar of a full-term rhesus monkey (Fig. 20.21), one would experience no difficulty in distinguishing it from that of a human or a gorilla. It would seem that the genes that control the development of the molars up to the stage of enamel formation are almost the same in man, chimp, and gorilla, but those controlling enamel formation are different; in the monkey it is the earlier development, prior to calcification, that has changed.

In the last century von Baer claimed that embryos pass through stages reminiscent of the embryonic forms of their ancestors. This means that the more closely related two species are, the more alike are their later developmental stages. Human teeth develop in essentially the same way as the teeth of other mammals. Thus, the mesiobuccal cusp of the molars (paracone or protoconid) is always the first to form and calcify; on upper molars the distolingual cusp (hypocone) is the last to develop, and on lower molars the talonid develops later than the trigonid. Human molars resemble those of other primates in de-

Figure 20.20

The mandibular first permanent molars of human, gorilla, and chimpanzee at eruption.

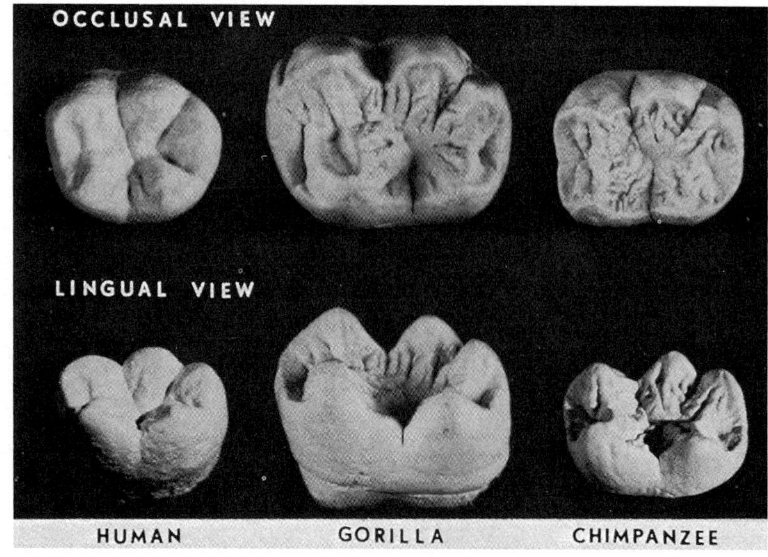

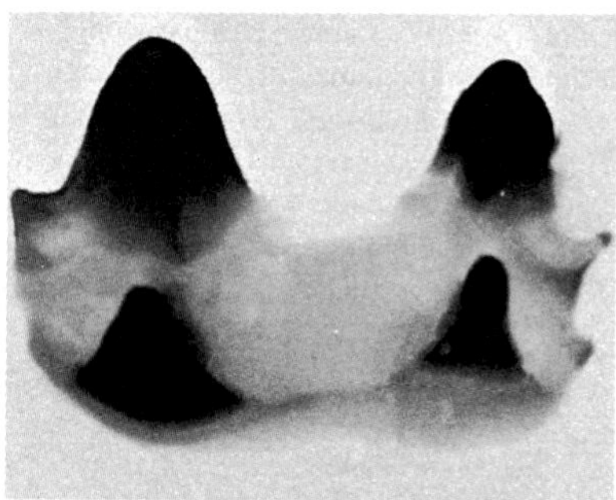

Figure 20.21
The mandibular first permanent molar of a rhesus monkey at time of birth.

veloping a large talonid, whereas the paraconid is small and appears late. As in other hominoids, the protocone and metacone become joined by an oblique ridge, but the conules remain undeveloped, and on lower molars the hypoconulid usually becomes large. Thus the development of teeth reveals the position of mankind in the animal kingdom. The genes that control the developmental processes must have been selected at various times in past evolutionary history, some far back and others, such as those responsible for enamel thickness, at a more recent date.

References

Korenhof CAW. The enamel dentine border. A new morphological factor in the study of the human molar pattern. Netherlands Dent J 1963; 70 (Suppl):30–57.

Kraus B, Jordan R. The human dentition before birth. Philadelphia: Lea & Febiger, 1965.

Oöe T. Human tooth and dental arch development. Tokyo: Ishiyaku, 1981.

Sasaki T. Cell biology of tooth enamel formation. Basel: Karger, 1990.

Slaukin HC. Molecular determinants of tooth development. Critical Rev Oral Biol Med 1990; 1:1–16.

Sperber GH. Craniofacial embryology. 4th ed. London: Wright/Butterworths, 1989.

Van der Linden FPGM, Duterloo HS. Development of the human dentition. An Atlas. Hagerstown: Harper and Row, 1976.

21

Normal and Abnormal Crown Structure

If this book were limited to conveying only one concept to the student, that concept would be one of *variability* in tooth structure as opposed to *stereotypy.* If we were to be allowed another, it would be to define *normality.* If, generally, all mandibular first molars were identical, it would be a simple thing to define normality, since every tooth that looks like every other tooth is normal, and any one that is noticeably different would be abnormal. Since variability in every trait in every species is a fundamental law of nature, and since the various forms or dimensions of any trait conform more or less to a "normal curve," it is obvious that any definition of what is abnormal is an arbitrary matter. If we were to decide that any mandibular first molar crown is abnormal if it occurs with a frequency of less than 1 percent in the population, then this standard of abnormality is a *statistical definition* and can be used, like any definition, as a tool for sorting and classifying data.

On the other hand an abnormality can also be defined on the basis of function; i.e., any trait that interferes with the proper functioning of the tooth or dentition in its usual masticatory, speech, or cosmetic roles is abnormal (*viz.*, pathological). In the statistical sense, a shovel-shaped incisor found in a caucasoid might be regarded as an abnormality, but in a mongoloid the converse would be true. In some mongoloid populations the frequency of the shovel-shape trait is as high as 99 percent and in most caucasoid populations it ranges from 1 to 5 percent. If, therefore, in a randomly selected sample from a caucasoid population, one were to find 60 percent with shovel-shaped incisors, one might suspect that the population from which the sample was drawn was abnormal. This is precisely the case when the incisors of a sample of persons with trisomy 21 (Down) syndrome are examined. These persons are characterized by a syndrome of effects, including mental retardation, as well as certain physical traits, such as shovel-shaped incisors and epicanthic eyefold, which are normal for mongolid populations (Chinese, Japanese, Mongolians, Eskimos).

This association of shovel-shaped teeth with a chromosomal abnormality (trisomy) has long been established. However, it now appears that abnormalities of dental crown structure, both statistically and functionally defined, are associated with many different kinds of congenital anomalies. Before surveying the recent findings in this area, it is important first to speculate still further about other aspects of dental embryology.

The human period of gestation is commonly divided into two parts: the *embryonic* period, which encompasses the first 8 weeks, and the *fetal* period, which includes the next 32 weeks. It is during the first 8 weeks that the human embryo passes through the various stages that seem to recapitulate the evolution of the species. At first, of course, the zygote recalls the time when life on earth consisted of protozoans, single-celled animals. The morula stage suggests the hypothetical period when colonial aggregates of cells represented the first step toward organization of cells into a single organism. And so, in successive days and weeks of gestation the embryo develops through forms that are almost identical to the embryos of fish, amphibians, reptiles, generalized mammals, generalized primates, and anthropoid apes. At 5 weeks the human and rhesus embryos cannot be distinguished on the basis of gross inspection (Fig. 21.1), but soon thereafter, the human embryo resembles more the chimpanzee or gorilla embryo. Finally, by the end of the seventh week, the human embryo has taken on those characteristics of external structure that identify it as a member of the species *Homo sapiens.* Henceforth, throughout the remaining 7 months of gestation, the organism, now a fetus, develops mainly in terms of increase in size, change in proportions, and achievement of greater physiological integration. Figure 21.2 compares gorilla, rhesus, and human fetuses, each approximately 15 weeks of age.

There is one organ, or system, however, that does not follow these lines of development. The dentition, consisting of 52 separate structures, *has an embryonic period that includes the entire prenatal span of time as well as the first 16 or 17 years of postnatal life!* We might define the embryonic period of a single tooth as beginning with the zygote (the genetic constitution controlling tooth development is already present) and terminating with the final calcification of the crown, before eruption. Its fetal period would be completion of root formation after eruption. It is thus

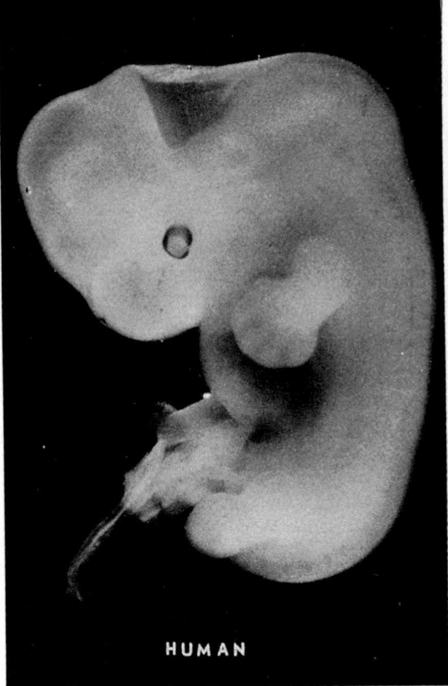

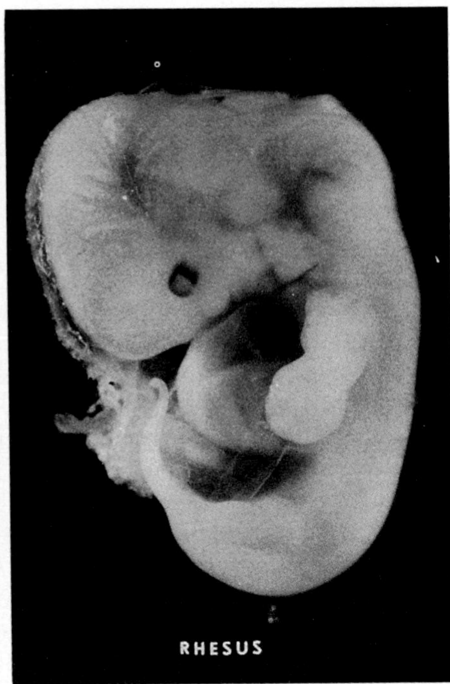

Figure 21.1
Human and rhesus embryos at 5 weeks' gestational age.

apparent that each tooth has its own characteristic embryonic period. To appreciate this significant fact, Table 21.1 examines the duration of the embryonic stages of several teeth, considering, for the sake of convenience, that odontogenesis is marked by Stage I in tooth development. These dates, particularly those pertaining to final calcification of the crowns, are only approximate. Nevertheless, it can readily be seen that different teeth take quite different lengths of time to achieve their final crown form. This suggests, among other things, that calcification does not proceed at a fixed rate but at various rates depending upon the tooth. Obviously the rates are faster for the primary teeth; possibly selection of these faster calci-

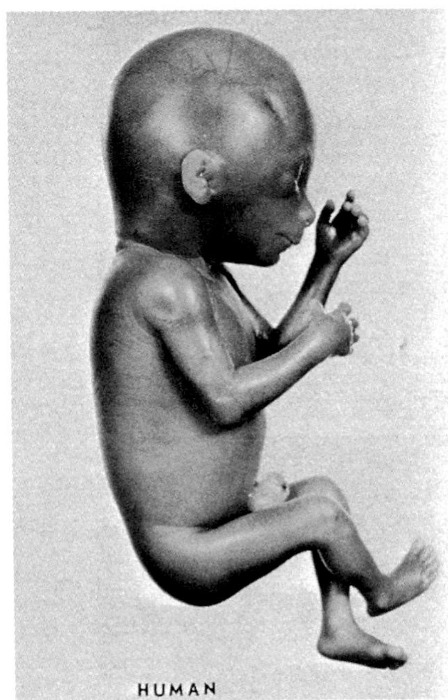

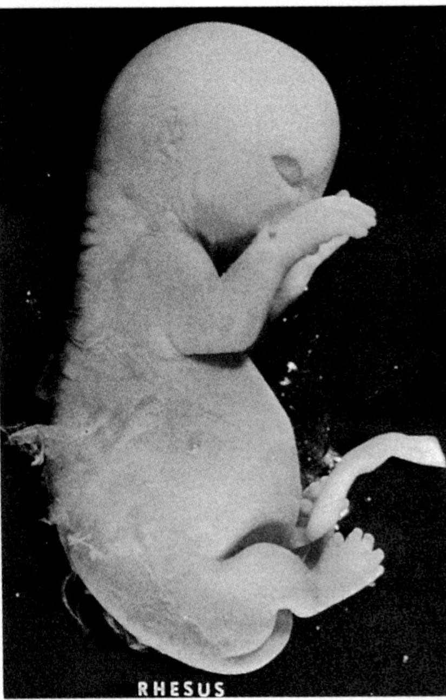

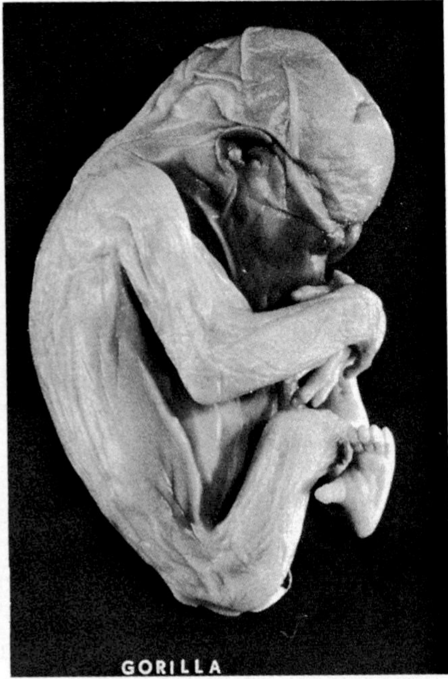

Figure 21.2
Human, rhesus, and gorilla fetuses at 15 weeks' gestational age.

Table 21.1
Duration of the Embryonic Stages of Some Primary and Permanent Teeth

Tooth	Stage I	Final Calcification of Crown	Duration of Embryology (mo)
Primary 1st molar	12th week (prenatal)	6th month (postnatal)	12
Primary 2nd molar	13th week (prenatal)	12th month (postnatal)	18
Permanent 1st molar	16th week (prenatal)	36th month (postnatal)	40
First premolar	2 years (postnatal)	7th year (postnatal)	60
Permanent 3rd molar	8 years (postnatal)	16th year (postnatal)	96

fication rates took place during early mammalian evolution because of the need for early eruption of the primary teeth.

Having established that the usual divisions of gestation into embryonic and fetal periods do not apply to the dentition, we now must consider the peculiar vulnerability of the various tissues and organs of the body to interferences with their development during the embryonic period. There is a multitude of events that customarily take place in an orderly progression beginning with penetration of the membrane of the ovum by the sperm until the fetal stage is reached. These events include, to name but a few, the separation of the three germinal layers, ectoderm, mesoderm, and endoderm; the migration of ectoderm forward to form the primitive streak; thickening, separation, and folding of epithelial layers to begin the formation of organs; aggregation of neural crest cells into spinal ganglia; migration of neural crest cells to the arches and their differentiation; and fusion of cell masses to form the nostrils, palate, and lip. The entire multiplicity of developmental events is so timed and coordinated that the introduction of any abnormal endogenous (mutant allele) or exogenous (virus or antibody) agent at any point is apt to upset the balance and sequence of normal development, leading to one or more malformed organs or tissues. Environmental agents that interfere with normal development to produce congenital anomalies are called *teratogens*. Many teratogenic agents are known, both those that occur spontaneously (*viz.*, rubella virus) and those that have been used experimentally to induce certain abnormalities in animals (*viz.*, cortisone, to induce cleft palate in mice).

There is more and more evidence accumulating to indicate that viruses are an important etiologic factor in many congenital malformations. Other known teratogens are alcohol, retinoic acid, folic acid, hypervitaminosis, anoxia, thalidomide, metabolic upsets in the mother, irradiation, trypan blue, and cytomegalic inclusion viruses. Of course, genetic factors must not be overlooked; they include point mutations, polyploidy and aneuploidy, trisomy and monosomy, chromosome breakages, translocations, and deletions.

Any given teratogen will be effective in disturbing normal development only within a certain range of time, the so-called "critical period," for a given organ or tissue relative to that particular teratogen. A given tissue is susceptible to a given teratogen only at a specific stage in its development and the degree of susceptibility is determined to a large extent by the genotype. In general, the age of the embryo at the time a teratogenic agent is introduced determines which tissues and organs will be affected. However, after organogenesis is complete (end of the embryonic period) teratogenic effects seldom can occur since the embryonic processes have terminated. As Wilson (1965) has pointed out, "human embryogenesis is completed about the end of the eighth week of intrauterine life and, with the exception of external genitalia, developmental defects for the most part cannot be produced after this time." Apparently Wilson forgot about the dentition and the fact that embryological processes involved in tooth development are taking place long after the embryonic period is ended, in fact, for 16 years after birth! Theoretically, and in practice, certain teratogenic agents introduced during the fetal period or even after birth could interfere with the normal developmental processes of specific teeth. As this is true, then the possibility exists for demonstrating through dental "markers" the occurrence of teratogenic disturbances in the body, and for dating the introduction of the teratogen such as tetracycline.

Evidence that the teeth might play an important role in future investigations of the mechanisms and causes of congenital anomalies is now beginning to accumulate. It has been shown that in all forms of cleft lip and/or palate in man, there is an unusual number of malformed dental crowns. Approximately 55 percent of a sample of cleft subjects showed one or more dental malformations, or an average of 2.5 abnormalities. In this study (Jordan et al, 1966), only the permanent teeth were studied, and it was readily shown that the affected teeth were not only those in the immediate region of the cleft but in the posterior segments of the quadrants as well as in the mandibular dentition. An additional serial study of both the primary and permanent dentitions of 39 cleft subjects showed that teeth in both sets were affected but not in any predictable way (Kraus et al, 1966). In aborted human fetuses exhibiting cleft lip and/or palate, abnormal tooth buds were consistently found. Some of the common crown abnormalities found in cleft subjects are illustrated in Figure 21.3.

Teratogenic effects in the dentition are not confined, however, to cases of cleft lip and/or palate. In cases of trisomy 21 (Down syndrome) the number of affected teeth per patient and the proportion of those affected are even greater than in cleft subjects. What is more, there are many kinds of crown abnormalities found in trisomy 21 that are not found in individuals with clefts (Kraus et al, 1968). In the case of cleft lip and/or palate, the etiology is unknown but is probably multifactorial and may involve genes in some cases and environmental factors in many others. In trisomy 21 the high correlation between mental retardation, physiognomic characteristics, and body build, on the one hand, and trisomy 21 on the other is additional indication of the genetic basis of this malformation. In both types of malformation, however, the teeth are involved, although to different degrees and perhaps in different ways. Examples of dental crown malformations found in trisomy 21 are presented in Figure 21.4.

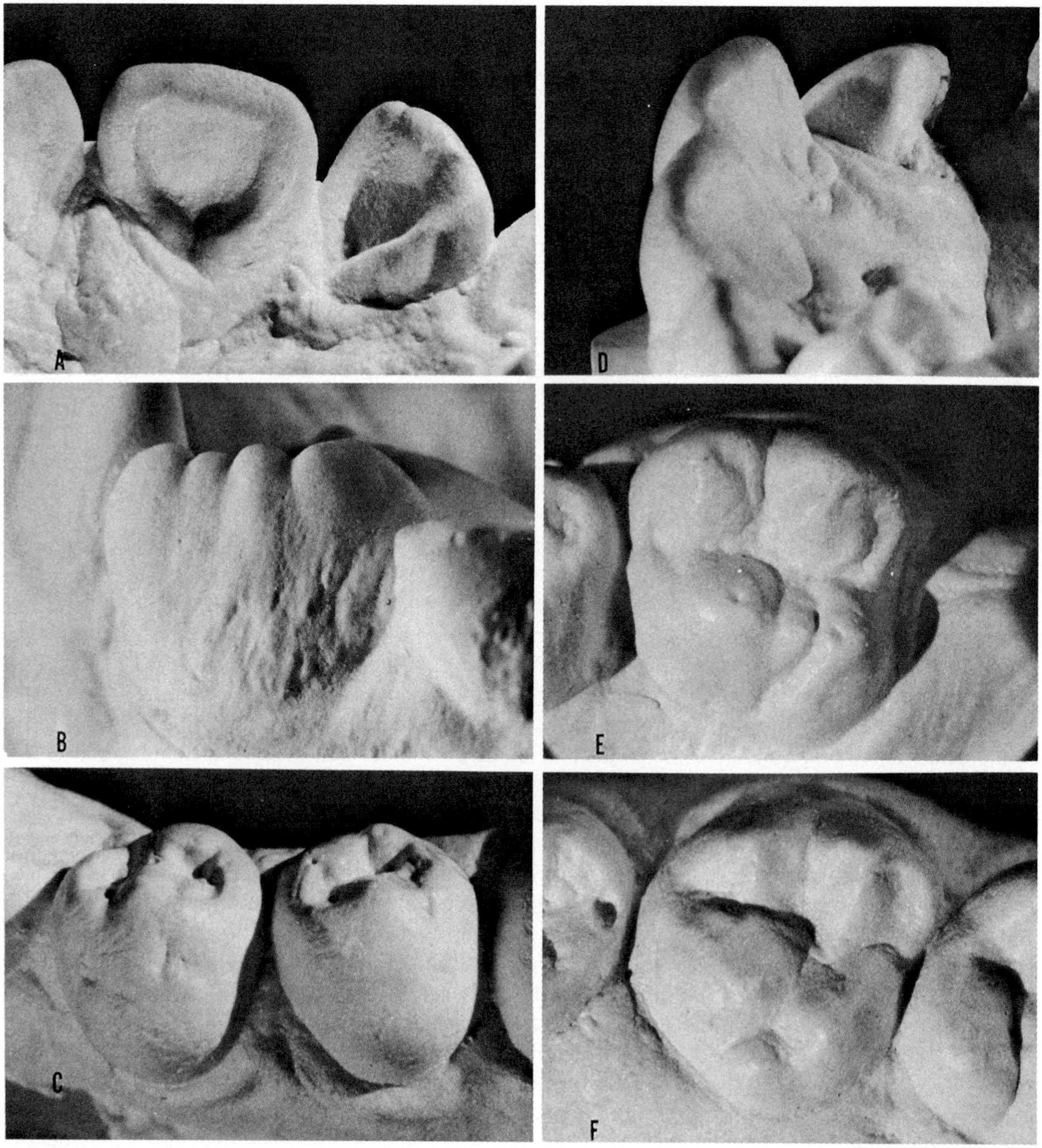

Figure 21.3
Abnormalities of dental crown structure in cleft lip and/or palate subjects.

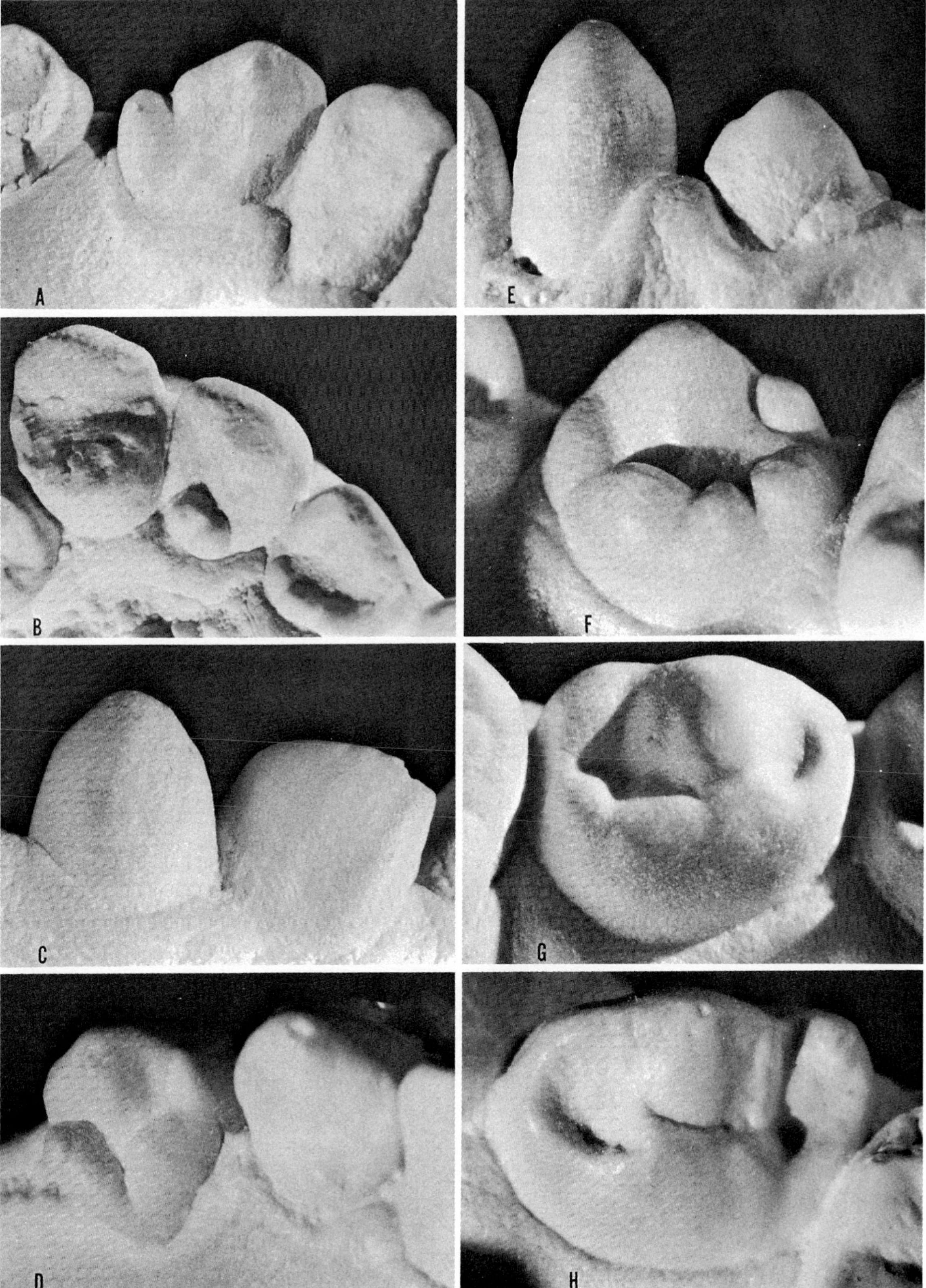

Figure 21.4

Abnormalities of dental crown structure found in trisomy 21 (Down syndrome).

Other congenital anomalies in which malformed teeth are involved include: holoprosencephaly, trisomy 13, culturofamilial cases of mental retardation, Sturge-Weber syndrome, superfemales (XXX and XXXX), amyotonia congenita, neurofibromatosis, and partial albinism. When sufficient data have been accumulated in these various categories, it should be possible to determine if the types of teeth and the kinds of crown abnormalities are specific to each kind of congenital anomaly. There is already some indication that the time when a malformation of the developing crown of a tooth occurred can be pinpointed. This has led to the postulation of a new dental science called *dentochronology,* the dating of the action of a teratogen on one or more tooth buds. Presumably if the onset of a tooth malformation can be fixed in time, this would also determine the time when the general congenital malformation was initiated.

References

Beere D, Hargreaves JA, Sperber GH, Cleaton-Jones P. Mirror-image supplemental primary incisors in twins. J Pediatric Dent 1990; 12.

Fitzgerald LR, Oberman K, Harris EF, McKnight JT. Incisor mamelon morphology: diagnostic indicators of abnormal development. J Am Dent Assoc 1983; 107:63–66.

Jordan R, Kraus B, Neptune C. Dental abnormalities associated with cleft lip and/or palate. Cleft Palate J 1966; 3:22–25.

Kraus B, Clark G, Oka S. Mental retardation and abnormalities of the dentition. Am J Ment Defic 1968; 72:905–917.

Kraus B, Jordan R, Pruzansky S. Dental abnormalities in the deciduous and permanent dentitions of individuals with cleft lip and palate. J Dent Res 1966; 45:1736–1746.

Nystrom M, Ranta R. Dental age and asymmetry in the formation of mandibular teeth in twins concordant or discordant for oral clefts. Scand J Dent Res 1988; 96:393–398.

Sperber GH, Honoré L. Anodontia totalis fetalis in a trisomy 13 mosais. J Dent Assoc S Afr 1988; 43:265–269.

22

The Human Dentition: A Biological Appraisal

In Chapters 15 to 21 we have reviewed some of the ways in which teeth concern the anthropologist, the paleontologist, the geneticist, the zoologist, the embryologist, and the teratologist. In the evolution of the hominids the dentition lost its adaptive value, perhaps for the first time in the history of life on earth. But in losing its significance for the selective forces of nature, it retained and even gained new importance in a historical sense. Like the relics found on a battlefield or the footprints of the long vanished dinosaurs or early hominids, teeth are records of the past. In their embryological processes they recall the many successive stages of dental development that were reached only after millions of years of biological evolution. On the other hand, each variation in ridge, groove, or cusp structure reminds us of the underlying genetic constitution that controls in so many ways the warp and woof of our lives. In the teeth of monozygotic twins is mirrored the miracle of genetic identity, whereas the uniqueness of the dentition of the rest of us attests to the fundamental theme of bisexual reproduction: the individuality of each member of the species.

With evidence steadily accumulating that teeth reflect disturbances in the organism, whether of endogenous or exogenous nature, whether in embryonic, fetal, or postnatal life, there is the likelihood that the dentition may prove to be of great importance in diagnosis and in research into the mechanisms and etiology of congenital anomalies.

It is true that in mankind teeth have lost their evolutionary adaptiveness and some of their original biological functions. Nevertheless, we each have teeth, and having them, we use them. The fact that they have no adaptive value does not alter the equally valid fact that they can cause us many days of anguish, discomfort, inefficiency, and economic loss. The paleontologist and geneticist cannot relieve a toothache, nor can the anthropologist alleviate the temporomandibular joint pain that may accompany a malocclusion. The dentist will remain with us and will become increasingly more important as the variability of the human dentition increases in all aspects: chemically, structurally, morphologically, developmentally, and occlusion-wise.

The human dentition, like the human brain, has its roots in the evolutionary beginnings of life on earth. It is at one with the teeth of all vertebrates. But like the brain, it is, at the same time, unique. It persists without a reason. It is apparently as unnecessary as the appendix. The brain, on the other hand, has become the most important human organ, with infinite possibilities for altering human evolutionary destiny, just as it has robbed the dentition of its original biological function, that of food acquisition.

There is much more to tell about teeth. This book only opens the door to broader understanding and, it is hoped, whets the appetite for more knowledge.

Suggested Reading

Aiello L, Dean C. An introduction to human evolutionary anatomy. San Diego: Academic Press, 1990.

Butler PM. The ontogeny of molar pattern. Biol Rev 1956; 31:30–70.

Butler PM, Joysey KA, eds. Development, function and evolution of teeth. New York: Academic Press, 1978.

Calow P. Evolutionary principles. Glasgow and London: Blackie, 1983.

Conroy CG. Primate evolution. New York: WW Norton & Co., 1990.

Dahlberg AA, ed. Dental morphology and evolution. Chicago: University of Chicago Press, 1971.

DeBeer G. Embryos and ancestors. London: Oxford University Press, 1962.

Dobzhansky T. Genetics and the origin of species. New York: Columbia University Press, 1961.

Edey MA, Johanson DC. Blueprints. Solving the mystery of evolution. Boston: Little, Brown, 1989.

Gregory W. Our face from fish to man. New York: Capricorn Books, 1965.

Grine FE. Evolutionary history of the "robust" Australopithecines. New York: Aldine, 1988.

Hillson S. Teeth (Cambridge Manuals in Archeology). Cambridge, England: Cambridge University Press, 1986.

Hoffman A. Arguments on evolution. A paleontologist's perspective. New York: Oxford University Press, 1989.

Johanson DC, Edey MA. Lucy: the beginnings of humankind. New York: Simon and Schuster, 1981.

Kemp TS. Mammal-like reptiles and the origin of mammals. New York: Academic Press, 1982.

Kraus B, Jordan R. The human dentition before birth. Philadelphia: Lea & Febiger, 1965.

Kurten B, ed. Teeth: form, function and evolution. New York: Columbia University Press, 1982.

Lambert D. The Cambridge guide to prehistoric man. Cambridge, England: Cambridge University Press, 1987.

Mayr E. Populations, species and evolution. Cambridge, MA: Harvard University Press, 1970.

Mellars P, Stringer C, eds. The origins and dispersal of modern humans: behavioral and biological perspectives. Edinburgh: Edinburgh University Press, 1990.

Miles AEW. The evolution of dentitions in the more recent ancestors of man. Proc R Soc Med 1972; 65:396–399.

Moorrees C. The dentition of the growing child. Cambridge, MA: Harvard University Press, 1959.

Osborn HF. The evolution of the mammalian molars to and from the tritubercular type. Am Natur 1967; 21.

Osborn JW. The evolution of dentitions. Am Scient 1973; 61:548.

Oöe, T. Human tooth and dental arch development. Tokyo: Ishyaku, 1981.

Pedersen PO, Dahlberg AA, Alexandersen V, eds. Proceedings of the International Symposium on Dental Morphology. J Dent Res 1965; 46 (Suppl): 769–992.

Peyer B. Comparative odontology. Chicago: University of Chicago Press, 1968.

Reader J. Missing links. The hunt for earliest man. 2nd ed. London: Penguin Books, 1988.

Robinson J. The dentition of the Australopithecinae. Memoir No. 9. Pretoria, South Africa: Transvaal, 1956.

Romer, A. Vertebrate paleontology. Chicago: University of Chicago Press, 1966.

Scott GR, Turner CG. Dental anthropology. Ann Rev Anthropol 1988; 17:99–126.

Simons EL. Human origins. Science 1989; 245:1343–1350.

Simpson SW, Lovejoy CO, Meindl RS. Hominoid dental maturation. J Hum Evol 1990; 19:285–297.

Skinner MF, Sperber GH. Atlas of radiographs of early man. New York: Alan R. Liss, 1982.

Slavkin HC. Molecular biology of dental development: a review. In: Davidovitch Z, ed. Biological mechanisms of tooth eruption and root resorption. Birmingham, AL: EBSCO Media, 1988.

Slavkin HC. Splice of life: toward understanding genetic determinants of oral diseases. Adv Dent Res 1989; 3:42–57.

Smith BH. Dental development in *Australopithecus* and early *Homo*. Nature 1986; 323:327–330.

Sperber GH. Tusks. J Can Dent Assoc 1976; 42:257–268.

Sperber GH. Paleodontopathology and paleodontotherapy. J Can Dent Assoc 1986; 52: 835–838.

Sperber GH. The phylogeny and ontogeny of dental morphology. In: Sperber GH, ed. From apes to angels: essays in anthropology. New York: Wiley/Liss, 1990, pp. 215–219.

Tattersall I, Delson E, Van Couvering J, eds. Encyclopedia of human evolution and prehistory. New York: Garland Publishing, 1988.

Tobias PV. Tooth material in the *Hominidae*. J Dent Assoc S Afr 1988; 43:557–560.

Tobias PV. Delineation and dating of some major phases in hominidization and hominization since the Middle Miocene. S Afr J Sci 1986; 82:92–94.

Tobias PV, ed. Hominid evolution: past, present and future. New York: Alan R. Liss, 1985.

Tobias PV. Olduvai Gorge. Vols. 4A and 4B. The skulls, endocasts and teeth of *Homo habilis*. Cambridge, England: Cambridge University Press, 1990.

Weidenreich F. The dentition of *Sinanthropus pekinensis*: a comparative odontography of the hominids. New Series D, No. 1. Peking: Palaeontologia Sinica, 1937.

Wilson J. Embryological considerations in teratology. In: Wilson J, Warkany J, eds. Teratology, principles and techniques. Chicago: University of Chicago Press, 1965.

Wood B, Martin L, Andrews P, eds. Major topics in primate and human evolution. Cambridge, England: Cambridge University Press, 1986.

Young WG, Jupp R, Kruger BJ. Evolution of the skull, jaws and teeth in vertebrates. St. Lucia, Qld., Australia: University of Queensland Press, 1989.

Index

Page numbers in italics indicate figures; page numbers followed by a "t" indicate tables.

Numerical Nomenclature Code

1 Mesioincisal Angle
2 Distoincisal Angle
3 Mesiolabial Line Angle
4 Distolabial Line Angle
5 Mesiobuccal Angle
6 Distobuccal Angle
7 Mesiolingual Angle
8 Distolingual Angle
9 Root Apex
10 Cusp Apex
11 Axial Root Center
12 Cervix
13 Cingulum
14 Proximal Root Concavity
15 Mesial Concavity
16 Contact Area
17 Buccal Cusp
18 Lingual Cusp
19 Mesiobuccal Cusp
20 Mesiolingual Cusp
21 Distobuccal Cusp
22 Distolingual Cusp
23 Distal Cusp
24 Carabelli Cusp
25 Mesial Marginal Ridge Cusp
26 Lingual Fossa
27 Mesiolingual Fossa
28 Distolingual Fossa
29 Mesial Triangular Fossa
30 Distal Triangular Fossa
31 Central Fossa
32 Distal Fossa
33 Mesiolabial Groove
34 Distolabial Groove
35 Mesial Marginal Groove
36 Supplemental Groove
37 Mesial Groove
38 Distal Groove
39 Central Groove
40 Mesiobuccal Groove
41 Distobuccal Groove
42 Mesiolingual Groove
43 Distolingual Groove
44 Lingual Groove
45 Buccal Groove
46 Carabelli Groove
47 Height of Contour
48 Cervical Line
49 Buccal Verticle Apex Line
50 Lingual Verticle Apex Line
51 Mesial Lobe
52 Middle Lobe
53 Distal Lobe
54 Mesial Mamelon
55 Middle Mamelon
56 Distal Mamelon
57 Median Longitudinal Axis
58 Lingual Pit
59 Mesial Pit
60 Distal Pit
61 Buccal Pit
62 Central Pit
63 Carabelli Pit
64 Incisal Ridge
65 Mesial Marginal Ridge
66 Distal Marginal Ridge
67 Mesial Cusp Ridge
68 Distal Cusp Ridge
69 Distal Transverse Ridge
70 Transverse Ridge
71 Buccal Ridge
72 Lingual Ridge
73 Oblique Ridge
74 Anterior Transverse Ridge
75 Triangular Ridge
76 Buccal Root
77 Lingual Root
78 Mesiobuccal Root
79 Distobuccal Root
80 Mesial Root
81 Distal Root
82 Root Bifurcation
83 Root Trunk (base)
84 Lingual Tubercle